Critical Findings in Neuroradiology

Renato Hoffmann Nunes
Ana Lorena Abello • Mauricio Castillo
Editors

Critical Findings in Neuroradiology

Springer

Editors
Renato Hoffmann Nunes
Division of Neuroradiology
Santa Casa de São Paulo
São Paulo
Brazil

Ana Lorena Abello
Research Fellow in Neuroradiology
Department of Radiology
University of North Carolina
Chapel Hill, NC
USA

Mauricio Castillo
James H. Scatliff Distinguished
Professor of Radiology
Chief, Division of Neuroradiology
University of North Carolina
Chapel Hill, NC
USA

ISBN 978-3-319-27985-5 ISBN 978-3-319-27987-9 (eBook)
DOI 10.1007/978-3-319-27987-9

Library of Congress Control Number: 2016933483

Printed on acid-free paper

This Springer imprint is published by Springer Nature
The registered company is Springer International Publishing AG Switzerland

To my lovely family, especially to my mother, and to my wonderful friends who have supported me throughout this and other projects. You have given me love and inspiration. Thank you.

Ana Lorena Abello

This book is dedicated to my wife Fernanda for her love and understanding and to my family for their unconditional support.

Renato Hoffmann Nunes

Contents

Part II Head and Neck

Part III Spine

Introduction

Important decisions that require immediate actions are made every day in almost every line of work. These types of issues have to be addressed with the highest priority and usually require close follow-up and are called "critical findings." For example, engineers of the National Bridge Inspection Standards follow a checklist of critical findings to find and prevent structural damage of a bridge. A critical finding for them is a structural- or safety-related deficiency that requires immediate follow-up inspection or action and includes instances where an entire bridge, one lane, or a shoulder is closed to assure public safety due to the condition of a bridge element or damage sustained by one of its elements. Bridge engineers know that once a critical finding is discovered, it is vital to act immediately in a prudent manner to protect public safety and infrastructure investments [1].

The word "critical" has different meanings in different occupations. In healthcare, it is usually defined as having a decisive or crucial importance in the success, failure, or existence of a condition and its treatment [2]. Based on this, in radiology, a critical finding is something detected on a study that could be a turning point in the patient's therapy and outcome and that requires immediate communication between healthcare providers [3].

Diagnostic errors occur in all branches of medicine, but they are especially critical in diagnostic radiology and neuroradiology, where misinterpretation or misidentification may significantly delay medical or surgical treatments and adversely affect patient outcomes. Approximately 4 % of all radiologic interpretations in daily practice contain errors [4]. Fortunately, most of them are minor errors or, if serious, are promptly discovered and corrected. So many individuals looked at diagnostic studies that even if a radiologist initially misses a finding, someone else may notice it. Although human errors are inevitable in medicine, including neuroradiology, it is important to distinguish medical errors from medical malpractice. A medical error is a failure of a planned action to be completed as intended, while medical malpractice is defined as a failure of the physician to exercise that degree of skill and knowledge commonly applied under similar circumstances in the community resulting in injury to the patient [5]. Lack of recognition and communication of critical findings may lead to medical errors and ultimately legal actions.

Elimination of preventable medical errors continues to be a major issue in healthcare. It is enough to compare the rate of medical errors (still very high) to that of the commercial air transport business (very low) to see that in medicine, we still have considerable space for improvement. Ineffective communication between healthcare providers has been identified as a major culprit resulting in poor patient outcomes. Patient safety initiatives have been implemented worldwide aiming to improve the system [6].

The Joint Commission (a nonprofit agency which accredits over 20,000 healthcare organizations) recommends to "report critical results of test and diagnostic procedures on a timely basis" [3]. Failure to communicate critical imaging findings in a timely manner is often the subject of medical malpractice claims against radiologists and can contribute significantly to patient mortality and morbidity. Since the Institute of Medicine's report on preventable medical errors, ineffective physician-to-physician and physician-to-patient communications have been identified as major contributors to poor patient outcome [7]. In 2012, 59 % of healthcare-related "sentinel events" in the United States reported to the Joint Commission resulted from communication errors and failed communication which was the number one reason for delay in treatment [6]. In radiology, timely communication of critical imaging findings has been emphasized by the American College of Radiology and recently has become a Joint Commission requirement for successful practice accreditation [3, 8, 9]. In order to improve patient safety and ensure quick and satisfactory communications between radiologists and referring physicians, healthcare organizations are encouraged to develop algorithmic approaches to report and communicate critical findings based on lists of them. Recently this issue was specifically addressed by scientific publications revealing that the need of this kind of approach (lists) is not well known by radiologists and training programs and often the critical findings lists are usually heterogeneous and non-reproducible across institutions [10, 11].

Therefore, the goal of this book is to provide a practical and illustrative approach that easily demonstrates what to look for, how to report it, and what and when follow-up is needed as well as the most common differential diagnoses of the main critical findings in neuroradiology. For this purpose we have selected those conditions considered as critical findings in our institutions, and although we understand that these may vary from institution to institution, we hope to have covered most if not all those that will affect patient outcomes.

Chapel Hill, NC, USA

Renato Hoffmann Nunes, MD
Ana Lorena Abello, MD
Mauricio Castillo, MD, FACR

References

1. Federal Highway Administration. Summary Report of Critical Findings – Reviews for the National Bridge Inspection Program. 2011. http://www.fhwa.dot.gov/bridge/nbip/critical.pdf. Accessed 10 Sept 2015.
2. Oxford Learner's Dictionaries. Oxford University Press. http://www.oxfordlearnersdictionaries.com/us/. Accessed 11 Sept 2015.
3. The Joint Commission website. National patient safety goals. http://www.jointcommission.org/standards_information/npsgs.aspx. Accessed 10 Sept 2015.
4. Borgstede JP, Lewis RS, Bhargavan M, Sunshine JH. RADPEER quality assurance program: a multifacility study of interpretive disagreement rates. J Am Coll Radiol. 2004;1(1):59–65. doi:10.1016/S1546-1440(03)00002-4.

5. Caranci F, Tedeschi E, Leone G, Reginelli A, Gatta G, Pinto A, Squillaci E, Briganti F, Brunese L. Errors in neuroradiology. Radiol Med. 2015;120(9):795–801. doi:10.1007/s11547-015-0564-7.
6. Babiarz LS, Lewin JS, Yousem DM. Continuous practice quality improvement initiative for communication of critical findings in neuroradiology. Am J Med Qual. 2015;30(5):447–53. doi:10.1177/1062860614539188.
7. Institute of Medicine. To err is human: building a safer health system. 1999.
8. Garvey CJ, Connolly S. Radiology reporting – where does the radiologist's duty end? Lancet. 2006;367(9508):443–5. doi:10.1016/S0140-6736(06)68145-2.
9. American College of Radiology. ACR practice guideline for communication of diagnostic imaging findings. Revised 2014. http://www.acr.org/~/media/C5D1443C9EA4424AA12477D1AD1D927D.pdf. Accessed 10 Sept 2015.
10. Trotter SA, Babiarz LS, Viertel VG, Nagy P, Lewin JS, Yousem DM. Determination and communication of critical findings in neuroradiology. J Am Coll Radiol. 2013;10(1):45–50. doi:10.1016/j.jacr.2012.07.012.
11. Babiarz LS, Trotter S, Viertel VG, Nagy P, Lewin JS, Yousem DM. Neuroradiology critical findings lists: survey of neuroradiology training programs. AJNR Am J Neuroradiol. 2013;34(4):735–9. doi:10.3174/ajnr.A3300.

Part I

Brain

Cerebral Edema

1

Juan Manuel González, Florencia Alamos,
and Ana Lorena Abello

Abstract

Brain edema is a pathologic increase in the amount of brain water as a result of several etiologies, either cellular damage and ionic pump dysfunction, blood–brain barrier disruption, or increased transependymal flow from the intraventricular compartment to the brain parenchyma. Brain edema can have focal or global distribution.

Diagnostic imaging can help detect the onset or progression of edema in patients with worsening clinical condition. CT is the modality of choice as the initial study to evaluate injuries that may require intervention. MRI is very sensitive to detect edema and has excellent tissue contrast to detect underlying lesions and may be used when the cause of the edema is not readily apparent on CT.

Background

Cerebral edema may be defined as a pathologic increase in the amount of total brain water content leading to an increase in brain volume [1]. It can be the consequence of a heterogeneous group of diseases, which typically fall under the categories of metabolic, infectious, neoplastic, cerebrovascular, and traumatic brain injury [2–9].

Symptoms of cerebral edema are nonspecific and related to mass effect, vascular compromise, and herniations. Clinical and imaging changes are usually reversible in the early stages as long as the underlying cause is corrected. Rapidly progressive edema overwhelms cerebral autoregulatory mechanisms, resulting in structural

J.M. González, MD
Department of Radiology, Hahnemann University Hospital, Drexel University College of Medicine, 230 North Broad Street, Philadelphia, PA 19102, USA
e-mail: Juan_m_gg@hotmail.com

F. Alamos, MD, PhD
Department of Neuroscience, School of Medicine, Universidad Católica de Chile, Luz larrain, 3946 Lo Barnechea, Santiago, Chile
e-mail: flopi1987@yahoo.com

A.L. Abello, MD (✉)
Department of Radiology, University of North Carolina, Chapel Hill, NC, USA
e-mail: anaabellop@hotmail.com

R. Hoffmann Nunes et al. (eds.), *Critical Findings in Neuroradiology*,
DOI 10.1007/978-3-319-27987-9_1

compression, cerebral ischemia, and ultimately fatal cerebral herniation [10].

Most fundamental pathophysiological processes following brain injury start with brain edema followed by increased intracranial pressure (ICP) leading to the reduction of cerebral blood flow, inadequate oxygen delivery, energy failure, and further edema. One of the treatment goals is to interrupt this vicious cycle by controlling swelling and maintaining an adequate blood and oxygen supply [11].

Glucocorticoids are very effective in ameliorating vasogenic edema that accompanies tumors or inflammatory conditions [12]. Drainage of cerebrospinal fluid (CSF) by ventriculostomy is also an effective alternative to control brain swelling in patients with interstitial edema due to hydrocephalus. Decompressive (hemi)craniectomy is sometimes the only treatment option when others less invasive have failed [11].

Table 1.1 Pathophysiology of edema

Cytotoxic
Arterial infarction
Small vessel disease
Vasogenic
Neoplasm
Hemorrhage
Venous thrombosis
Arteriovenous shunts
Interstitial
Hydrocephalus
Combined
Trauma
Hypoxic–ischemic encephalopathy
Osmotic
Hydrostatic
Infection or inflammation

Key Points

Etiology

According to its location, cerebral edema may be classified as:

Focal: Generates a pressure gradient in adjacent regions and may result in tissue shifts and herniations. Examples of focal edema can be found around tumors, hematomas, and infarctions [13].

Global: Diffusely affects the whole brain and, when critical, may cause intracranial hypertension and compromised perfusion and lead to generalized ischemia. Cardiopulmonary arrest, severe traumatic injury, multisystem organ failure, hypertensive crisis, infection or inflammation, hypoxic–ischemic injury, and toxic and metabolic conditions are common causes of global cerebral edema [10, 13].

Edema in the brain may be also classified according to its pathophysiological mechanisms (Table 1.1) as follows [1, 10, 13, 14]:

Cytotoxic edema: Cytotoxic edema is defined as a cellular process, where extracellular Na^+ and other cations enter neurons and astrocytes and accumulate due to failure of energy-dependent mechanisms. This incapacity to maintain cellular homeostasis is called "cytotoxic edema." Ischemia and profound metabolic derangements are the most common causes [15].

Vasogenic edema: It is caused by breakdown of the tight endothelial junctions comprising the blood–brain barrier, secondary to either physical disruption or release of vasoactive compounds. As a result, intravascular proteins and fluid escape into the extracellular space [10]. It accompanies tumors, inflammatory lesions, and traumatic tissue damage, among others [13].

Interstitial edema: Results from increased transependymal flow from the intraventricular compartment to the brain parenchyma. It typically occurs in the setting of obstructive hydrocephalus [13].

Best Imaging Modality

Non-enhanced computed tomography (CT) CT is the modality of choice for initial assessment of suspected cerebral edema because it can be promptly performed, is widely available, and is highly accurate in detecting associated injuries (tumors, hemorrhage, fractures) and in evaluating injuries that require intervention [10, 16–18].

Magnetic resonance imaging (MRI) MRI is highly sensitive to detect edema and provides excellent soft tissue contrast resolution to evaluate for underlying lesions. On MRI, edema produces high signal on T2-weighted image (T2WI) and low signal on T1-weighted image (T1WI). Diffusion-weighted images (DWI) and apparent diffusion coefficient (ADC) maps distinguish between cytotoxic edema (restricted diffusion) and vasogenic or interstitial edema (increased or facilitated diffusion) [10, 19].

Major Findings

Global Edema

CT and MRI show generalized loss of gray–white matter differentiation, effacement of sulci, ventricles, and basal cisterns. If the cause is not addressed, these findings can progress to transtentorial and fatal brain herniations [10].

The *pseudo-subarachnoid hemorrhage* appearance in non-enhanced CT makes reference to diffuse brain edema associated with increased attenuation of the basal cisterns and subarachnoid space, the falx, and the tentorium probably as consequence of slow venous blood circulation (Fig. 1.1) [20]. The *white cerebellum sign* is a relative hyperdensity of the cerebellum when compared with the supratentorial compartment that can be seen in patients with anoxic-ischemic encephalopathy [21]. CT evidence of global edema predicts a poor outcome [22].

Cytotoxic Edema

Infarction is the most common cause of cytotoxic edema. In acute arterial infarction, the gray matter is the first to be affected because of its high metabolic activity and greater cellular density; later, both the gray and white matter become involved. CT shows edema as decreased density compared to the surrounding normal parenchyma, which can be more readily visualized using a narrow stroke window (width, 30 HU and level, 30 HU) [10].

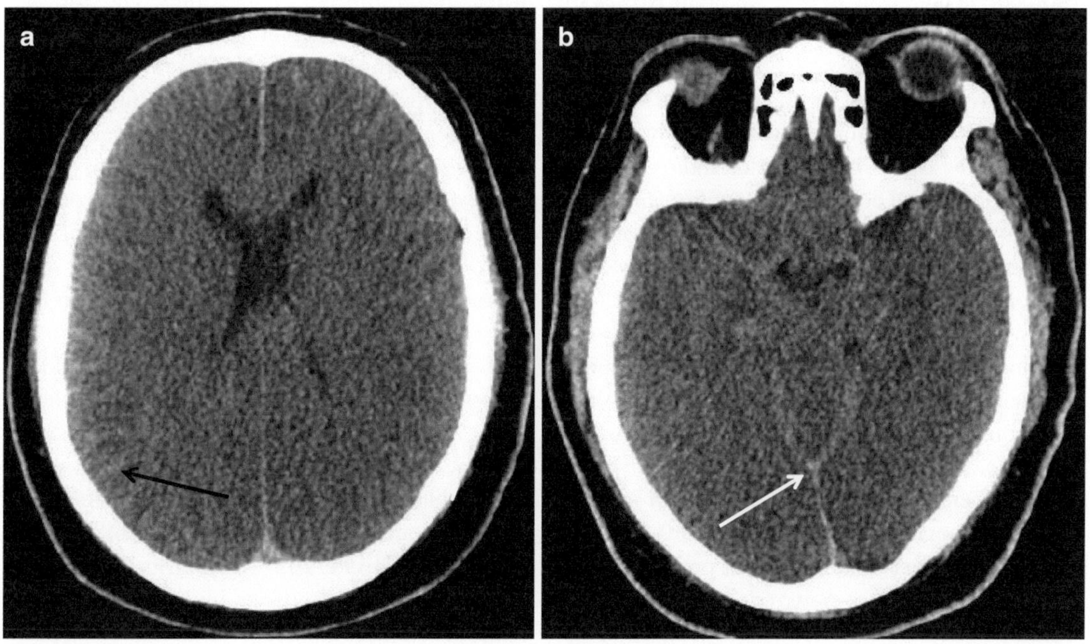

Fig. 1.1 Global edema. Axial NECT shows diffuse global hypodensity of the brain parenchyma with loss of gray–white matter differentiation and relative increase density of the subarachnoid spaces (*black arrow* in **a**), posterior falx, and tentorium (*white arrow* in **b**) compatible with a pseudo-subarachnoid hemorrhage appearance

DWI MRI demonstrates restricted diffusion resulting in regional high signal on DWI and low signal on ADC maps. This sequence is most sensitive for detection of hyperacute infarction (<30 min after presentation), preceding the identification of changes on CT (6 h) and T2WI (6–12 h). As infarcts evolve into the subacute stage, there is progression to vasogenic edema. This is reflected by progressive increase in T2/FLAIR intensity, with concomitant normalization of diffusivity at around 10–14 days after the infarction [10]. T1WI is usually normal within the first 6 h and subtle gyral swelling and hypointensity begins to develop within 12–24 h and are seen as blurring of the gray matter–white matter interfaces (Fig. 1.2) [23].

Vasogenic Edema

Expanded extracellular fluid yields decreased T1 signal and increased T2 signal. The white matter is preferentially affected because of its lower cellular density with multiple unconnected parallel axonal tracts. In the early stages, vasogenic edema may be reversible with reconstitution of the blood–brain barrier. Excess fluid can be resorbed via bulk flow of CSF and lymphovascular clearance [10].

Neoplasm: Both benign and malignant neoplasms are associated with vasogenic edema, which results from tumor angiogenesis with disruption of the blood–brain barrier and/or secondary to parenchymal compression and ischemia and necrosis that persist even after tumor removal. On CT, vasogenic edema appears as regional hypodensity confined to the white matter. T2 and FLAIR imaging show high signal. T1WI pre- and post-gadolinium, DWI, and perfusion MRI sequences are useful for tumor characterization but do not allow differentiation between vasogenic edema and tumoral infiltration. Diffusion tensor images (DTI) may enable one to distinguish tumor infiltration from vasogenic edema (Fig. 1.3) [10, 24, 25].

There are other conditions that produce vasogenic edema, such as *hemorrhage* with edema around the hemorrhagic foci. *Venous thrombosis* results in a form of infarction in which there is obstruction of venous outflow, leading to parenchymal congestion and breakdown of the normal blood–brain barrier [10]. Some authors consider that venous thrombosis produces combined vasogenic and cytotoxic processes based on its variable presentation on DWI and ADC (with increased ADC values presumably related to venous congestion) or cytotoxic edema (with decreased ADC values related to cellular energy disruption) [26, 27]. *Arteriovenous shunts* result in impaired venous drainage, arterial steal phenomena, and blood vessel rupture with hemorrhage. Although the primary pattern of edema in these shunts is vasogenic, hemodynamically significant lesions may produce ischemia with associated cytotoxic edema [10].

Posterior reversible encephalopathy syndrome (PRES): Initially described in association with eclampsia, immunosuppressive drugs, and acute hypertensive crisis, PRES is now recognized as a disorder that can be induced by a wide number of diseases including thrombotic microangiopathies, disseminated intravascular coagulation, uremic encephalopathies, sepsis, drugs, and tumor lysis syndromes. The etiology of PRES is not completely understood; hypertension leading to failed cerebral autoregulation, hyperperfusion, blood–brain barrier disruption, and breakthrough vasogenic edema are the most common explanations [23]. However, PRES may occur without hypertension. It is proposed that direct endothelial dysfunction and/or hypoalbuminemia leading to an increase in permeability of the blood–brain barrier may be an additional mechanism responsible for parenchymal fluid extravasation. In MRI, the lesions are usually isointense to hypointense on T1WI and hyperintense on T2WI and FLAIR sequences. There is more involvement of white matter than gray matter which is consistent with vasogenic edema. Lesions are mostly hemispheric and bilaterally symmetric. With more severe disease, extensive involvement of the brain occurs along with involvement of atypical

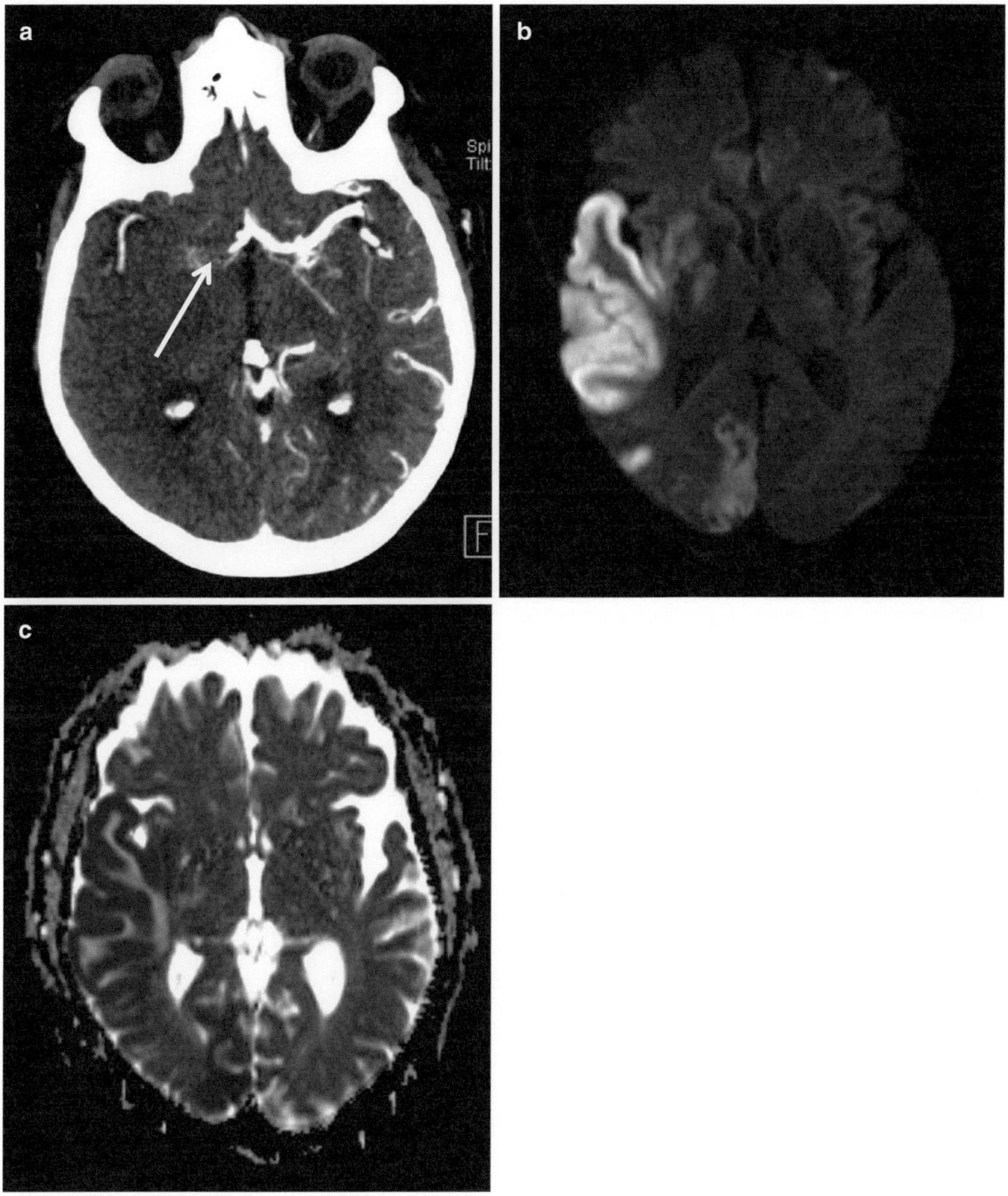

Fig. 1.2 Cytotoxic edema. (**a**) CT angiogram of the brain demonstrates hypodensity and loss of the gray–white matter interfaces of the right cerebral hemisphere. The M1 segment of middle cerebral artery is occluded (*white arrow*) and there are no collateral blood vessels. (**b**, **c**) DWI and ADC map demonstrate restricted diffusion in the temporal and occipital lobes corresponding to cytotoxic edema due to embolic infarcts in the middle and posterior cerebral artery territories

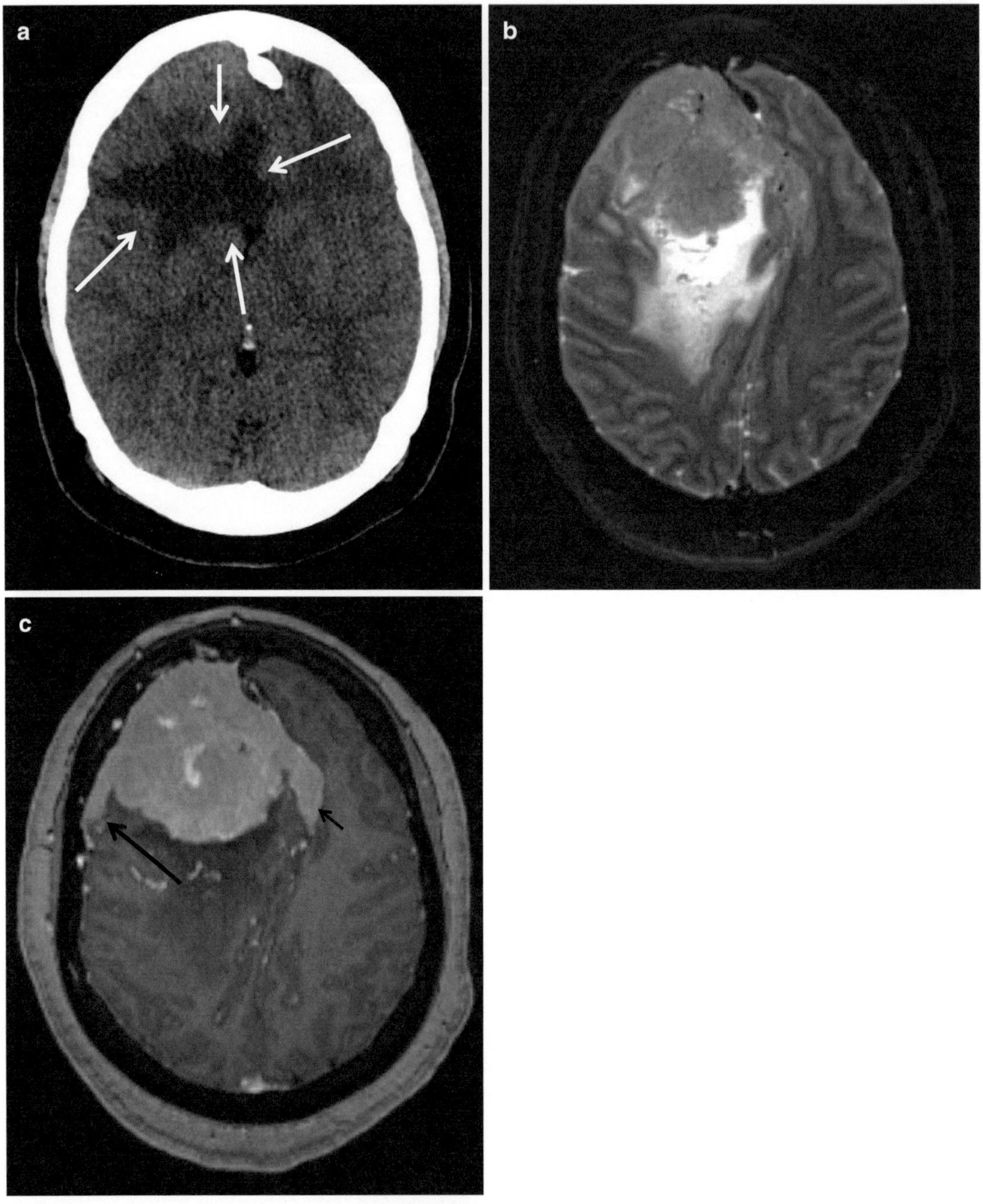

Fig. 1.3 Vasogenic edema associated with meningioma. (**a**) NECT depicts a hypodense area in the frontal white matter with fingerlike projections characteristic of vasogenic edema (*white arrows*). (**b**) T2WI shows white matter high signal associated with an extraaxial lesion. (**c**) Postcontrast T1WI demonstrates frontal lobe tumor (*short arrow*) with intense enhancement and dural tail (*long arrow*) compatible with a meningioma. About 30–60 % of meningiomas show underlying vasogenic edema

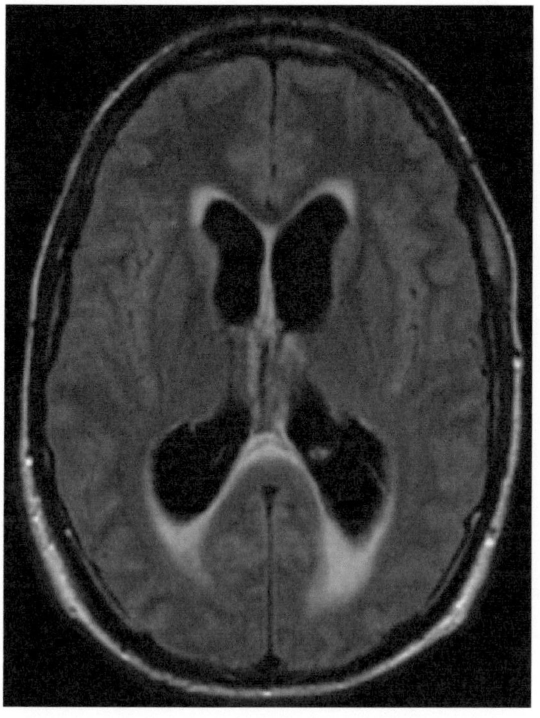

Fig. 1.4 Interstitial edema. Axial FLAIR image from a patient with acute obstructive hydrocephalus reveals dilated lateral ventricles and bilateral ill-defined periventricular hyperintensity of the white matter secondary to transependymal fluid migration and interstitial edema

areas like the frontal lobes, temporal lobes, corpus callosum, cerebellum, brainstem, basal ganglia, and thalami. DWI helps to differentiate vasogenic edema of PRES from cytotoxic edema [28, 29]. Junewar et al. in 2014 found a higher incidence of atypical distribution and cytotoxic edema than previously thought (cytotoxic edema was seen in 33 % of patients with eclampsia). They also found that an atypical presentation of PRES was associated with poor outcome [29].

Interstitial Edema

Interstitial edema occurs in the setting of increased intraventricular pressure, which causes rupture of the ventricular ependymal lining. This allows transependymal migration of CSF into the extracellular space most commonly in the periventricular white matter. On CT, the combination of ventriculomegaly and increased periventricular hypodensity is suggestive of interstitial edema. MRI is a more sensitive imaging modality showing hypointensity on T1WI and periventricular hyperintensity on T2WI and FLAIR (Fig. 1.4) [10].

Imaging Follow-Up

Cytotoxic edema: Contrast-enhanced CT angiography, MR angiography, and arteriography are useful for characterizing vascular abnormalities that accompany edema. In the setting of an acute stroke, CT or MRI perfusion is useful to define the ischemic areas and penumbra [10].

Vasogenic edema in tumors: MRI is the technique of choice to assess progression of tumors. Different and more sophisticated techniques are used together to determine the evolution of the disease even though most of the time histopathology is necessary to rule out tumor recurrence or progression.

Main Differential Diagnosis

Excitotoxic brain injury: Excitotoxic brain injury is considered a final common pathway for many conditions. It is characterized by excessive glutamate release in the synaptic clefts that bind with N-methyl-D-aspartate (NMDA) receptors allowing entry of Ca^{++} to the postsynaptic neurons and adjacent glial cells causing necrotic cell death or apoptosis [30]. The following conditions is associated with excitotoxic injury:

- *Status epilepticus*: Neuronal injury results primarily from an excitotoxic mechanism. During status epilepticus, neuronal seizure activity

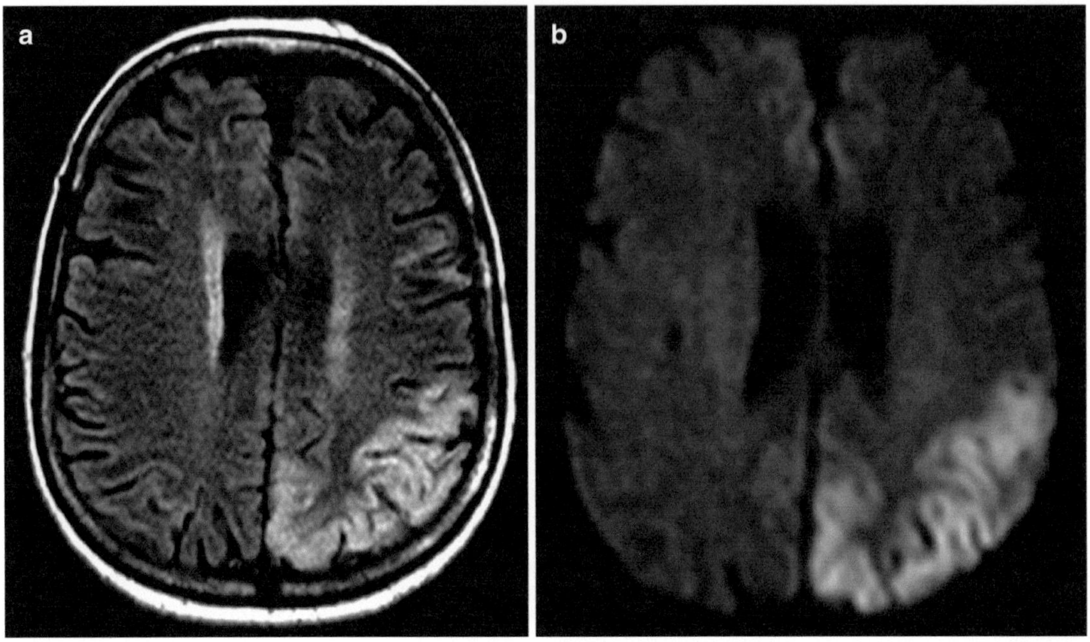

Fig. 1.5 Seizure-induced brain edema. (**a**) FLAIR and (**b**) DWI show cytotoxic edema probably caused by excitotoxic mechanisms involving the occipital and parietal cortex. These findings may mimic an acute stroke; however, the injury is not restricted to one vascular territory as is commonly in infarction. Two weeks later, the MRI study was unremarkable (not shown), confirming the diagnosis of seizure-induced edema

increases the release of glutamate from the presynaptic terminals of neuronal axons which causes cytotoxic edema in neurons and glial cells. Encephalopathy with status epilepticus often involves the hippocampus, other parts of the limbic system, the thalami, the cerebellum, and different cortical areas than can simulate an acute stroke (Fig. 1.5) [30, 31].

- *Transient lesion in the splenium of the corpus callosum* (*CC*): A unique focal area of diffusion abnormality may be observed in the splenium of the CC in the immediate postictal period. Transhemispheric connection of seizure activity may be the cause of this transient focal edema. Other speculations as to the causes of the focal lesion in the CC are the withdrawal of antiepileptic medications and some types of encephalitis. Seizure activity, effects of medications, or some infectious encephalitis can lead to excitotoxic injury, resulting in reversible cytotoxic edema. T2WI imaging shows a hyperintense lesion in the splenium of the CC, which is slightly hypointense in T1WI and has restricted diffusion on DWI (Fig. 1.6) [30, 32].

Ependymitis granularis: This normal anatomic variant around the tips of the frontal horns of the lateral ventricles results from regionally decreased myelin, increased extracellular fluid, or focal breakdown of the ependymal lining with gliosis which should not be mistaken with transependymal CSF resorption in hydrocephalus [10].

Tips

- It is important to characterize edema in terms of type, location, gray–white matter junction involvement, and associated mass effect (midline shift; ventricular, sulcal, and cisternal effacement; and cerebral herniations).
- Comparison with previous imaging studies is useful to determinate progression or regression.
- Determining the underlying cause of edema is imperative to guide the adequate management.

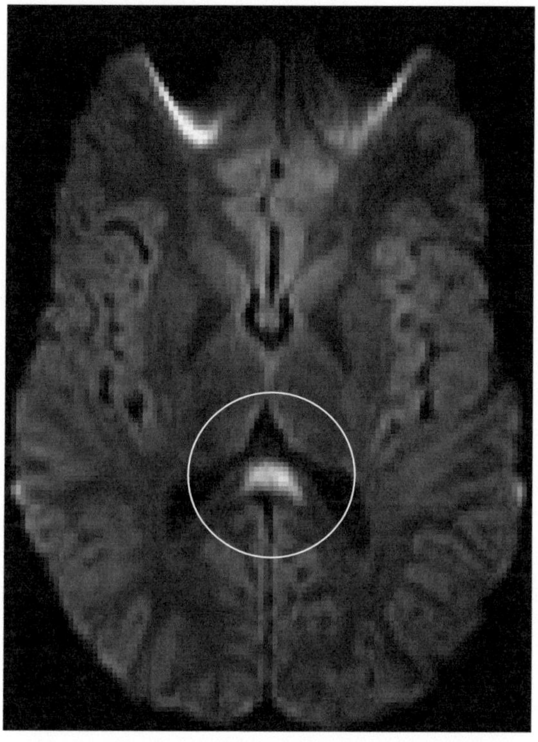

Fig. 1.6 Transient lesion of the splenium of the corpus callosum in a child with seizures. DWI demonstrates a high signal lesion (*circle*) which on ADC map showed restricted diffusion and that disappeared 3 months later (not shown)

- Some conditions like infarctions due to venous thrombosis, PRES, and arteriovenous shunts can present in a combination of cytotoxic and vasogenic edema.
- Remember the mechanism and locations responsible for excitotoxic edema to avoid confusion with other lesions.

References

1. Fishman RA. Brain edema. N Engl J Med. 1975; 293(14):706–11.
2. Glaser N, Barnett P, McCaslin I, Nelson D, Trainor J, Louie J, et al. Risk factors for cerebral edema in children with diabetic ketoacidosis. The Pediatric Emergency Medicine Collaborative Research Committee of the American Academy of Pediatrics. N Engl J Med. 2001;344(4):264–9.
3. Matsuzaki M, Takahashi R, Nakayama T, Shishikura K, Suzuki H, Hirayama Y, et al. Disruption of endothelial tight junctions in a patient with mitochondrial encephalomyopathy, lactic acidosis and stroke-like episodes (MELAS). Neuropediatrics. 2010;41(2): 72–4.
4. Gerstner ER, Duda DG, di Tomaso E, Ryg PA, Loeffler JS, Sorensen AG, et al. VEGF inhibitors in the treatment of cerebral edema in patients with brain cancer. Nat Rev Clin Oncol. 2009;6(4):229–36.
5. Hofmeijer J, Algra A, Kappelle LJ, van der Worp HB. Predictors of life-threatening brain edema in middle cerebral artery infarction. Cerebrovasc Dis. 2008; 25(1–2):176–84.
6. Hofmeijer J, Kappelle LJ, Algra A, Amelink GJ, van Gijn J, van der Worp HB, et al. Surgical decompression for space-occupying cerebral infarction (the Hemicraniectomy After Middle Cerebral Artery infarction with Life-threatening Edema Trial [HAMLET]): a multicentre, open, randomised trial. Lancet Neurol. 2009;8(4):326–33.
7. Simard JM, Sahuquillo J, Sheth KN, Kahle KT, Walcott BP. Managing malignant cerebral infarction. Curr Treat Options Neurol. 2011;13(2):217–29.
8. Wilde EA, McCauley SR, Hunter JV, Bigler ED, Chu Z, Wang ZJ, et al. Diffusion tensor imaging of acute mild traumatic brain injury in adolescents. Neurology. 2008;70(12):948–55.
9. Donkin JJ, Vink R. Mechanisms of cerebral edema in traumatic brain injury: therapeutic developments. Curr Opin Neurol. 2010;23(3):293–9.
10. Ho ML, Rojas R, Eisenberg RL. Cerebral edema. AJR Am J Roentgenol. 2012;199(3):W258–73.
11. Hutchinson P, Timofeev I, Kirkpatrick P. Surgery for brain edema. Neurosurg Focus. 2007;22(5):E14.
12. French LA, Galicich JH. The use of steroids for control of cerebral edema. Clin Neurosurg. 1964;10: 212–23.
13. Rabinstein AA. Treatment of cerebral edema. Neurologist. 2006;12(2):59–73.
14. Klatzo I. Presidential address. Neuropathological aspects of brain edema. J Neuropathol Exp Neurol. 1967;26(1):1–14.
15. Liang D, Bhatta S, Gerzanich V, Simard JM. Cytotoxic edema: mechanisms of pathological cell swelling. Neurosurg Focus. 2007;22(5):E2.
16. Le TH, Gean AD. Neuroimaging of traumatic brain injury. Mt Sinai J Med. 2009;76(2):145–62.
17. Andriessen TM, Jacobs B, Vos PE. Clinical characteristics and pathophysiological mechanisms of focal and diffuse traumatic brain injury. J Cell Mol Med. 2010;14(10):2381–92.
18. Krieger DW, Demchuk AM, Kasner SE, Jauss M, Hantson L. Early clinical and radiological predictors of fatal brain swelling in ischemic stroke. Stroke. 1999;30(2):287–92.
19. Foerster BR, Petrou M, Lin D, Thurnher MM, Carlson MD, Strouse PJ, et al. Neuroimaging evaluation of non-accidental head trauma with correlation to clinical outcomes: a review of 57 cases. J Pediatr. 2009;154(4):573–7.
20. Given 2nd CA, Burdette JH, Elster AD, Williams 3rd DW. Pseudo-subarachnoid hemorrhage: a potential

imaging pitfall associated with diffuse cerebral edema. AJNR Am J Neuroradiol. 2003;24(2):254–6.
21. Chalela JA, Rothlisberger J, West B, Hays A. The white cerebellum sign: an under recognized sign of increased intracranial pressure. Neurocrit Care. 2013;18(3):398–9.
22. Claassen J, Carhuapoma JR, Kreiter KT, Du EY, Connolly ES, Mayer SA. Global cerebral edema after subarachnoid hemorrhage: frequency, predictors, and impact on outcome. Stroke. 2002;33(5):1225–32.
23. Osborn AG. Osborn's brain : imaging, pathology, and anatomy. 1st ed. Salt Lake City: Amirsys; 2013.
24. Provenzale JM, McGraw P, Mhatre P, Guo AC, Delong D. Peritumoral brain regions in gliomas and meningiomas: investigation with isotropic diffusion-weighted MR imaging and diffusion-tensor MR imaging. Radiology. 2004;232(2):451–60.
25. Sternberg EJ, Lipton ML, Burns J. Utility of diffusion tensor imaging in evaluation of the peritumoral region in patients with primary and metastatic brain tumors. AJNR Am J Neuroradiol. 2014;35(3):439–44.
26. Yoshikawa T, Abe O, Tsuchiya K, Okubo T, Tobe K, Masumoto T, et al. Diffusion-weighted magnetic resonance imaging of dural sinus thrombosis. Neuroradiology. 2002;44(6):481–8.
27. Lovblad KO, Bassetti C, Schneider J, Ozdoba C, Remonda L, Schroth G. Diffusion-weighted MRI suggests the coexistence of cytotoxic and vasogenic oedema in a case of deep cerebral venous thrombosis. Neuroradiology. 2000;42(10):728–31.
28. Feske SK. Posterior reversible encephalopathy syndrome: a review. Semin Neurol. 2011;31(2): 202–15.
29. Junewar V, Verma R, Sankhwar PL, Garg RK, Singh MK, Malhotra HS, et al. Neuroimaging features and predictors of outcome in eclamptic encephalopathy: a prospective observational study. AJNR Am J Neuroradiol. 2014;35(9):1728–34.
30. Moritani T, Smoker WR, Sato Y, Numaguchi Y, Westesson PL. Diffusion-weighted imaging of acute excitotoxic brain injury. AJNR Am J Neuroradiol. 2005;26(2):216–28.
31. Cianfoni A, Caulo M, Cerase A, Della Marca G, Falcone C, Di Lella GM, et al. Seizure-induced brain lesions: a wide spectrum of variably reversible MRI abnormalities. Eur J Radiol. 2013;82(11): 1964–72.
32. Gallucci M, Limbucci N, Paonessa A, Caranci F. Reversible focal splenial lesions. Neuroradiology. 2007;49(7):541–4.

Cerebral Herniation

2

Natalí Angulo Carvallo, Prabhumallikarjun Patil, and Ana Lorena Abello

Abstract

Cerebral herniation refers to the displacement of the brain tissues from their normal compartments into adjacent spaces, and are the most common secondary manifestation of any space-occupying intracranial mass regardless of its etiology. Several types of herniations have been described following anatomical basis (subfalcine, descending transtentorial, ascending transtentorial, transalar, and transcranial). The availability and speed of CT make it very useful in critically ill patients who may not tolerate either the wait for or duration of an MRI examination; however, MRI allows better characterization of brain herniations as well as early diagnosis of ischemic and hemorrhagic complications.

Background

Cerebral herniation is the displacement of brain tissue from its normal compartment into an adjacent space. Cerebral herniation is the most common secondary manifestation of any space-occupying intracranial mass regardless of its etiology and depends upon many factors including patient age, size, location, and progression rate of the mass lesion [1, 2].

The sum of the volumes of the brain, cerebrospinal fluid (CSF), and intracranial blood is constant in an intact skull. Accordingly, any increase in intracranial volume requires a compensatory and equal decrease in other contents (the Monro–Kellie hypothesis). CSF in sulci and subarachnoid cisterns is initially squeezed out when extra volume is added. The mass effect eventually

N. Angulo Carvallo, MD
Departamento de Radiología, Instituto Nacional de Enfermedades Neoplasicas, Universidad Nacional Mayor de San Marcos, AV. Sergio Bernales 124 apto, 1002 Surquillo, Lima, Peru
e-mail: natyangulo15@gmail.com

P. Patil, MBBS, MD
Bangalore Medical College and Research Institute, Mallikarjun Sadan Station Rd, Bijapur, Karnataka 586101, India
e-mail: prabhupatil16@gmail.com

A.L. Abello, MD (✉)
Department of Radiology, University of North Carolina, Chapel Hill, NC, USA
e-mail: anaabellop@hotmail.com

R. Hoffmann Nunes et al. (eds.), *Critical Findings in Neuroradiology*,
DOI 10.1007/978-3-319-27987-9_2

exceeds the brain's compensatory capacity, and intracranial pressure (ICP) begins to rise and causes displacement of brain tissues resulting in one or more cerebral herniations [1–3].

Several types of herniations have been described following anatomical basis (Table 2.1).

Symptoms of cerebral herniation depend on the part of the brain affected, the structures compressed, and other underlying conditions such as hydrocephalus or infarct.

Subfalcine herniation (*SFH*) results in unilateral hydrocephalus because the contralateral foramen of Monro is obstructed. If SFH becomes severe, the herniated anterior cerebral artery can be pinned against the inferior "free" margin of the falx cerebri and then occluded causing an infarct. *In unilateral descending transtentorial* (*uncal*) *herniation*, pupillary dilatation and ophthalmoplegia (due to third cranial nerve compression) followed by ipsilateral hemiplegia (the "false-localizing" sign) are due to the contralateral cerebral peduncle being forced against the edge of the tentorium inducing ischemia (Kernohan's notch phenomenon). This may be followed by an irregular respiratory pattern, fixed and dilated pupils, coma, and cardiorespiratory collapse [1, 4]. *Bilateral cerebral herniation or central herniation* is a condition whose manifestations consist in progressive syndromes that develop in the brainstem from top to bottom [5].

Table 2.1 Classification of brain herniations

1. Subfalcine herniation
2. Descending transtentorial herniation
Unilateral DTH or uncal herniation
Bilateral DTH or central herniation
3. Ascending transtentorial herniation
4. Transalar herniation
Ascending
Descending
5. Tonsillar herniation
6. Transcranial herniation

Key Points

Etiology

Cerebral herniations developed due to several factors that produce mass effect within the skull and increase the intracranial pressure. The most common causes include hematomas, infarctions, infection, cerebral edema, tumors, or hemorrhages (Table 2.2) [1, 2, 6, 7].

Best Imaging Modality

Non-enhanced computed tomography (*CT*): The availability and speed of CT are very useful in critically ill patients who may not tolerate either the wait for or duration of an MRI examination. CT is useful to diagnose subfalcine, transalar, and transcranial herniation and the effacement of the suprasellar cisterns in transtentorial herniations [8, 9].

Magnetic resonance imaging (*MRI*): Allows better characterization of brain herniations and early diagnosis of ischemic and hemorrhagic complications [8, 9]. It may be dangerous to place patients with herniations in the MRI units

Table 2.2 Etiology of brain herniations

Type	Causes
Traumatic	Epidural/subdural hematoma
	Pneumocephalus
	Brain contusion
Infectious	Empyema
	Encephalitis
	Brain abscess
	Focal inflammatory lesions
Metabolic	Hepatic encephalopathy
	Toxic–metabolic encephalopathy
Vascular	Intracerebral hemorrhage
	Stroke
	Hypertensive encephalopathy
	Vascular malformations
Neoplastic	Benign, malignant, primary, and metastatic tumors

as monitoring is more complex than when the examinations are done with CT.

Major Findings

Subfalcine Herniation

When subfalcine herniation occurs, the anterior falx, although rigid, will tilt away from the mass lesion. The posterior falx is wider, more rigid, and more resistant to displacement. This explains why subfalcine herniations only occur anteriorly. Displacement from midline involving the cingulate gyrus, anterior cerebral arteries, ipsilateral lateral ventricle, and internal cerebral veins occurs below the interhemispheric falx. Contralateral ventricle enlargement and transependymal edema develop if the foramen of Monro is obstructed and the ipsilateral ventricle is compressed because of mass effect. As the brain is displaced beneath the free margin of the falx, branches of the ipsilateral anterior cerebral artery may become trapped, resulting in infarction of the anterior cerebral artery territory. Ross et al. reported that greater midline shift on CT scans correlates with a significantly lower likelihood of recovery in patients with acute intracranial hematomas. All patients in their series with a septal shift over 15 mm had a poor outcome. Conversely, no patient with septal shift less than 5 mm shift had a poor outcome (Figs. 2.1 and 2.2) [1, 8–12].

Descending Transtentorial Herniation (DTH)

Transtentorial herniation occurs when the brain tissue is displaced into the tentorial notch [11]. It can be of the following types:

- *Unilateral descending transtentorial herniation or uncal herniation*: This type of herniation is usually generated by a hemispheric mass-like lesion. Axial CT/MRI images show the uncus displaced medially and the ipsilateral suprasellar cistern to be effaced. As DTH progresses, the hippocampus herniates medially over the edge of the tentorium compressing the quadrigeminal/ambient cistern and pushing the midbrain toward the contralateral edge of the incisura. The posterior cerebral artery may be displaced inferomedially and can eventually be occluded as it passes back up over the medial edge of the tentorium causing an occipital infarction. Perforating arteries that arise from the top of the basilar artery may be compressed and become occluded causing a secondary hemorrhagic midbrain infarct known as *Duret hemorrhages* (Figs. 2.2 and 2.3) [1, 9, 13].
- *Bilateral descending transtentorial herniation*: Also called "complete" or "central" descending herniation. This occurs when the supratentorial mass effect becomes severe in the frontal, parietal, and occipital lobes. On axial CT/MR images, the temporal lobes are herniated medially into the tentorial hiatus,

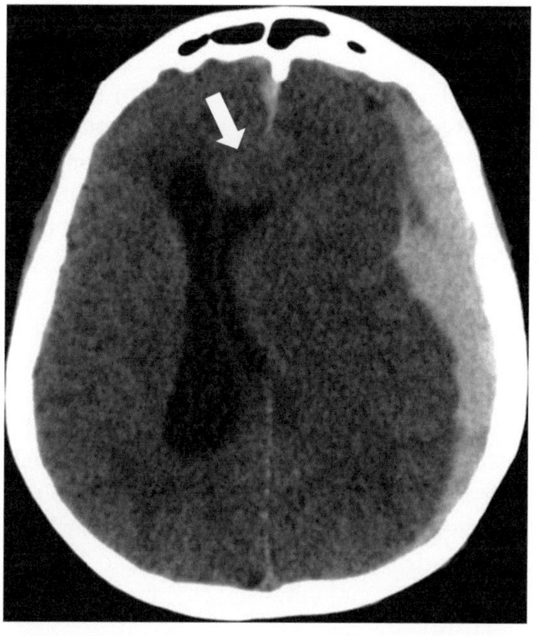

Fig. 2.1 Patient with history of trauma and a left-sided acute subdural hematoma. Axial NECT shows a left subdural hematoma with mass effect generating left lateral ventricle effacement, right midline shift, unilateral right lateral ventricle dilatation, and subfalcine herniation of the left cingulate gyrus (*arrow*)

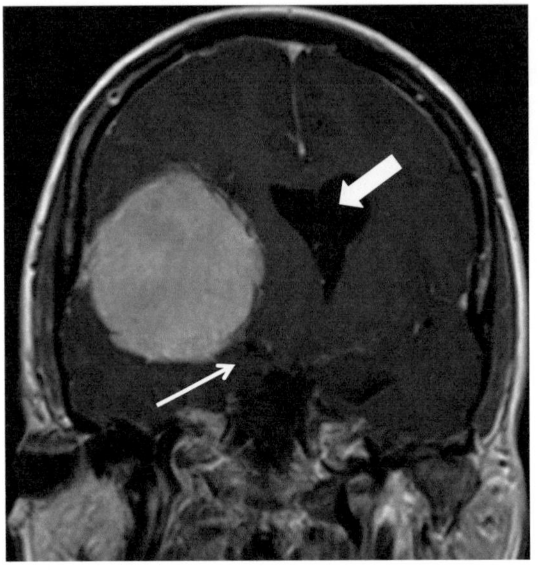

Fig. 2.2 Postcontrast coronal T1WI MRI in a patient with right Sylvian fissure meningioma producing mass effect and secondary subfalcine herniation and left midline shift (*thick arrow*). Unilateral descending transtentorial herniation with uncus effacement of the right side of the suprasellar cistern is seen (*thin arrow*)

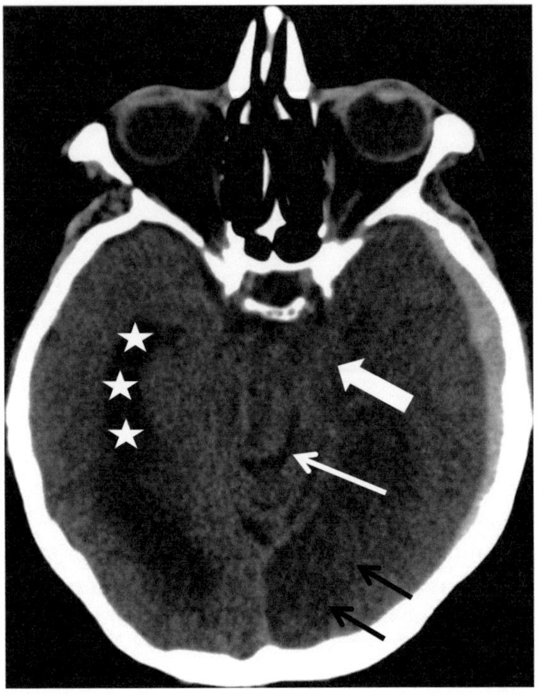

Fig. 2.3 Patient with a left acute subdural hematoma. Axial NECT shows left unilateral descending transtentorial herniation. The uncus is displaced medially and the ipsilateral perimesencephalic cistern is effaced (*thick white arrow*). Brainstem is rotated and displaced to the opposite side and caudally producing widening of the ipsilateral ambient cistern (*thin white arrow*). Compression of the contralateral posterior temporal horn results in dilatation of its anterior aspect (*stars*). Note left occipital lobe infarction (*thin black arrows*) secondary to left posterior cerebral artery compression

and there is complete effacement of the basal cisterns. The midbrain is compressed and squeezed medially from both sides, and the pons is displaced inferiorly and compressed against the clivus. Caudal displacement of the third ventricle and the thalami may be seen. Hydrocephalus develops because of distortion and obstruction of the cerebral aqueduct, further increasing the volume and pressure of supratentorial contents. Perforating arteries that arise from the circle of Willis may be compressed and become occluded causing hypothalamic and basal ganglia infarctions. Duret hemorrhages are also frequent and are better demonstrated on gradient-echo MRI, as well as susceptibility-weighted imaging [1, 9, 11, 14].

Ascending Transtentorial Herniation (ATH)

It is caused by expanding lesions in the posterior fossa. In most cases, it is bilateral and results in symmetric obliteration of the perimesencephalic cisterns [15]. The vermis and medial portions of cerebellar hemispheres are pushed upward through the tentorial incisura leading to effacement of the superior vermian, ambient, and quadrigeminal cisterns and flattening and compression of the tectal plate and midbrain. The cerebral aqueduct of Sylvius is generally compressed causing hydrocephalus. Ascending tentorial herniation can compress the posterior cerebral arteries or superior cerebellar arteries against the tentorium, resulting in infarctions (Figs. 2.4 and 2.6) [8, 9, 11, 13].

Transalar Herniation

- *Ascending transalar herniation*: Is better depicted on off-midline sagittal MRI/CT

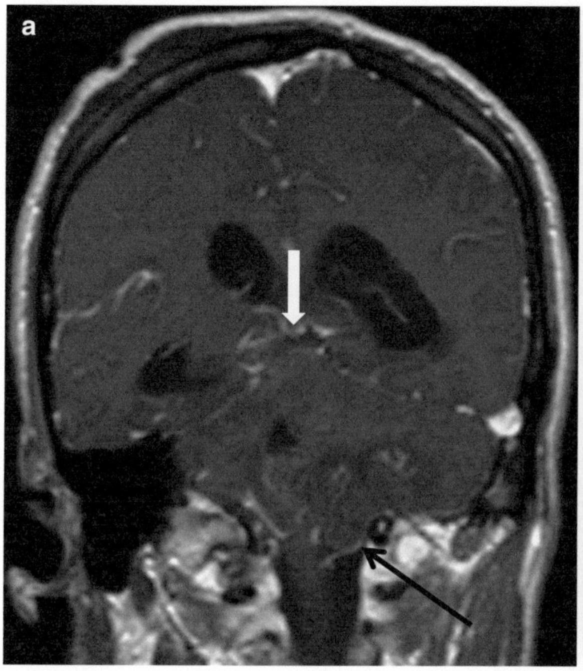

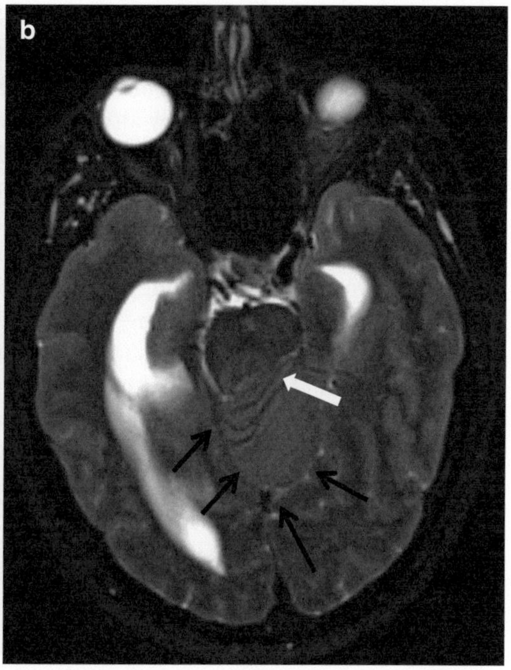

Fig. 2.4 Patient with left subacute cerebellar infarct. (**a**) Coronal postcontrast T1WI MR illustrates left tonsillar herniation (*thin black arrow*) and left cerebellar hemisphere extension across the posterior edge of the tentorial notch, constituting an ascending transtentorial herniation (*thick white arrow*). Compression and displacement of the fourth ventricle is also seen. (**b**) Axial T2WI MR shows the vermis and left cerebellar hemisphere (*thin black arrows*) pushed upward through the tentorial incisura with a flattened and compressed tectal plate (*thick white arrow*). There is lateral ventricle enlargement due infratentorial ventricular system compression

images. In this type of herniation, a large middle cranial fossa mass (intra-/extra-axial) generally displaces the temporal lobe, the Sylvian fissure and middle cerebral artery superiorly and anteriorly, and over the greater sphenoid wing [8, 9]. Superior displacement of the temporal lobe can compress the supraclinoid internal carotid artery against the anterior clinoid process and result in infarction of the anterior and middle cerebral artery territories (Fig. 2.5) [15].

- *Descending transalar herniation*: In this situation, a large anterior cranial fossa mass displaces the gyrus rectus posteroinferiorly over the greater sphenoid wing displacing the Sylvian fissure. Shifting the middle cerebral artery backward results in a middle cerebral artery infarction due to its compression against the sphenoid ridge [8, 9, 15].

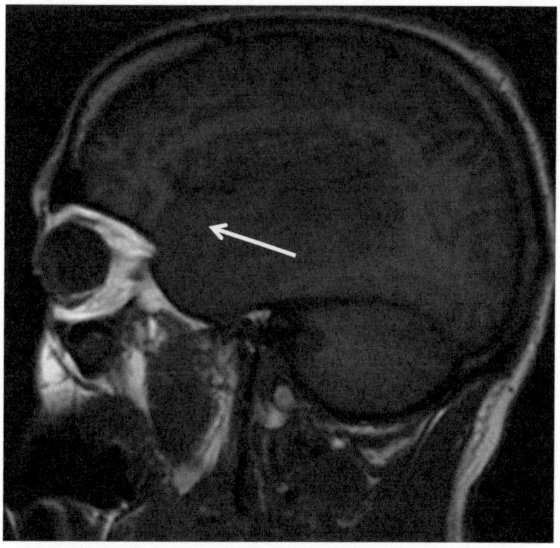

Fig. 2.5 Sagittal T1WI MR in a patient with left temporal lobe low-grade glioma shows ascending transalar herniation. Note that the middle cranial fossa mass displaces the left temporal lobe and Sylvian fissure into the anterior cranial fossa (*thin white arrow*)

Tonsillar Herniation

Caudal herniation of the cerebellar tonsils into the foramen magnum is most commonly caused by an infratentorial mass but may also occur as a result of an expanding supratentorial mass. In fact, tonsillar herniation occurs in association with descending transtentorial herniation in 20–50 % of cases. The tonsils are impacted into the foramen magnum obliterating CSF space in the cisterna magna and displacing the medulla anteriorly. Sagittal plane images show vertically oriented tonsils and displacement of over 5 mm below the foramen magnum. Perhaps, more important than strict quantitative criteria of tonsillar displacement are the morphologic appearances of the brainstem and surrounding CSF spaces. When the tonsils extend below the foramen magnum, anterior displacement of the lower brainstem and loss of CSF space surrounding the brainstem are important in distinguishing tonsillar herniation from normal variations. The main complications are obstructive hydrocephalus and tonsillar necrosis (Figs. 2.4 and 2.6) [1, 9, 11, 13, 16].

Transcranial Herniation

Surgery or trauma can be the cause of calvarial defects, these providing an easy pathway through which swollen brain tissues may herniate and extrude through them into the subgaleal space [15]. The disrupted dura is better seen in MRI as a discontinuous black line on T2WI. The herniated brain tissue adopts a similar morphology to that of a mushroom [1, 8, 9] (Fig. 2.7).

Imaging Follow-Up

- Compare brain herniation with previous studies to detect rapid progression and prevent a fatal outcome.
- If MRI must be obtained it should include diffusion-weighted imaging, SWI, and contrast are recommended to rule out early ischemic and hemorrhagic complications as well as to appropriately assess the probable cause [8, 9].

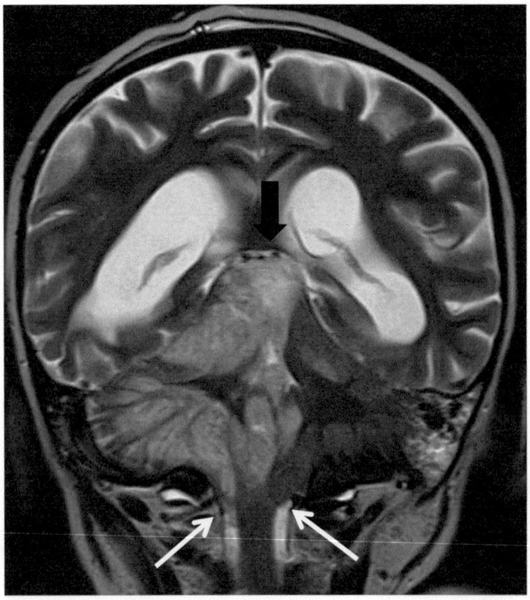

Fig. 2.6 Patient with basilar artery infarct. Coronal T2WI MR shows ascending transtentorial herniation (*thick black arrow*) and bilateral tonsillar herniation (*thin white arrows*)

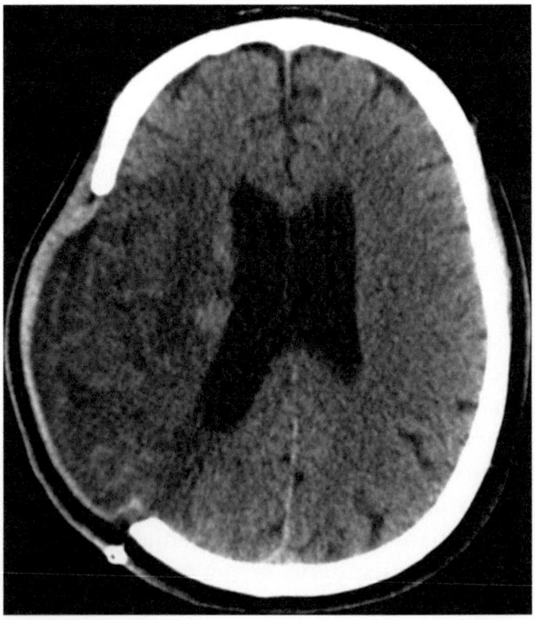

Fig. 2.7 Axial NECT in a patient with extensive right middle cerebral artery stroke, and a decompressive hemicraniectomy, shows transcranial herniation with the brain tissue through the skull defect

Main Differential Diagnosis

Intracranial hypotension: The brain is sagging but not pushed down and the suprasellar cisterns are effaced, in this situation other signs help to differentiate it from bilateral transtentorial brain herniation. These include diffuse dural thickening, engorgement of the dural sinuses, pituitary gland enlargement, and the absence of a lesion that produces the herniation [8]. In intracranial hypotension, symptoms are chronic, and in many patients, there is a history of lumbar puncture or surgery.

Congenital tonsillar herniation associated with Chiari I malformation could be misdiagnosed for acute tonsillar herniation; however, Chiari I patients have chronic symptoms and the absence of mass effect.

Tips

- Look for midline shift, ventricle displacement, obliteration of basilar cisterns, or CSF spaces at the foramen magnum and effacement of sulci.
- Mention the degree of herniation (i.e., how many millimeters are shifted off the midline in subfalcine herniation) and the structures involved.
- Look for secondary complications such as hydrocephalus, transependymal edema, infarctions, Duret hemorrhages, and others [9].
- Diagnose the primary cause of the herniation.

References

1. Osborn AG. Osborn's brain: imaging, pathology, and anatomy. 1st ed. Salt Lake City: Amirsys Pub; 2013. xi, 1272 p.
2. Cruz J, Minoja G, Okuchi K. Improving clinical outcomes from acute subdural hematomas with the emergency preoperative administration of high doses of mannitol: a randomized trial. Neurosurgery. 2001;49(4):864–71.
3. Mokri B. The Monro-Kellie hypothesis: applications in CSF volume depletion. Neurology. 2001;56(12): 1746–8.
4. Pourmand R. Practicing neurology: what you need to know, what you need to do. 2nd ed. Totowa: Humana Press; 2008. xii, 222 p.
5. Sekula Jr RF, Marchan EM, Baghai P, Jannetta PJ, Quigley MR. Central brain herniation secondary to fulminant acute disseminated encephalomyelitis: implications for neurosurgical management. Case report. J Neurosurg. 2006;105(3):472–4.
6. Jain G, Yadav G, Varshney R. Brain herniation. In: Ltd. iP, editor. Neurological disorders: clinical methods. USA: iConcept Press Ltd; 2014.
7. Weinberg JS, Rhines LD, Cohen ZR, Langford L, Levin VA. Posterior fossa decompression for life-threatening tonsillar herniation in patients with gliomatosis cerebri: report of three cases. Neurosurgery. 2003;52(1):216–23. discussion 23.
8. Osborn AG, Salzman KL, Barkovich AJ. Diagnostic imaging. Brain. 2nd ed. Salt Lake City: Amirsys; 2010.
9. Naidich TP. Imaging of the brain. Philadelphia: Saunders/Elsevier; 2013. xv, 1052 p.
10. Wu H, Yang SF, Qiu YM, Dai J, Li SQ, Zhang XH, et al. The diagnosis and surgical treatment of central brain herniations caused by traumatic bifrontal contusions. J Craniofac Surg. 2014;25(6):2105–8.
11. Johnson PL, Eckard DA, Chason DP, Brecheisen MA, Batnitzky S. Imaging of acquired cerebral herniations. Neuroimaging Clin N Am. 2002;12(2):217–28.
12. Ross DA, Olsen WL, Ross AM, Andrews BT, Pitts LH. Brain shift, level of consciousness, and restoration of consciousness in patients with acute intracranial hematoma. J Neurosurg. 1989;71(4):498–502.
13. Yousem DM, Grossman RI. Neuroradiology: the requisites. 3rd ed. Philadelphia: Mosby/Elsevier; 2010. xvii, 619 p.
14. Swingler RJ. Controversial treatments for spinal-cord injuries. Lancet. 2005;365(9462):841–2.
15. Laine FJ, Shedden AI, Dunn MM, Ghatak NR. Acquired intracranial herniations: MR imaging findings. AJR Am J Roentgenol. 1995;165(4): 967–73.
16. Reimer P. Clinical MR imaging: a practical approach. 3rd ed. Heidelberg: Springer; 2010. xx, 820 p.

3 Intracranial Hypotension (Hypovolemia) Syndrome

Juan Manuel González and Florencia Álamos

Abstract

Intracranial hypotension syndrome (IHS) consists of decreased cerebrospinal fluid (CSF) volume resulting in compensatory distention of vascular structures and downward traction of richly innervated structures. Clinical presentation can vary from orthostatic headache, cranial nerve neuropathy, tonsillar herniation, coma, to demise. Magnetic resonance of the brain is the study of choice demonstrating several characteristic features that suggest the diagnosis. Management consists of supportive measures with symptom resolution in most cases; in more severe cases, therapeutic procedures to close the leaking defect are required.

Background

IHS is a clinical syndrome in which low CSF volume results in orthostatic or postural headaches that improves in recumbent position [1]. The diagnosis of IHS can be confirmed by demonstrating a cerebrospinal fluid (CSF) opening pressure less than 60 mm H_2O [2].

J.M. González, MD (✉)
Department of Radiology, Hahnemann University Hospital, Drexel University College of Medicine, 230 North Broad Street, Philadelphia, PA 19102, USA
e-mail: Juan_m_gg@hotmail.com

F. Álamos, MD, PhD
Department of Neuroscience, School of Medicine, Universidad Católica de Chile, Luz larrain, 3946, Lo Barnechea, Santiago, Chile
e-mail: Flopi1987@yahoo.com

One hypothesis suggests that orthostatic headaches in IHS are most likely caused by downward displacement of the brain resulting in downward traction of the richly innervated dura [3–6]. Another hypothesis advocates dilatation of vascular venous structures as the cause of headaches. According to the Monro–Kellie hypothesis, acute CSF loss is compensated with increase in intracranial blood volume, and the intracranial pressure suffers an additional decrease during upright position inducing vascular dilatation generating additional distention of venous structures [3, 4, 6, 7].

IHS can be classified as primary or secondary [2–4, 6, 8–10]. The incidence of spontaneous IHS is 5 per 100,000 individuals per year while the estimated prevalence is 1:50.000 per year. It can occur at any age, but peak prevalence is during the third and fourth decades of life [9, 11, 12].

R. Hoffmann Nunes et al. (eds.), *Critical Findings in Neuroradiology*,
DOI 10.1007/978-3-319-27987-9_3

Women are more often affected than men (2:1) and IHS is unusual in children [6, 9, 13–15].

The most common symptom in IHS is orthostatic headaches which are generally gradual in onset and vary in severity from mild to debilitating [4, 7, 9, 16–19]. Secondary symptoms are seen in 50 % of patients and include posterior neck pain or stiffness, nausea, and vomiting, all attributable to meningeal irritation. IHS is sometimes accompanied by photophobia, dizziness, horizontal diplopia, galactorrhea, facial numbness or weakness, and radicular symptoms involving upper extremities, all of which are orthostatic in nature and less commonly by hypoacusia and tinnitus attributable to either vestibulocochlear nerve traction associated with the sagging brain or transmission of low CSF pressure to the perilymph [18]. Although very uncommon, stupor or coma rarely progressing to demise from tonsillar herniation and brainstem compression can be the initial presentation of severe IHS [16]. Atypical presentations include parkinsonism, frontotemporal dementia, syringomyelia, hypopituitarism, seizures, coma, and death [3–5, 9].

In most patients, symptoms resolve spontaneously in 2 weeks to 6 months and can be treated with analgesics [5, 6]. CSF pressure decreases in recumbent position allowing the leaking meningeal defect to seal [3, 9]. Therapies directed to increase CSF volume include intravenous or oral hydration, increased salt intake, carbon dioxide inhalation, and steroid therapy; however, these therapies are empirical and their efficacy remains unclear [3, 6]. Some patients develop persistent symptomatic intracranial hypotension that does not respond to simple measures, and in them an epidural blood patch can be performed and is being effective in 80–90 % and in 98 % of patients undergoing repeated patches [3, 5, 6, 20]. If IHS presents with downward brain herniation with progressive mental status decline, increasing the intracranial and intraspinal pressure by means of intrathecal infusion of artificial CSF or preservative-free saline can be lifesaving if instituted rapidly [21, 22]. If all treatment measures are unsuccessful, surgical correction of dural tears or meningeal diverticula may be indicated [3, 6].

Key Points

Etiology

Although causes of IHS are diverse, they can be classified as *spontaneous* (*primary*) or *secondary* [2–4, 6, 8–10]. In both spontaneous and secondary types of intracranial hypotension, the cause is generally persistent CSF leakage through a dural defect. Causes of secondary IHS include therapeutic and diagnostic spinal puncture, craniotomy, spinal surgery, craniospinal trauma, ventriculoperitoneal shunt, and medical conditions such as dehydration, diabetic coma, uremia, severe systemic illness, and connective tissue abnormalities (e.g., Marfan, Ehlers–Danlos).

In addition to meningeal diverticula, direct mechanical perforation of the dura secondary to osteophytes is a cause of IHS [23–27]. Approximately one-third of patients with IHS have a history of recent minor trauma although its significance is not certain, and two-thirds have clinical features suggestive of an underlying connective tissue disorder [2, 17, 18, 28–31].

Best Imaging Modality

Magnetic resonance imaging (*MRI*): Cranial MRI with contrast is the imaging study of choice. It demonstrates signs of IHS which have been reported to have a specificity and sensitivity of nearly 94 % [32]. On the other hand, the spectrum of findings is variable and rarely all signs are found in the same patient [9].

Computed tomography (*CT*): Headache evaluation usually starts with non-contrast head CT to detect other intracranial causes; however, it is not a sensitive study for the detection of IHS and the brain may appear normal [9].

Spinal MRI: Findings suggesting the leaking defect include extra-arachnoid fluid collections, spinal meningeal enhancement, and dilatation of the anterior internal epidural venous plexus. Spinal MRI can give the location of the leaking defect even if leakage is not active, because it can detect fluid accumulation using T2-weighted images (T2WI) [3].

Computerized tomography myelography: CT slices are obtained after administering intrathecal iodine contrast agent. The advantages of the study include higher resolution, more precise localization of the defect, and visualization of anatomic defects such as meningeal diverticula. CT myelography demonstrates the leaking level more often than spinal magnetic resonance or radioisotope cisternography [3].

The suggested protocol to study IHS is depicted in Diagram 3.1.

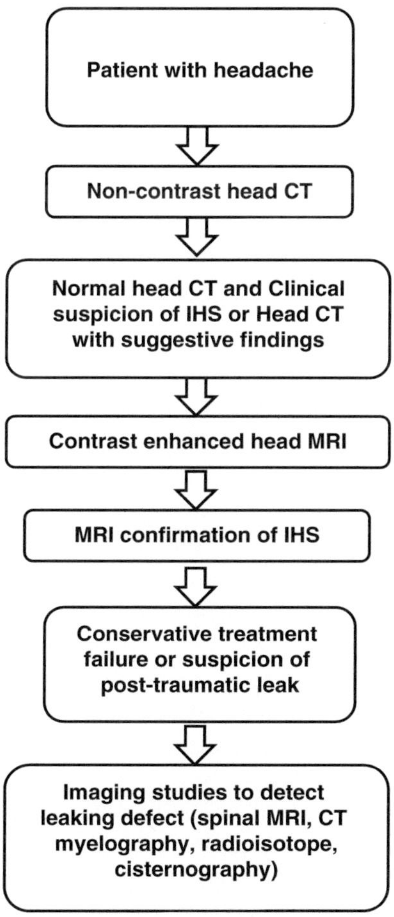

Diagram 3.1 Workup protocol for intracranial hypotension syndrome

Major Findings

CT may demonstrate obliteration of basilar cisterns from brain sagging, temporal lobe herniation into the tentorial incisura, subdural fluid collections in 15 % of patients, subdural hemorrhages, small ventricles with medial deviation of atria, and a "fat-appearing" pons [3, 9].

In *MRI*, the most constant finding is linear diffuse pachymeningeal thickening and enhancement in the supra- and infratentorial compartments without the involvement of leptomeninges on postcontrast T1-weighted images (T1WI) which is detected in 85 % of patients (Figs. 3.1 and 3.4). This finding was also seen on fluid-attenuated inversion recovery imaging (FLAIR) as high signal of the meninges [3, 5–7, 19, 33].

Other findings include engorgement of venous sinuses and flow voids in them and enlargement of arteries and medullary and cortical veins.

An outwardly convex inferior margin of the dominant transverse sinus is a sign of IHS with sensitivity and specificity close to 94 % (Fig. 3.2) [3, 5–7, 9, 19, 33].

Downward displacement of the brain is seen in 50 % of patients. On sagittal T1WI, the midbrain is displaced caudally with the angle between cerebral peduncles and pons measuring less than 90°. In IHS, the midbrain is usually located more than 1.8 mm below the incisural line (a line connecting the anterior tuberculum sellae to the point of confluence of straight and inferior sagittal sinus with the great cerebral vein) (Fig. 3.3) [3, 5–7, 9, 19, 33].

Enlargement of the pituitary gland, flattening of the pons against clivus, reduction in the width of the prepontine cistern, and downward descent of cerebellar tonsils 3 mm below the McRae line (line connecting the most caudal portion of the clivus to the posterior border of the foramen magnum) are other typical signs (Fig. 3.3) [3, 5–7, 9, 19, 33].

Recently described is enlargement of the inferior intercavernous sinus that is almost never seen in the normal adult population. It appears as enlargement of the sellar contents and has been described as an adjunctive sign for the diagnosis of IHS [34].

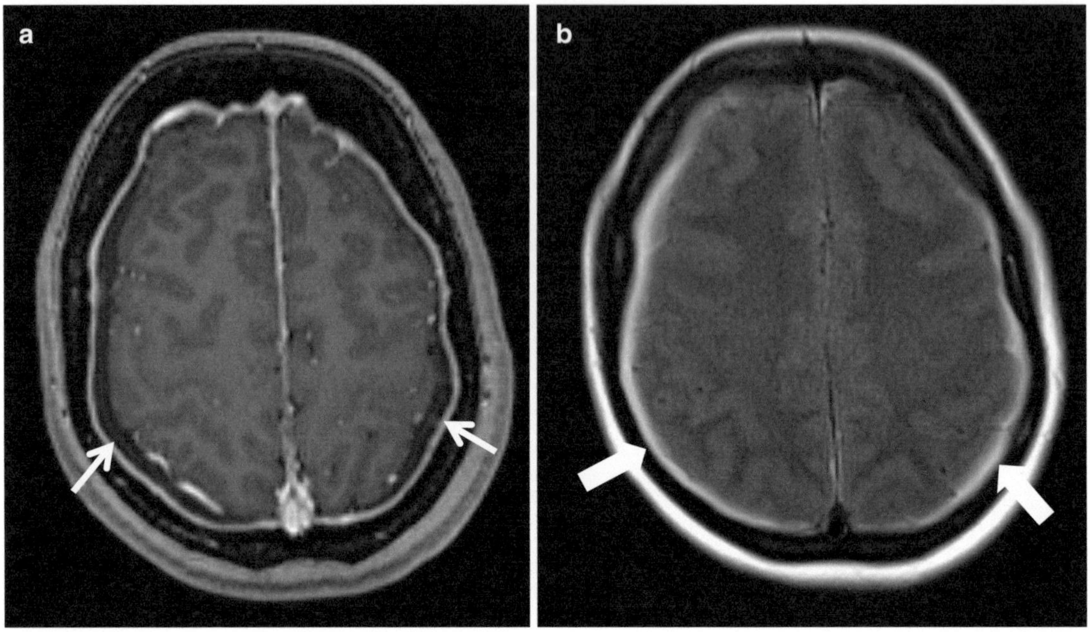

Fig. 3.1 Pachymeningeal thickening and subdural collections. (**a**) Axial postcontrast T1WI and (**b**) axial FLAIR demonstrate diffuse smooth pachymeningeal thickening (*thin arrows* in **a**) and bilateral subdural collections (*thick arrows* in **b**). The subdural collections are also seen in (**a**) as areas of low signal intensity medially

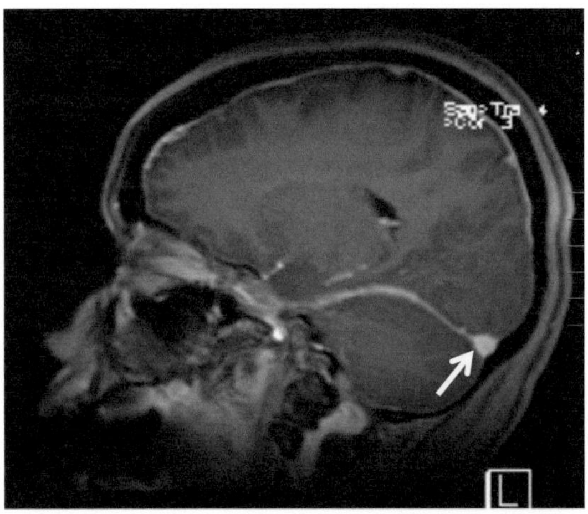

Fig. 3.2 Sagittal postcontrast T1WI shows dilated transverse sinus with outward bowing of its borders (*white arrow*). The tentorium is thick and enhances

Additional signs include inferior displacement of the optic chiasm, a hypothalamus draped around the sella, effacement of the chiasmatic cistern, and a callosal splenium displacing downward the junction of the internal cerebral veins with the great vein of Galen (Figs. 3.3 and 3.4) [3, 5–7, 9, 19, 33].

Subdural collections or hygromas usually bilateral and less than 7 mm thick without mass effect are commonly found (Figs. 3.1 and 3.4) [3, 5–7, 9, 19, 33].

IHS has also been associated with superficial siderosis, which has been hypothesized to be secondary to microtrauma of the venous plexus, dural defects, or vascular engorgement related to the hypovolemia [35].

On coronal images, the lateral ventricles have a diminished diameter, and the angle between the roofs of both lateral ventricles can be below 120° [3, 5–7, 9, 19, 33].

Dural sinus and cortical vein thrombosis have been described as uncommon complications of IHS and are believed to be secondary to slow blood flow in a dilated dural sinus [36]. Their risk is increased in patients with thrombotic preconditions [37].

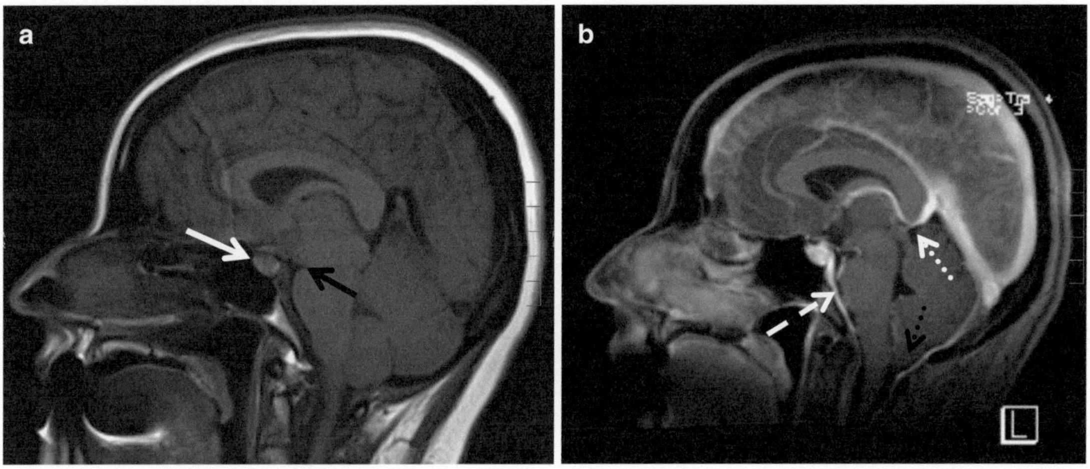

Fig. 3.3 Brain sagging and enlargement of the pituitary gland. (**a**) Sagittal T1WI demonstrates the obliterated suprasellar cistern, draped optic chiasm, hypophyseal enlargement (*white arrow*), and brainstem sagging with decreased cerebral peduncle–pons angle due to compression of the interpeduncular cistern (*black arrow*). (**b**) Sagittal postcontrast T1WI demonstrates dilated venous sinuses, downward displacement of the splenium pushing on the junction of the internal cerebral veins with the great vein of Galen (*dotted white arrow*), obliteration of the prepontine cistern with "fat pons" sign (*dashed white arrow*), and caudal displacement of cerebellar tonsils (*dotted black arrow*)

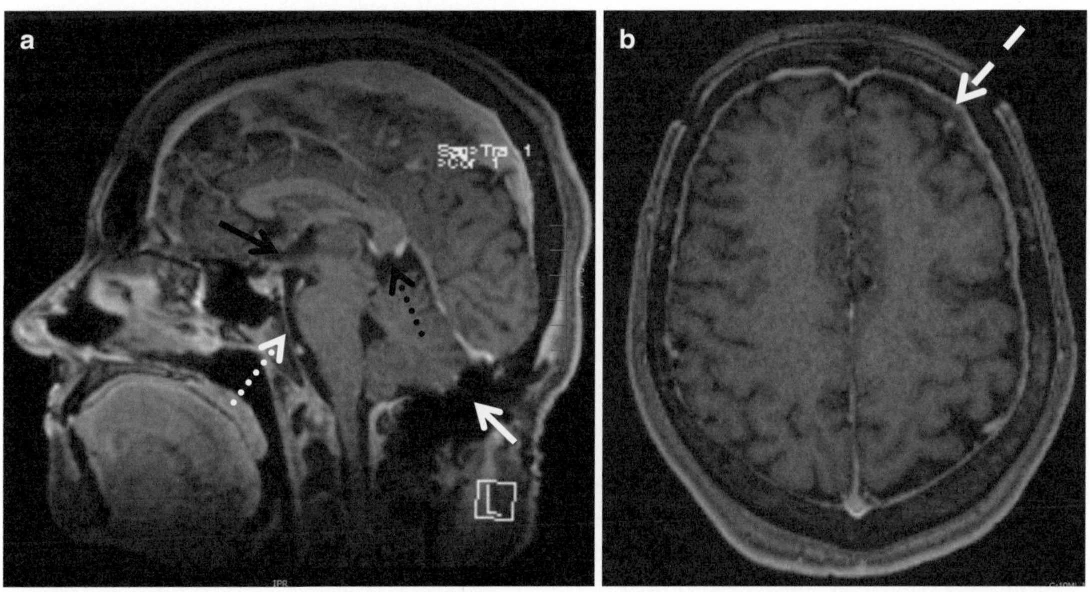

Fig. 3.4 Brain sagging and pachymeningeal thickening in a patient post-craniectomy and orthostatic headache. (**a**, **b**) Sagittal and axial postcontrast T1WI. (**a**) Obliteration of a suprasellar cistern, an optic chiasm, and a hypothalamus draped over the sella (*black arrow*). The brainstem is sagging with an obliterated prepontine cistern (*dotted white arrow*). Downward displacement of the callosal splenium is also seen (*dotted black arrow*). *White arrow* points to the suboccipital craniectomy. (**b**) Diffuse pachymeningeal thickening and enhancement with small right frontal subdural collection (*dashed white arrow*)

Spinal imaging studies: Spinal MRI reveals pachymeningeal contrast enhancement and nerve root sleeve thickening, the site of CSF leakage, and engorged enhancing cervical epidural plexuses giving the aspect of a "draped curtain" narrowing the spinal canal on axial images. Thickened dura mater may mimic sarcoid or metastases [6, 8, 9].

When MRI is unable to detect the site of leaking, a fluoroscopy-guided myelogram or a dynamic CT myelogram is best for accurate localization of the dural defect [35].

Imaging Follow-Up

The majority of IHS cases are managed with supportive measures achieving total resolution of symptoms; less often the condition continues requiring therapeutic procedures including surgery, for which spinal imaging is required to find the site of fluid leak.

Main Differential Diagnoses

Chiari type I malformation in which the findings are limited to caudal displacement and peg-like appearance of the cerebellar tonsils without other findings of IHS. Surgery for this condition may worsen IHS if the patient is incorrectly diagnosed [5, 9].

Idiopathic hypertrophic cranial pachymeningitis has dural hypointensity or slight hyperintensity on T2WI. Pachymeningeal thickening is less diffuse than IHS and may show bone invasion, and headaches do not have an orthostatic nature [4, 5].

Meningitis usually presents with leptomeningeal enhancement, while IHS demonstrates pachymeningeal enhancement [5]. The diagnosis of meningitis is a clinical one.

Metastases and meningeal carcinomatosis have nodular meningeal thickening more frequently than diffuse linear thickening [4–6].

Dural sinus thrombosis can present with dilated venous structures in non-contrast head CT; however, it can be differentiated from IHS by the identification of the thrombus ("empty delta sign") in CT and MRI with contrast [4, 9].

Diffuse dural thickening has also been described in rheumatoid arthritis, sarcoid, Wegener granulomatosis, syphilis, and mucopolysaccharidosis [5]. Most of the time, diffuse dural thickening is idiopathic and of little clinical significance. Dural enhancement is normally seen at 3.0 T and above.

Tips

- It is important to make an early diagnosis of IHS because performing a therapeutic or diagnostic lumbar puncture can aggravate the clinical picture.
- Do not confuse IHS with a Chiari type I malformation as performing decompressive surgery in IHS may aggravate the symptoms and even results in cerebellar infarcts and death.
- The most prevalent sign of IHS is dural thickening and contrast enhancement. The dural abnormalities should be diffuse and smooth and not nodular.
- Always look for other signs of IHS and remember that they are nonspecific; thus, their number increases the possibility of an accurate diagnosis.
- Lack of findings does not exclude the diagnosis, and it is important to keep IHS in the differential diagnosis in the correct clinical setting.

References

1. Yuh EL, Dillon WP. Intracranial hypotension and intracranial hypertension. Neuroimaging Clin N Am. 2010;20(4):597–617.
2. Inamasu J, Guiot BH. Intracranial hypotension with spinal pathology. Spine J: Off J N Am Spine Soc. 2006;6(5):591–9.
3. Paldino M, Mogilner AY, Tenner MS. Intracranial hypotension syndrome: a comprehensive review. Neurosurg Focus. 2003;15(6):ECP2.
4. Barahona ML, Mora-Encinas JP, Gonzalez-Montano VM, Pozo-Zamorano T, Fernandez-Gil MA. Intracranial hypotension syndrome: a review of the magnetic resonance findings. Rev Neurol. 2011;52(11):676–80.
5. Ferrante E, Riva M, Gatti A, Brioschi AM, Guccione A, Colombo N, et al. Intracranial hypotension syndrome: neuroimaging in five spontaneous cases and

etiopathogenetic correlations. Clin Neurol Neurosurg. 1998;100(1):33–9.
6. Sousa R, Gouveia R, Lopes L, Ruivo N, Henriques N, Sa G, et al. Spontaneous intracranial hypotension syndrome. Acta Med Port. 2003;16(3):197–202.
7. Gonzalez-Gonzalez C, Crisostomo J, Perez J, Martin-Garcia V. Radiological findings in intracranial hypotension syndrome. Rev Neurol. 2009;49(2):100–1.
8. Yousem DM, Grossman RI. Neuroradiology: the requisites. 3rd ed. Philadelphia: Mosby/Elsevier; 2010. xvii, 619 p. p.
9. Osborn AG. Osborn's brain: imaging, pathology, and anatomy. 1st ed. Salt Lake City: Amirsys Pub; 2013. xi, 1272 p. p.
10. Chung SJ. CSF hypovolemia vs intracranial hypotension in "spontaneous intracranial hypotension syndrome". Neurology. 2003;61(10):1461–2. author reply 2.
11. Schwartz KM, Luetmer PH, Hunt CH, Kotsenas AL, Diehn FE, Eckel LJ, et al. Position-related variability of CSF opening pressure measurements. AJNR Am J Neuroradiol. 2013;34(4):904–7.
12. Franzini A, Messina G, Nazzi V, Mea E, Leone M, Chiapparini L, et al. Spontaneous intracranial hypotension syndrome: a novel speculative physiopathological hypothesis and a novel patch method in a series of 28 consecutive patients. J Neurosurg. 2010;112(2):300–6.
13. Schievink WI, Maya MM, Louy C, Moser FG, Sloninsky L. Spontaneous intracranial hypotension in childhood and adolescence. J Pediatr. 2013;163(2):504–10.
14. Schievink WI, Meyer FB, Atkinson JL, Mokri B. Spontaneous spinal cerebrospinal fluid leaks and intracranial hypotension. J Neurosurg. 1996;84(4):598–605.
15. Schievink WI, Morreale VM, Atkinson JL, Meyer FB, Piepgras DG, Ebersold MJ. Surgical treatment of spontaneous spinal cerebrospinal fluid leaks. J Neurosurg. 1998;88(2):243–6.
16. Headache Classification Subcommittee of the International Headache. The international classification of headache disorders: 2nd edition. Cephalalgia: Int J Headache. 2004;24 Suppl 1:9–160.
17. Schievink WI. Spontaneous spinal cerebrospinal fluid leaks. Cephalalgia: Int J Headache. 2008;28(12):1345–56.
18. Schievink WI. Spontaneous spinal cerebrospinal fluid leaks and intracranial hypotension. JAMA. 2006;295(19):2286–96.
19. Matias-Guiu JA, Ramos-Levi A, Casas-Limon J, Cuadrado-Perez ML, Porta-Etessam J. Spontaneous intracranial hypotension syndrome: importance of magnetic resonance findings. Rev Neurol. 2012;54(7):445.
20. Darof RB, Bradley WG, et al. In: Daroff RB, editor. Bradley's neurology in clinical practice. Philadelphia: Elsevier/Saunders; 2012. Available from: http://getitatduke.library.duke.edu/?sid=sersol&SS_jc=TC0000630111&title=Bradley%27s%20Neurology%20in%20Clinical%20Practice.
21. Aghaei Lasboo A, Hurley MC, Walker MT, Surdell D, Song JK, Rosenow JM, et al. Emergent image-guided treatment of a large CSF leak to reverse "in-extremis" signs of intracranial hypotension. AJNR Am J Neuroradiol. 2008;29(9):1627–9.
22. Binder DK, Dillon WP, Fishman RA, Schmidt MH. Intrathecal saline infusion in the treatment of obtundation associated with spontaneous intracranial hypotension: technical case report. Neurosurgery. 2002;51(3):830–6; discussion 6–7.
23. Binder DK, Sarkissian V, Dillon WP, Weinstein PR. Spontaneous intracranial hypotension associated with transdural thoracic osteophyte reversed by primary. dural repair. Case report. J Neurosurg Spine. 2005;2(5):614–8.
24. Eross EJ, Dodick DW, Nelson KD, Bosch P, Lyons M. Orthostatic headache syndrome with CSF leak secondary to bony pathology of the cervical spine. Cephalalgia: Int J Headache. 2002;22(6):439–43.
25. Rapport RL, Hillier D, Scearce T, Ferguson C. Spontaneous intracranial hypotension from intradural thoracic disc herniation. Case report. J Neurosurg. 2003;98(3 Suppl):282–4.
26. Vishteh AG, Schievink WI, Baskin JJ, Sonntag VK. Cervical bone spur presenting with spontaneous intracranial hypotension. Case report. J Neurosurg. 1998;89(3):483–4.
27. Winter SC, Maartens NF, Anslow P, Teddy PJ. Spontaneous intracranial hypotension due to thoracic disc herniation. Case report. J Neurosurg. 2002;96(3 Suppl):343–5.
28. Fernandez E. Headaches associated with low spinal fluid pressure. Headache. 1990;30(3):122–8.
29. Hadizadeh DR, Kovacs A, Tschampa H, Kristof R, Schramm J, Urbach H. Postsurgical intracranial hypotension: diagnostic and prognostic imaging findings. AJNR Am J Neuroradiol. 2010;31(1):100–5.
30. Mokri B. Low cerebrospinal fluid pressure syndromes. Neurol Clin. 2004;22(1):55–74, vi.
31. Raskin NH. Lumbar puncture headache: a review. Headache. 1990;30(4):197–200.
32. Farb RI, Forghani R, Lee SK, Mikulis DJ, Agid R. The venous distension sign: a diagnostic sign of intracranial hypotension at MR imaging of the brain. AJNR Am J Neuroradiol. 2007;28(8):1489–93.
33. Labiano-Fontcuberta A, Benito-Leon J. Intracranial hypotension syndrome: a review of the magnetic resonance findings. Rev Neurol. 2011;53(8):512.
34. Bonneville JF, Cattin F, Bonneville F. Enlargement of the inferior intercavernous sinus: a new sign for the diagnosis of craniospinal hypotension. AJNR Am J Neuroradiol. 2011;32(10):E194.
35. Kumar N. Beyond superficial siderosis: introducing "duropathies". Neurology. 2012;78(24):1992–9.
36. Savoiardo M, Armenise S, Spagnolo P, De Simone T, Mandelli ML, Marcone A, et al. Dural sinus thrombosis in spontaneous intracranial hypotension: hypotheses on possible mechanisms. J Neurol. 2006;253(9):1197–202.
37. Kate MP, Thomas B, Sylaja PN. Cerebral venous thrombosis in post-lumbar puncture intracranial hypotension: case report and review of literature. F1000Research. 2014;3:41.

Ischemic Stroke in Adults

4

Felipe Torres Pacheco and Antônio José da Rocha

Abstract

Stroke is a neurological deficit attributed to an acute injury of the central nervous system. Imaging plays a key role in evaluating acute stroke patients, guiding treatment and clinical management. Before treatment, it is necessary to exclude intracranial hemorrhage. Imaging of the acute stroke patient before endovascular therapy is necessary to determine the presence of an embolus/thrombus that is amenable to intra-arterial thrombolysis and/or mechanical thrombectomy. Brain perfusion imaging provides information on cerebral hemodynamics

Background

The word "stroke" was likely first introduced into medicine in 1689 by William Cole in *A Physico-Medical Essay Concerning the Late Frequencies of Apoplexies* [1]. Before Cole, the common term used to describe acute nontraumatic brain injuries was "apoplexy." Hippocrates used the term "apoplexy" circa 400 BC [1].

F.T. Pacheco, MD, PhD (✉) • A.J. da Rocha, MD, PhD
Division of Neuroradiology,
Hospital Santa Casa de Misericórdia de São Paulo,
Rua Dr. Cesário Motta Junior 112, Vila Buarque,
Sao Paulo, SP 01221-020, Brazil

Division of Neuroradiology, Grupo Fleury,
Sao Paulo, SP, Brazil
e-mail: felipetorrespacheco@hotmail.com;
antonio.rocha@grupofleury.com.br

Stroke is defined as a neurological deficit attributed to acute cerebral, spinal, or retinal infarctions [1]. It is a common and serious disorder, with an incidence of approximately 795,000 each year in the United States. Worldwide, stroke is a leading cause of death and disability [2].

Thrombolysis with recombinant tissue plasminogen activator (rtPA) and endovascular thrombectomy are the only approved therapies for acute ischemic stroke [3, 4]. Before any treatment it is necessary to exclude intracranial hemorrhage and severe stroke which is defined by an NIHSS score higher than 20 or an affected area larger than one-third of the middle cerebral artery territory as demonstrated on imaging [3, 5–8].

Intravenous thrombolytic is the most widespread therapy for acute ischemic stroke. However, in patients with proximal occlusions of the anterior circulation, intra-arterial treatment

R. Hoffmann Nunes et al. (eds.), *Critical Findings in Neuroradiology*,
DOI 10.1007/978-3-319-27987-9_4

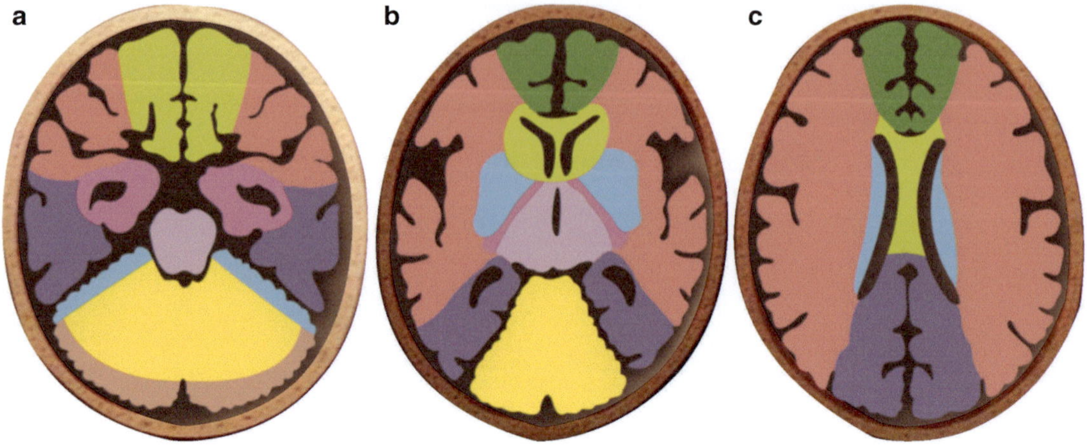

Fig. 4.1 (**a–c**) Schematically representation of the intracranial vascular territories. The anterior cerebral artery territory is demonstrated by the areas in *light green* (proximal branches) and *dark green* (distal branches). The middle cerebral artery territory is demonstrated by the areas in *light blue* in the basal ganglia (deep branches) and *salmon* (superficial branches). The posterior cerebral artery territory is demonstrated by the areas in *light purple* (deep branches) and *purple* (superficial branches). The choroidal artery territory is represented in *dark pink*. The areas in *yellow*, *tuscan*, and *light blue* in the cerebellum are irrigated respectively by the superior cerebellar arteries, posterior inferior cerebellar arteries, and the anterior inferior cerebellar arteries

within 6 h after stroke onset is more effective than intravenous therapy alone [5–8].

Key Points

Etiology

The etiologies of acute ischemic stroke are diverse, making it difficult to include all subtypes within a single classification system [9]. Therefore, an appropriate classification based upon the causative mechanisms is essential for guiding treatment and determining prognosis [10]. The Trial of Org 10172 in Acute Stroke Treatment (TOAST) classification system is widely used to categorize stroke subtypes [11]. It was developed in the early 1900s using the available diagnostic and clinical information at that time.

Based on the TOAST classification system [11], five etiologies are considered:

1. *Large-artery atherosclerosis*: patients with clinical and brain imaging findings of significant (>50 %) stenosis or occlusion of a major brain artery or cortical branch presumably due to atherosclerosis.
2. *Cardioembolism*: patients with arterial occlusion presumably due to an embolus arising in the heart.
3. *Small-artery occlusion* (*lacunae*): patients have normal brain imaging or a relevant brain stem or subcortical hemispheric lesion with a diameter of less than 1.5 cm.
4. *Stroke of other determined etiology*: includes patients with rare causes of stroke such as nonatherosclerotic vasculopathy, hypercoagulable states, cervical arterial dissection, or hematologic disorders.
5. *Stroke of undetermined etiology*: the cause of a stroke cannot be determined with any degree of certainty. This category also includes patients with two or more potential causes of stroke.

The boundaries between vascular distributions (Fig. 4.1) are determined by anatomic variations and by hemodynamic conditions that govern flow in leptomeningeal anastomoses connecting the different arterial territories [12]. Arterial cerebral circulation can be divided into two systems: (1) leptomeningeal also known as superficial or pial arterial system and (2) perforating or deep penetrating arterial system.

Table 4.1 Topographic pattern of brain infarction

Leptomeningeal system	
Malignant infarct	Complete or almost complete MCA infarction
Large infarct	Covering at least two of the three MCA territories
Limited infarct	Covering one of the three MCA territories
Centrum ovale infarcts	
Large	>1.5 cm
Small	<1.5 cm
Lacunar infarcts	<2.0 cm in the acute phase and <1.5 cm in the chronic stage
Watershed infarcts	Junction between two or three arterial territories

Despite these variabilities, brain imaging can accurately locate an ischemic stroke to a specific vascular distribution in the majority of patients [13, 14]. Therefore, in 1991, the Oxfordshire Community Stroke Project (OCSP) proposed four easily defined subgroups of cerebral infarction based on the infarction topography (Table 4.1) [15]. The topographic imaging patterns correlate well with the underlying pathophysiology and imaging findings [12].

Best Imaging Modality

The greatest importance of brain imaging in acute ischemic stroke is to exclude intracranial hemorrhage and detect a large infarct before rtPA administration. Different imaging technologies deliver information regarding the stroke subtype, tissue perfusion, and vessel patency [16].

Magnetic resonance imaging (MRI) provides better visualization of the brain parenchyma than computed tomography (CT) and fewer artifacts in the infratentorial brain and earlier detection of ischemia. The recommended protocol for MRI should include the following sequences: fluid-attenuated inversion recovery (FLAIR), diffusion-weighted imaging (DWI), and T2*-weighted sequences such as gradient recalled-echo (GRE) or susceptibility-weighted imaging (SWI) [17].

DWI has a high sensitivity (88–100 %) and specificity (95–100 %) for detecting acutely infarcted regions even within minutes of symptom onset. DWI can detect relatively small lesions which are often poorly seen or not diagnosed on CT [18–20].

T2*-weighted sequences have been used for detection of acute and chronic hemorrhage in stroke patients. The accuracy of these for detection of intracranial hemorrhage in the acute stroke setting (within 6 h) has been reported as equivalent to that of non-contrast computed tomography (NCCT). Additionally, T2*-weighted sequences, including GRE and SWI, have superior accuracy in the detection of small hemorrhages. SWI is an MRI sequence that is exquisitely sensitive to paramagnetic substances, such as deoxygenated blood, blood products, iron, and calcium [21]. This sequence allows detection of acute intraparenchymal as well as subarachnoid hemorrhage, which may contraindicate therapy of acute ischemic stroke [17, 22].

Despite these clear advantages, NCCT remains the "workhorse" [23] of acute stroke care in most hospitals as it is fast and available and confidently excludes intracranial hemorrhage and large infarctions. Imaging in patients who are potential candidates for IV thrombolysis should not delay administration of IV thrombolysis as "time is brain." Therefore, the decision to give IV rtPA should be made immediately after NCCT is completed [24]. The use of narrow window and level CT settings centered at approximately 35–45 HU width and 35–45 HU level aids to identify early ischemic changes by accentuating hypodense zones [2, 22].

Vascular imaging of the acute stroke patient before endovascular therapy is necessary to determine whether an embolus/thrombus is present and if it is amenable to intra-arterial thrombolysis and/or mechanical thrombectomy. Imaging of the intracranial vessels can be performed quickly and noninvasively by using computed tomography angiography (CTA) and magnetic resonance angiography (MRA). There are several different MRA techniques that have been used for imaging intracranial vessels and the most used is time of flight (TOF). Even though catheter angiography (DSA) is considered the gold standard for detection of vascular

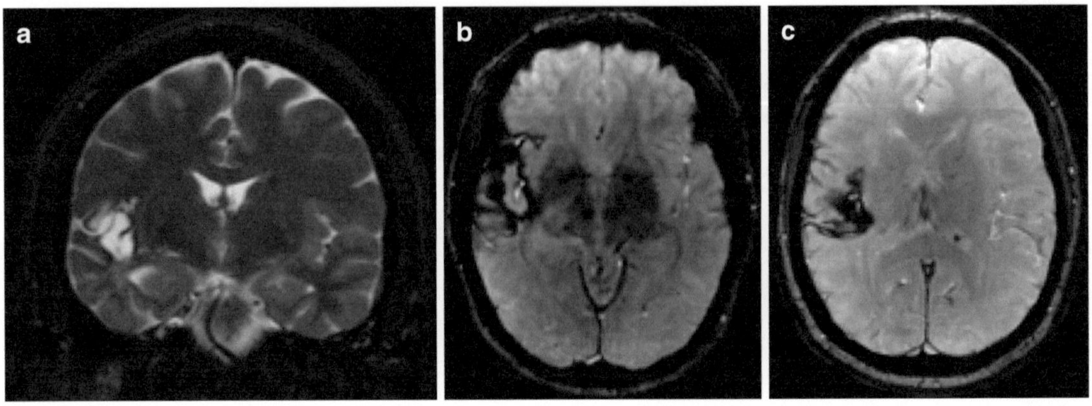

Fig. 4.2 Chronic infarction in the right MCA territory that suffered previous hemorrhagic transformation. (**a**) Coronal T2WI shows an area of encephalomalacia involving the right insula and superior temporal gyrus. (**b**, **c**) Axial SWI depicts blood products (blooming effect) in the right opercular region and along the Sylvian fissure

stenosis and occlusions, CTA and MRA have a high sensitivity (97–100 %) and specificity (98–100 %) for these purposes. CTA is slightly superior to MRA, especially for distal vascular lesions. Another advantage of CTA is that it can be obtained immediately following NCCT, after initiation rtPA in the CT scanner, avoiding delays in treatment [17, 22].

Brain perfusion imaging provides information on cerebral hemodynamics. Additionally, much research has been devoted to demonstrating that perfusion imaging can identify the infarct core and its penumbra and that perfusion imaging is useful for identifying patients who are candidates for interventional therapy [17, 22]. Perfusion CT may be added to the stroke CT protocol and may help distinguish the penumbra from infarcted tissue core in acute stroke patients [22]. Perfusion MRI does not have the same radiation exposure issues as CT and demonstrates the extent of potentially salvageable tissue ("penumbra" vs the volume of "ischemic core") when analyzed together with DWI [17, 22].

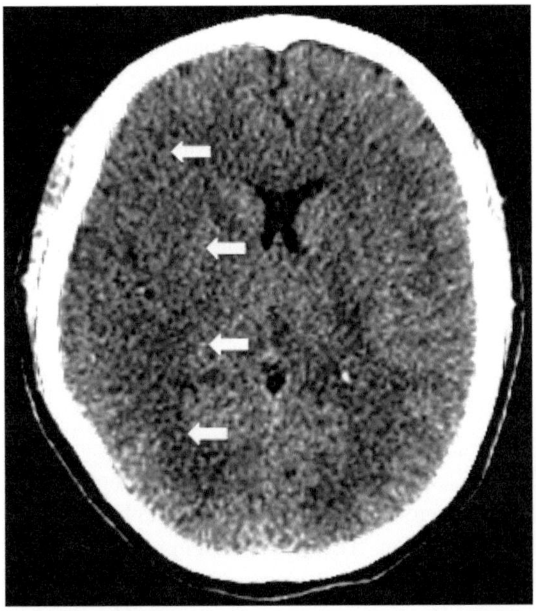

Fig. 4.3 Large stroke. Axial NCCT shows an extensive hypoattenuated area (*arrows*) affecting more than 1/3 right middle cerebral artery territory, corresponding to early ischemic changes

Major Findings

Brain Imaging

Besides the exclusion of intracranial hemorrhage (Fig. 4.2) and detection of a large stroke (Fig. 4.3), NCCT may demonstrate early signs of hyperacute ischemia (Fig. 4.4) as follows [2, 22]:

1. *Cortical ribbon sign*: represents cortical cytotoxic edema causing blending of the densities of the cortex and underlying white matter,

leading to loss of gray-white matter differentiation.

2. *Insular ribbon sign*: it is a subtype of cortical ribbon sign specifically involving the insula.
3. *Loss of basal ganglia definition*: also due to cytotoxic edema in the deep gray matter, resulting in loss of gray-white matter differentiation.
4. *Focal swelling with sulcal effacement*: narrowing of the cerebrospinal fluid spaces between the sulci as a result of compression by an abnormal and swollen brain parenchyma usually displaying loss of gray-white matter differentiation.

Alberta Stroke Program Early CT Score (ASPECTS) was developed to assess parenchymal hypo-attenuation on NCCT as a simple, reliable, and systematic approach [25]. Any ischemic lesion on axial NCCT at the level of the caudate head or below is adjudicated to a ganglionic ASPECTS region (M1–M3, insula, caudate nucleus, lentiform nucleus, internal capsule); ischemic lesions above the level of the caudate head are adjudicated to a supraganglionic ASPECTS region (M4–M6). The caudate nucleus is assessed in both the ganglionic level (head of caudate) and supraganglionic level (body and tail of caudate). To compute the ASPECTS, a single point is subtracted from a total of 10 for evidence of ischemic lesions in each of the ten ASPECTS regions. A score of 10 reflects a normal CT scan and a score of 0 diffuse ischemic involvement throughout the complete MCA territory. Scores of 7 or less, indicating extensive cerebral hypo-attenuation in the MCA territory, correlate with both poor functional outcomes and higher ASPECTS values (ASPECT 8–10) are associated with greater benefits from rtPA (Fig. 4.5) [26].

Hyperacute ischemia is demonstrated on DWI which is the most sensitive and specific sequence for stroke patients (Fig. 4.6) [18–20]. The area of acute infarction (cytotoxic edema) is hyperintense on DWI and hypointense on apparent diffusion coefficient (ADC) maps. DWI detects relatively small cortical lesions and small deep or subcortical lesions, including those in the brain stem and cerebellum which are often poorly or not seen on NCCT (Fig. 4.7). DWI abnormalities are sometimes reversible. However, reversal of a DWI abnormality is unusual. When DWI reversal does occur, it usually involves only a small part of the original lesion. Most times the apparent DWI reversal is actually a pseudo-reversal in that the tissue involved proceeds to infarction anyway [17].

Intracranial Large Vessel Imaging

NCCT is useful to demonstrate an intravascular thrombus seen as increased density within an occluded artery. The "hyperdense vessel" sign (Fig. 4.8) is, however, seen in only 30–50 % of patients with angiographically proven thromboses [27]. Another NCCT sign is the hyperdense vessel "dot" sign that represents a clot within a Sylvian branch of the middle cerebral artery (MCA). The "susceptibility vessel sign" is the MRI correlate of the "hyperdense vessel" sign seen on NCCT, and in it the occluded artery appears of low signal intensity [28]. Calcified emboli are rare but potentially devastating causes of acute ischemic stroke and may be the first manifestation of vascular or cardiac disease [29].

CTA and MRA can be used to demonstrate the following findings [2, 22]:

1. *Arterial filling defect*: a filling defect within an artery (Fig. 4.8) representing an intraluminal fresh thrombus [30].
2. *Collateral circulation*: collateral vessels provide blood flow to preserve viable tissue and can potentially extend the time window for treatment-induced recanalization. Collateral circulation limits the growth of the infarct core by irrigating the penumbral tissue during acute ischemia. The collateral circulation includes convexity leptomeningeal vessels and vascular communications from the circle of Willis (anterior and posterior communicating arteries).

The clot burden score (CBS) is a scoring system that defines the extent of thrombus found in the proximal anterior circulation by location and is scored on a scale of 0–10 [31]. A score of 10 is

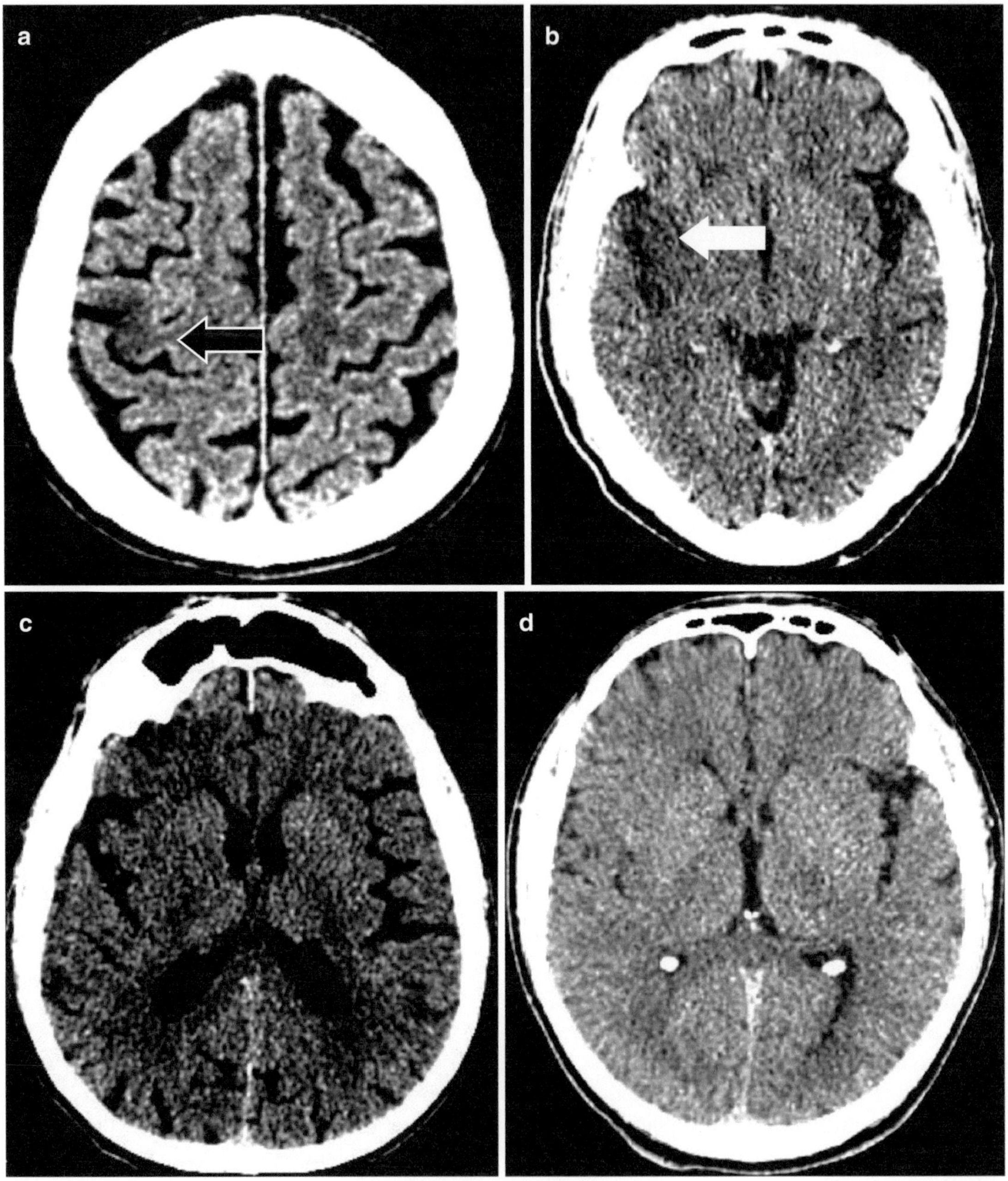

Fig. 4.4 Early signs of hyperacute brain ischemia in different patients. **a–d**. Axial NCCT demonstrate the cortical ribbon sign in the right motor cortex on A (*black arrow*), the insular ribbon sign on **b** (*white arrow*), loss of basal ganglia definition on the right side on **c** and focal gyri swelling with right Sylvian fissure effacement on **d**

normal, implying no clot. A score of 0 implies complete multi-segmental vessel occlusion. In order to define CBS, a score of 2 is subtracted if thrombus is found in each of the supraclinoid ICAs, the proximal half of the MCA trunk, and the distal half of MCA trunk. A score of 1 is subtracted if thrombus is found in the infraclinoid ICA, ACA, and for each affected M2 branch.

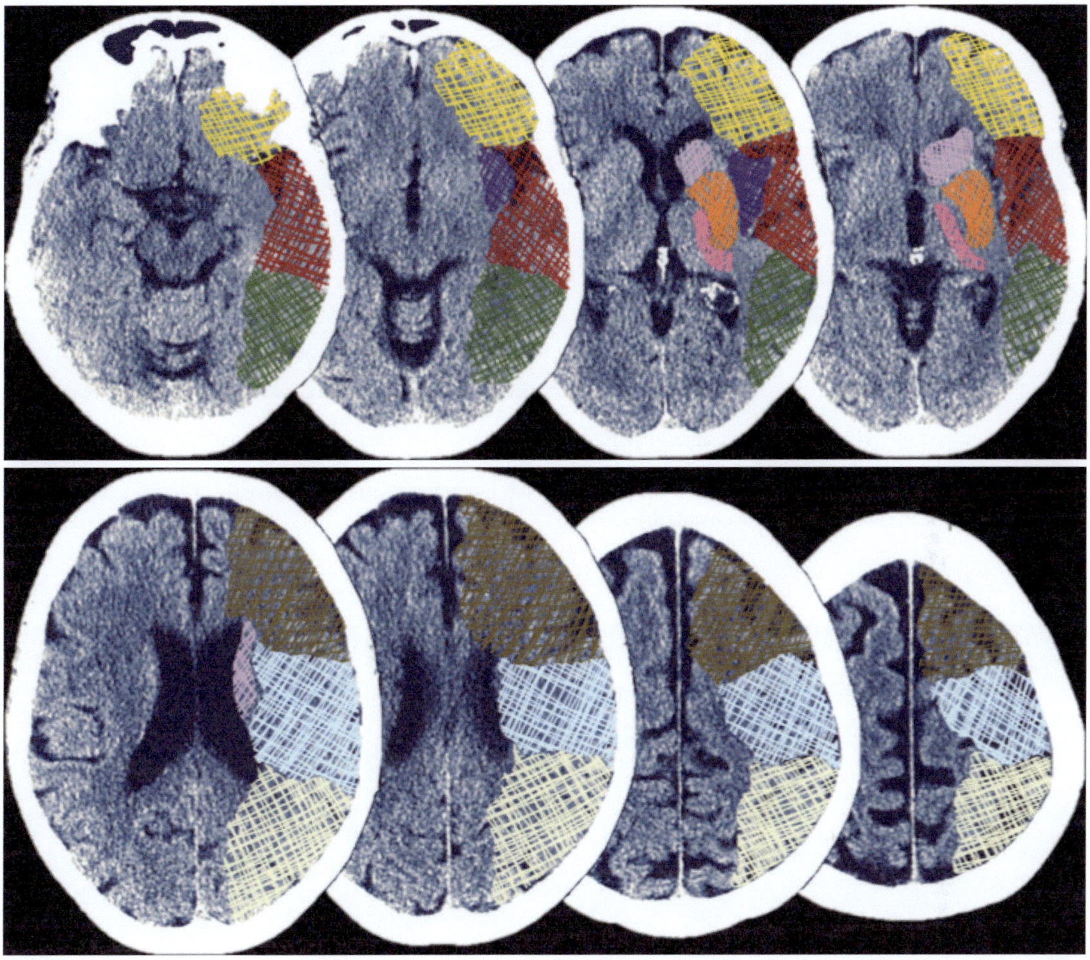

Fig. 4.5 ASPECTS scoring scheme. The upper row demonstrates axial CT slices of the ganglionic ASPECTS level [M1–M3, insula (in *purple*), lentiform nucleus (in *orange*), caudate nucleus (in *light pink*), posterior limb of the internal capsule (in pink)]. The lower row demonstrates CT slices of the supraganglionic ASPECTS level (M4–M6) that can be divided in anterior (in *brown*), middle (in *light blue*), and posterior (in *light yellow*) regions irrigated by the MCA. The caudate nucleus (in *light pink*) is assessed in both the ganglionic level (head of caudate) and supraganglionic level (body and tail of caudate)

The thrombus can be partially or completely occlusive.

The collateral score scale quantifies the degree of collateral supply through peripheral leptomeningeal sources and correlates with a smaller final infarct volume [32]. Various methods have been described for the assessment of intracranial collaterals on CTA in patients with acute ischemic stroke [33–36]. Only the Miteff scoring system [33] is reliable for predicting favorable outcome in acute ischemic stroke. However, poor outcomes can be predicted by most existing methods for scoring intracranial collaterals. The Maas system scoring system [34] is the most widespread used and grades the leptomeningeal vascularity as follows: (1) absent, (2) less than the contralateral unaffected side, (3) equal to the contralateral unaffected side, (4) more than the contralateral unaffected side, and (5) exuberant (Fig. 4.9).

Perfusion Imaging

Even though brain perfusion imaging is not mandatory in acute ischemic stroke evaluation, it

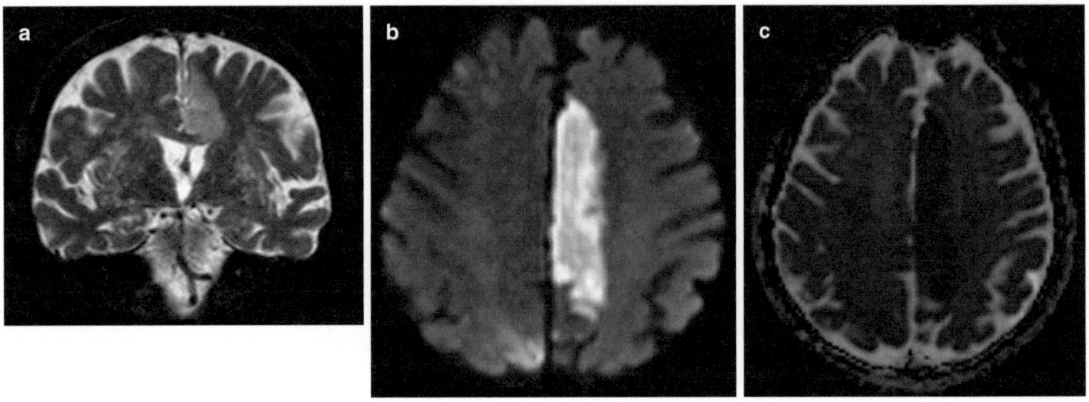

Fig. 4.6 Acute stroke affecting the left anterior circulation. (**a**) Coronal T2WI image shows areas of hypersignal involving the cortex and the white matter of the left cyngulate gyrus with subtle sulcal effacement. (**b**) and (**c**). DWI and ADC map images demonstrate areas of increased signal on DWI and decreased signal on ADC map in the left cyngulate gyrus, characteristic of restricted diffusion

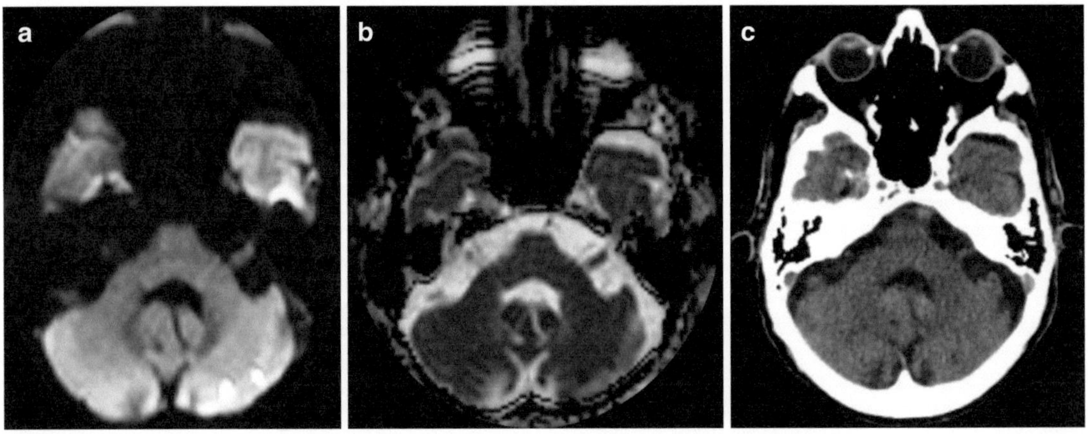

Fig. 4.7 Acute lacunar stroke. (**a**) and (**b**). DWI and ADC map images demonstrate lacunar lesions in the left cerebellar hemisphere with increased signal on DWI and decreased signal on ADC map consistent with acute infarction that was not detected on NCCT (**c**)

provides information about regional brain hemodynamics in the form of parameters such as cerebral blood flow (CBF), cerebral blood volume (CBV), and mean transit time (MTT). The quantification of these parameters is based on the equation CBF = CBV/MTT. Perfusion MRI or perfusion CT imaging allows delineation of the ischemic penumbra (core/penumbra mismatch) as follows [37–41]:

CBV: defined as the total volume of blood in a given unit volume of the brain. CBV map depicts similar size/extension lesions to the ones with restricted diffusion helping to predict the infarcted brain tissue that is not salvageable despite reperfusion.

CBF: defined as the volume of blood moving through a given unit volume of brain per unit time. CBF map depicts areas of slow flow which are considered ischemic zones. It is the most physiological measure of ischemia but sometimes difficult to appreciate on MR perfusion.

MTT: defined as the average of the transit time of blood through a given brain region. Since the

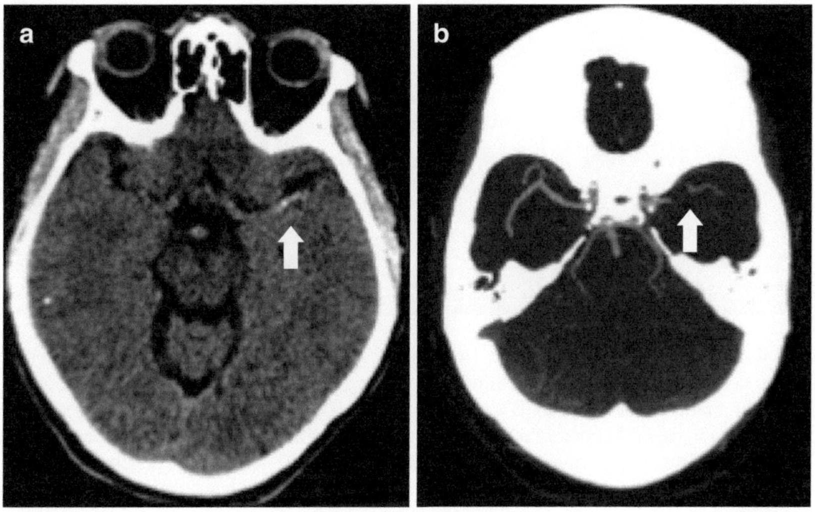

Fig. 4.8 Hyperdense vessel sign. A hyperattenuation is seen within the left M1 segment (*arrow*) on axial NCCT image (**a**). A filling defect is confirmed in the same region (*arrow*) on axial CTA image (**b**)

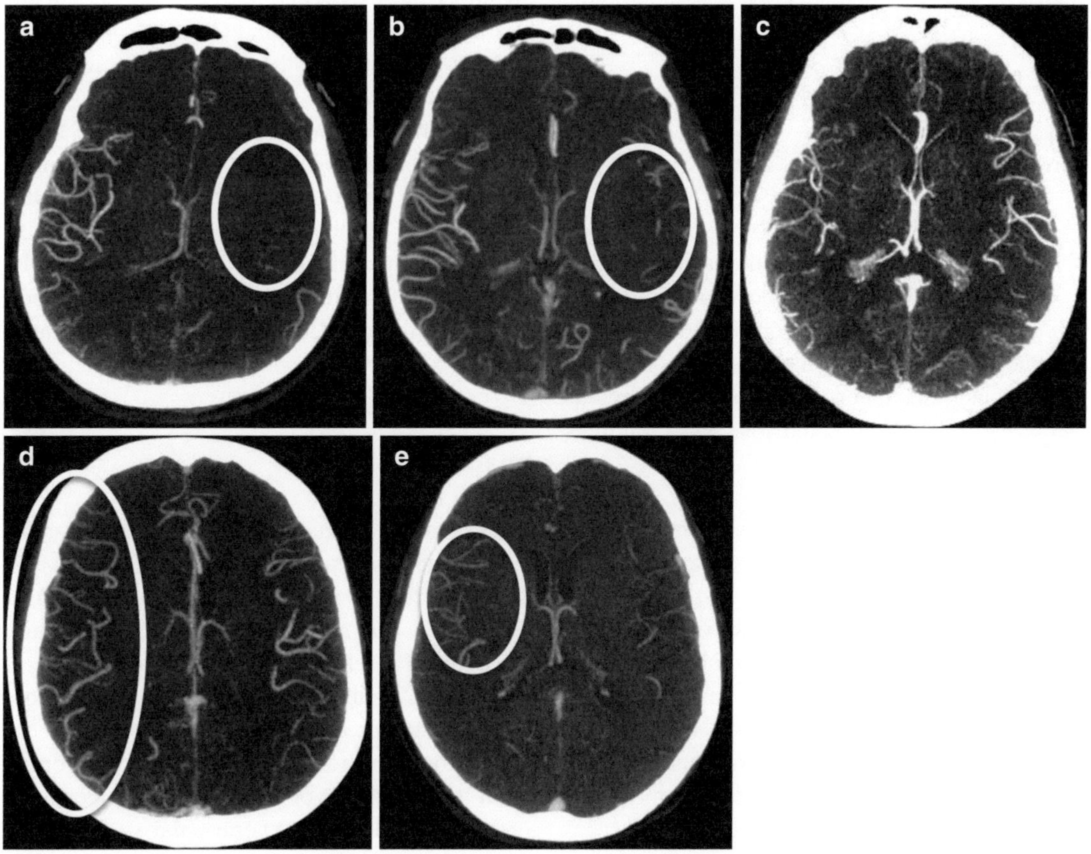

Fig. 4.9 Leptomeningeal vascularity score. (**a–e**) Examples of the leptomeningeal vascularity score are demonstrated on axial CTA MIP images of different patients with occlusion of the middle cerebral artery (*circles*). (**a**) *1* (absent in the affected side). (**b**) *2* (less than the contralateral unaffected side). (**c**) *3* (equal to the contralateral unaffected side). (**d**) *4* (more than the contralateral unaffected side). (**e**) *5* (exuberant in the affected side)

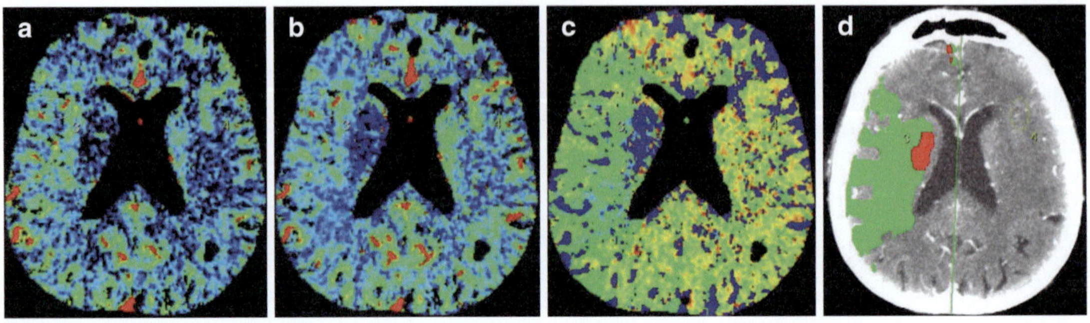

Fig. 4.10 Perfusion CT mismatch (**a**) Axial CBV map image demonstrates in the right putaminal region a small area with markedly decreased CBV values (<2 ml × 100 g) and an area in the right opercular zone surrounding it with slightly increased CBV values. (**b**) Axial CBF map image shows decreased CBF values in the right putaminal region and slightly decreased values in the opercular region surrounding it. (**c**) Axial MTT map image depicts increased MTT values in the putaminal region and mildly increased MTT values in the regions surrounding it. (**d**) Computed generated schematic figure (**d**) demonstrates the expected salvageable brain tissue on green and the core on *red*

Table 4.2 Perfusion CT analysis of hyperacute ischemic stroke

	MTT	CBF	CBV
Penumbra	↑ (>145 %)	↓	↑
Ischemic core	↑	↓	↓ (<2.0 mL × 100 g)

blood velocity is slower in the ischemic area, the MTT map shows areas of slow flow ischemic area which are considered ischemic zones. Although not the best physiological parameter, the abnormalities are very obvious on visual inspection, and thus MTT findings must be correlated with CBF and CBV.

The "core" is typically defined as brain likely to be irreversibly infarcted at presentation despite early recanalization. "Penumbra" is the functionally ischemic and potentially salvageable "at-risk" brain parenchyma. "Mismatch" is defined as the difference in volume and extension between core and penumbra (Fig. 4.10).

Ischemic tissue (penumbra) presents increased MTT, decreased CBF, and normal or increased CBV (due to secondary to autoregulatory mechanisms in the early stage of ischemia or presence of collateral circulation), whereas the infarcted tissue (core) shows markedly decreased CBF and CBV and increased MTT (Table 4.2). The salvageable brain tissue (mismatch) is equivalent to the area of low CBF and normal CBV subtracted by the area of low CBF and CBV [41, 42].

MRI demonstrates the "core" of the infarcted tissues on DWI as restricted diffusion areas, whereas the perfusion images despite the "penumbra" providing similar delay-based parameters, such as Tmax and TTP (time to peak of the deconvolved tissue residue function and raw concentration–time curve, respectively) [43]. To define "target mismatch," a recent study described a mismatch ratio >1.8 and an absolute mismatch volume >15 ml [44].

Imaging Follow-Up

Strokes may be classified and dated as early hyperacute, a stroke that is 0–6 h old; late hyperacute, a stroke that is 6–24 h old; acute, 24 h to 7 days old; subacute, 1–3 weeks; and chronic, more than 3 weeks old [45].

On NCCT subacute and chronic strokes show hypodensity in the affected areas. Subacute stroke does not show significant mass or atrophy. With the passing of time, atrophy becomes prominent and adjacent ventricular system compensatory dilatation and sulcal enlargement occurs.

Signal intensity on ADC maps is said to be lowest (most restricted) 2–3 days after an infarct and persists for about 7–14 days. Afterwards a

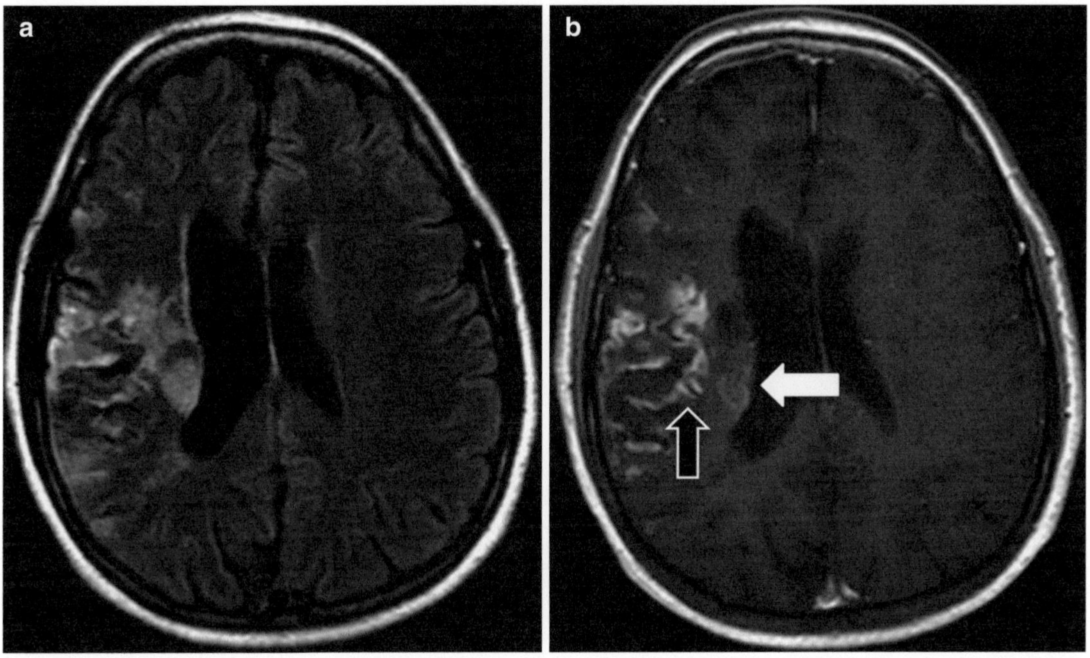

Fig. 4.11 Subacute infarct. (**a**) Axial FLAIR image shows a corticosubcortical hyperintense lesion affecting part of the right MCA territory. (**b**) Axial postcontrast T1WI depicts a gyriform pattern of parenchymal enhancement in the cortex of the right opercular region (*black arrow*) and a slightly ringlike enhancement in the right periventricular region (*white arrow*)

phenomenon called "pseudonormalization" occurs with DWI/ADC returning to normal but signal intensity remaining high on T2WI [46]. Similarly, a "fogging" effect may be seen on T2WI around 1–4 weeks after stroke and appears as an area of isointensity relative to the brain and is thought to result from infiltration of inflammatory cells into infarcted tissue [47].

In most subacute infarcts, parenchymal contrast enhancement is seen usually between 1 week and 2 months after the stroke. In cortical infarctions, parenchymal contrast enhancement may be gyriform, and in the basal ganglia and brainstem, it may be generalized or ringlike (Fig. 4.11). However, if parenchymal contrast enhancement persists longer than 8–12 weeks, a diagnosis other than ischemic stroke should be entertained [45].

Cortical laminar and pseudolaminar necrosis cause serpiginous cortical T1 shortening (Fig. 4.12) which is not due to presence of calcium or blood products but possibly to the presence of lipid-laden macrophages [48, 49]. High cortical signal intensity may be seen on T1WI 3–5 days after stroke, and in many patients, it is present 2 weeks after the stroke. Thereafter, it increases in intensity and fades after about 3 months, but in some patients, it may persist for over 1 year [50]. In patients with suspected cortical laminar necrosis, SWI may help differentiate it from hemorrhagic transformation as the former shows no signal drop while blood at any stage is hypointense [51, 52].

An important complication of ischemic stroke that may be identified by imaging follow-up is hemorrhagic transformation. The European Cooperative Acute Stroke Study (ECASS) [53] classified hemorrhagic infarction 1 (HI1) as small petechiae along the periphery of the infarct, hemorrhagic infarction 2 (HI2) as confluent petechiae within the infarct without space-occupying effect, parenchymal hemorrhage 1 (PH1) as bleeding $\leq 30\ \%$ of the infarcted area with mild space-occupying effect, and parenchymal hemorrhage 2 (PH2) as bleeding $>30\ \%$ of the infarcted area with space-occupying effect (Fig. 4.13).

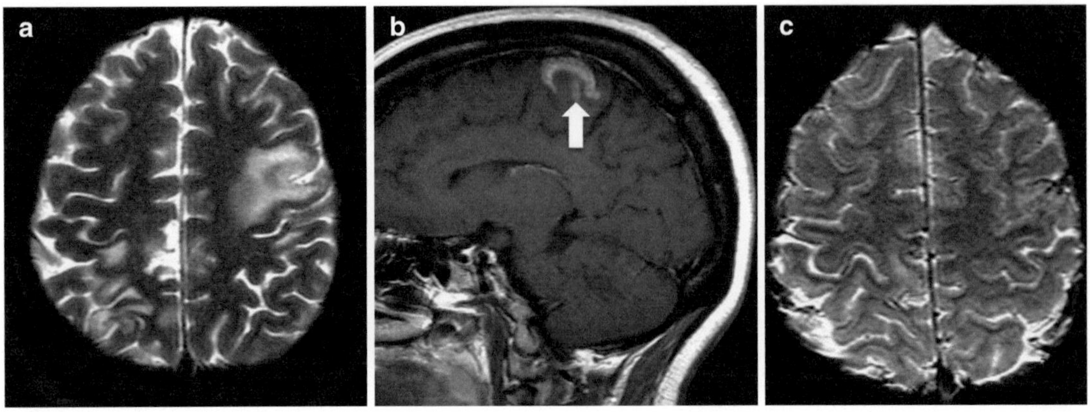

Fig. 4.12 Cortical laminar necrosis. An area of ischemia affecting the left frontal lobe is demonstrated on axial T2WI (**a**). There is serpiginous cortical T1 shortening (*arrow*) on a sagittal T1WI (**b**) which is not caused by calcium or hemoglobin products as blooming effect is not visualized on axial T2* image (**c**)

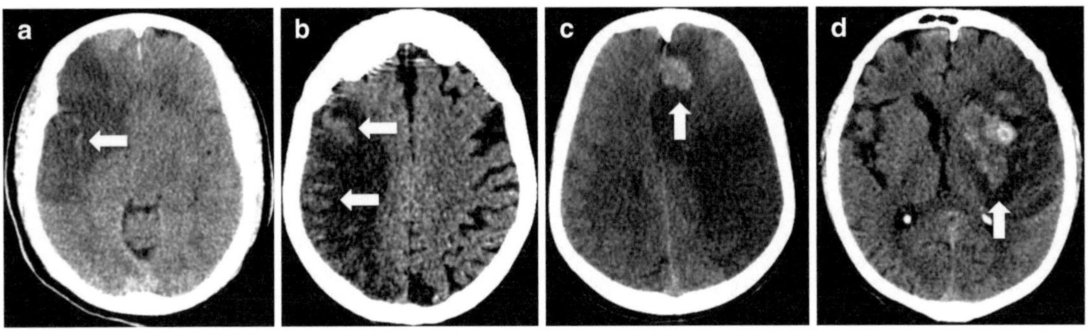

Fig. 4.13 Hemorrhagic transformation classification. (**a–d**) Different examples of hemorrhagic transformation subtypes (*arrows*) are demonstrated on axial NCCT images of different patients. HI1: small petechiae in the infarct region (**a**). HI2: confluent petechiae within the infarct, without space-occupying effect. PH1: bleeding affecting less than 30 % of the infarcted area, with mild mass effect. PH2: bleeding affecting more than 30 % of the infarcted area, with mass effect

Hemorrhagic transformation is rare in the first 12 h after stroke onset. When it occurs, it is usually within the first 24–48 h, and in almost all patients, it occurs 4–5 days after stroke [54, 55]. Late hemorrhagic transformation is less common but may occur 1 week after stroke. Today, the most common cause of acute hemorrhagic transformation is previous administration of thrombolytic medications.

Main Differential Diagnosis

*TIA*s are brief episodes of neurological dysfunction that result from focal cerebral ischemia not associated with permanent cerebral infarction. Therefore, the main differentiation between a true acute ischemic stroke and a TIA is the exclusion of brain infarction that can be demonstrated DWI [56].

In cases of atypical clinical presentations, *brain hemorrhage*, *venous infarct*, *cerebritis*, *demyelination*, and, especially, *neoplastic lesions* may mimic an ischemic stroke. The presence of a lesion affecting exclusively an arterial territory narrows the differential diagnosis. Infarctions show progressive decrease in mass effect starting late in the first week and increasing contrast enhancement peaking in the second week which is not the case with the entities mentioned above except for venous infarction [45, 48, 49].

Enlarged *perivascular spaces* should not be misinterpreted as lacunar strokes. They are most commonly located in the lower half of the basal ganglia especially along the line of the anterior commissure and follow the cerebrospinal fluid signal on all MRI pulse sequences. Besides, when small, the adjacent white matter is normal, thus helping to distinguish them from lacunar infarcts which have edema and later gliosis. When they are large, a thin halo of increased T2WI intensity may be seen. On T2WI and other MRI sequences, a blood vessel traversing the perivascular space may be seen.

Tips

All patients presenting with an acute stroke syndrome after receiving a neurological evaluation should be evaluated with NCCT followed by CTA. If NCCT does not demonstrate hemorrhage or a large hypodensity and the patient is within the appropriate time window for treatment, IV tPA may be infused while the CTA is performed. If the patient has a distal ICA and/or proximal middle cerebral artery, intra-arterial treatment must be considered. Perfusion imaging with CT or MRI may be performed in this setting and relevant clinical information may be provided (Flow chart 4.1). In many centers, to expedite treatment, only NCCT and CTA are done. The aim is an admission to angiography time of less than 30 min.

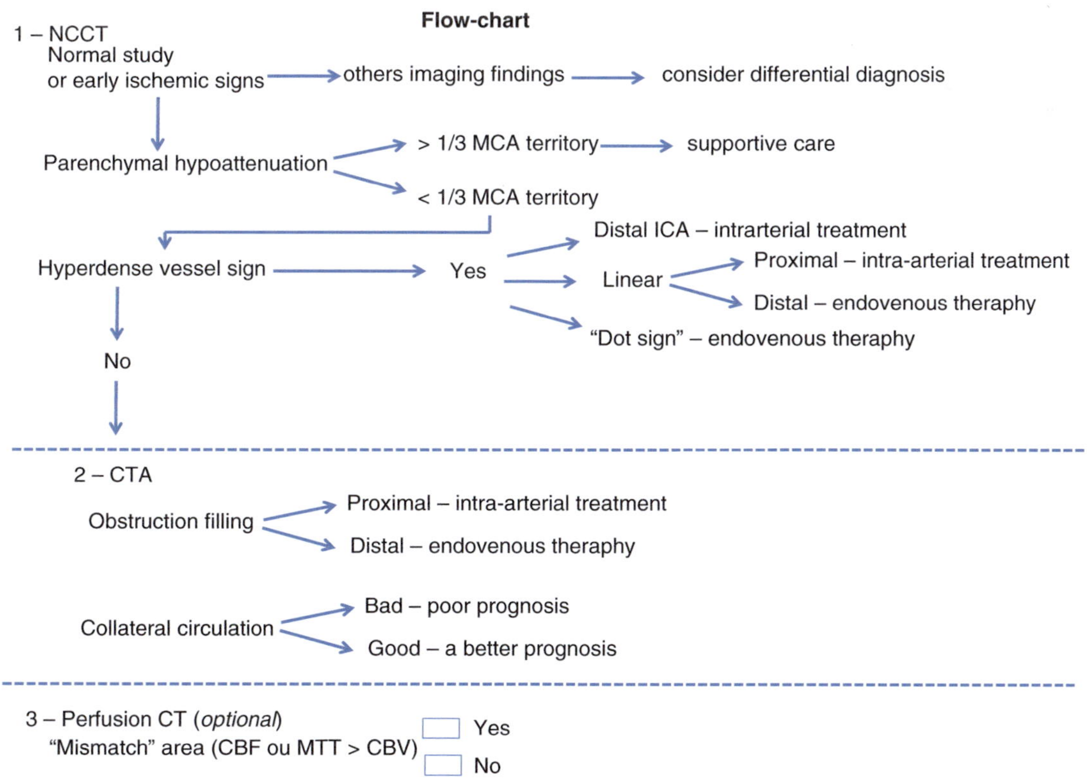

Flow chart 4.1 Acute stroke: CT findings (Adapted by Pacheco et al. (2013) [57])

References

1. Sacco RL, Kasner SE, Broderick JP, Caplan LR, Connors JJ, Culebras A, et al. An updated definition of stroke for the 21st century: a statement for healthcare professionals from the American Heart Association/American Stroke Association. Stroke: J Cereb Circ. 2013;44(7):2064–89.
2. Latchaw RE, Alberts MJ, Lev MH, Connors JJ, Harbaugh RE, Higashida RT, et al. Recommendations for imaging of acute ischemic stroke: a scientific statement from the American Heart Association. Stroke: J Cereb Circ. 2009;40(11):3646–78.
3. Hacke W, Kaste M, Bluhmki E, Brozman M, Davalos A, Guidetti D, et al. Thrombolysis with alteplase 3 to 4.5 hours after acute ischemic stroke. N Engl J Med. 2008;359(13):1317–29.
4. Penumbra Pivotal Stroke Trial I. The penumbra pivotal stroke trial: safety and effectiveness of a new generation of mechanical devices for clot removal in intracranial large vessel occlusive disease. Stroke: J Cereb Circ. 2009;40(8):2761–8.
5. Berkhemer OA, Fransen PS, Beumer D, van den Berg LA, Lingsma HF, Yoo AJ, et al. A randomized trial of intraarterial treatment for acute ischemic stroke. N Engl J Med. 2015;372(1):11–20.
6. Goyal M, Demchuk AM, Menon BK, Eesa M, Rempel JL, Thornton J, et al. Randomized assessment of rapid endovascular treatment of ischemic stroke. N Engl J Med. 2015;372(11):1019–30.
7. Saver JL, Goyal M, Bonafe A, Diener HC, Levy EI, Pereira VM, et al. Stent-retriever thrombectomy after intravenous t-PA vs. t-PA alone in stroke. N Engl J Med. 2015;372:2285–95.
8. Campbell BC, Mitchell PJ, Kleinig TJ, Dewey HM, Churilov L, Yassi N, et al. Endovascular therapy for ischemic stroke with perfusion-imaging selection. N Engl J Med. 2015;372(11):1009–18.
9. Muir KW. Heterogeneity of stroke pathophysiology and neuroprotective clinical trial design. Stroke: J Cereb Circ. 2002;33(6):1545–50.
10. Kim BJ, Kim JS. Ischemic stroke subtype classification: an asian viewpoint. J Stroke. 2014;16(1):8–17.
11. Adams Jr HP, Bendixen BH, Kappelle LJ, Biller J, Love BB, Gordon DL, et al. Classification of subtype of acute ischemic stroke. Definitions for use in a multicenter clinical trial. TOAST. Trial of Org 10172 in Acute Stroke Treatment. Stroke: J Cereb Circ. 1993; 24(1):35–41.
12. van der Zwan A, Hillen B, Tulleken CA, Dujovny M, Dragovic L. Variability of the territories of the major cerebral arteries. J Neurosurg. 1992;77(6):927–40.
13. Tatu L, Moulin T, Bogousslavsky J, Duvernoy H. Arterial territories of the human brain: cerebral hemispheres. Neurology. 1998;50(6):1699–708.
14. Takahashi S, Suzuki M, Matsumoto K, Ishii K, Higano S, Fukasawa H, et al. Extent and location of cerebral infarcts on multiplanar MR images: correlation with distribution of perforating arteries on cerebral angiograms and on cadaveric microangiograms. AJR Am J Roentgenol. 1994;163(5):1215–22.
15. Bamford J, Sandercock P, Dennis M, Burn J, Warlow C. Classification and natural history of clinically identifiable subtypes of cerebral infarction. Lancet. 1991;337(8756):1521–6.
16. Audebert HJ, Fiebach JB. Brain imaging in acute ischemic stroke-MRI or CT? Curr Neurol Neurosci Rep. 2015;15(3):526.
17. Gonzalez RG, Copen WA, Schaefer PW, Lev MH, Pomerantz SR, Rapalino O, et al. The Massachusetts general hospital acute stroke imaging algorithm: an experience and evidence based approach. J NeuroInterventional Surg. 2013;5 Suppl 1:i7–12.
18. Mohr JP, Biller J, Hilal SK, Yuh WT, Tatemichi TK, Hedges S, et al. Magnetic resonance versus computed tomographic imaging in acute stroke. Stroke: J Cereb Circ. 1995;26(5):807–12.
19. Fiebach JB, Schellinger PD, Jansen O, Meyer M, Wilde P, Bender J, et al. CT and diffusion-weighted MR imaging in randomized order: diffusion-weighted imaging results in higher accuracy and lower interrater variability in the diagnosis of hyperacute ischemic stroke. Stroke: J Cereb Circ. 2002;33(9):2206–10.
20. Gonzalez RG, Schaefer PW, Buonanno FS, Schwamm LH, Budzik RF, Rordorf G, et al. Diffusion-weighted MR imaging: diagnostic accuracy in patients imaged within 6 hours of stroke symptom onset. Radiology. 1999;210(1):155–62.
21. Santhosh K, Kesavadas C, Thomas B, Gupta AK, Thamburaj K, Kapilamoorthy TR. Susceptibility weighted imaging: a new tool in magnetic resonance imaging of stroke. Clin Radiol. 2009;64(1):74–83.
22. Wintermark M, Sanelli PC, Albers GW, Bello J, Derdeyn C, Hetts SW, et al. Imaging recommendations for acute stroke and transient ischemic attack patients: a joint statement by the American Society of Neuroradiology, the American College of Radiology, and the Society of NeuroInterventional Surgery. AJNR Am J Neuroradiol. 2013;34(11):E117–27.
23. Kaste M. Reborn workhorse, CT, pulls the wagon toward thrombolysis beyond 3 hours. Stroke: J Cereb Circ. 2004;35(2):357–9.
24. Saver JL. Time is brain – quantified. Stroke: J Cereb Circ. 2006;37(1):263–6.
25. Barber PA, Demchuk AM, Zhang J, Buchan AM. Validity and reliability of a quantitative computed tomography score in predicting outcome of hyperacute stroke before thrombolytic therapy. ASPECTS Study Group. Alberta Stroke Programme Early CT Score. Lancet. 2000;355(9216):1670–4.
26. Menon BK, Puetz V, Kochar P, Demchuk AM. ASPECTS and other neuroimaging scores in the triage and prediction of outcome in acute stroke patients. Neuroimaging Clin N Am. 2011;21(2):407–23. xii.
27. Tomsick T, Brott T, Barsan W, Broderick J, Haley EC, Spilker J, et al. Prognostic value of the hyperdense

middle cerebral artery sign and stroke scale score before ultraearly thrombolytic therapy. AJNR Am J Neuroradiol. 1996;17(1):79–85.
28. Hermier M, Nighoghossian N. Contribution of susceptibility-weighted imaging to acute stroke assessment. Stroke: J Cereb Circ. 2004;35(8): 1989–94.
29. Walker BS, Shah LM, Osborn AG. Calcified cerebral emboli, a "do not miss" imaging diagnosis: 22 new cases and review of the literature. AJNR Am J Neuroradiol. 2014;35(8):1515–9.
30. Saarinen JT, Rusanen H, Sillanpaa N. Collateral score complements clot location in predicting the outcome of intravenous thrombolysis. AJNR Am J Neuroradiol. 2014;35(10):1892–6.
31. Puetz V, Dzialowski I, Hill MD, Subramaniam S, Sylaja PN, Krol A, et al. Intracranial thrombus extent predicts clinical outcome, final infarct size and hemorrhagic transformation in ischemic stroke: the clot burden score. Int J Stroke Off J Int Stroke Soc. 2008;3(4):230–6.
32. Bozzao L, Fantozzi LM, Bastianello S, Bozzao A, Fieschi C. Early collateral blood supply and late parenchymal brain damage in patients with middle cerebral artery occlusion. Stroke: J Cereb Circ. 1989;20(6):735–40.
33. Miteff F, Levi CR, Bateman GA, Spratt N, McElduff P, Parsons MW. The independent predictive utility of computed tomography angiographic collateral status in acute ischaemic stroke. Brain. 2009;132(Pt 8):2231–8.
34. Maas MB, Lev MH, Ay H, Singhal AB, Greer DM, Smith WS, et al. Collateral vessels on CT angiography predict outcome in acute ischemic stroke. Stroke: J Cereb Circ. 2009;40(9):3001–5.
35. Tan IY, Demchuk AM, Hopyan J, Zhang L, Gladstone D, Wong K, et al. CT angiography clot burden score and collateral score: correlation with clinical and radiologic outcomes in acute middle cerebral artery infarct. AJNR Am J Neuroradiol. 2009;30(3): 525–31.
36. Menon BK, Smith EE, Modi J, Patel SK, Bhatia R, Watson TW, et al. Regional leptomeningeal score on CT angiography predicts clinical and imaging outcomes in patients with acute anterior circulation occlusions. AJNR Am J Neuroradiol. 2011;32(9): 1640–5.
37. Warach S. Measurement of the ischemic penumbra with MRI: it's about time. Stroke: J Cereb Circ. 2003;34(10):2533–4.
38. Albers GW, Thijs VN, Wechsler L, Kemp S, Schlaug G, Skalabrin E, et al. Magnetic resonance imaging profiles predict clinical response to early reperfusion: the diffusion and perfusion imaging evaluation for understanding stroke evolution (DEFUSE) study. Ann Neurol. 2006;60(5):508–17.
39. Goyal M, Menon BK, Derdeyn CP. Perfusion imaging in acute ischemic stroke: let us improve the science before changing clinical practice. Radiology. 2013; 266(1):16–21.
40. Wintermark M, Reichhart M, Thiran JP, Maeder P, Chalaron M, Schnyder P, et al. Prognostic accuracy of cerebral blood flow measurement by perfusion computed tomography, at the time of emergency room admission, in acute stroke patients. Ann Neurol. 2002;51(4):417–32.
41. Wintermark M, Flanders AE, Velthuis B, Meuli R, van Leeuwen M, Goldsher D, et al. Perfusion-CT assessment of infarct core and penumbra: receiver operating characteristic curve analysis in 130 patients suspected of acute hemispheric stroke. Stroke: J Cereb Circ. 2006;37(4):979–85.
42. Wintermark M, Meuli R, Browaeys P, Reichhart M, Bogousslavsky J, Schnyder P, et al. Comparison of CT perfusion and angiography and MRI in selecting stroke patients for acute treatment. Neurology. 2007; 68(9):694–7.
43. Campbell BC, Macrae IM. Translational perspectives on perfusion-diffusion mismatch in ischemic stroke. Int J Stroke Off J Int Stroke Soc. 2015;10(2):153–62.
44. Lansberg MG, Straka M, Kemp S, Mlynash M, Wechsler LR, Jovin TG, et al. MRI profile and response to endovascular reperfusion after stroke (DEFUSE 2): a prospective cohort study. Lancet Neurol. 2012;11(10):860–7.
45. Allen LM, Hasso AN, Handwerker J, Farid H. Sequence-specific MR imaging findings that are useful in dating ischemic stroke. RadioGraphics Rev Publ Radiol Soc N Am Inc. 2012;32(5):1285–97. discussion 97–9.
46. Copen WA, Schwamm LH, Gonzalez RG, Wu O, Harmath CB, Schaefer PW, et al. Ischemic stroke: effects of etiology and patient age on the time course of the core apparent diffusion coefficient. Radiology. 2001;221(1):27–34.
47. O'Brien P, Sellar RJ, Wardlaw JM. Fogging on T2-weighted MR after acute ischaemic stroke: how often might this occur and what are the implications? Neuroradiology. 2004;46(8):635–41.
48. Kinoshita T, Ogawa T, Yoshida Y, Tamura H, Kado H, Okudera T. Curvilinear T1 hyperintense lesions representing cortical necrosis after cerebral infarction. Neuroradiology. 2005;47(9):647–51.
49. Kesavadas C, Santhosh K, Thomas B, Gupta AK, Kapilamoorthy TR, Bodhey N, et al. Signal changes in cortical laminar necrosis-evidence from susceptibility-weighted magnetic resonance imaging. Neuroradiology. 2009;51(5):293–8.
50. Siskas N, Lefkopoulos A, Ioannidis I, Charitandi A, Dimitriadis AS. Cortical laminar necrosis in brain infarcts: serial MRI. Neuroradiology. 2003;45(5): 283–8.
51. Niwa T, Aida N, Shishikura A, Fujita K, Inoue T. Susceptibility-weighted imaging findings of cortical laminar necrosis in pediatric patients. AJNR Am J Neuroradiol. 2008;29(9):1795–8.

52. Tsui YK, Tsai FY, Hasso AN, Greensite F, Nguyen BV. Susceptibility-weighted imaging for differential diagnosis of cerebral vascular pathology: a pictorial review. J Neurol Sci. 2009;287(1–2):7–16.
53. Renou P, Sibon I, Tourdias T, Rouanet F, Rosso C, Galanaud D, et al. Reliability of the ECASS radiological classification of postthrombolysis brain haemorrhage: a comparison of CT and three MRI sequences. Cerebrovasc Dis. 2010;29(6):597–604.
54. Alexandrov AV, Black SE, Ehrlich LE, Caldwell CB, Norris JW. Predictors of hemorrhagic transformation occurring spontaneously and on anticoagulants in patients with acute ischemic stroke. Stroke: J Cereb Circ. 1997;28(6):1198–202.
55. Boulanger JM, Coutts SB, Eliasziw M, Gagnon AJ, Simon JE, Subramaniam S, et al. Cerebral microhemorrhages predict new disabling or fatal strokes in patients with acute ischemic stroke or transient ischemic attack. Stroke: J Cereb Circ. 2006;37(3):911–4.
56. Easton JD, Saver JL, Albers GW, Alberts MJ, Chaturvedi S, Feldmann E, et al. Definition and evaluation of transient ischemic attack: a scientific statement for healthcare professionals from the American Heart Association/American Stroke Association Stroke Council; Council on Cardiovascular Surgery and Anesthesia; Council on Cardiovascular Radiology and Intervention; Council on Cardiovascular Nursing; and the Interdisciplinary Council on Peripheral Vascular Disease. The American Academy of Neurology affirms the value of this statement as an educational tool for neurologists. Stroke: J Cereb Circ. 2009;40(6):2276–93.
57. Pacheco FT, Rocha AJ, Littig IA, Maia Jr ACMM, Gagliardi RJ, Multiparametric multidetector computed tomography scanning on suspicion of hyperacute ischemic stroke: validating a standardized protocol. Arq Neuropsiquiatr. 2013;71(6):349–56.

Ischemic Stroke in Children

5

Felipe Torres Pacheco and Antônio José da Rocha

Abstract

Stroke in children is being increasingly recognized as a significant source of morbidity and mortality. Children and adolescents with stroke have remarkable differences in presentation compared with adults. Sickle cell disease is a major risk factor of overt and silent strokes in children. Cervicocephalic arterial dissection is an important but probably under-recognized cause of stroke in children. Cerebral vasculitis may be considered in children with either ischemic or hemorrhagic stroke, especially recurrent strokes. Cardiac disease is present in 10–30 % of children with stroke. Owing to the frequency of stroke mimics in childhood, the diagnosis requires the imaging confirmation of an ischemic lesion.

Background

Stroke has been increasingly recognized in children in recent years. Children and adolescents with stroke have remarkable differences in clinical presentation compared with older patients [1]. Approximately 80–85 % of strokes in adults are ischemic and the remaining are hemorrhagic. In children, around 55 % of strokes are ischemic [1].

Arterial ischemic stroke in children and infants encompasses those occurring during the perinatal period, defined as 1 month before delivery to 1 month after it, and pediatric stroke, defined as that occurring between 1 month and 18 years of age with a peak at about the age of 5 years [2].

Data from the National Hospital Discharge Survey from 1980 to 1998 indicate that the risk of ischemic stroke in individuals from birth through 18 years of age is 7.8 per 100,000, with a hemorrhagic stroke risk of 2.9 per 100,000 [3].

Results of outcome studies show a high rate of lifelong morbidity as follows: 10 % of children who have a stroke die, 20 % have further strokes, and 70 % have seizures or other chronic neurological deficits [4, 5].

F.T. Pacheco, MD, PhD (✉) • A.J. da Rocha, MD, PhD
Division of Neuroradiology, Hospital Santa Casa de Misericórdia de São Paulo, Rua Dr. Cesário Motta Junior 112, Vila Buarque, Sao Paulo, SP 01221-020, Brazil

Division of Neuroradiology, Grupo Fleury, Sao Paulo, SP, Brazil
e-mail: felipetorrespacheco@hotmail.com; antonio.rocha@grupofleury.com.br

R. Hoffmann Nunes et al. (eds.), *Critical Findings in Neuroradiology*,
DOI 10.1007/978-3-319-27987-9_5

Key Points

Etiology

Almost half of children with stroke are known to have a risk factor at the time of infarction, and more than one vascular risk factor can be identified in at least two-thirds of such children after a thorough evaluation. But, after extensive clinical investigations, no cause can be discovered in up to 30 % of children [6].

Sickle cell disease: Sickle cell disease (SCD) is a major risk factor for overt and silent strokes in children [7]. Eleven percent of patients with SCD have clinically overt strokes by the age of 20 years [8]. SCD is associated with a progressive occlusive arteriopathy (moyamoya syndrome) that involves the supraclinoid internal carotid arteries (ICAs) and proximal middle cerebral arteries (MCAs), relatively sparing the posterior circulation and completely sparing the cerebellum [9].

Moyamoya disease and moyamoya syndrome: An angiographic pattern called moyamoya is characterized by chronic progressive stenosis of the distal intracranial ICAs and, less often, stenosis of the proximal anterior cerebral artery (ACA) and middle cerebral arteries (MCA), the basilar artery, and the posterior cerebral arteries [1]. Moyamoya pattern can be either primary (idiopathic moyamoya disease) or secondary to underlying disorders such as SCD (moyamoya syndrome) [10]. Ischemic strokes are often multiple and recurrent, involving predominantly the anterior circulation [1].

Cervicocephalic arterial dissections: It is an important but probably under-recognized cause of stroke in children [11, 12]. In adults, most arterial dissections occur in the extracranial ICA, typically in the pharyngeal portion of the ICA, while in children, the site of dissection is often intracranial [11]. Furthermore, although up to one-half of arterial dissections in adults are diagnosed before an ischemic event [13], children usually have a history of an ischemic event (stroke or transient ischemic attack) before the diagnosis of arterial dissection [10]. The failure to detect dissections in children before an ischemic event may be related to the low incidence of related pain in this population [14].

Vasculitis: Cerebral vasculitis should be considered in children with either ischemic or hemorrhagic strokes, patients with recurrent strokes, strokes associated with encephalopathic abnormalities, as well as strokes accompanied by fever, multifocal neurological events, unexplained skin lesions, glomerulopathy, or elevated sedimentation rate [15]. CNS vasculitis may be infectious or noninfectious and the latter can be either primary or secondary to systemic diseases. Vasculitis may accompany intracranial infections and up to one-third of the stroke patients between 2 and 10 years of age have post-varicella angiopathy occurring weeks to months after uncomplicated chickenpox [16].

Cardiac disease: Cardiac disease is present in 10–30 % of children with strokes [17]. The majority of children with a cardiac cause for their stroke have a previous diagnosis of heart disease and it is rare for stroke to be the initial presentation of cardiac disease. Although any heart abnormality confers an increased risk of stroke, complex anatomic abnormalities have the highest risk [10].

Best Imaging Modality

Owing to the frequency of stroke mimics in childhood, the diagnosis requires imaging confirmation of an ischemic lesion. Computed tomography (CT) may miss early or small lesions as well as lesions in the posterior fossa; therefore, magnetic resonance imaging (MRI) is recommended although it may require sedation of young and uncooperative patients [10].

Brain MRI and magnetic resonance angiography (MRA) of the cervical and intracranial arteries are sensitive and noninvasive imaging modalities that should be the first step when investigating a suspected stroke in a child. Vascular imaging is important, owing to the high incidence of underlying cerebral arteriopathy in patients with stroke and the value of such imaging to predict the risk of stroke recurrence [10].

Perfusion MRI can be useful to identify regions of relative ischemia that are at risk for infarction. An increase in mean transit time (MTT) associated with reduced cerebral blood flow (CBF) is suggestive of tissue at risk. Perfusion imaging is also useful to assess changes in after therapy in moyamoya disease. (For more information, see chapter on adult acute stroke.)

Major Findings

Sickle cell disease: Often presents with large ischemic infarctions in the MCA and watershed (border-zone) territories. Small infarctions are common and typically involve the basal ganglia and deep white matter within the anterior circulation. Border-zone infarctions are not as common as large infarctions but both are due to large artery disease. Large infarctions within the ACA or posterior cerebral artery territories occur less often. Approximately 20 % of children with SCD have "silent" brain infarctions on MRI predominantly in frontal and parietal cortical, subcortical, and watershed locations (Fig. 5.1) [18]. These so-called silent infarcts are important because they are associated with deterioration in cognitive function with effects on learning and behavior [19].

Moyamoya disease and moyamoya syndrome: For the diagnosis of moyamoya, the following signs must be present: (1) stenosis involving the distal ICA bifurcation (C6 segment) and proximal portions of the ACA (A1 segment) and MCA (M1 segment), (2) dilated basal ganglia collateral arteries, and (3) bilateral abnormalities which may be asymmetrical or symmetrical (Fig. 5.2). If any of these findings are present and the angiographic pattern is unilateral, only a probable diagnosis of moyamoya can be entertained. Ischemic strokes often are multiple and recurrent, predominantly involving the anterior circulation. Infarctions may be superficial or deep and often are found in watershed territories.

The term "moyamoya" in Japan is used to describe irregular vascular networks that resemble a "puff or spiral of smoke" (cloud-like

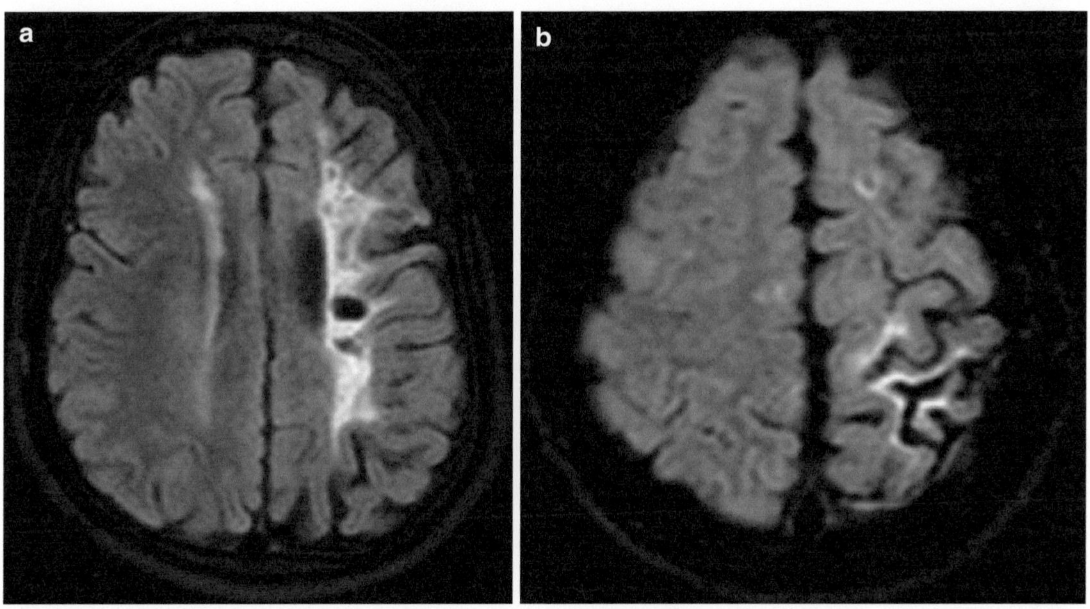

Fig. 5.1 Subtypes of sickle cell infarctions. (**a–d**) Axial FLAIR images demonstrate border-zone infarctions in the left hemisphere on A and a large ischemic infarction in the left MCA territory on B which were related to large artery disease. A lacunar infarction in the left cerebellar hemisphere is depicted on C (*dashed arrow*) and small "silent" ischemic brain lesions are shown on D (*arrows*). (**e**) Complete obstruction involving the region of the left distal ICA and proximal portions of the ACA and MCA is revealed on MRA TOF 3D reconstruction image. (**f**) Mean transit time perfusion MRI map identifies increase in mean transit time in the left hemisphere suggestive of tissue at risk

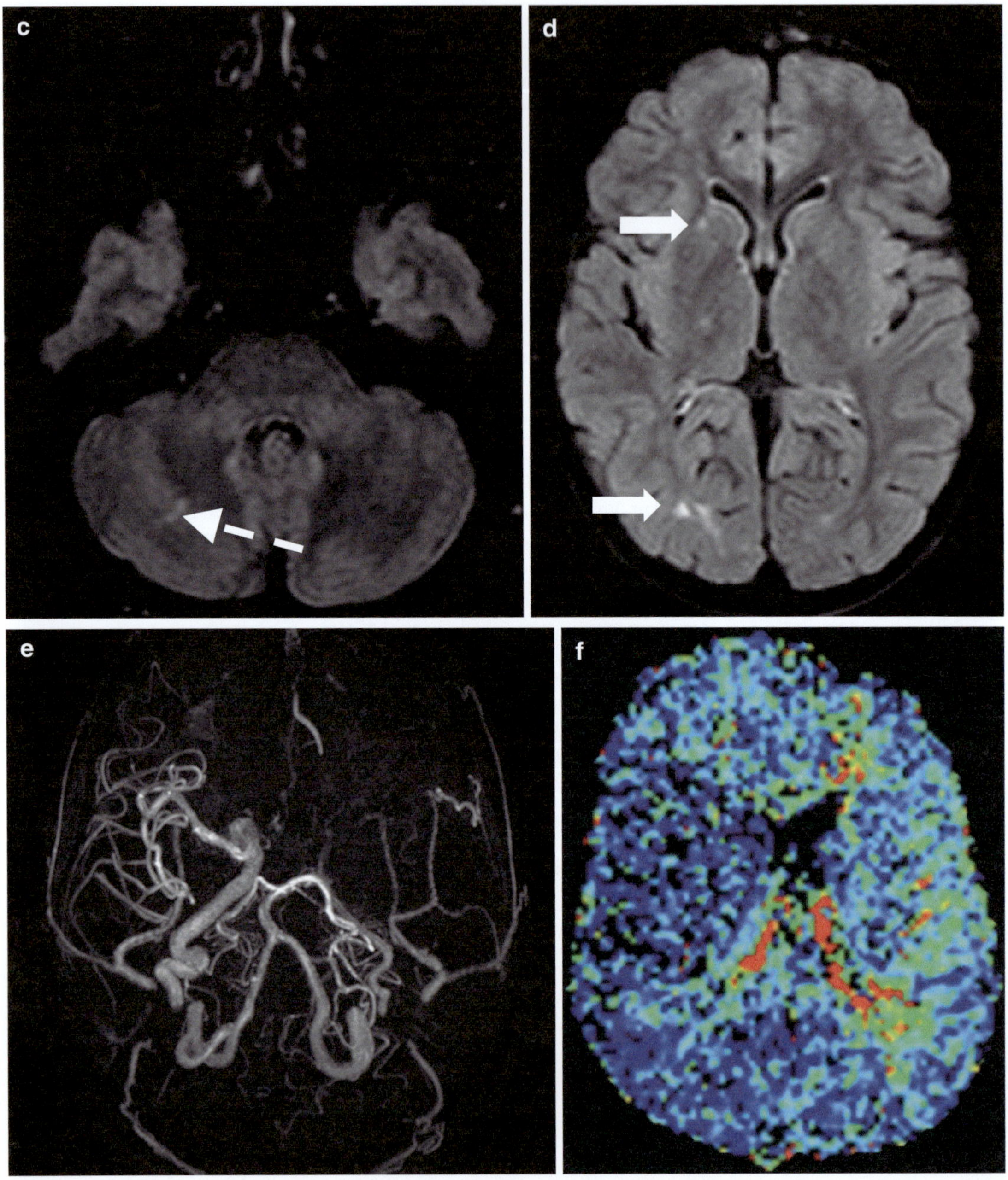

Fig. 5.1 (continued)

lenticulostriate and thalamostriate collaterals on angiography) [20]. This, in reality, is a misnomer and it was employed to describe the disease when imaging resolution was insufficient to detect individually enlarged collateral arteries. After the guidelines for diagnosing moyamoya disease with MRI and MRA were published in 1997 [21], 3D time-of-flight MRA has become widely accepted

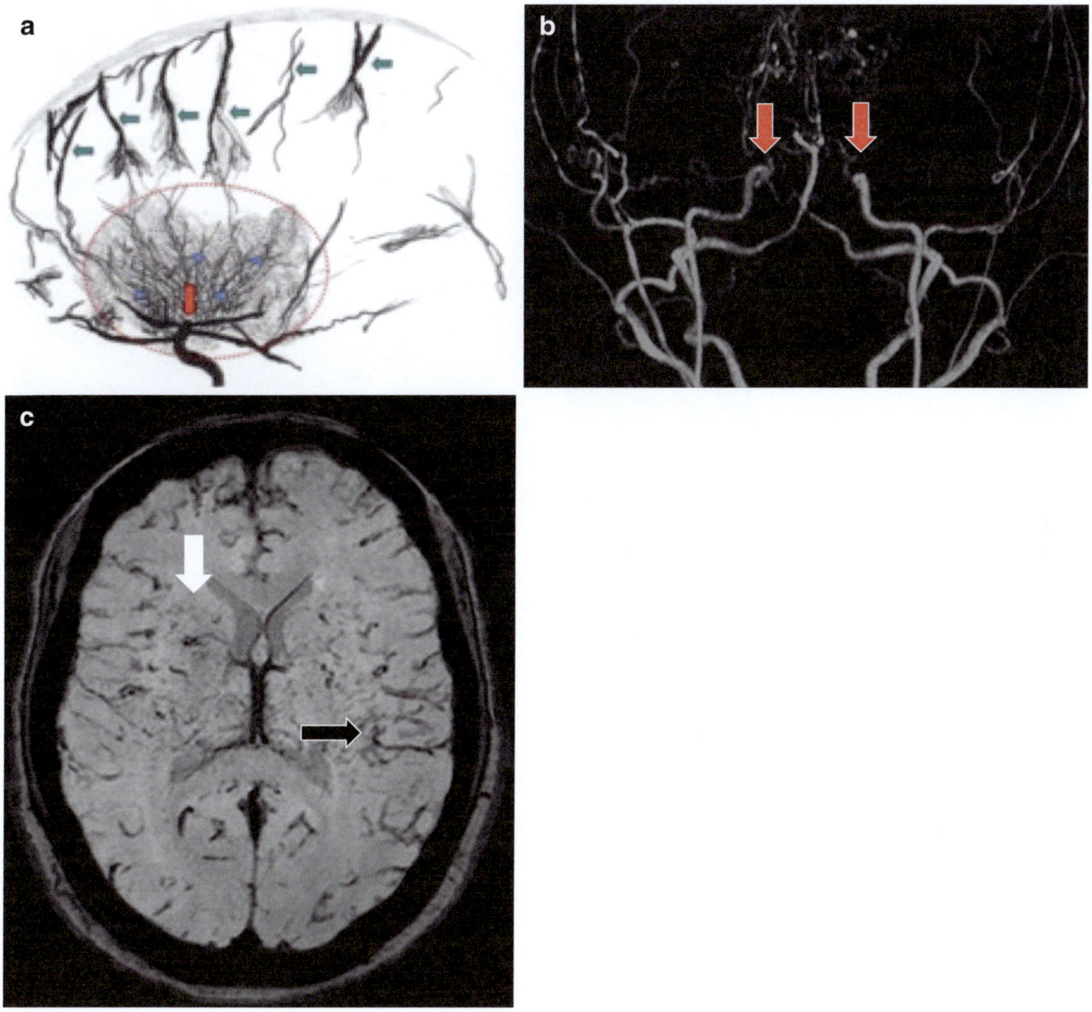

Fig. 5.2 Collateral circulation. (**a**) A schematic drawing demonstrates ICA distal obstruction (*red arrow*) with dilated basal collateral (*blue arrows*) and leptomeningeal collateral circulation (*green arrows*). (**b**) MRA TOF 3D reconstruction image shows bilateral severe stenosis involving the distal ICAs bifurcations (*red arrows*) and proximal portions of the ACA and MCA. (**c**) Axial SWI image shows the presence of dilated deep medullary veins (*white arrow*) and leptomeningeal collateral circulation (*black arrow*)

as an excellent noninvasive diagnostic modality to diagnose this disease. If intravenous contrast has been administered, contrast enhancement of the basal ganglia can occur due to the presence of abnormal collateral vessels. Furthermore, SWI is now accepted as a method useful in the evaluation of deep venous flow in acute or chronic ischemia and to demonstrate increased oxygen extraction in focal cerebral ischemia [22]. The increased conspicuity of deep medullary veins known as "brush sign" using SWI may predict the severity of moyamoya disease (Fig. 5.3) [23].

Another important finding is the leptomeningeal high signal intensity on FLAIR images that is depicted as a continuous linear or focal increased signal intensity along the cortical sulci and

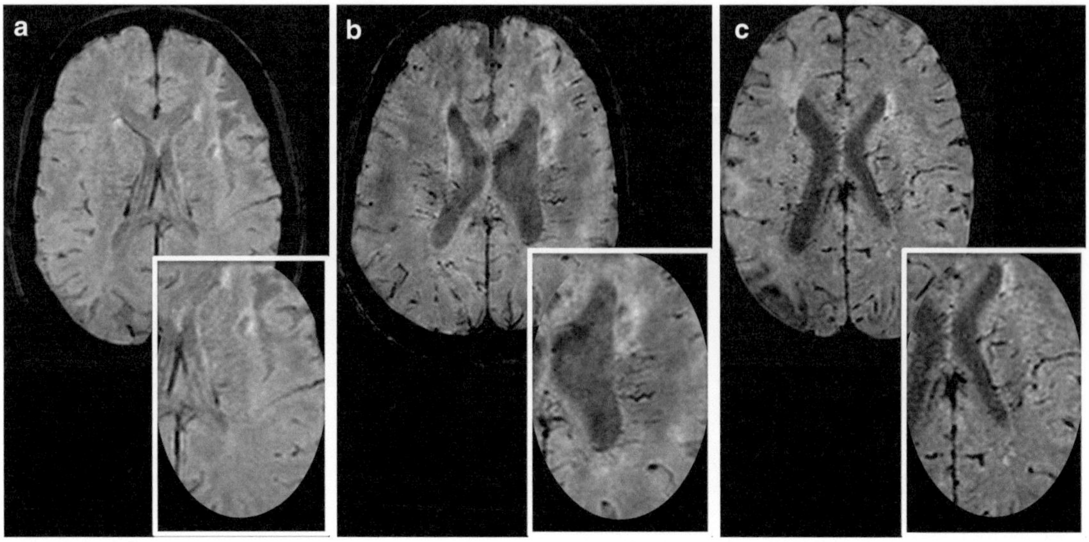

Fig. 5.3 "Brush sign" in moyamoya syndrome. (**a**–**c**) Axial SWI images demonstrate the different stages of conspicuity of the abnormally dilated deep medullary veins (mild (**a**), moderate (**b**), and severe or "brushlike" (**c**) stages). These dilated veins indicate parenchymal ischemia

subarachnoid spaces reflecting slow vascular flow and has been named the "ivy sign" (Fig. 5.4) [24].

Recent evidence suggests that symptomatic hyperperfusion may occur after revascularization surgery in 15–31.5 % of patients with moyamoya disease [25]. This hyperperfusion may lead to transient neurological deterioration, seizures, or even delayed intracerebral hemorrhage, and therefore the early detection and careful clinical management of hyperperfusion is mandatory after bypass surgery for moyamoya disease [26].

Cervicocephalic arterial dissections: MRA and MRI demonstrate incomplete or complete occlusion in the compromised vessel with residual patent vessel lumen ("string" sign). T1-weighted fat-suppressed axial image demonstrates the "methemoglobin crescent" sign that represents the intramural hematoma [11, 12].

Vasculitis: Abnormalities seen in vasculitis include narrowings/stenoses ranging from mild to complete occlusions, irregularities, concentric bands of narrowings, and vasospasm. Gadolinium-enhanced studies may reveal wall thickening and contrast enhancement of the affected vessel wall. The typical presentation is generally unilateral and the anterior circulation is predominantly involved, especially the proximal segments of the MCA and ACA. This pattern of vascular involvement is typical and explains the higher frequency of basal ganglia strokes in this condition because the lenticulostriate arteries, the sole source of blood supply for the basal ganglia, arise from them. The term unilateral intracranial arteriopathy has been proposed to describe a transient cerebral arteriopathy, different from the progressive pattern of moyamoya disease and vasculitis. It is characterized by lenticulostriate infarctions due to nonprogressive unilateral arterial disease affecting the supraclinoid ICA and its proximal branches [27]. When transient cerebral arteriopathy is preceded by varicella zoster (VZV) infection up to 12 months prior to the strokes, the arteriopathy is called post-varicella angiopathy. In general, VZV vasculopathy is related to a broad spectrum of central nervous system injuries, including ischemic infarction of the brain and spinal cord, aneurysms, subarachnoid and cerebral hemorrhages, as well as dissection in immunocompetent or immunocompromised individuals leading to unifocal or multifocal deep-seated and superficial infarctions (Fig. 5.5) [28].

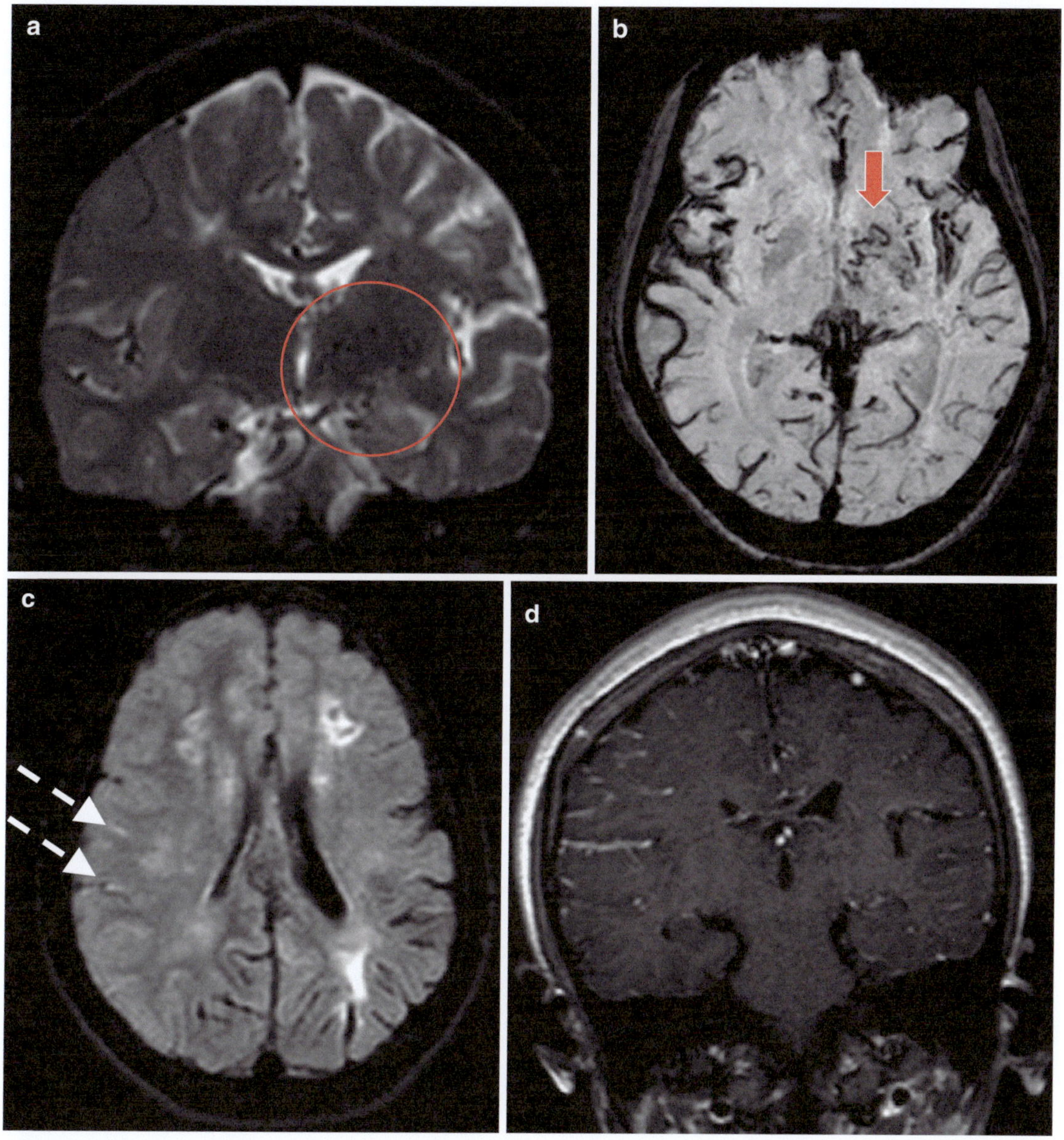

Fig. 5.4 Abnormal collateral vessels in moyamoya disease. (**a**) Coronal T2WI shows the dilated basal collateral circulation on the left (*circle*). (**b**) SWI better depicts dilated deep medullary veins (*arrow*). (**c**) Axial FLAIR image reveals leptomeningeal high signal intensities in the right hemisphere (*arrows*), representing the "ivy sign" which may reflect slow cerebral blood flow. (**d**) The ivy sign correlate is also shown on postcontrast T1WI where the slow-flowing arteries enhance

Cardiac disease: These patients present with thromboembolic strokes that can affect more than one arterial territory in the same event or in a recurrent form. Usually the infarction is extensive because the embolic thrombus is larger [10].

Main Differential Diagnosis

The differential diagnosis for acute hemiparesis in a child includes complicated *migraine*, *focal encephalitis*, and a *focal seizure*, mainly a postictal Todd's paresis [29]. Because seizures and

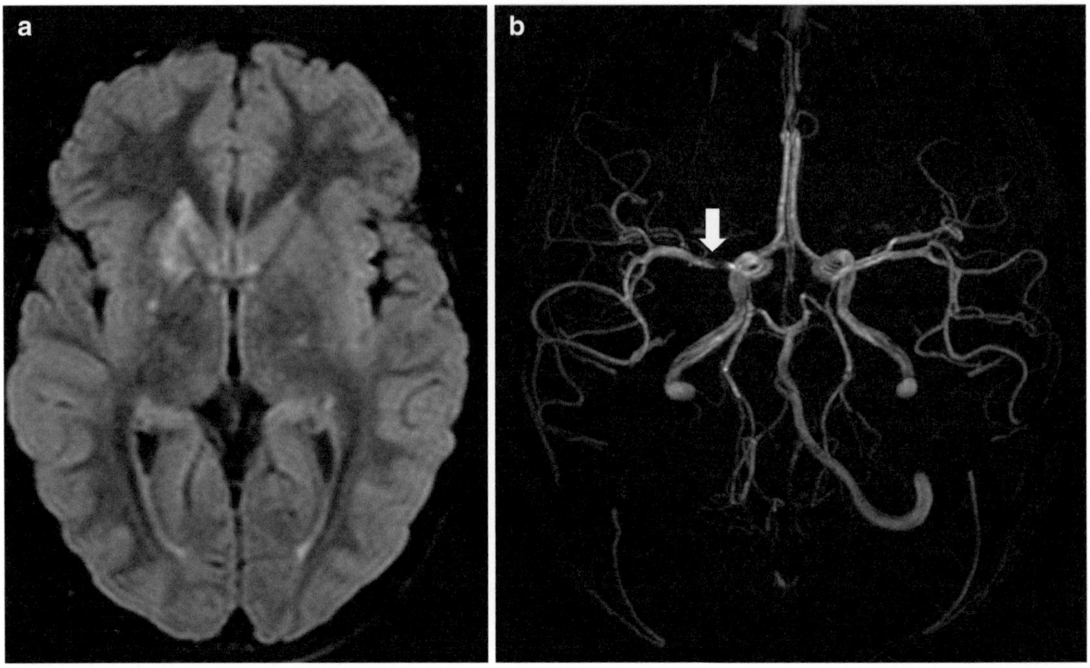

Fig. 5.5 A 9-year-old girl presenting with left-sided hemiparesis. (**a**) Axial FLAIR image demonstrated foci of high signal intensity in the right basal ganglia suggesting ischemic infarctions. (**b**) MRA TOF 3D reconstruction image showed narrowing in the right middle cerebral artery (*white arrow*). VZV-DNA was detected by polymerase chain reaction in the CSF, and VZV vasculopathy-related stroke was thus diagnosed

headaches are common stroke manifestations in children, head imaging is often indispensible to help in their differentiation. The presence of a lesion affecting exclusively an arterial territory narrows the differential diagnosis. Infarctions show progressive decrease in mass effect, starting late in the first week and increasing contrast enhancement peaking during the second postictus week which is not observed in the other entities [10, 29].

Tips

- Border-zone infarctions should heighten suspicion of an ICA abnormality. Look for the cavernous carotid artery signal intensity on T2WI to confirm its normal flow void. Absence of flow void may indicate occlusion.
- T2* or SWI may help to identify dilated collateral arteries for the diagnosis of moyamoya.
- Question about a history of varicella infection in the presence of children stroke, especially involving the basal ganglia unilaterally or an MCA territory.
- Keep in mind that axial T1-weighted fat-suppressed images are essential to make the diagnosis cervicocephalic arterial dissection.

References

1. Roach ES, Golomb MR, Adams R, et al. Management of stroke in infants and children: a scientific statement from a Special Writing Group of the American Heart Association Stroke Council and the Council on Cardiovascular Disease in the Young. Stroke; J Cereb Circ. 2008;39:2644–91.
2. Goodman S, Pavlakis S. Pediatric and newborn stroke. Curr Treat Options Neurol. 2008;10:431–9.
3. Lynch JK, Hirtz DG, DeVeber G, Nelson KB. Report of the National Institute of Neurological Disorders

and Stroke workshop on perinatal and childhood stroke. Pediatrics. 2002;109:116–23.
4. deVeber GA, MacGregor D, Curtis R, Mayank S. Neurologic outcome in survivors of childhood arterial ischemic stroke and sinovenous thrombosis. J Child Neurol. 2000;15:316–24.
5. Ganesan V, Hogan A, Shack N, Gordon A, Isaacs E, Kirkham FJ. Outcome after ischaemic stroke in childhood. Dev Med Child Neurol. 2000;42:455–61.
6. Ganesan V, Prengler M, McShane MA, Wade AM, Kirkham FJ. Investigation of risk factors in children with arterial ischemic stroke. Ann Neurol. 2003;53: 167–73.
7. Earley CJ, Kittner SJ, Feeser BR, et al. Stroke in children and sickle-cell disease: Baltimore-Washington Cooperative Young Stroke Study. Neurology. 1998;51:169–76.
8. Ohene-Frempong K, Weiner SJ, Sleeper LA, et al. Cerebrovascular accidents in sickle cell disease: rates and risk factors. Blood. 1998;91:288–94.
9. Stockman JA, Nigro MA, Mishkin MM, Oski FA. Occlusion of large cerebral vessels in sickle-cell anemia. N Engl J Med. 1972;287:846–9.
10. Amlie-Lefond C, Sebire G, Fullerton HJ. Recent developments in childhood arterial ischaemic stroke. Lancet Neurol. 2008;7:425–35.
11. Fullerton HJ, Johnston SC, Smith WS. Arterial dissection and stroke in children. Neurology. 2001;57:1155–60.
12. Rafay MF, Armstrong D, Deveber G, Domi T, Chan A, MacGregor DL. Craniocervical arterial dissection in children: clinical and radiographic presentation and outcome. J Child Neurol. 2006;21:8–16.
13. Silbert PL, Mokri B, Schievink WI. Headache and neck pain in spontaneous internal carotid and vertebral artery dissections. Neurology. 1995;45: 1517–22.
14. Chabrier S, Husson B, Lasjaunias P, Landrieu P, Tardieu M. Stroke in childhood: outcome and recurrence risk by mechanism in 59 patients. J Child Neurol. 2000;15:290–4.
15. Moharir M, Shroff M, Benseler SM. Childhood central nervous system vasculitis. Neuroimaging Clin N Am. 2013;23:293–308.
16. Askalan R, Laughlin S, Mayank S, et al. Chickenpox and stroke in childhood: a study of frequency and causation. Stroke; J Cereb Circ. 2001;32:1257–62.
17. Pavlakis SG, Levinson K. Arterial ischemic stroke: common risk factors in newborns and children. Stroke; J Cereb Circ. 2009;40:S79–81.
18. Moser FG, Miller ST, Bello JA, et al. The spectrum of brain MR abnormalities in sickle-cell disease: a report from the Cooperative Study of Sickle Cell Disease. AJNR Am J Neuroradiol. 1996;17:965–72.
19. Armstrong FD, Thompson Jr RJ, Wang W, et al. Cognitive functioning and brain magnetic resonance imaging in children with sickle Cell disease. Neuropsychology Committee of the Cooperative Study of Sickle Cell Disease. Pediatrics. 1996;97: 864–70.
20. Suzuki J, Takaku A. Cerebrovascular "moyamoya" disease. Disease showing abnormal net-like vessels in base of brain. Arch Neurol. 1969;20:288–99.
21. Fukui M. Guidelines for the diagnosis and treatment of spontaneous occlusion of the circle of Willis ('moyamoya' disease). Research Committee on Spontaneous Occlusion of the Circle of Willis (Moyamoya Disease) of the Ministry of Health and Welfare, Japan. Clin Neurol Neurosurg. 1997;99 Suppl 2:S238–40.
22. Tong KA, Ashwal S, Obenaus A, Nickerson JP, Kido D, Haacke EM. Susceptibility-weighted MR imaging: a review of clinical applications in children. AJNR Am J Neuroradiol. 2008;29:9–17.
23. Horie N, Morikawa M, Nozaki A, Hayashi K, Suyama K, Nagata I. "Brush Sign" on susceptibility-weighted MR imaging indicates the severity of moyamoya disease. AJNR Am J Neuroradiol. 2011;32: 1697–702.
24. Maeda M, Tsuchida C. "Ivy sign" on fluid-attenuated inversion-recovery images in childhood moyamoya disease. AJNR Am J Neuroradiol. 1999;20:1836–8.
25. Uchino H, Kuroda S, Hirata K, Shiga T, Houkin K, Tamaki N. Predictors and clinical features of postoperative hyperperfusion after surgical revascularization for moyamoya disease: a serial single photon emission CT/positron emission tomography study. Stroke; J Cereb Circ. 2012;43:2610–6.
26. Horie N, Morikawa M, Morofuji Y, et al. De novo ivy sign indicates postoperative hyperperfusion in moyamoya disease. Stroke; J Cereb Circ. 2014;45:1488–91.
27. Braun KP, Bulder MM, Chabrier S, et al. The course and outcome of unilateral intracranial arteriopathy in 79 children with ischaemic stroke. Brain. 2009;132: 544–57.
28. Gilden D, Cohrs RJ, Mahalingam R, Nagel MA. Varicella zoster virus vasculopathies: diverse clinical manifestations, laboratory features, pathogenesis, and treatment. Lancet Neurol. 2009;8:731–40.
29. Shellhaas RA, Smith SE, O'Tool E, Licht DJ, Ichord RN. Mimics of childhood stroke: characteristics of a prospective cohort. Pediatrics. 2006; 118:704–9.

Hypoxic–Ischemic Injuries

6

Francisco José Chiang and Ana Lorena Abello

Abstract

Hypoxic–ischemic injury to the brain is usually a devastating event and an important cause of morbidity and mortality. Neuroimaging plays a pivotal role in diagnosis, treatment, and long-term prognosis determination for these patients. The correct diagnosis is made on the basis of different imaging modalities requires knowledge of the different manifestations of this type of injury. Some of the factors that contribute to the different findings are brain maturity, duration and severity of the insult, underlying cause, and associated disorders. Advanced magnetic resonance imaging (MRI) techniques such as diffusion-weighted image (DWI) and proton spectroscopy are useful in making the diagnosis especially in the acute setting where conventional MRI and CT are be less sensitive.

Background

Hypoxic–ischemic injury (HII) is often a devastating event that occurs when the entire brain lacks an adequate oxygen supply. HII is considered the third leading cause of death in the United States with approximately half a million new victims per year. Death will occur in nearly one-third of these patients, while another third will end up suffering severe neurologic deficits with important functional impairment. The last third will recover with mild or no neurologic deficits [1].

Key Points

Etiology

This serious condition is most often caused by insults such as cardiac arrest, asphyxia, seizures, poisoning (drug overdose or carbon monoxide

F.J. Chiang, MD (✉)
Department of Radiology, School of Medicine, Universidad de Los Andes, Monseñor Alvaro del Portillo, 12455, Las Condes, Santiago, Chile
e-mail: franciscochiang@gmail.com

A.L. Abello, MD
Department of Radiology, University of North Carolina, Chapel Hill, NC, USA
e-mail: anaabellop@hotmail.com

R. Hoffmann Nunes et al. (eds.), *Critical Findings in Neuroradiology*,
DOI 10.1007/978-3-319-27987-9_6

intoxication), and head trauma, with infants and small children more inclined to suffer asphyxia, while chronic cerebrovascular disease and/or cardiac arrest with secondary hypoxemia are the leading causes in older adults [1].

Pathophysiology: There are important pathophysiological concepts that must be taken into account when analyzing the imaging pattern of HII. First, some areas of the brain are more susceptible to ischemic injury than others because of their concentrations of glutamate and other excitatory amino acid receptors (primarily located in the gray matter), a concept known as *selective vulnerability*. Second, there are some areas of the brain with more energy demand than others. In these, energy will be depleted faster, and therefore, the injury will ensue earlier, and finally due to delayed neuron death (apoptosis). Thus, not all of the injury may be evident until days after the initial insult [2].

The sites of the brain that are most vulnerable and are first affected by HII will be determined by the degree of maturity of the brain, which depends on the age of the patient. This is one of the reasons why HII manifestations in the perinatal period (up to 1 month of age) differ from those seen in older infants [3]. For this reason, we divide this review of the different manifestations of HII in imaging studies in preterm babies, term babies, and older children/adults.

Best Imaging Modality

Neuroimaging plays a pivotal role in diagnosis, treatment, and long-term prognosis determination for these patients. The correct diagnosis made on the basis of different imaging modalities requires knowledge of the different manifestations of this type of injury. It is necessary to emphasize that findings in HII are variable. They depend on many different factors such as age (brain maturity), duration, severity, and exact type of insult and also modality and timing of the imaging studies.

Ultrasonography (US): US is the preferred initial study in neonates as it is a noninvasive, bedside examination and can easily be used in the intensive care unit as a screening tool.

Magnetic Resonance Imaging (MRI): MRI is the most sensitive imaging modality, especially DWI in the first 24 h. The MRI protocol should include DWI, apparent diffusion coefficient map (ADC map), T1-weighted image (TIWI), and T2-weighted image (T2WI). Spectroscopy can be useful when in the acute phase DWI is negative and there is a high clinical suspicion for HII.

Computed Tomography (CT): CT is usually avoided in neonates and small children because of the exposure to ionizing radiation, and also it does not provide much more information than US and MRI. CT could be helpful in confirming periventricular leukomalacia (PVL) end-stage injury later in life.

Major Findings in Preterm Neonates

Severe Injury

The injury pattern in preterm neonates suffering a severe but brief hypoxic event includes lesions in basal ganglia, thalami, brain stem structures, cerebellum, and corticospinal tracts, as well as decreased cerebral hemispheric white matter in the chronic stages. Although acute basal ganglia injury is frequent, it is less severe than involvement of the thalami in this age group and especially among those less than 32 weeks of age. When involved, the basal ganglia tend to atrophy without scarring with passing time. Overall, the thalami, anterior vermis, and dorsal brainstem are the most commonly involved structures when profound asphyxia happens [2, 4].

Mild-to-Moderate Injury

Germinal matrix hemorrhage (GMH) is the most characteristic pattern of injury in mild-to-moderate asphyxia in preterm babies. It is caused by direct injury and hemorrhage of the germinal matrix. Neonatal cerebral hemorrhages are divided in four grades reflecting their locations and degree of dilatation of the ventricles (Table 6.1) [2].

A common manifestation that can be seen in mild-to-moderate asphyxia in preterm babies is white matter injury of prematurity, which appears to be inversely related to gestational age at birth. PVL is most commonly seen in the peritrigonal regions and adjacent to the foramina of Monro [5, 6]. Chronically, the injury may be

Table 6.1 Germinal matrix hemorrhage (GMH) – intraventricular hemorrhage grading

Grade I
Subependymal GMH (mostly in the caudothalamic groove)
Grade II
GMH and IVH with or without mild ventriculomegaly
Grade III
GMH and IVH with ventriculomegaly
Grade IV
Above + periventricular parenchymal hemorrhagic infraction (not true GMH)

cavitary or non-cavitary presentation, this last type being more frequent.

US is usually used as the first examination in evaluating suspected acute HII cases. Nevertheless, it lacks the sensitivity and positive predictive value, and the study can be normal in patients who eventually develop PVL. Conversely in other cases, US shows increased echogenicity in the periventricular areas of normal neonates. The presence of hyperechogenicity of the periventricular white matter has a fairly low sensitivity and positive predictive value for the detection of PVL [7]. Serial US examinations improve substantially the detection of transient cystic lesions and can be better than MRI studies for this purpose. This has an important prognostic value as most of patients with cystic changes present neurologic sequelae [8]. For these reasons, the primary role of US is to detect germinal matrix hemorrhages in the immediate postnatal period and the detection of cystic changes later in perinatal life [2]. In US, the major acute findings include hyperechogenicity in periventricular areas and GMH (Fig. 6.1).

MRI allows better visualization of the periventricular white matter lesions and is a useful complement to cranial US especially among patients without cystic lesions. It also allows better depiction of hemorrhages and/or white matter volume loss which has prognostic value [8]. In MRI, early injury to the white matter appears as foci of T1 hyperintensity in larger areas of T2 hyperintensity. These T1 hyperintense foci must be distinguished from hemorrhages and they do not produce T2 shortening. These T1WI abnormalities may represent focal areas of mineralization [9]. These changes are usually evident at the third to fourth day post-injury, and then they give way to a mild T2 shortening of the white matter at days 6–7. The high T2 signal is most evident in the peritrigonal regions (Fig. 6.2) (Table 6.2).

Major Findings in Term Neonates

Severe Injury

Severe injury results mainly in a central pattern of lesions that usually involves the deep gray matter including the putamina, ventrolateral thalami, hippocampi, dorsal brainstem, and lateral geniculate nuclei. Occasionally, the perirolandic cortex is also involved [2].

Mild-to-Moderate Injury

In insults of short duration, there may be little or no injury [3]. When the autoregulatory mechanisms are exceeded, the result is injury to the watershed zones which become relatively hypoperfused [2].

US: In term neonates, transfontanelle US is the first imaging study to be obtained when HII is suspected. Although some abnormalities can be detected by US, it has a low sensitivity, and therefore a negative study should not be used as a definite evidence of absence of hypoxic injury. If there is strong clinical suspicion of HII and US is negative, MRI should be obtained to evaluate the presence and severity of the injury.

MRI: In MRI, it is important to remember that the biochemical and histological features of HII that influence the imaging findings vary with time so that a study performed only hours after the event will be different from one done several days later.

DWI in the first 24 h is most sensitive to detect injuries which may not be visible in conventional T1WI and T2WI. In severe asphyxia, DWI shows high signal (with corresponding low ADC values) in the ventrolateral thalami and basal ganglia (particularly the posterior putamina), perirolandic regions, and along the corticospinal tracts (Fig. 6.3). In mild or moderate insults, DWI shows hyperintensity with corresponding low ADC values (restricted diffusion) in the watershed territories. T1WI and T2WI may be normal

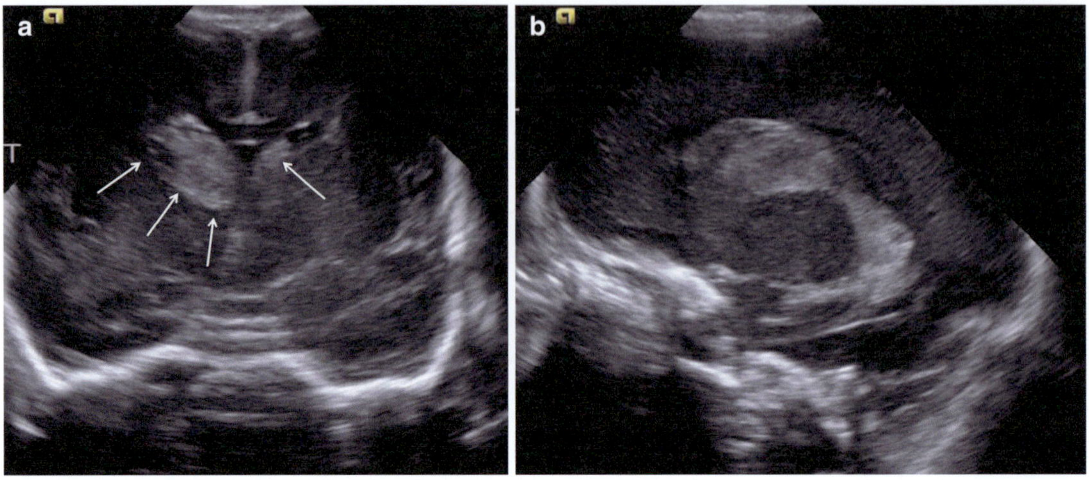

Fig. 6.1 US image in a preterm patient with GMH grade II. (**a**) Coronal and (**b**) sagittal images demonstrate bilateral areas of subependymal echogenicity right greater than left corresponding with hematomas (*arrows*). The sagittal image confirms the location in the caudothalamic groove with extension in a ventricle but no hydrocephalus

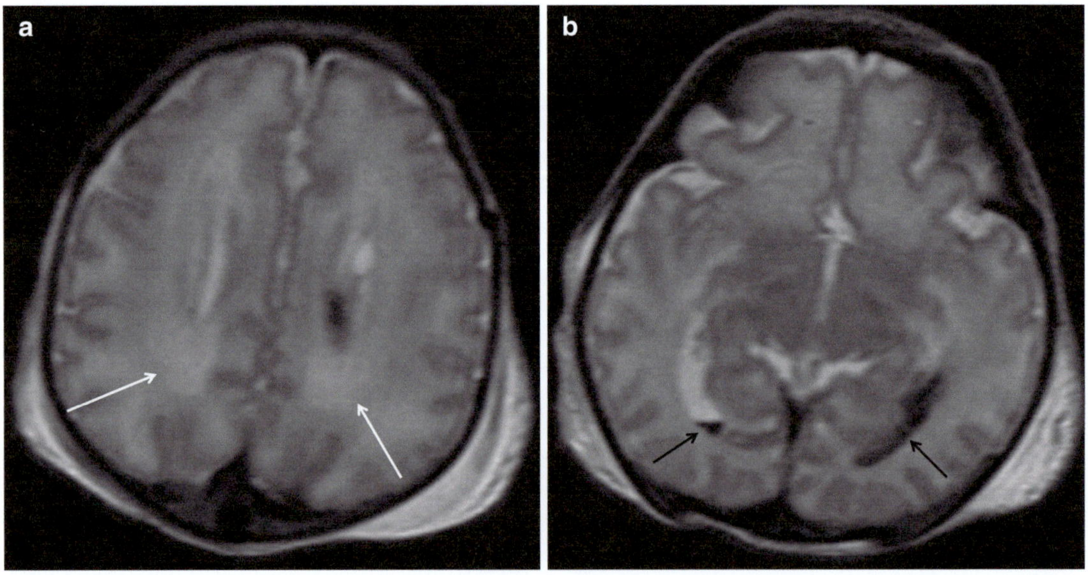

Fig. 6.2 Preterm neonate who suffered mild-to-moderate asphyxia. (**a, b**) Axial T2WI at the semiovale center and more caudal level show T2 hyperintensity in the periventricular white matter in the setting of acute PVL (*white arrows* in **a**). Also dark fluid levels can be seen inside lateral ventricles compatible with intraventricular hemorrhage (*black arrows* in **b**)

in the first 24 h, but by the second day, they show T2 hyperintensity in the involved areas. Also, loss of normal hyperintensity on T1WI and hypointensity on T2WI in the posterior limb of the internal capsule with respect to the lateral ventral thalami may present "absent posterior limb sign" (Fig. 6.4) (Table 6.3) [10].

Major Findings in Postnatal Infants and Young Children

Severe Injury

Severe episodes of asphyxia in infants between 1 and 2 years of age result in injuries to the caudate nuclei, putamina, lateral geniculate nuclei, hippocampi, and cerebral cortex. The anterior frontal and parieto-occipital cortex will be most affected with relative sparing of the perirolandic cortex and thalami [11].

In patients who experience asphyxia after the immediate perinatal period but before 1 year of age, findings are often a mixture between those of neonatal asphyxia and later infantile asphyxia and result in involvement of the basal ganglia in particular the posterior putamina and lateral thalami and also in involvement of the dorsal midbrain and cortex.

Table 6.2 HII in preterm neonates

Severity	Best imaging modality	Key manifestations
Severe	MRI	Injury in the deep gray matter, mostly thalami but also basal ganglia, dorsal brain stem, cerebellum, and corticospinal tracts as well as diminished volume of cerebral hemispheric white matter
Mild to moderate	US, MRI	Germinal matrix hemorrhage
		Intraventricular hemorrhage
		Periventricular leukomalacia

Mild-to-Moderate Injury

Mild hypoxic insults to older infants, watershed zone abnormalities in the cortex, and subcortical white matter are seen.

US: With the anterior fontanelle closure (4 months), US cannot be used anymore.

CT: CT is the study of choice. However, CT examinations that are done too early, before 24 h, can show only subtle hypodensity in the deep gray matter structures or be negative. In severe asphyxia, CT demonstrates diffuse basal ganglia abnormalities along with diffuse cortical hypoattenuation with loss of gray–white matter differentiation and sulcal and cisternal effacement all of which are a consequence of cerebral edema. The perirolandic cortex may be relatively spared [4, 12, 13]. At 4–6 days, hemorrhagic infarcts may be evident in the basal ganglia. In some patients, the "reversal sign" can be seen. The reversal sign refers to a reversal in the normal CT attenuation patterns between gray and white matter probably due to congestion of deep

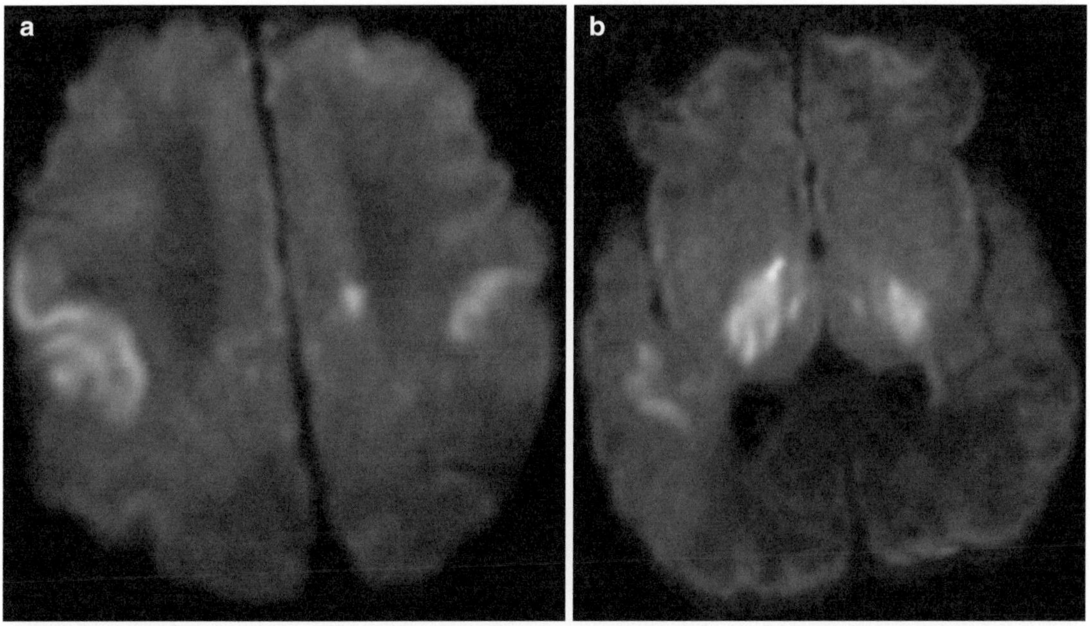

Fig. 6.3 Term neonate with severe asphyxia. Axial DWI (**a**) at the level of semiovale centrum and (**b**) at the level of the basal ganglia demonstrate high signal predominantly in the ventrolateral thalami and perirolandic cortex

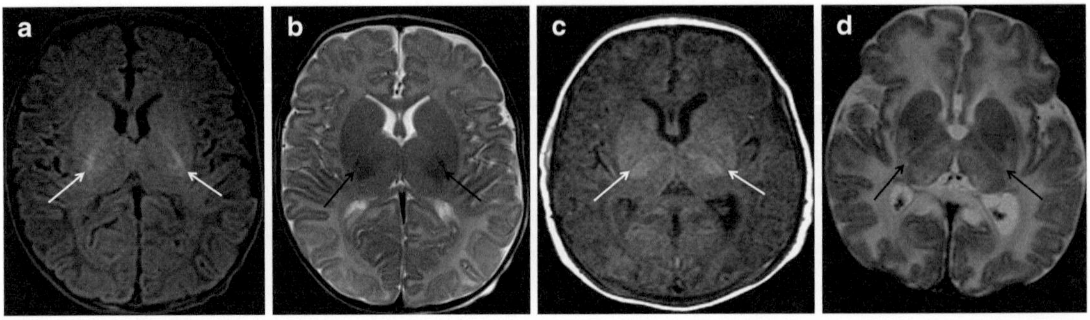

Fig. 6.4 "Absent posterior limb sign" in a term neonate with severe asphyxia. (**a**) Axial T1WI and (**b**) axial T2WI in a normal patient show normal myelination with the arrows pointing the posterior limb of the internal capsule which is hyperintense in T1WI and hypointense in T2WI, respectively. (**c**) Axial T1WI and (**d**) axial T2WI show loss of hyperintensity on T1WI and hypointensity on T2WI of the posterior limb of the internal capsule (*arrows*). Note linear T1 hyperintensity and T2 hypointensity in lateral thalami that should not be confused with the normal internal capsule

Table 6.3 HII in term neonates

Severity	Best imaging modality	Key manifestations
Severe	MRI	Injury of the deep gray nuclei (putamina, ventrolateral thalami), hippocampi, dorsal brainstem, and lateral geniculate nuclei
		Occasionally perirolandic cortex
Partial or less severe asphyxia	MRI	Cortical watershed zones

medullary veins secondary to obstruction of venous outflow by cerebral edema and subsequent compression of them; thus, the white matter will appear denser than the gray matter. The other sign in CT studies is the "white cerebellum sign" (Fig. 6.5), in which the cerebral hemispheres are hypodense due to diffuse edema, making the cerebellum and brainstem appear relatively hyperdense. Both the reversal and white cerebellum signs are associated with poor outcome.

MRI: If early imaging studies are done, MRI is more useful, since the abnormalities on DWI are evident in the first 12–24 h. In cases of severe injury, the initial MRI studies show high intensity in the posterolateral lentiform nuclei, and if the thalami are involved, usually the ventrolateral nuclei will be most affected. In the next 48 h, there is progression and involvement of the rest of the basal ganglia and cortex. Conventional T1WI and T2WI are usually normal during the first day and may remain normal for up to 48 h [14]. After this, T2WI shows diffuse basal ganglia and cortical hyperintensities with relative sparing of thalami and perirolandic cortex (Fig. 6.6).

In mild hypoxic insults to older infants, watershed zone abnormalities in the cortex and subcortical white matter are seen. White matter lesions may also be seen but are more common in younger children (under 1 year of age) [15]. Relative sparring of the periventricular white matter is common (Table 6.4) [16].

Major Findings in Older Children

Severe Injury

Severe insults have deleterious effects in the cortical gray matter and deep gray structures. The cortex is usually diffusely affected predominantly in the perirolandic and visual areas, and the cerebellum and hippocampi may also be affected.

Mild-to-Moderate Injury

In this group of patients, mild-to-moderate injury will manifest as watershed infarcts.

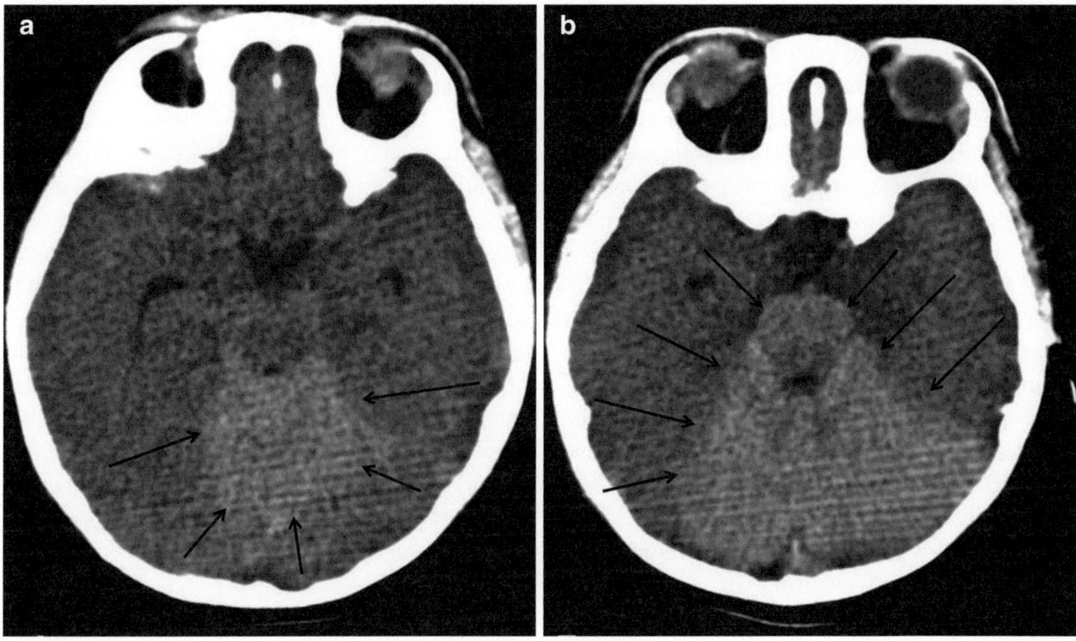

Fig. 6.5 Severe HII in a postnatal infant. (**a**) Axial NECT at the level of the midbrain (**a**) and the cerebellar hemispheres (**b**) show diffuse hyperdensity of the cerebellum and brainstem when compared with the supratentorial parenchyma. This appearance is compatible with the "white cerebellum sign" (*arrows*) described in HII

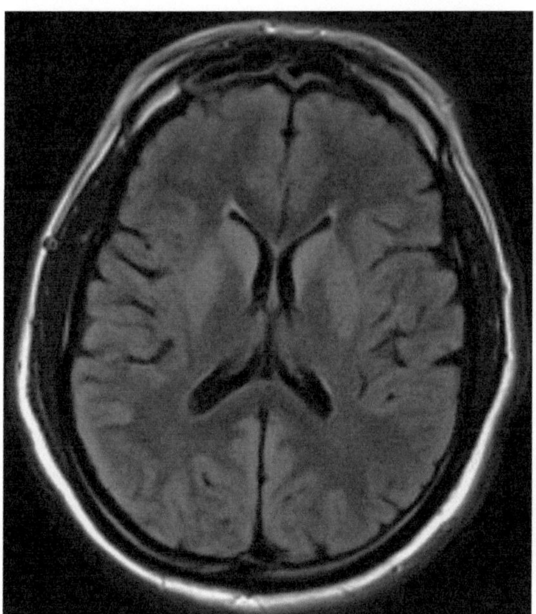

Fig. 6.6 Older child with severe HII. Axial FLAIR demonstrates hyperintensity of the basal ganglia with sparing of the thalami. The occipital cortex is also involved

Table 6.4 HII in postnatal infants and young children

Severity	Best imaging modality	Key manifestations
Severe	MRI	1–2 years: injury to caudate nuclei, putamina, lateral geniculate nuclei, hippocampi, and cerebral cortex (especially anterior frontal and parieto-occipital)
		<1 year: mixture of features of neonatal asphyxia and later infantile asphyxia
Mild to moderate	MRI	Cortical watershed zones

In older patients, the first imaging study performed for a suspected brain anoxic injury is commonly a CT. However, as in other age groups, MRI, in particular DWI, is the earliest to show abnormalities usually starting after a few hours after the injury.

CT: The most common findings are diffuse hypoattenuation of the cortex and basal ganglia, consistent with edema, effacement of the CSF-containing spaces, and loss of gray–white matter differentiation (Fig. 6.7). In older patients, as in children, the "reversal sign" and "white cerebellum" sign may be present and also indicate a poor prognosis.

MRI: During the first 24 h, hyperintensity in DWI is evident in basal ganglia, cerebellar hemispheres, and cerebral cortex (especially in perirolandic and occipital areas), and the thalami, brainstem, and basal ganglia may also be involved (Fig. 6.8) [15, 17, 18]. Abnormalities on T1WI and T2WI may be delayed in comparison with DWI. After the first 24 h, T2WI begins to show abnormalities that consist of hyperintensity and swelling of gray matter structures that may persist until the end of the second week (Fig. 6.9). DWI usually pseudonormalizes by the end of the first week to 10 days. In the chronic stage, T2WI demonstrates some residual hyperintensity in basal ganglia, and the T1WI may show hyperintensity in the affected cortex representing cortical laminar necrosis in addition to diffuse atrophy (Fig. 6.10) (Table 6.5) [18].

Imaging Follow-Up

In neonates, if subtle abnormalities are present on MRI in the acute setting, follow-up imaging at the end of the first week is recommended to define progression and overall extent of injury [19]. MRI is also helpful in depicting the last stage of PVL, in which there is a characteristic loss of volume of the periventricular white matter and centrum semiovale with secondary enlargement of the lateral ventricles and a characteristic irregular outline and wavy appearance of the outer wall of the lateral ventricles. MRI can also show loss of volume in the corpus callosum, particularly in the posterior aspect of the body and splenium [16]. CT can also be used in confirming PVL end-stage injury later in life.

Main Differential Diagnosis

Hypoglycemia: Predominantly has a posterior distribution.

Arterial ischemic stroke: Involves typical vascular territories.

Mitochondrial disorders: Search for typical patterns (e.g., MELAS with posterior stroke-like

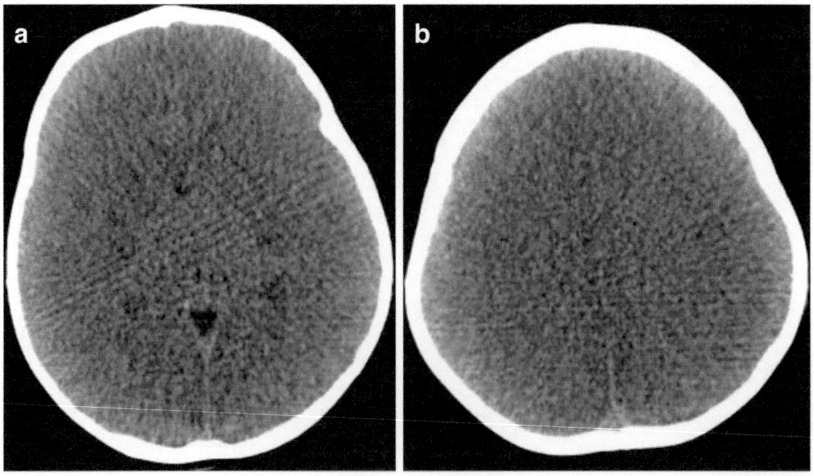

Fig. 6.7 An 8-year-old patient with severe HII injury after a cardiac arrest. NECT (**a**) at the level of basal ganglia and (**b**) at the level of semiovale centrum show total loss of gray–white matter differentiation with hypoattenuation of the cortex and basal ganglia. There is also effacement of all of the CSF-containing spaces

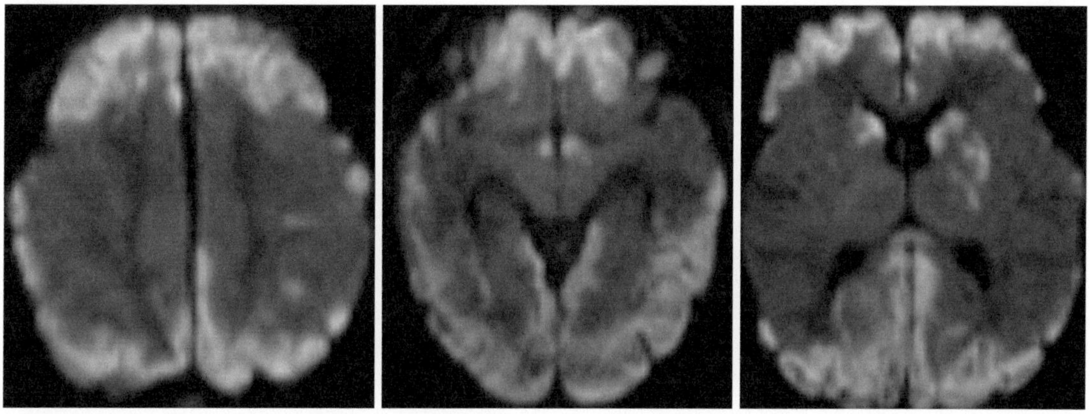

Fig. 6.8 Child with severe HII. DWI at different levels shows diffusion restriction in the cerebral cortex and basal ganglia. Note that cortex is affected in a nearly watershed distribution

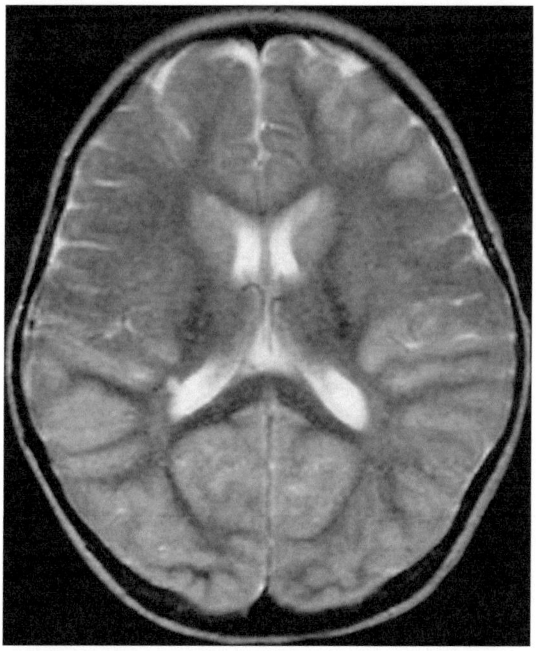

Fig. 6.9 HII in a pediatric patient. Axial FLAIR shows hyperintensity and swelling of the parieto-occipital cortex and to a lesser degree in the frontal cortex and head of the caudate nuclei

cortical lesions crossing vascular territories or Leigh syndrome with more striatum involvement than globus pallidus).

Infectious encephalitis: Abnormal T2WI hyperintensity of gray and white matter and deep gray nuclei and may have areas of hemorrhage.

Status epilepticus: The entire cortex may show high T2 signal and even restricted diffusion. The basal ganglia tend to be normal, but the medial thalami may be abnormal.

Tips

- DWI is more sensitive in the first 24 h; however, it can be normal initially and become abnormal within next few days. Pseudonormalization of DWI occurs at about 7–10 days after the insult but T1WI and T2WI will remain abnormal.
- US is a noninvasive and easy to perform, especially in the intensive care units. The major limitations of US are operator dependence and low sensitivity (especially in some areas such as the convexities). When US is positive for HII, it is very helpful, but if is negative, an MRI study may be required.
- Spectroscopy can be useful in the acute phase when DWI is negative and there is a high clinical suspicion for HII. Look for lactate peak in voxels positioned in the basal ganglia and centrum semiovale. Generally, all other metabolites (choline, creatine, n-acetyl aspartate) show low concentrations.

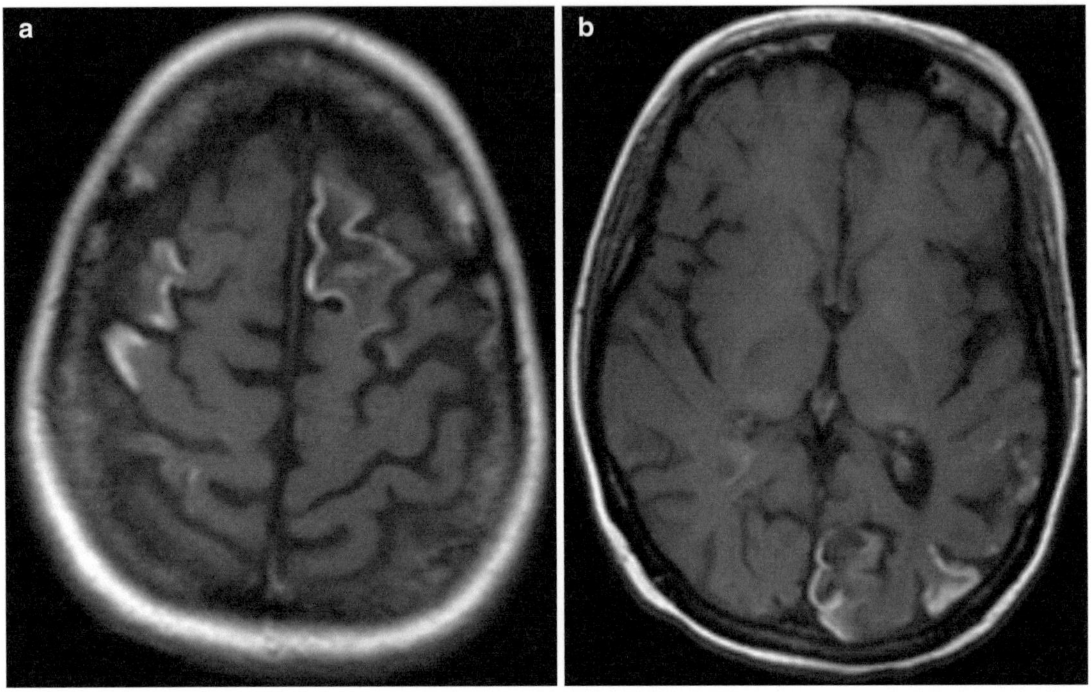

Fig. 6.10 Cortical laminar necrosis. Axial T1WI in the same patient as Fig. 6.9, 3 weeks later. (**a**) At the convexity and (**b**) at the basal ganglia levels images show areas of hyperintense cortex representing cortical laminar necrosis

Table 6.5 HII in older children

Severity	Best imaging modality	Key manifestations
Severe	MRI, CT	Cortex usually diffusely affected, deep gray structures (basal ganglia and thalami), hippocampi, and cerebellum
Mild to moderate	MRI, CT	Cortical watershed zones

References

1. Dugan LL, Choi DW, et al. Hypoxia-ischemia and brain infarction. In: Siegel GJ, Agranoff BW, Albers RW, editors. Basic neurochemistry: molecular, cellular and medical aspects. 6th ed. Philadelphia: Lippincott-Raven; 1999. Available from: http://www.ncbi.nlm.nih.gov/books/NBK28046/.
2. Huang BY, Castillo M. Hypoxic-ischemic brain injury: imaging findings from birth to adulthood. Radiographics. 2008;28(2):417–39. doi:10.1148/rg.282075066, quiz 617.
3. Barkovich AJ. Brain and spine injuries in infancy and childhood. In: Barkovich AJ, editor. Pediatric neuroimaging. 4th ed. Philadelphia: Lippincott Williams & Wilkins; 2005. p. 190–290.
4. Castillo M. Selective vulnerability and the cerebellum in neonates. AJNR Am J Neuroradiol. 2007;28:20–1.
5. Martinez-Biarge M, Diez-Sebastian J, Wusthoff CJ, Mercuri E, Cowan FM. Antepartum and intrapartum factors preceding neonatal hypoxic-ischemic encephalopathy. Pediatrics. 2013;132(4):e952–9. doi:10.1542/peds.2013-0511.
6. Blankenberg F, Loh N, Bracci P, D'Arceuil H, et al. Sonography, CT, and MR imaging: a prospective comparison of neonates with suspected intracranial ischemia and hemorrhage. AJNR Am J Neuroradiol. 2000;21:213–8.
7. Inder TE, Anderson NJ, Spencer C, Wells S, Volpe JJ. White matter injury in the premature infant: a comparison between serial cranial sonographic and MR findings at term. AJNR Am J Neuroradiol. 2003;24:805–9.
8. Murgo S, Avni EF, David P, Muller MF, Golzarian J, Balériaux D, Struyven J. Periventricular leukomalacia in premature infants: prognostic role of ultrasonography and MRI. J Radiol. 1999;80(7):715–20.
9. Felderhoff-Mueser U, Rutherford MA, Squier WV, et al. Relationship between MR imaging and histopathologic findings of the brain in extremely sick preterm infants. AJNR Am J Neuroradiol. 1999;20:1349–57.

10. Ghei S, Zan E, Choudhri A, et al. MR imaging of hypoxic-ischemic injury in term neonates: Pearls and pitfalls. RadioGraphics. 2014;34:1047–61.
11. Barkovich AJ. MR and CT evaluation of profound neonatal and infantile asphyxia. AJNR Am J Neuroradiol. 1992;13:959–72.
12. Harwood-Nash DC. Abuse to the pediatric central nervous system. AJNR Am J Neuroradiol. 1992;13: 569–75.
13. Bird CR, Drayer BP, Gilles FH. Pathophysiology of "reverse" edema in global cerebral ischemia. AJNR Am J Neuroradiol. 1989;10:95–8.
14. Dubowitz DJ, Bluml S, Arcinue E, Dietrich RB. MR of hypoxic encephalopathy in children after near drowning: correlation with quantitative proton MR spectroscopy and clinical outcome. AJNR Am J Neuroradiol. 1998;19:1617–27.
15. Christophe C, Fonteyne C, Ziereisen F, et al. Value of MR imaging of the brain in children with hypoxic coma. AJNR Am J Neuroradiol. 2002;23:716–23.
16. Barkovich AJ, Truwit CL. Brain damage from perinatal asphyxia: correlation of MR findings with gestational age. AJNR Am J Neuroradiol. 1990;11: 1087–96.
17. Arbelaez A, Castillo M, Mukherji S. Diffusion weighted MR imaging of global cerebral anoxia. AJNR Am J Neuroradiol. 1999;20:999–1007.
18. Takahashi S, Higano S, Ishii K, et al. Hypoxic brain damage: cortical laminar necrosis and delayed changes in white matter at sequential MR imaging. Radiology. 1993;189:449–56.
19. Grant PE, Yu D. Acute injury to the immature brain with hypoxia with or without hypoperfusion. Radiol Clin North Am. 2006;44:63–77, viii.

Intraparenchymal Hemorrhage 7

Marcos Rosa Jr., Renato Hoffmann Nunes, and Antônio José da Rocha

Abstract

Intracerebral hemorrhage is a spontaneous extravasation of blood into the brain parenchyma. It represents 10–15 % of all clinical strokes in the Western world and is associated with a higher mortality rate compared to ischemic stroke and subarachnoid hemorrhage. It is classified as primary or secondary according to its etiologies. More than one-half of primary bleeds are related to hypertension and one-third are associated with cerebral amyloid angiopathy. Secondary hemorrhages are due to drugs, vascular malformations, coagulopathy, neoplasms, trauma, vasculitis, moyamoya disease, and sinus venous thrombosis. An abrupt onset of focal neurological symptoms is presumed to be vascular in origin until proven otherwise; however, it is impossible to know whether symptoms are caused by ischemia or hemorrhage on the basis of clinical characteristics alone, and thus neuroimaging is needed to ascertain their cause.

M. Rosa Jr., MD (✉)
Department of Radiology, Universidade Federal do Espírito Santo, Avenida Marechal Campos, 1468, 29043-900 Vitoria, Espirito Santo, Brazil
e-mail: marcosrosajr@hotmail.com

R. Hoffmann Nunes, MD
Division of Neuroradiology, Santa Casa de São Paulo, São Paulo, Brazil
e-mail: renatohn@hotmail.com

A.J. da Rocha, MD, PhD
Division of Neuroradiology, Hospital Santa Casa de Misericórdia de São Paulo, Rua Dr. Cesário Motta Junior 112, 01221-020 Sao Paulo, SP, Brazil

Division of Neuroradiology, Grupo Fleury, Sao Paulo, SP, Brazil
e-mail: antonio.rocha@grupofleury.com.br

R. Hoffmann Nunes et al. (eds.), *Critical Findings in Neuroradiology*,
DOI 10.1007/978-3-319-27987-9_7

Background

Spontaneous nontraumatic intraparenchymal hemorrhage (IPH) is responsible for about 10–15 % of clinical strokes in the United States [1–3]. An abrupt onset of focal neurological symptoms is presumed to be vascular in origin until proven otherwise; however, it is impossible to ascertain if these symptoms are caused by ischemia or hemorrhage on the basis of clinical characteristics alone, and thus neuroimaging techniques help to differentiate between them [4, 5]. Furthermore, the clinical presentations of IPH are varied, given the wide range of locations in which IPH can occur and the diversity of its causes. Common symptoms include nausea, vomiting, seizure, focal neurologic deficits, headache, and altered mental status [1]. It is important to know the patient's previous clinical history including hypertension, drug use, anticoagulation, and prior hemorrhage [5].

Signs and symptoms of an IPH can be subtle and less specific in infants and neonates than in older children, especially with smaller hemorrhages. Consequently, it is likely that some smaller hemorrhages in neonates go unrecognized. Older children and adolescents present much like adults, with seizures, whereas some infants develop hydrocephalus, particularly with posterior fossa bleeds [6].

IPH treatment includes supportive care, blood pressure control, and correction of a coagulopathy if present [7, 8]. Surgical evacuation has a limited role but may be necessary in some patients. Hemostatic therapies aiming to reduce hematoma expansion such as recombinant activated factor VII or intensive blood pressure reduction may decrease morbidity and mortality especially in patients with active bleeding demonstrated on computed tomography angiography (CTA) [9–11].

The prognosis of IPH is grave with a mortality of 50 % and high rates of neurological disabilities in survivors [12]. Larger volumes of IPH [13–17], intraventricular extension, posterior fossa location, and/or presence of active extravasation of contrast within a hemorrhage carry a poor prognosis [18].

Key Points

Etiology

IPH are divided into primary and secondary hemorrhages. Systemic arterial hypertension and cerebral amyloid angiopathy (CAA) are the most common primary causes of IPH in adults (box) [1–3]. The main causes of hemorrhage in children are vascular anomalies (arterial aneurysm, cavernous malformation, AVM, or arteriovenous fistula) and congenital or acquired coagulation defects [6].

Box: Common Causes of Intraparenchymal Hemorrhage (all ages)

Primary
- Hypertension
- Cerebral amyloid angiopathy

Secondary
- Neoplastic hemorrhage
- Vascular malformations
  - Aneurysms
  - Arteriovenous malformations
  - Developmental venous anomaly
  - Cavernous angioma
- Drugs (amphetamines and cocaine)
- Medication (warfarin and heparin)
- Coagulation disorders

Hypertensive Hemorrhage

Systemic arterial hypertension is considered the most common cause in adults accounting for 50 % of all IPH. Underlying lipophyalinosis of the arterial walls is their cause. Hypertensive hemorrhages usually occur in the basal ganglia (especially the putamina), thalami, central portions (dentate nuclei) of the cerebellum, and pons [1–3, 9].

Cerebral Amyloid Angiopathy

In adults, CAA is the second cause of nontraumatic IPH and is considered to be responsible for 10 % of all hemorrhagic strokes and is the most common cause of IPH in normotensive elderly individuals. CAA occurs due to amyloid accumulation in the walls of peripheral cerebral arteries within the cortex and leptomeninges and generally affects individuals older than 55 years. There are three clinical manifestations of the disease. The first consists in deposits of amyloid in the vessel walls in asymptomatic patients. The second is related to vessel wall weakness, leading to delamination and rupture and subsequent IPH. The third and rarest clinical manifestation is obliteration of the vascular lumen leading to ischemia and leukoencephalopathy [1].

Secondary Hemorrhage

Secondary IPH occurs as a result of venous thrombosis, underlying neoplasm, vascular malformations, aneurysms, or inflammatory lesions and is more prevalent in children and young adults [1–3, 9]. Early diagnosis of underlying vascular abnormalities influences clinical management and prognosis. Patient's clinical profile and non-contrast CT (NCCT) findings may raise suspicion for secondary causes of IPH. The patient's age is one of the most important variables, since up to 40 % of IPH found in patients younger than 45 years of age are related to an underlying vascular lesion. Other risk factors for underlying vascular abnormalities are female sex, nonsmoker, lobar hematoma, intraventricular hemorrhage extension, and absence of a history of hypertension or coagulopathy [8].

Best Imaging Modality

Computed tomography (CT) and magnetic resonance imaging (MRI) are both reasonable techniques for initial evaluation, but unstable patients are better examined with CT which is faster. CT is very sensitive for identifying acute hemorrhage and is considered the "gold standard"; however, gradient-echo T2* and susceptibility-weighted imaging (SWI) are as sensitive as CT for detection of acute hemorrhage and are more sensitive for identification of prior hemorrhage. Time, cost, proximity to the emergency room, patient tolerance, clinical status, and MRI availability preclude emergent MRI in many patients [8].

The high rate of early neurological deterioration after IPH is related mostly to active bleeding that may continue for hours after symptom onset. Although CT angiography (CTA) is not routinely used for uncomplicated acute IPH, it helps to identify patients at high risk of IPH expansion based on the presence of contrast within the hematoma termed the "spot sign" [18–22]. CTA sensitivity for detection of vascular causes of IPH ranges from 89–96 % and allows a rapid identification of potential causes of secondary IPH [9]. Magnetic resonance angiography (MRA) may also identify specific causes of hemorrhage, including arteriovenous malformations, tumors, and moyamoya; however, CTA has been more widely used acutely [3, 8, 9, 22].

Catheter angiogram may be considered if clinical suspicion is high or noninvasive studies are suggestive of an underlying lesion and better pretreatment mapping of a lesion is needed [8].

Major Findings

An acute IPH on CT appears as a hyperdense lesion compared with the normal brain tissue in all patients with hemoglobin concentrations greater than 9 g/dL (Fig. 7.1). One should keep in mind that acute IPH may not be significantly hyperdense in patients with lower hemoglobin levels. CT is also able to determine the approximate age of hematomas by evaluating for their density measured in Hounsfield units (blood normally measures between 30–60 units). At onset, an acute hematoma is commonly seen as uniform, smooth, and dense on CT (Fig. 7.1). Over the course of the first 48 h, large hematomas may show fluid levels indicating that they are not yet fully contracted. Fluid blood levels in acute IPH are moderately sensitive and highly specific (98 %) for presence of an underlying coagulopathy. Fluid levels are also frequent in thrombolysis-related IPH and are associated with higher hemorrhage volumes. In the first 72 h, a hypodense region can be detected around lesions, as a result of edema l [3]. The hematoma loses approximately 1.5 Hounsfield units per day

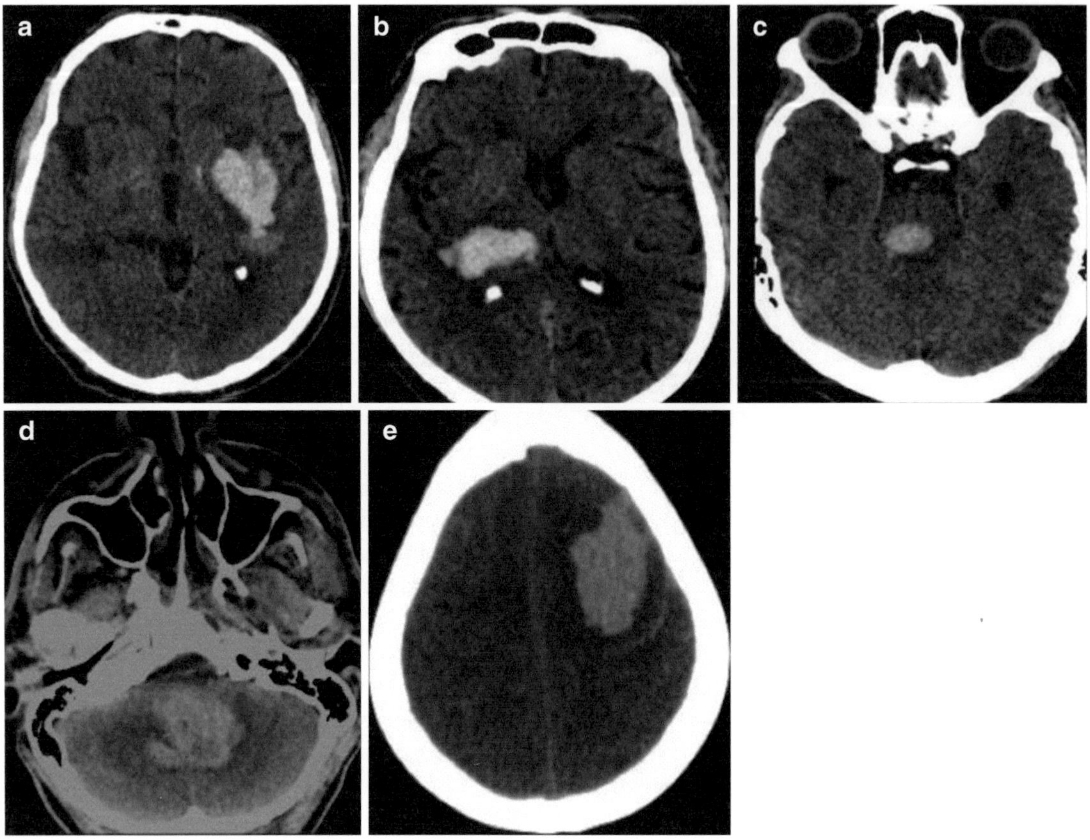

Fig. 7.1 Acute hypertensive hemorrhage. Axial noncontrast CT images demonstrate common presentations of acute hypertensive hemorrhage in five different patients and sites. (**a**) Left lateral putamen/external capsule hematoma. (**b**) Right thalamic hematoma. (**c**) Pontine hematoma. (**d**) Cerebellar hemorrhage with extension into the fourth ventricle. (**e**) Lobar hematoma

starting at the periphery and progressing toward its center. This appearance has been called the "melting ice cube" (Fig. 7.2) [23]. The periphery of the lesion tends to take on an uneven profile and acquires a pseudo-abscess (ringlike) appearance after contrast administration (Fig. 7.2). Reductions in edema and mass occur up until the ninth week when only a region of hypodensity remains [3].

CTA is able to identify patients at high risk of hemorrhage enlargement by revealing a spot sign (Fig. 7.3) which is a contrast medium extravasation within the hematoma. The spot sign is a strong predictor of hematoma expansion, poor prognosis, and mortality in primary [18, 19, 24, 25] and secondary IPH [21].

On MRI, the appearance of the IPH changes as the blood products evolve from oxyhemoglobin to ferritin and hemosiderin (Table 7.1). Patients with acquired or congenital coagulopathy may also display a fluid–fluid level within the IPH [1].

Hypertensive Hemorrhage

An IPH centrally located in the brain (in the basal ganglia, thalami, central cerebellum, and pons) seen in an adult patient is probably caused by a vascular injury due to hypertension (Figs. 7.1, 7.2, and 7.3). Lobar hemorrhage may also occur with hypertension. On MRI, presence of microbleeds on SWI or T2* images (appearing

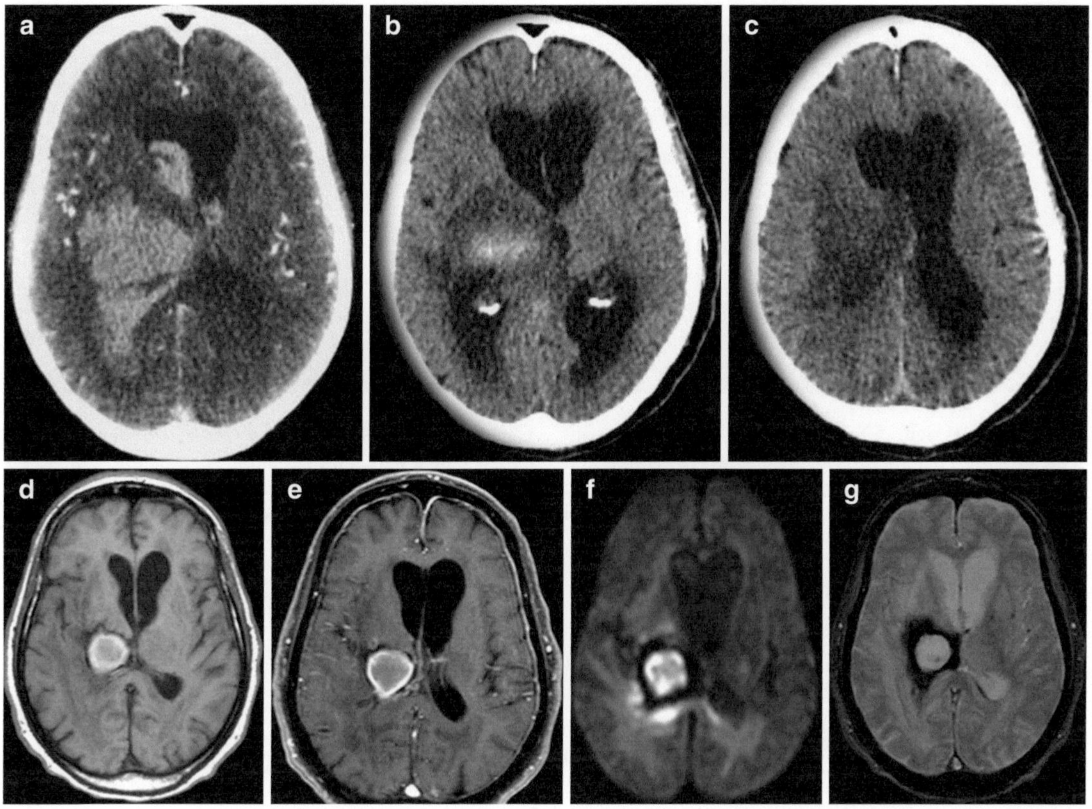

Fig. 7.2 Evaluation of intraparenchymal hematoma. 42-year-old man presenting unconscious to the emergency room. (**a**) Axial postcontrast CT image reveals a large hemorrhage involving the deep gray matter structures on the right with intraventricular extension. There is no sign of abnormal enhancement within the lesion or contrast extravasation. (**b**) Axial non-contrast CT image performed 1 week later demonstrates signs of hydrocephalus and a decrease of the attenuation within the hemorrhage ("melting ice cube" appearance due to clot retraction). (**c**) Axial non-contrast CT image performed 2 weeks after demonstrates persistent hydrocephalus and a hypoattenuating lesion. MRI was performed 1 day after the last CT confirming hydrocephalus and demonstrating the typical "pseudo-abscess" appearance of a late hematoma characterized by a hyperintense lesion in the right thalamus on axial T1WI (**d**), with peripheral enhancement on postcontrast T1WI (**e**) and hyperintensity on diffusion-weighted imaging (**f**). GRE T2* depicts the typical hypointense rim surrounding the hyperintense core of the lesion, compatible with a hematoma in reabsorption stages (**g**). The completely surrounding hypointense rim also suggests the absence of underlying lesions

as small dots with low signal intensity) in the brainstem and deep gray nuclei supports the diagnosis of hypertensive-related microhemorrhages (Fig. 7.4) [1–3, 9].

Cerebral Amyloid Angiopathy

CAA usually presents as lobar, cortical, or corticosubcortical IPH affecting normotensive individuals usually older than 55 years which may suffer multiple and recurrent hemorrhages often extending to the subarachnoid space. Their diagnosis is greatly facilitated by the presence of multiple microbleeds identified on SWI or T2*-weighted MRI typically located in the periphery of the cerebellum and of the cerebral hemispheres (Figs. 7.5 and 7.6) [26].

An unusual presentation of CAA is cerebral amyloid inflammatory vasculopathy which shows focal regions of vasogenic edema with fingerlike hyperintensities on T2WI and FLAIR. Usually,

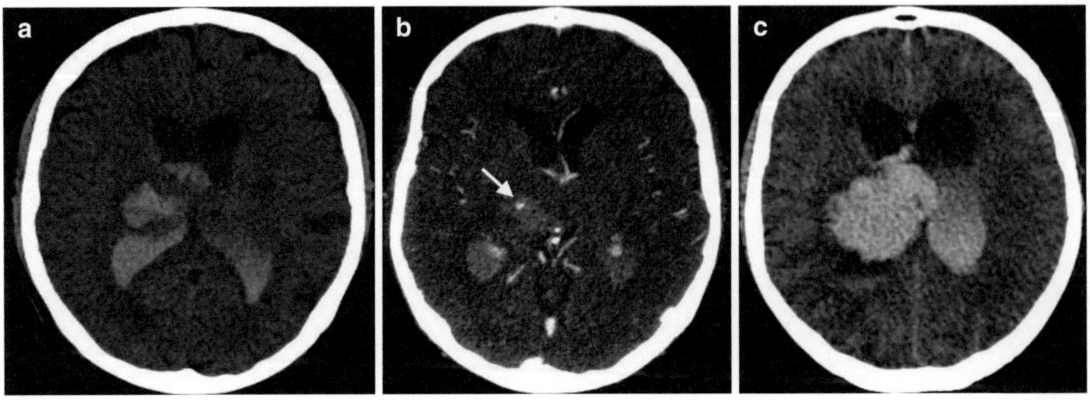

Fig. 7.3 Spot sign. 52-year-old man presenting with acute onset left hemiparesis and headache. (**a**) Axial non-contrast CT image shows a right heterogeneous thalamic hemorrhage extending to the lateral ventricles. (**b**) Axial CTA image shows a small dot (*white arrow*) of contrast enhancement within the hematoma compatible with a spot sign. (**c**) Follow-up non-contrast CT performed 24 h later demonstrates hemorrhage expansion

Table 7.1 Intensity of signal on MRI of hemorrhage

Stage	Time	Hemoglobin	T1WI	T2WI
Hyperacute	<6 h	Oxyhemoglobin	iso/↓	↑
Acute	6–72 h	Deoxyhemoglobin	iso/↓	↓
Early subacute	3–10 days	Methemoglobin intracellular	↑	↓
Late subacute	1 week to months	Methemoglobin extracellular	↑	↑
Chronic[a]	Months to years	Hemosiderin and ferritin	↓	↓

[a]May be differentiated from the acute stage by imaging as initially hemorrhage is surrounded by vasogenic edema that is not expected in late stages

changes are confined to the subcortical white matter, but involvement of the cortex may be present and predisposes to seizures. Faint leptomeningeal enhancement may also be seen. White matter changes commonly surround the microhemorrhages [27, 28].

Secondary Hemorrhage

Patient's clinical profile and CT findings may raise suspicion for secondary causes of IPH. Imaging evidence suggestive of vascular abnormalities as causative factors for IPH includes presence of subarachnoid hemorrhage, enlarged blood vessels or calcifications (Fig. 7.7), hyperattenuation within a dural venous sinus or cortical veins, unusual hematoma shape, presence of edema out of proportion to the time/size of the IPH, unusual location, and presence of abnormal contrast-enhancing structures [8]. A secondary IPH score was proposed in an attempt to stratify the risk of a hemorrhage as secondary and especially a possible vascular cause (Tables 7.2 and 7.3). The score ranges from 0 to 6. Lower scores (0 and 1) are usually related to hypertensive hemorrhages, while higher scores (5 and 6) are commonly related to secondary lesions. Female patients, younger than 46 years, without history of arterial hypertension or impaired coagulation receive the highest score. Patients with intermediate scores (1–5) should have other diagnostic studies such as MRI or catheter angiography [9].

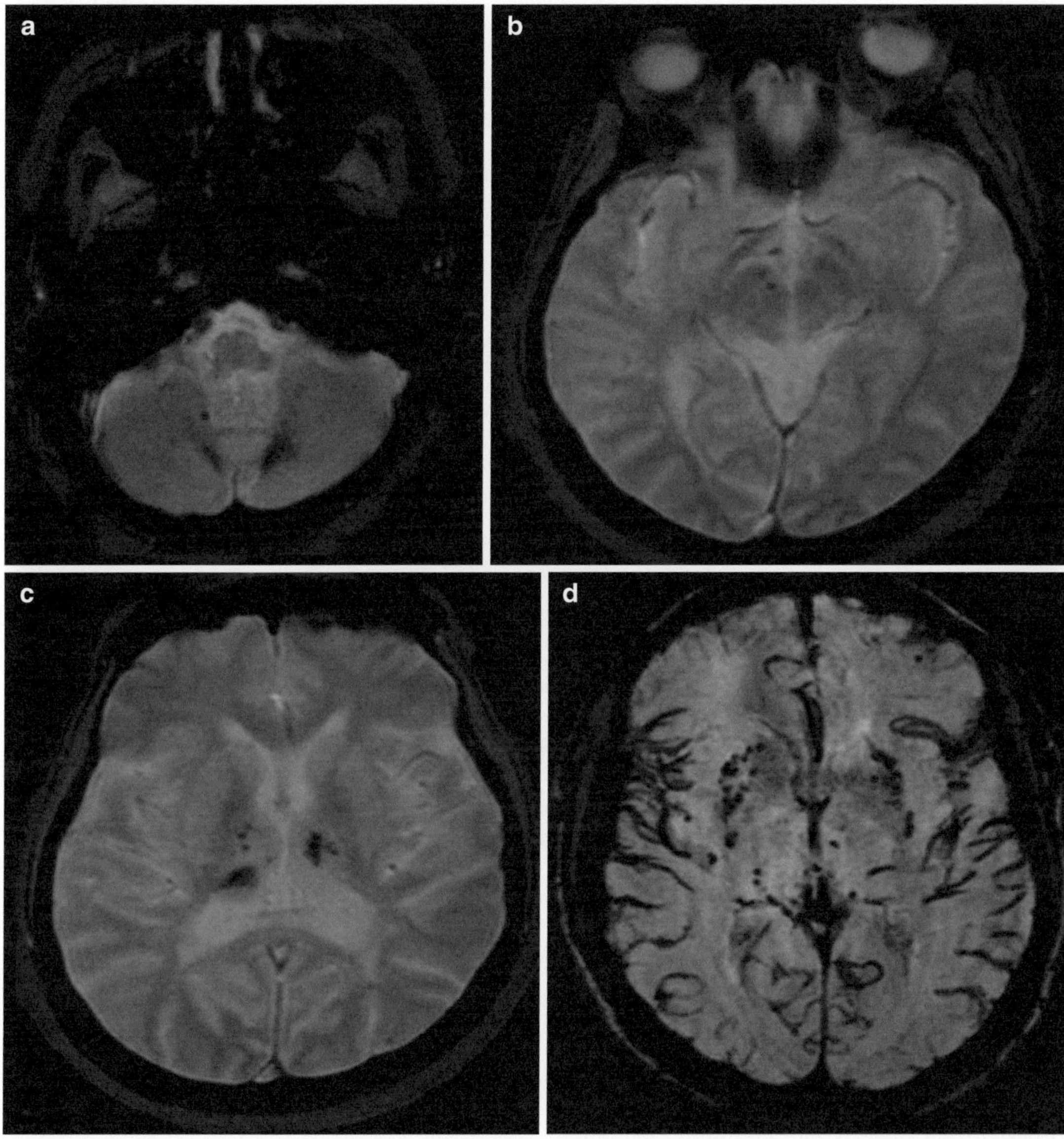

Fig. 7.4 Hypertensive hemorrhages. 68-year-old man with mild cognitive decline. Axial GRE T2* images through the posterior fossa show multiple dark spots in the medial cerebellum (**a**), midbrain (**b**), and thalami (**c**), compatible with multifocal microhemorrhages related to chronic hypertension. (**d**) Axial SWI filtered-phase images from a different patient with systemic arterial hypertension show multiple *dark spots* throughout the central areas of the brain, compatible with hypertensive microbleeds

Imaging Follow-Up

Children, patients with secondary IPH score higher than 1, presence of subarachnoid hemorrhage, atypical shaped hematomas, edema out of proportion at admission, unusual location, and/or presence of masses are all distinctive features of secondary ICH. In these patients, MRI is necessary to better characterize the hematoma. If a vascular malformation is diagnosed or MRI is

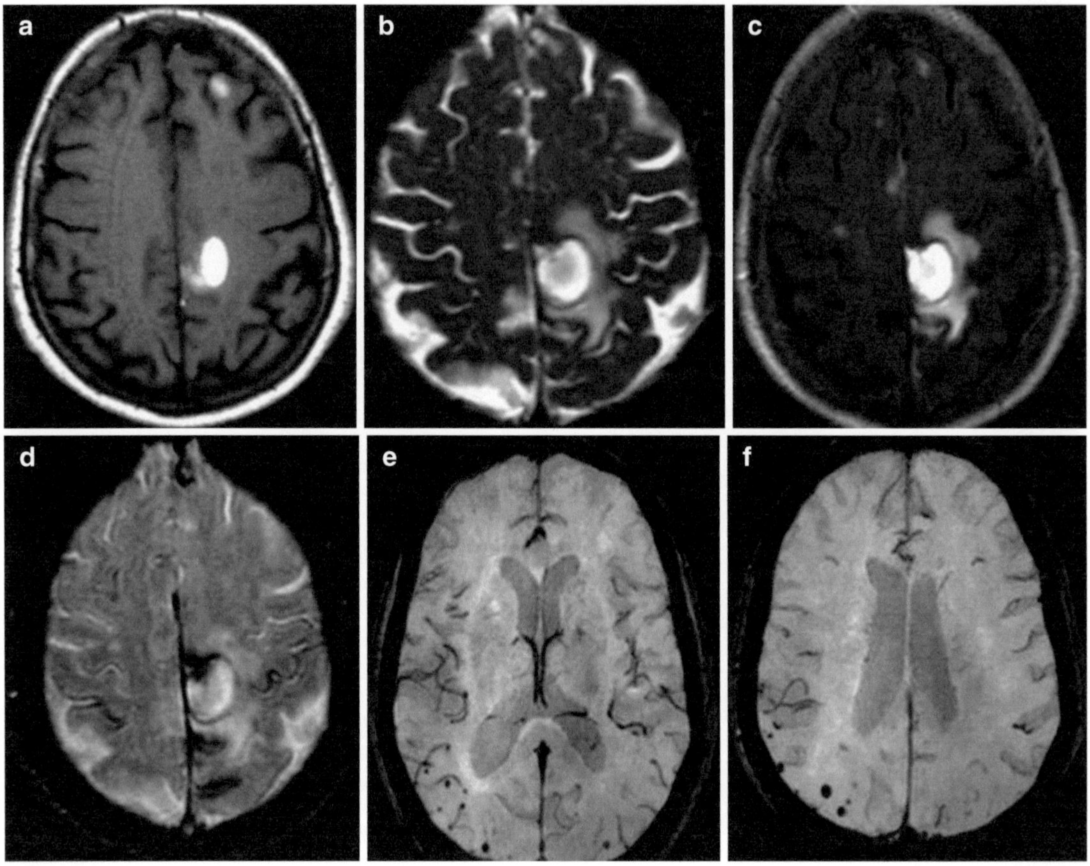

Fig. 7.5 Cerebral amyloid angiopathy. 72-year-old man presenting with right-side paresis and seizures. Axial T1WI (**a**), T2WI (**b**), FLAIR (**c**), and GRE T2* (**d**) images show a left posterior parasagittal late subacute lobar hematoma containing extracellular methemoglobin. There are also signs of superficial siderosis within the adjacent sulci seen on (**d**). Axial SWI filtered images (**e** and **f**) demonstrate dark spots located posteriorly in the periphery of the cerebral hemispheres compatible with multifocal microbleeds related to cerebral amyloid angiopathy. A smaller intra-axial hematoma is seen in the left frontal lobe

not diagnostic, a catheter angiogram is necessary to best reveal underlying conditions, including arteriovenous malformations, moyamoya disease, tumors, vasculitis, reversible cerebral vasoconstriction syndrome, and cerebral venous thrombosis. Angiography is also indicated in patients with no obvious cause of bleeding. Follow-up angiography should be considered for patients with a negative first angiogram, and if negative again, a later follow-up angiography or a MR angiogram is recommended after the complete resolution of the IPH (4–6 weeks) [3].

Main Differential Diagnosis

Diffuse axonal injury: It refers to severe parenchymal trauma usually seen in closed head injuries and it is a difficult diagnosis to make on CT, resulting in severe neurological impairment. MRI is the best imaging approach and characterizes regions of restricted diffusion and/or susceptibility artifacts at the gray–white matter junctions, the corpus callosum and in severe cases in the brainstem. Typically, the microbleed distribution is different from that of hypertensive hemorrhages and CAA [29].

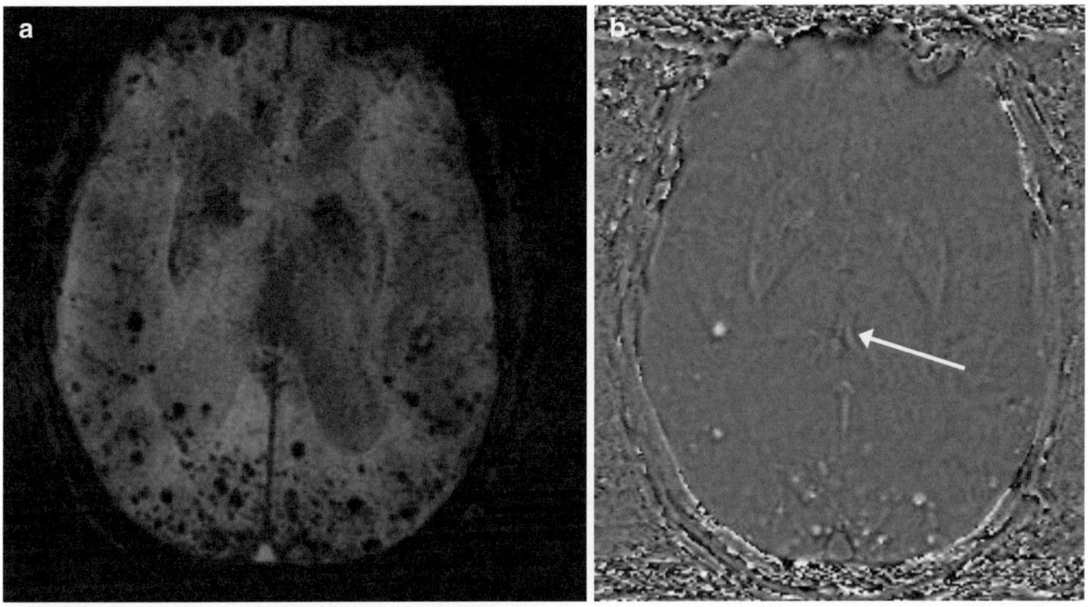

Fig. 7.6 Cerebral amyloid angiopathy. An 84-year-old man with mild cognitive decline. (**a**) SWI filtered-phase image shows subcortical *black spot* periphery located in the parietal/occipital regions. (**b**) SWI phase image demonstrates that the spots have similar signal to that of the deep venous structures (*white arrow*) indicating that they correspond to blood

Cavernoma: These malformations are composed of abnormal capillary-like vessels with intermingled connective tissue whose rupture may lead to IPH. Cavernomas have a typical hyperintense popcorn-like appearance on T2WI. Their central component is hyperintense and indicates recent bleeding, while their hypointense halos consist of hemosiderin and are the sequelae of remote bleeding [3].

Calcifications: Distinguishing between calcification and blood products is not possible on post-processed SWI images as both demonstrate signal dropout and blooming. However, filtered phase images are able to distinguish between them as diamagnetic (deoxyhemoglobin, ferritin, and hemosiderin) and paramagnetic (bone minerals and dystrophic calcifications) compounds affect phase differently appearing of opposite signal intensity. Grayscale inversion-filtered phase images are not uniformly windowed or presented equally by all manufacturers; therefore, care must be taken to ensure correct interpretation. A simple step to make sure that you always view the images in the same way is to look at venous structures and compare them with the lesions. The lesions containing blood have the same signal as veins (Fig. 7.6) [30].

Venous thrombosis: MR venography or CT venography should be performed if hemorrhage location, relative edema volume, or abnormal signal/density in the cerebral sinuses to suggest cerebral sinus/vein thrombosis. Nontraumatic IPH located in the parieto-occipital region or in a parasagittal location close to the venous sinuses, vein of Labbé or vein of Trolard, may be the result from thrombosis [8].

Ischemic injury with secondary hemorrhagic transformation: Most hemorrhagic transformations are smaller than their corresponding infarctions, and thus, MRI provides valuable information as a primary hematoma tends to be round in shape and have more surrounding edema

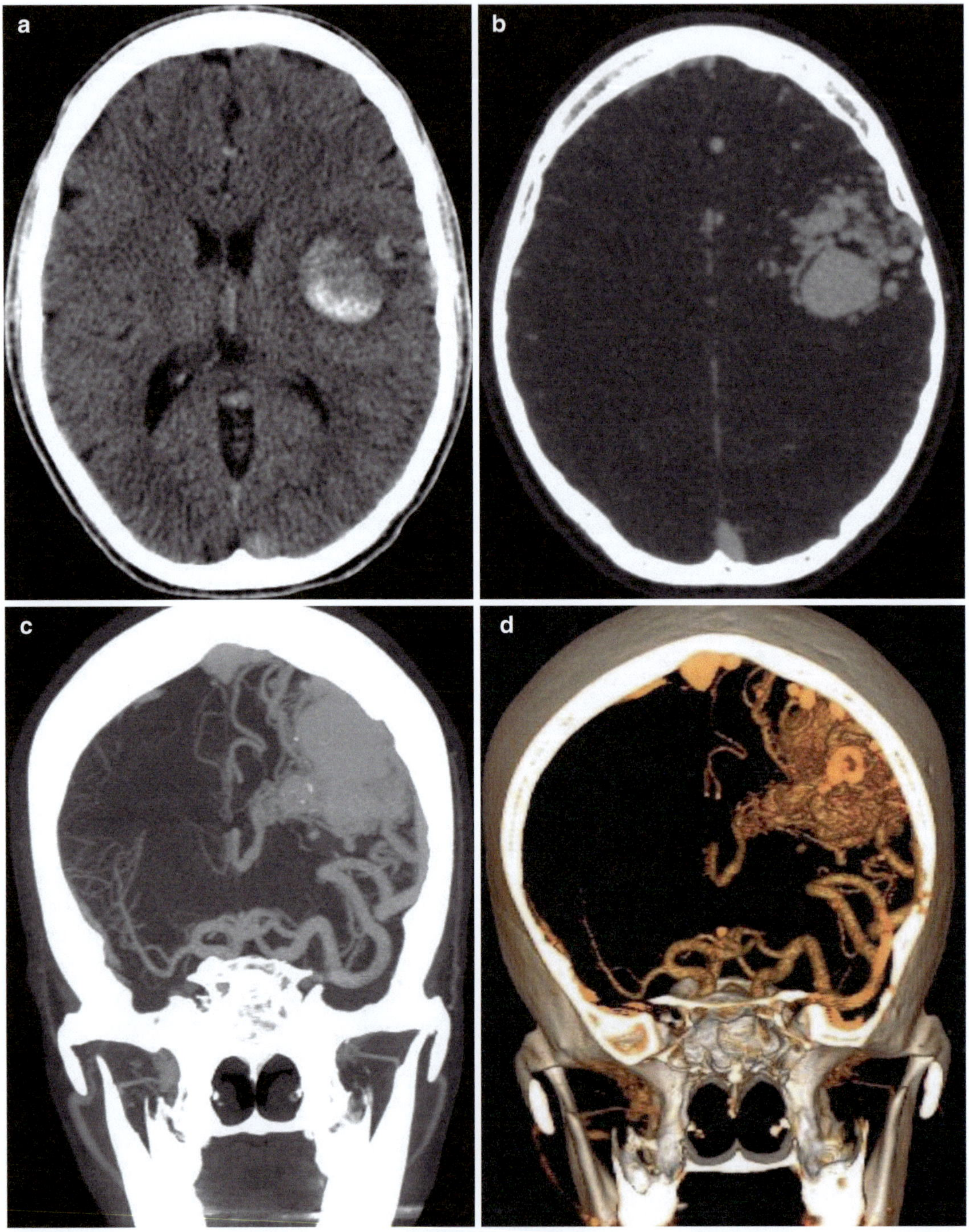

Fig. 7.7 Secondary cerebral hemorrhage due to AVM. An 16-year-old boy presenting with seizures and acute headache. (**a**) Axial non-contrast CT image shows a left frontal heterogeneous hematoma. Axial (**b**) and coronal (**c**) maximum intensity projection CTA images demonstrate prominent vascular structures within the hemorrhage. (**d**) Coronal volume rendering CT image shows a large-size AVM adjacent to the hemorrhage

Table 7.2 Calculation of the secondary IPH score

Parameter	Points
NCCT	
High probability[a]	2
Indeterminate[b]	1
Low probability[c]	0
Age group (years)	
18–45	2
46–70	1
≥71	0
Sex	
Female	1
Male	0
Neither known hypertension or impaired coagulation	
Yes	1
No	0

Adapted from Delgado-Almandoz et al. [9]

[a]High-probability NCCT was defined as enlarged vessels or calcifications along the margins of the IPH, or hyperdensity within a dural venous sinus or cortical vein

[b]Indeterminate NCCT was defined as a study that did not meet the criteria for a high- or low-probability NCCT, usually a lobar or cerebellar IPH

[c]Low-probability NCCT was defined as IPH located at the typical sites of hypertensive hemorrhage (basal ganglia, thalamus, or brainstem) not displaying any of the findings of a high-probability NCCT

Table 7.3 Secondary IPH score

Score	% vascular cause of IPH
0	0 %
1	1.4 %
2	5.1 %
3	18.5 %
4	39 %
5	84.2 %
6	100 %

than a secondary hemorrhagic transformation of an infarction. Idiopathic hematomas do not necessarily respect vascular territories [3].

Neoplasia: Presence of an IPH that does not follow the organized evolution of a hematoma and/or shows contrast should raise the possibility of underlying tumor. Hematocrit fluid–fluid levels are also associated with tumors (especially metastases) and coagulation disorders [3].

Aneurysmal IPH: Nontraumatic IPH located at the base of the frontal lobes and in temporal lobes poles close to the circle of Willis associated with subarachnoid hemorrhage should raise the possibility of aneurysm rupture [3].

Tips

- Report the location of the IPH, volume, shape (regular vs. irregular), and the attenuation of the hematoma (homogeneous vs. heterogeneous).
- Look for signs of secondary IPH on noncontract CT as follows: presence of subarachnoid hemorrhage, atypical (noncircular) hematoma configuration, edema out of proportion, unusual hemorrhage location, enlarged vessels or calcifications in the IPH, or hyperdensity within a dural venous sinus or cortical vein.
- A spot or swirl sign within the hemorrhage as seen on CTA means extravasation or presence of associated aneurysms and arteriovenous malformations.
- Hypertensive hemorrhages are centrally located in the brain in the basal ganglia, thalami, central portions of the cerebellum, and pons. Conversely, CAA is usually peripherally located.
- Distinguishing between calcification and blood products is not possible on post-processed SWI images. On filtered-phase SWI, the hemorrhage has the same signal intensity as the veins.

References

1. Fischbein NJ, Wijman CA. Nontraumatic intracranial hemorrhage. Neuroimaging Clin N Am. 2010;20(4):469–92. doi:10.1016/j.nic.2010.07.003.
2. Steiner T, Petersson J, Al-Shahi Salman R, Christensen H, Cordonnier C, Csiba L, Harnof S, Krieger D, Mendelow D, Molina C, Montaner J, Overgaard K,

Roine RO, Schmutzhard E, Tatlisumak T, Toni D, Stapf C, European Research Network on Intracerebral H. European research priorities for intracerebral haemorrhage. Cerebrovasc Dis. 2011;32(5):409–19. doi:10.1159/000330653.

3. Macellari F, Paciaroni M, Agnelli G, Caso V. Neuroimaging in intracerebral hemorrhage. Stroke. 2014;45(3):903–8. doi:10.1161/STROKEAHA.113.003701.
4. Qureshi AI, Tuhrim S, Broderick JP, Batjer HH, Hondo H, Hanley DF. Spontaneous intracerebral hemorrhage. N Engl J Med. 2001;344(19):1450–60. doi:10.1056/NEJM200105103441907.
5. Kidwell CS, Wintermark M. Imaging of intracranial haemorrhage. Lancet Neurol. 2008;7(3):256–67. doi:10.1016/S1474-4422(08)70041-3.
6. Roach ES, Golomb MR, Adams R, Biller J, Daniels S, Deveber G, Ferriero D, Jones BV, Kirkham FJ, Scott RM, Smith ER, American Heart Association Stroke C, Council on Cardiovascular Disease in the Y. Management of stroke in infants and children: a scientific statement from a Special Writing Group of the American Heart Association Stroke Council and the Council on Cardiovascular Disease in the Young. Stroke. 2008;39((9):2644–91. doi:10.1161/STROKEAHA.108.189696.
7. Pontes-Neto OM, Oliveira-Filho J, Valiente R, Friedrich M, Pedreira B, Rodrigues BC, Liberato B, Freitas GR, Comite Executivo da Sociedade Brasileira de Doencas C, Departamento Cientifico de Doencas Cerebrovasculares ABdN. Brazilian guidelines for the management of intracerebral hemorrhage. Arq Neuropsiquiatr. 2009;67(3B):940–50.
8. 3rd Hemphill JC, Greenberg SM, Anderson CS, Becker K, Bendok BR, Cushman M, Fung GL, Goldstein JN, Macdonald RL, Mitchell PH, Scott PA, Selim MH, Woo D, American Heart Association Stroke C, Council on C, Stroke N, Council on Clinical C. Guidelines for the management of spontaneous intracerebral hemorrhage: a guideline for healthcare professionals from the American Heart Association/American Stroke Association. Stroke. 2015;46(7):2032–60. doi:10.1161/STR.0000000000000069.
9. Delgado Almandoz JE, Romero JM. Advanced CT imaging in the evaluation of hemorrhagic stroke. Neuroimaging Clin N Am. 2011;21(2):197–213. doi:10.1016/j.nic.2011.01.001. ix.
10. Mayer SA, Brun NC, Begtrup K, Broderick J, Davis S, Diringer MN, Skolnick BE, Steiner T, Investigators FT. Efficacy and safety of recombinant activated factor VII for acute intracerebral hemorrhage. N Engl J Med. 2008;358(20):2127–37. doi:10.1056/NEJMoa0707534.
11. Anderson CS, Huang Y, Wang JG, Arima H, Neal B, Peng B, Heeley E, Skulina C, Parsons MW, Kim JS, Tao QL, Li YC, Jiang JD, Tai LW, Zhang JL, Xu E, Cheng Y, Heritier S, Morgenstern LB, Chalmers J, Investigators I. Intensive blood pressure reduction in acute cerebral haemorrhage trial (INTERACT): a randomised pilot trial. Lancet Neurol. 2008;7(5):391–9. doi:10.1016/S1474-4422(08)70069-3.
12. Dennis MS, Burn JP, Sandercock PA, Bamford JM, Wade DT, Warlow CP. Long-term survival after first-ever stroke: the Oxfordshire Community Stroke Project. Stroke. 1993;24(6):796–800.
13. Broderick JP, Brott TG, Duldner JE, Tomsick T, Huster G. Volume of intracerebral hemorrhage. A powerful and easy-to-use predictor of 30-day mortality. Stroke. 1993;24(7):987–93.
14. Zimmerman RD, Maldjian JA, Brun NC, Horvath B, Skolnick BE. Radiologic estimation of hematoma volume in intracerebral hemorrhage trial by CT scan. AJNR Am J Neuroradiol. 2006;27(3):666–70.
15. Kothari RU, Brott T, Broderick JP, Barsan WG, Sauerbeck LR, Zuccarello M, Khoury J. The ABCs of measuring intracerebral hemorrhage volumes. Stroke. 1996;27(8):1304–5.
16. Divani AA, Majidi S, Luo X, Souslian FG, Zhang J, Abosch A, Tummala RP. The ABCs of accurate volumetric measurement of cerebral hematoma. Stroke. 2011;42(6):1569–74. doi:10.1161/STROKEAHA.110.607861.
17. Kosior JC, Idris S, Dowlatshahi D, Alzawahmah M, Eesa M, Sharma P, Tymchuk S, Hill MD, Aviv RI, Frayne R, Demchuk AM, investigators PRSCIs. Quantomo: validation of a computer-assisted methodology for the volumetric analysis of intracerebral haemorrhage. Int J Stroke. 2011;6(4):302–5. doi:10.1111/j.1747-4949.2010.00579.x.
18. Rosa Junior M, Rocha AJ, Saade N, Maia Junior AC, Gagliardi RJ. Active extravasation of contrast within the hemorrhage (spot sign): a multidetector computed tomography finding that predicts growth and a worse prognosis in non-traumatic intracerebral hemorrhage. Arq Neuropsiquiatr. 2013;71(10):791–7. doi:10.1590/0004-282X20130124.
19. Murai Y, Ikeda Y, Teramoto A, Goldstein JN, Greenberg SM, Smith EE, Lev MH, Rosand J. Contrast extravasation on CT angiography predicts hematoma expansion in intracerebral hemorrhage. Neurology. 2007;69(6):617. doi:10.1212/01.wnl.0000278894.44311.0b. author reply 617.
20. Wada R, Aviv RI, Fox AJ, Sahlas DJ, Gladstone DJ, Tomlinson G, Symons SP. CT angiography "spot sign" predicts hematoma expansion in acute intracerebral hemorrhage. Stroke. 2007;38(4):1257–62. doi:10.1161/01.STR.0000259633.59404.f3.
21. Delgado Almandoz JE, Kelly HR, Schaefer PW, Brouwers HB, Yoo AJ, Stone MJ, Goldstein JN, Rosand J, Lev MH, Gonzalez RG, Romero JM. CT angiography spot sign predicts in-hospital mortality in patients with secondary intracerebral hemorrhage. J NeuroInterventional Surg. 2012;4(6):442–7. doi:10.1136/neurintsurg-2011-010061.
22. Du FZ, Jiang R, Gu M, He C, Guan J. The accuracy of spot sign in predicting hematoma expansion after

intracerebral hemorrhage: a systematic review and meta-analysis. PLoS One. 2014;9(12), e115777. doi:10.1371/journal.pone.0115777.
23. Zimmerman RD, Jou AD. Intracranial hemorrhage. In: Naidich TP, Castillo M, Cha S, Smirniotopoulos JG, editors. Imaging of the brain, vol. 1. Philadelphia: Saunders; 2012. p. 387–98.
24. Demchuk AM, Dowlatshahi D, Rodriguez-Luna D, Molina CA, Blas YS, Dzialowski I, Kobayashi A, Boulanger JM, Lum C, Gubitz G, Padma V, Roy J, Kase CS, Kosior J, Bhatia R, Tymchuk S, Subramaniam S, Gladstone DJ, Hill MD, Aviv RI, Group PRSICs. Prediction of haematoma growth and outcome in patients with intracerebral haemorrhage using the CT-angiography spot sign (PREDICT): a prospective observational study. Lancet Neurol. 2012;11(4):307–14. doi:10.1016/S1474-4422(12)70038-8.
25. Becker KJ, Baxter AB, Bybee HM, Tirschwell DL, Abouelsaad T, Cohen WA. Extravasation of radiographic contrast is an independent predictor of death in primary intracerebral hemorrhage. Stroke. 1999;30(10):2025–32.
26. Knudsen KA, Rosand J, Karluk D, Greenberg SM. Clinical diagnosis of cerebral amyloid angiopathy: validation of the Boston criteria. Neurology. 2001;56(4):537–9.
27. Caulo M, Tampieri D, Brassard R, Christine Guiot M, Melanson D. Cerebral amyloid angiopathy presenting as nonhemorrhagic diffuse encephalopathy: neuropathologic and neuroradiologic manifestations in one case. AJNR Am J Neuroradiol. 2001;22(6):1072–6.
28. Barakos J, Sperling R, Salloway S, Jack C, Gass A, Fiebach JB, Tampieri D, Melancon D, Miaux Y, Rippon G, Black R, Lu Y, Brashear HR, Arrighi HM, Morris KA, Grundman M. MR imaging features of amyloid-related imaging abnormalities. AJNR Am J Neuroradiol. 2013;34(10):1958–65. doi:10.3174/ajnr.A3500.
29. Davis PC, Expert Panel on Neurologic I. Head trauma. AJNR Am J Neuroradiol. 2007;28(8):1619–21.
30. Haacke EM, Mittal S, Wu Z, Neelavalli J, Cheng YC. Susceptibility-weighted imaging: technical aspects and clinical applications, part 1. AJNR Am J Neuroradiol. 2009;30(1):19–30. doi:10.3174/ajnr.A1400.

Remote Cerebellar Hemorrhages

8

Ana Lorena Abello and Florencia Álamos

Abstract

Remote cerebellar hemorrhage is a rare complication of a variety of neurosurgical procedures, mainly supratentorial craniotomies, which occur frequently distant to the site of surgery. The precise mechanisms by which remote cerebellar hemorrhage occurs are unknown; however, two facts are known: it is of venous origin and is the result of intra- and postoperative loss of cerebrospinal fluid. Non-enhanced CT is the modality of choice and shows superficial linear hyperdense bleeds in the superior surface of the cerebellar hemispheres. Although MRI is more sensitive than CT in detection of small hemorrhages, this does not affect treatment, and therefore, MRI is not the first modality of choice to image patients in which this condition is suspected.

Background

Remote cerebellar hemorrhage (RCH) is a rare complication of a variety of neurosurgical procedures, mainly supratentorial craniotomies, which occur distant to the site of surgery [1, 2].

RCH is more common between the ages of 30 and 60 years [1]. Common presenting symptoms of RCH are prolonged awakening from anesthesia, decreased level of consciousness, motor deficits, and gait ataxia [3]. However, RCH is frequently asymptomatic; consequently, it is probably under-recognized and underreported [4]. Authors report RCH after 0.6 % of all supratentorial craniotomies, 3.5 % after surgical repair of ruptured anterior communicating artery aneurysms, and 5 % after temporal lobectomies [5, 6]. It can also be a rare complication of spinal surgery [2].

Treatment is generally conservative or may be surgical (external ventricular drainage, hematoma evacuation, and suboccipital decompression). Treatment depends on the patient's

A.L. Abello, MD (✉)
Department of Radiology, University of North Carolina, Chapel Hill, NC, USA
e-mail: anaabellop@hotmail.com

F. Álamos, MD, PhD
Department of Neuroscience, School of Medicine, Universidad Católica de Chile, Luz larrain, 3946 Lo Barnechea, Santiago, Chile
e-mail: flopi1987@yahoo.com

R. Hoffmann Nunes et al. (eds.), *Critical Findings in Neuroradiology*,
DOI 10.1007/978-3-319-27987-9_8

condition and the degree of mass effect by the hematoma [4, 7].

Key Points

Etiology

The precise mechanisms by which cerebellar hemorrhage occurs are unknown; however, male sex, perioperative hypertension, and preoperative usage of anticoagulation are risk factors [1]. However, no specific etiological factors have been identified although most authors agree on two facts regarding RCH [4, 7].

- RCH is of venous origin.
- RCH is a result of intra- and even more likely postoperative loss of cerebrospinal fluid (CSF).

But despite the agreement that loss of CSF is an underlying reason for RCH, no consensus regarding the exact mechanisms has been reached. Some authors have suggested that it may be due to mechanical forces (shearing of cerebellar bridging veins) or hemodynamic causes (increase in venous blood pressure) [1, 2, 4]. Friedman et al. proposed that opening of cisterns and of the ventricular system causes CSF hypovolemia resulting in cerebellar sagging. This causes transient occlusion of the superior bridging veins in the posterior fossa leading to subsequent hemorrhagic infarction [5].

Best Imaging Modality

Non-enhanced computed tomography (CT). It is the modality of choice and shows superficial linear hyperdense areas related to hemorrhage in the cerebellum. These bleeds follow the configuration of the folia and fissures and have often been called "zebra stripes."

Other Imaging Techniques

Magnetic resonance imaging (MRI). Since MRI is more sensitive than CT in the evaluation of the posterior fossa, it can show smaller hemorrhages [8]. Because small amounts of blood and their localizations do not affect treatment, MRI is not the first modality of choice to image patients suspected of having RCH. When it is performed, findings vary with the age of the hematoma. Gradient-recalled echo (GRE) and susceptibility-weighted image (SWI) demonstrate "blooming effect" and make identification of hemorrhages easier [4].

Conventional catheter digital angiography is usually normal [4].

Major Findings

RCH is commonly bilateral (53.5 %) or unilateral (46.5 %). In CT, the classic associated bleeding pattern includes superficial blood extension into the subarachnoid space of the cerebellar fissures/folia and vermis, producing alternating hyperdense (blood) and hypodense (cerebellum) curvilinear slightly irregular stripes that are similar to a zebra's coat and gave the "*zebra sign*" its name (Figs. 8.1 and 8.2). Hemorrhages that are somewhat irregular rather than purely curvilinear should raise the question of whether there could be a deeper intraparenchymal component. Additionally, *intracerebellar hemorrhage*, mainly in the upper parts of the cerebellum, may be observed [2, 8, 9]. The "zebra sign" can also be seen on MRI (Fig. 8.3).

It is important to establish the amount of blood as the bleed may be large enough to cause mass effect, leading to cerebellar herniation and obstructive hydrocephalus [1].

Imaging Follow-Up

Small bleeds with little or no mass effect seem to be self-limiting and do not require further workup in the face of clinical stability. If follow-up is indicated, CT is helpful in assessing the evolution of the bleeds [1, 4].

Main Differential Diagnosis

It is important to recognize this type of hemorrhage in a postsurgical state as an apparently sequela of surgery rather than as a result of

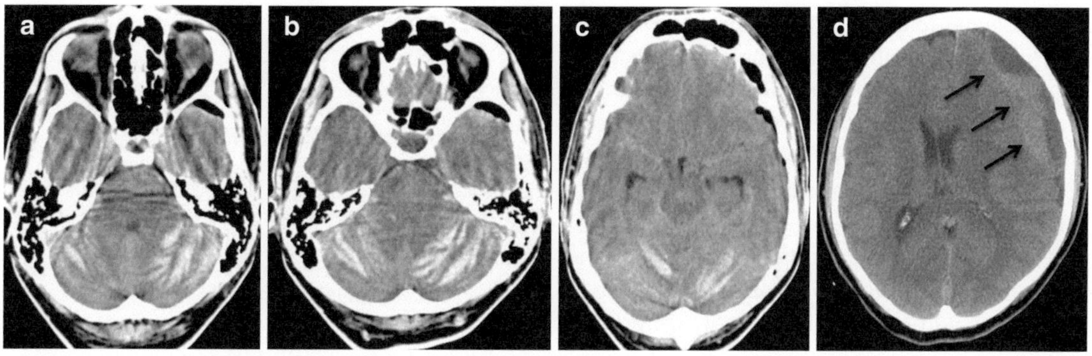

Fig. 8.1 Remote cerebellar hemorrhage post-craniotomy. (**a–c**) Non-enhanced CT depicts blood with curvilinear stripe appearance called "zebra sign" in the cerebellum. The patient developed this complication after surgical treatment of subdural hematoma (*black arrows* in **d**) (Courtesy of Sonia Bermudez MD, Bogotá – Colombia)

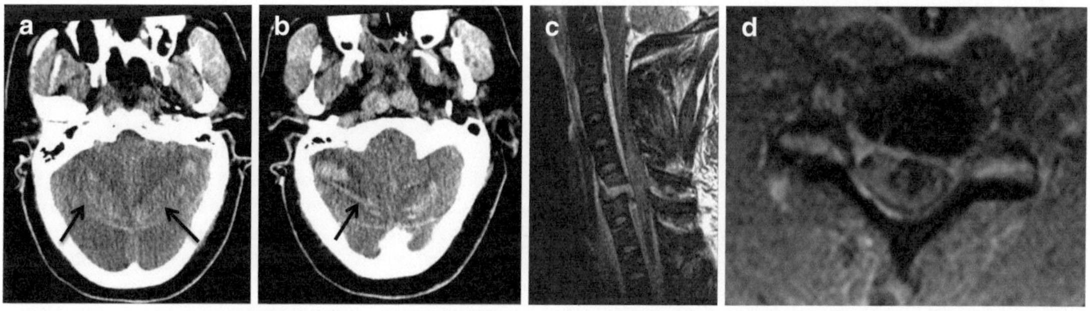

Fig. 8.2 Remote cerebral hemorrhage in a patient with recent spinal surgery. (**a**, **b**) Non-enhanced CT in two different levels shows blood in the posterior fossa with curvilinear and irregular hyperdense stripes, compatible with the "zebra sign" (*arrows*). (**c**, **d**) Sagittal and axial T2WI show C6–C7 dislocation with spinal cord injury and a hemorrhagic pattern. After surgery for stabilization, the patient developed RCH

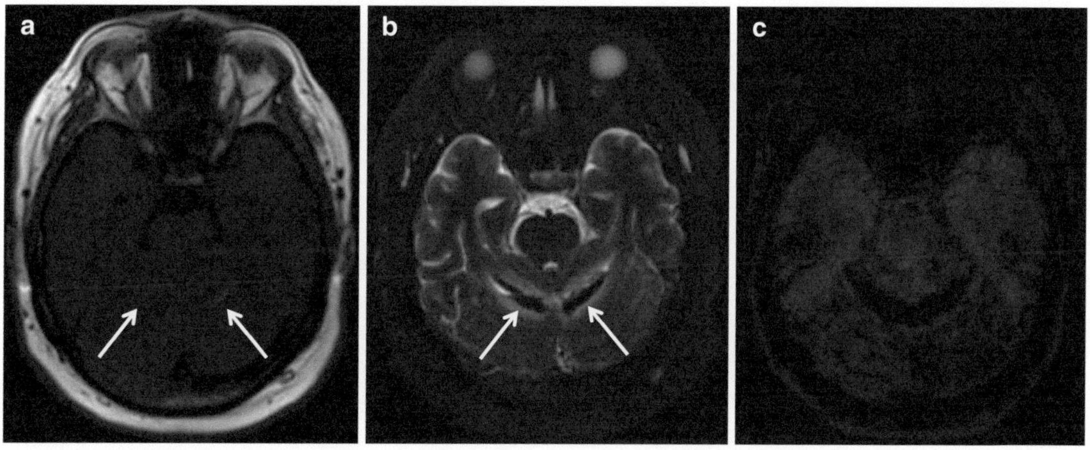

Fig. 8.3 "Zebra sign" in MRI. Patient with RCH after supratentorial craniectomy. (**a**) Axial TIWI and (**b**) axial T2WI show subacute hemorrhage with stripe appearance in the cerebellum (*arrows*). (**c**) SWI showing "blooming" effect and hemorrhages better seen

arterial hypertension, previously unrecognized vascular malformation, neoplasm, or subarachnoid bleeding from a ruptured aneurysm [8]. However, ruptured vascular malformations in the cerebellum may result in hemorrhages of similar appearance but such patients have no history of prior surgery.

Other postsurgical complications, such as *sinus venous thrombosis* leading to venous infarcts, should be considered in the differential diagnosis.

Tips

- Patients with unexplained and severe headaches, acute confusion, lethargy, and ataxic symptoms postoperatively should immediately undergo head CT.
- "Zebra sign" is the classical appearance of RCH in a patient with worsening neurological status after surgery.
- Establishing the size of the bleeds and degree of hydrocephalus has important prognostic value.
- Immediately report mass effect and possible cerebral herniation to allow for rapid intervention.

References

1. Amini A, Osborn AG, McCall TD, Couldwell WT. Remote cerebellar hemorrhage. AJNR Am J Neuroradiol. 2006;27(2):387–90.
2. Brockmann MA, Groden C. Remote cerebellar hemorrhage: a review. Cerebellum. 2006;5(1):64–8.
3. Brockmann MA, Nowak G, Reusche E, Russlies M, Petersen D. Zebra sign: cerebellar bleeding pattern characteristic of cerebrospinal fluid loss. Case report. J Neurosurg. 2005;102(6):1159–62.
4. Lehmann PS. Guillaume. Remote cerebellar haemorrhage. Eur J Radiol Ext. 2011;77(2):29–33.
5. Friedman JA, Piepgras DG, Duke DA, McClelland RL, Bechtle PS, Maher CO, et al. Zebra sign: cerebellar bleeding pattern characteristic of cerebrospinal fluid loss. Case report cerebellar hemorrhage after supratentorial surgery. Neurosurgery. 2001;49(6):1327–40.
6. Heros RC, Nelson PB. Intracerebral hemorrhage after microsurgical cerebral revascularization. Neurosurgery. 1980;6(4):371–5.
7. Honegger J, Zentner J, Spreer J, Carmona H, Schulze-Bonhage A. Cerebellar hemorrhage arising postoperatively as a complication of supratentorial surgery: a retrospective study. J Neurosurg. 2002;96(2):248–54.
8. Cloft HJ, Matsumoto JA, Lanzino G, Cail WS. Posterior fossa hemorrhage after supratentorial surgery. AJNR Am J Neuroradiol. 1997;18(8):1573–80.
9. Kaloostian PE, Kim JE, Bydon A, Sciubba DM, Wolinsky JP, Gokaslan ZL, et al. Intracranial hemorrhage after spine surgery. J Neurosurg Spine. 2013;19(3):370–80.

Brain Vascular Malformations

9

João Maia Jacinto and Isabel Ribeiro Fragata

Abstract

Brain vascular malformations (excluding dural arteriovenous fistulas) are mostly congenital lesions that are less common than cerebral aneurysms but also cause serious disabilities or death in a significant proportion of affected patients.

The group of lesions called "brain vascular malformations" is a heterogeneous one, clinically, histologically, and in terms of imaging. High-flow lesions such as arteriovenous malformations and slow-flow lesions such as cavernous malformations are included in this group.

Clinical manifestations range from headaches, seizures, to focal deficits due to intracranial hemorrhages. CT and CTA are commonly the first diagnostic modalities used in these patients, and MRI and MRA help in the diagnosis of smaller lesions and are helpful in surgical planning. Digital subtraction angiography is the gold standard for evaluation of arterial and venous malformations, allowing higher spatial and temporal resolution and also detailed evaluation before endovascular or surgical treatments.

Background

Brain vascular malformations are mostly congenital lesions that may pose imaging diagnostic challenges. They are less common than cerebral aneurysms and cause serious disabilities or death in a significant proportion of affected patients. Brain vascular malformations are divided based on anatomic features and also according to their hemodynamic characteristics (Table 9.1) [1–4].

Brain vascular malformations tend to be solitary (>95 % of patients) and sporadic, but when there are multiple, they may be a part of syndromic associations such as the Wyburn–Mason (cerebrofacial arteriovenous metameric syndrome) or Osler–Rendu–Weber (hereditary hemorrhagic telangiectasia) [5]. The most common vascular malformation is the developmental venous anomaly (DVA) representing up to 60 % of them followed by arteriovenous malformations (AVM) and cavernomas

J.M. Jacinto, MD (✉) • I.R. Fragata, MD
Department of Neuroradiology, Centro Hospitalar Lisboa Central, Rua José António Serrano, Lisboa 1150-199, Portugal
e-mail: jnmjacinto@gmail.com; isabelfragata@gmail.com

R. Hoffmann Nunes et al. (eds.), *Critical Findings in Neuroradiology*,
DOI 10.1007/978-3-319-27987-9_9

Table 9.1 Classification of brain vascular malformations

Classification based on the anatomic features	Classification based on hemodynamic characteristics
Arteriovenous malformation (AVM) Developmental venous anomaly (DVA) Cavernomas Capillary telangiectasias Mixed types (capillary venous)	*High flow* Parenchymal/pial AVM Dural arteriovenous fistula Mixed AVM *Low flow* Venous malformations Developmental venous anomaly Sinus pericranii Cavernomas Capillary telangiectasias Mixed vascular malformations (e.g., cavernoma with DVA) Previously and partially treated high-flow lesions

(cavernous malformations) which have an estimated incidence of 1.1 and 0.5 per 100,000 adults/year, respectively [6, 7].

The clinical manifestations can be as follows:

Asymptomatic: Some brain vascular malformations are incidentally discovered. Most DVAs, capillary telangiectasias, sinus pericranii, and cavernomas even with those with associated microhemorrhages tend to be asymptomatic [3, 5, 8].

Headaches: Headaches with parenchymal hemorrhage occur in about one-half of patients with AVMs and are rare with other brain vascular malformations [5].

Seizures and focal neurologic deficits: They occur in 50 % of patients with cavernomas and in 25 % of those with AVMs. Cortical-based cavernomas generally present with seizures.

Treatment options differ depending on the type of brain vascular malformations but consist mostly of conservative management. In high-flow or symptomatic lesions, surgery, endovascular embolization, and/or radiosurgery are employed. In AVMs, a randomized trial of unruptured brain arteriovenous malformations (the ARUBA trial) published in 2014 showed that medical management alone was superior to medical management with interventional therapy for the prevention of death or stroke in patients with unruptured brain AVMs followed up for 33 months [9].

Key Points

Etiology

AVM. Brain AVMs, or more specifically pial AVMs, are abnormal connections between arteries that normally supply the brain (i.e., pial vessels) and veins that normally drain it resulting in arteriovenous shunting with an intervening network of vessels within the brain parenchyma and lack of a true capillary bed. The transition between artery and vein can take place via a so-called nidus (a tangle of abnormal vessels located in the brain parenchyma) or can be direct (fistulous) without any intervening network of blood vessels. In the latter case, the term brain arteriovenous fistula or pial arteriovenous fistula is used. Although brain AVMs are congenital lesions, patients tend to present later in life, most commonly with intracranial hemorrhage or seizures [10]. Only 20 % are diagnosed before 20 years of age [11].

Cavernomas are vascular hamartomas, consisting of dilated sinusoidal vascular channels with no feeding arteries or draining veins and little or no flow.

Other brain vascular malformations. Capillary telangiectasias consist of enlarged capillaries embedded in normal brain tissue usually located in the pons. A *DVA* is not true vascular malformation; instead, it is a variation of venous development and drains normal brain tissue. They are sometimes associated with capillary telangiectasias, cavernomas, or even AVMs. About 10 % of DVAs are associated with gliosis, infarctions, and abnormal perfusion studies, and these are now thought to be somewhat atypical and not as benign as believed in the past. A *sinus pericranii* is an abnormal congenital venous communication between epicranial veins and intracranial dural sinuses. Usually, it has low flow and becomes symptomatic when the overlying skin is eroded and infected. It is generally found in children.

Best Imaging Modality

Non-contrast Computed Tomography (CT). CT is generally the first imaging study performed in patients with symptoms due to brain vascular malformations. Intracranial hemorrhage can be easily identified as well as its complications such as mass effect and herniations. In addition, abnormal enlarged vessels, parenchymal calcifications, and calvarial defects (in cases of sinus pericranii) may also be seen. Small uncomplicated brain vascular malformations are often invisible on CT particularly capillary telangiectasias and cavernomas.

CT Angiography (CTA). CTA is diagnostic for most AVMs. It allows for characterization of the AVM architecture but may be negative in the setting of acute rupture because of the mass effect of the hematoma collapsing the nidus or because the nidus is destroyed by the hemorrhage. Repeat CTA after 2–3 weeks after the hemorrhage is recommended [5]. Dynamic CTA has been developed in recent years as a technique that combines the noninvasive nature of CTA with the dynamic acquisition of digital subtraction angiography (DSA). The technique is also referred to as 4DCTA or time-resolved CTA and enables the noninvasive evaluation of flow dynamics of the intracranial vasculature by multiple subsequent CT acquisitions or a continuous volume CT acquisition for a progressive period of time. Studies show that intracranial vascular malformations can be adequately depicted and classified by 4DCTA [12].

CTA is generally negative for capillary telangiectasias and cavernomas (although larger cavernomas show stipple calcifications) [5].

Magnetic Resonance Imaging (MRI) and MR Angiography (MRA). MRI is the best noninvasive imaging option for lesion characterization and surrounding parenchymal evaluation. It can also help estimate the age of a hemorrhage. In addition, small undetectable brain vascular malformations by CT are generally seen on MRI (e.g., capillary telangiectasias and cavernomas). The utility of MRA is controversial as high-flow states result in artifacts and commonly incomplete lesion evaluation. Dynamic contrast-enhanced MRA (4D, also called time resolved) is emerging as a powerful resource for noninvasive hemodynamic characterization of AVMs, but its spatial resolution is limited [4, 13].

Digital Subtraction Angiography. DSA is the gold standard for evaluation of AVMs. It has higher spatial resolution, and most importantly, temporal resolution, allowing treatment selection. DSA does not show capillary telangiectasias and cavernomas, and thus these are commonly called "angiographically occult lesions" [3].

Major Findings

AVM. On CT, hyperdense serpentine vessels having a "bag of worms" appearance is a typical finding of AVMs. Calcifications are common but not always present (Figs. 9.1 and 9.2).

On MRI, findings vary with hemodynamics, presence and chronology of hemorrhages, and secondary changes in the surrounding parenchyma. A "honeycomb-appearing" mass with multiple serpiginous flow voids on both T1-weighted (T1WI) and T2-weighted images (T2WI) is characteristic of AVMs. The parenchyma surrounding an AVM can show hyperintensity on T2WI and in fluid-attenuated inversion recovery (FLAIR) related to gliosis and edema. Hemorrhagic components are detectable on all sequences but especially on T2* sequences or susceptibility-weighted images (SWI). Contrast enhancement is variable, but draining dilated veins usually enhance (Fig. 9.3).

Enlarged and tortuous feeding arteries toward the core of the lesion (nidus) with direct arteriovenous shunting to enlarged draining veins is the typical appearance of AVMs on DSA. Intranidal and prenidal aneurysms are present in up to 50 % and 15 % of lesions, respectively, and they represent risk factors for hemorrhage.

The Spetzler–Martin scale for AVMs (Table 9.2) provides accurate estimation of operative morbidity and mortality. The grade of the lesion is derived by adding the points assigned for three categories (1. size of the AVM, 2. pattern of venous drainage, and 3. neurological eloquence of

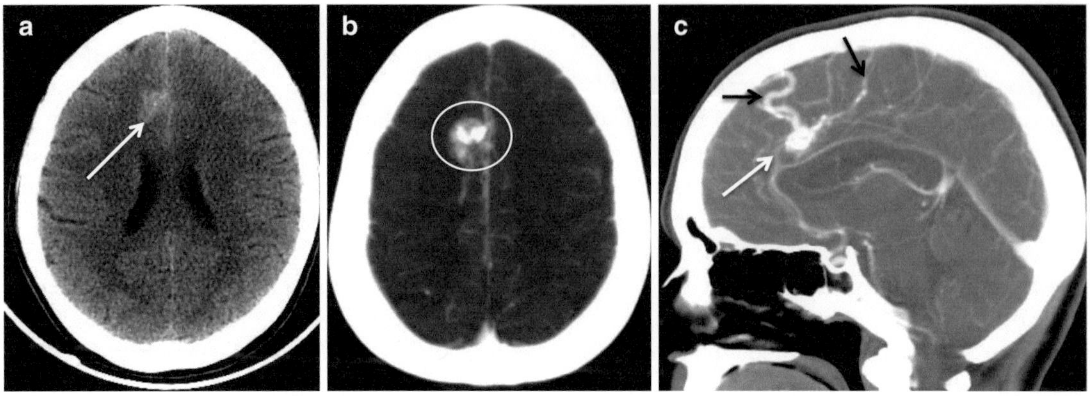

Fig. 9.1 Patient referred to the emergency department because of acute seizures. (**a**) Axial non-enhanced CT shows a parasagittal hyperdense ill-defined lesion without significant mass effect (*white arrow*). (**b**) Axial CTA and (**c**) sagittal CTA confirmed the diagnosis of AVM by virtue of showing a typical "bag of worms" appearance (*circle*). Arterial feeders (*white arrow*), nidus, and prominent cortical draining veins are seen in (**c**) (*black arrows*)

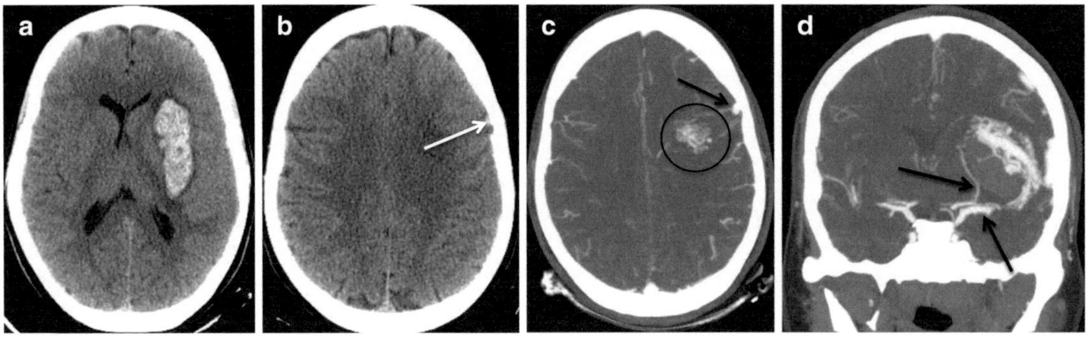

Fig. 9.2 A 22 year-old patient admitted to the emergency department with sudden headache and right hemiparesis. (**a**) Axial non-enhanced CT shows acute intracranial hematoma in the left basal ganglia which in absence of a clinical history of hypertension needs to be further evaluated. (**b**) Axial non-enhanced CT at superior level depicts small cortical hyperdensity compatible with enlarged vein (*white arrow*). (**c**) Axial CTA confirmed the presence of cortical draining vein (*black arrow*) and the AVM nidus (*circle*). (**d**) Coronal CTA shows cortical and lenticulostriate and middle cerebral artery supply to the nidus (*black arrows*)

the brain regions adjacent to the AVM). The lowest grade possible is Grade I; such a lesion is small (1 point), located in a non-eloquent region such as the anterior frontal lobe (0 points), and has exclusively superficial drainage (0 points). Complete surgical excision of such an AVM would present relatively minor technical difficulties and would entail little risk of resultant morbidity or mortality. The highest grade within this scheme is Grade V. An AVM of this type is larger than 6 cm (3 points), located within or immediately adjacent to eloquent brain (1 point), and a portion of the drainage is into the deep venous system (1 point). A Grade V lesion is associated with significant risk of surgical morbidity and mortality. These large, critically located malformations require extensive dissection in close proximity to important brain regions; their removal may be complicated by difficulties with controlling fragile deep veins. Obliteration of the large AVM shunt may lead to a sudden increase in perfusion that may result in vasogenic edema or hemorrhage (a phenomenon that has been termed "normal perfusion pressure breakthrough"). Various combinations of lesion size, location, and venous drainage pattern result in the intermediate grades of AVMs. There

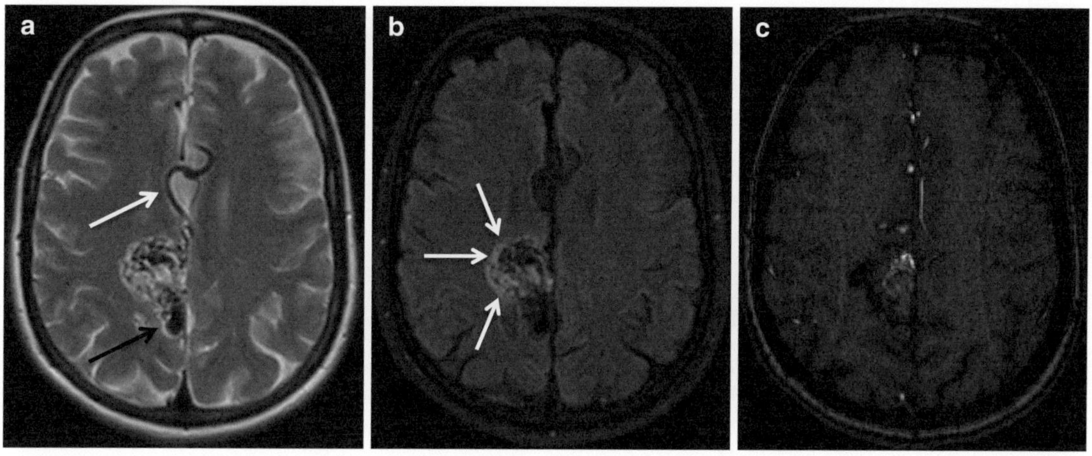

Fig. 9.3 MRI of an AVM presenting with seizures. (**a**) Axial T2WI image showing the typical "honeycomb" appearance of the nidus which contains multiple flow voids. A major arterial feeder from the anterior cerebral artery (*white arrow*) and a draining vein containing an aneurysm (*black arrow*) are seen. (**b**) Axial FLAIR shows gliotic parenchyma surrounding the nidus (*white arrows*). (**c**) TOF MRA shows hyperintense linear arterial structures and the presence of an arterialized draining vein. Note that due to flow artifacts, this MRA does not allow for full and detailed characterization of the lesion

Table 9.2 Spetzler–Martin grading scale for AVMs [14]

Size of nidus	Small (<3 cm) = 1
	Medium (3–6 cm) = 2
	Large (>6 cm) = 3
Eloquence of adjacent brain	Non-eloquent = 0
	Eloquent = 1
Venous drainage	Superficial only = 0
	Deep = 1

are certain lesions that should not currently be considered for surgery. Within this group are extremely large diffuse AVMs that are dispersed through critical neurologically eloquent areas or malformations with a diffuse nidus that encompasses critical structures such as the hypothalamus or brain stem. Surgical resection of such lesions would almost unavoidably be associated with significant disabling deficits or death; thus, these AVMs fall into a separate category that can be termed "Grade VI" or, more simply, "inoperable." This grading system has demonstrated a relationship to the technical difficulty of removing individual AVMs. Virtually all the Grade I and II AVMs can be removed without much difficulty in single-staged procedures. Grade IV and V lesions, however, often required pre- and intraoperative embolization and multistage surgical resection [14].

Cavernomas: On CT, they may be seen as hyperdense well-delineated lesions with subtle intralesional calcifications with or without mass effect. Often, an acute hemorrhage is the only CT sign of an underlying cavernoma that presents acutely.

On MRI, a "popcorn" or "berrylike" lesion with a low signal intensity rim and "blooming" effect on T2*/SWI is suggestive of a cavernoma. T1 and T2 signals are variable due to different stages of blood products present inside the lesions. Fluid–fluid levels and surrounding edema (especially if hemorrhage is recent) may be present. Contrast enhancement is unusual or faint. Yun et al. demonstrated that complete or nearly complete perilesional high signal intensity in T1WI around a hemorrhagic mass has high rate predicting the presence of a cavernous angioma and that this MRI finding may be helpful for differentiating cavernous angioma from hemorrhagic tumors and other intracerebral hemorrhages [15]. Multiple lesions may occur, particularly on familial cavernomatosis, and other vascular malformations can coexist especially DVAs (Fig. 9.4) [3–5, 8, 16, 17].

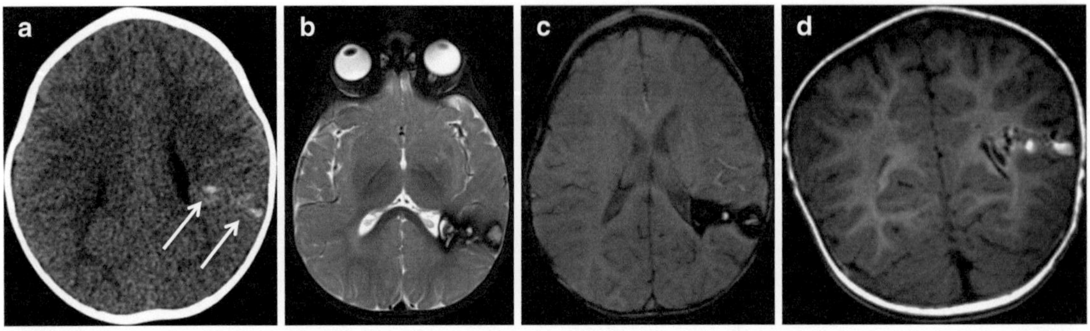

Fig. 9.4 Cavernoma. (**a**) Axial CT shows an irregular hyperdense lesion in the left hemisphere (*arrows*). (**b**) Axial T2WI depicts a lesion with blood in different ages. (**c**) Axial SWI demonstrates "blooming" effect, and (**d**) coronal T1WI shows high signal due to presence of methemoglobin suggestive of recent (early subacute) hemorrhage

MRA, CTA, and DSA are typically negative due to absence of arterial feeders or large venous drainage or to its very slow-flow hemodynamics.

Imaging Follow-Up

As state previously, brain vascular malformations comprise different lesions with a broad spectrum of epidemiologic, clinical, and imaging features as well as variable risks of complications. DSA was the golden standard follow-up imaging method, but due to its invasive nature and radiation, noninvasive techniques are preferred for follow-up. Dynamic 4DMRA and even dynamic 4DCTA are increasingly used in many centers for follow-up [4, 13].

AVMs have the highest risk of hemorrhage (2–4 %/year) [18]. Therefore, imaging follow-up, especially after treatment, is essential to assure complete obliteration of the nidus. Most authors agree that at least one posttreatment DSA should be performed followed by MRI and MRA for long-term follow-ups [19]. Arterial spin label (ASL) is a perfusion MRI sequence useful to detect high-flow vascular lesions and when available can be used for follow-up. Any high ASL signal in a treated lesion implies residual flow, and thus it has a sensitivity for the diagnosis of nidus patency after radiosurgery, surgery, and/or embolization [20].

Cavernomas are associated with a 2.4 % per patient/year risk of hemorrhage, rising to 4–13 % in familial cases [21]. However, hemorrhage risk is unpredictable on an individual basis. Lesion growth and repeat spontaneous and often asymptomatic hemorrhages are to be expected during lifetime, and thus symptoms that arise de novo should prompt imaging [5]. Empirically, yearly follow-up is suggested for asymptomatic ones (to judge lesion growth) or earlier if symptoms change or appear.

Main Differential Diagnosis

Mixed vascular malformations. Occasionally, it can be challenging to distinguish DVAs, AVMs, cavernomas, and capillary telangiectasias since they can coexist. Mixed vascular malformations should be considered in the differential diagnosis of DVAs with hemorrhages and cavernomas with prominent venous drainage [5, 6, 17]. The combination of cavernoma/DVA is the most common mixed type of malformations (also called transitional). It is estimated that this happens in nearly 30 % of cavernomas and DVAs and that most pontine cavernomas have an associated DVA.

Perfusion ASL MRI can differentiate vascular malformations with high-flow from the low-flow ones. Iv et al. found signal abnormalities in ASL only in 8 % of 248 DVAs evaluated. They concluded that DVAs with intrinsic ASL signal or signal in draining veins may be associated with arteriovenous shunting [22].

Neoplasms are an important differential diagnosis of brain vascular malformations. A glioblastoma may display prominent blood vessels that can mimic an AVM [5]. Giant cavernomas may simulate hemorrhagic tumors and they are commonly found in children than in adults.

Tips

- Keep in mind that some brain vascular malformations are frequently incidental findings.
- Suspect of a brain vascular malformation in the presence of intracranial hemorrhage, especially in atypical locations (e.g., cortical hematomas) or in different stages of organization even in the clinical context of hypertension or trauma.
- Perfusion ASL MRI is useful to follow-up AVMs and fistulas after treatment. It is also positive in untreated lesions.
- Signs of increased risk for future hemorrhage in AVMs include previous hemorrhage, intranidal or feeding vessel aneurysms, venous drainage stenosis, deep venous drainage, and deep location of the nidus.

References

1. McCormick WF. The pathology of vascular ("arteriovenous") malformations. J Neurosurg. 1966;24(4): 807–16.
2. Moussa R, Wong J, Awad I. Pathology and genetic factors. In Stieg P, Batjer HH, Samson D. Intracranial arteriovenous malformations. 1st ed, New York: Informa Healthcare USA, Inc; 2007. p. 21–6.
3. Berenstein AL, Pierre, Brugge K. Cerebral vascular malformations: incidence, classification, angioarchitecture and symptomatology of brain arteriovenous and venous malformations. In: Surgical neuroangiography. Springer-Verlag Berlin Heilderberg NewYork; 2004. p. 609–94.
4. Lowe LH, Marchant TC, Rivard DC, Scherbel AJ. Vascular malformations: classification and terminology the radiologist needs to know. Semin Roentgenol. 2012;47(2):106–17.
5. Osborn AG. Osborn's brain: imaging, pathology, and anatomy. 1st ed. Salt Lake City: Amirsys; 2013. xi, 1272 p.
6. Zimmer A, Hagen T, Ahlhelm F, Viera J, Reith W, Schulte-Altedorneburg G. Developmental venous anomaly (DVA). Radiologe. 2007;47(10):868. 70–4.
7. Hsu F, Rigamonti D, Huhn SL. Chapter 2 - Epidemiology of cavernous malformations. In Awad IA, Barrow DL. Cavernous malformations. Park Ridge - Illinois, USA: AANS Publications Comittee; 1993. p. 13–4.
8. Carpenter JS, Rosen CL, Bailes JE, Gailloud P. Sinus pericranii: clinical and imaging findings in two cases of spontaneous partial thrombosis. AJNR Am J Neuroradiol. 2004;25(1):121–5.
9. Mohr JP, Parides MK, Stapf C, Moquete E, Moy CS, Overbey JR, et al. Medical management with or without interventional therapy for unruptured brain arteriovenous malformations (ARUBA): a multicentre, non-blinded, randomised trial. Lancet. 2014;383(9917):614–21.
10. Geibprasert S, Pongpech S, Jiarakongmun P, Shroff MM, Armstrong DC, Krings T. Radiologic assessment of brain arteriovenous malformations: what clinicians need to know. Radiographics: Rev Publ Radiol Soc N Am Inc. 2010;30(2):483–501.
11. Albright L, Pollack I, Adelson D. Principles and practice of pediatric neurosurgery. 3rd ed. Stuttgart: Georg Thieme Verlag; 2015.
12. Kortman HG, Smit EJ, Oei MT, Manniesing R, Prokop M, Meijer FJ. 4D-CTA in neurovascular disease: a review. AJNR Am J Neuroradiol. 2015;36(6):1026–33.
13. Taschner CA, Gieseke J, Le Thuc V, Rachdi H, Reyns N, Gauvrit JY, et al. Intracranial arteriovenous malformation: time-resolved contrast-enhanced MR angiography with combination of parallel imaging, keyhole acquisition, and k-space sampling techniques at 1.5 T. Radiology. 2008;246(3):871–9.
14. Spetzler RF, Martin NA. A proposed grading system for arteriovenous malformations. J Neurosurg. 1986;65(4):476–83.
15. Yun TJ, Na DG, Kwon BJ, Rho HG, Park SH, Suh YL, et al. A T1 hyperintense perilesional signal aids in the differentiation of a cavernous angioma from other hemorrhagic masses. AJNR Am J Neuroradiol. 2008;29(3):494–500.
16. Greenberg M. Handbook of neurosurgery. 7th ed. New York: Thieme. Greenberg Graphics, Inc.Tampa Florida; 2010. 1352 p.
17. Atlas SW. Magnetic resonance imaging of the brain and spine. 4th ed. Philadelphia: Wolters Kluwer Health/Lippincott Williams & Wilkins; 2009.
18. Spetzler RF, Kondziolka D, Higashida RT, Kalani Y. Comprehensive management of arteriovenous malformations of the brain and spine. Available from: http://libproxy.lib.unc.edu/login?url=http://dx.doi.org/10.1017/CBO9781139523943.
19. International Radiosurgery Association. Stereoatactic radiosurgery for patients with intracranial arteriovenous malformations. Radiosurgery practice guideline report. 2009.
20. Blauwblomme T, Naggara O, Brunelle F, Grevent D, Puget S, Di Rocco F, et al. Arterial spin label-

ing magnetic resonance imaging: toward noninvasive diagnosis and follow-up of pediatric brain arteriovenous malformations. J Neurosurg Pediatr. 2015;15(4):451–8.
21. Gross BA, Lin N, Du R, Day AL. The natural history of intracranial cavernous malformations. Neurosurg Focus. 2011;30(6):E24.
22. Iv M, Fischbein NJ, Zaharchuk G. Association of developmental venous anomalies with perfusion abnormalities on arterial spin labeling and bolus perfusion-weighted imaging. J Neuroimaging: Off J Am Soc Neuroimaging. 2015;25(2):243–50.

Venous Thrombosis 10

Ingrid Aguiar Littig and Antônio José da Rocha

Abstract

Cerebral venous thrombosis is defined as the presence of a thrombus inside a venous sinus or inside a superficial or deep intracranial vein. The most commonly affected population is young females, and among children, neonates are known to have a higher risk of thrombotic events due to a maturing hemostatic system as well as perinatal and maternal risk factors. Early diagnosis leads to prompt and effective treatment and neuroimaging plays an important role providing early diagnosis since symptoms and clinical course are variable. Magnetic resonance imaging demonstrates the location and extension of the thrombus as well as the temporal evolution of the thrombosis. Imaging findings include intraluminal thrombosis associated with parenchymal alterations, venous congestion, and, sometimes, parenchymal and/or subarachnoid hemorrhage.

Background

Cerebral venous thrombosis (CVT) is defined as the presence of a thrombus inside a venous sinus or superficial or deep intracranial veins. CVT was first recognized at the beginning of the nineteenth century when it was thought to be an infectious disorder. At that time it was only diagnosed by autopsy, which usually showed hemorrhagic lesions leading to believe that anticoagulation was contraindicated. The use of neuroimaging modified our understanding of this disorder, and today, CVT is now recognized as a non-septic condition with 80 % of good neurological outcome and mortality below 10 % and commonly treated with anticoagulation [1, 2].

I.A. Littig, MD (✉)
Division of Neuroradiology, Hospital Santa Casa de Misericórdia de São Paulo, Rua Dr. Cesário Motta Junior 112, Vila Buarque, Sao Paulo, SP 01221-020, Brazil
e-mail: ingridlittig@globo.com

A.J. da Rocha, MD, PhD
Division of Neuroradiology, Hospital Santa Casa de Misericórdia de São Paulo, Rua Dr. Cesário Motta Junior 112, Vila Buarque, Sao Paulo, SP 01221-020, Brazil

Division of Neuroradiology, Grupo Fleury, Rua Dr. Cesário Motta Junior 112, Vila Buarque, Sao Paulo, SP 01221-020, Brazil
e-mail: antonio.rocha@grupofleury.com.br

R. Hoffmann Nunes et al. (eds.), *Critical Findings in Neuroradiology*,
DOI 10.1007/978-3-319-27987-9_10

The most frequently affected population is young females, which correlates with common prothrombotic states, such as the use of oral contraceptives and the peripartum period. This female predominance does not occur in children or in the elderly [2, 3].

Clinical manifestations depend on the CVT mechanism. One mechanism is the development of intracranial hypertension attributable to diffusely impaired venous drainage as the result of occlusion of the major venous sinuses. The other is the occlusion of cerebral veins, which may lead to parenchymal alterations, particularly vasogenic edema and hemorrhage (Fig. 10.1). Superficial venous thrombosis may present as seizures and also result in deep venous thrombosis affecting the level of consciousness. Both may manifest as focal brain lesions [2, 4, 5].

CVT is an underdiagnosed condition in children because of the subtle and usually nonspecific clinical presentation. It occurs in about one out of 100,000 children per year including neonates and accounts for one in four cases of pediatric stroke. CVT is associated with high mortality and morbidity, and pediatric CVT studies report mortality rates of 8–19 % and severe long-term neurological sequelae in 38–48 % of patients [6–8]. Neonates are the age group most commonly affected by CVT especially on the day of birth or within the first week of life [7, 8].

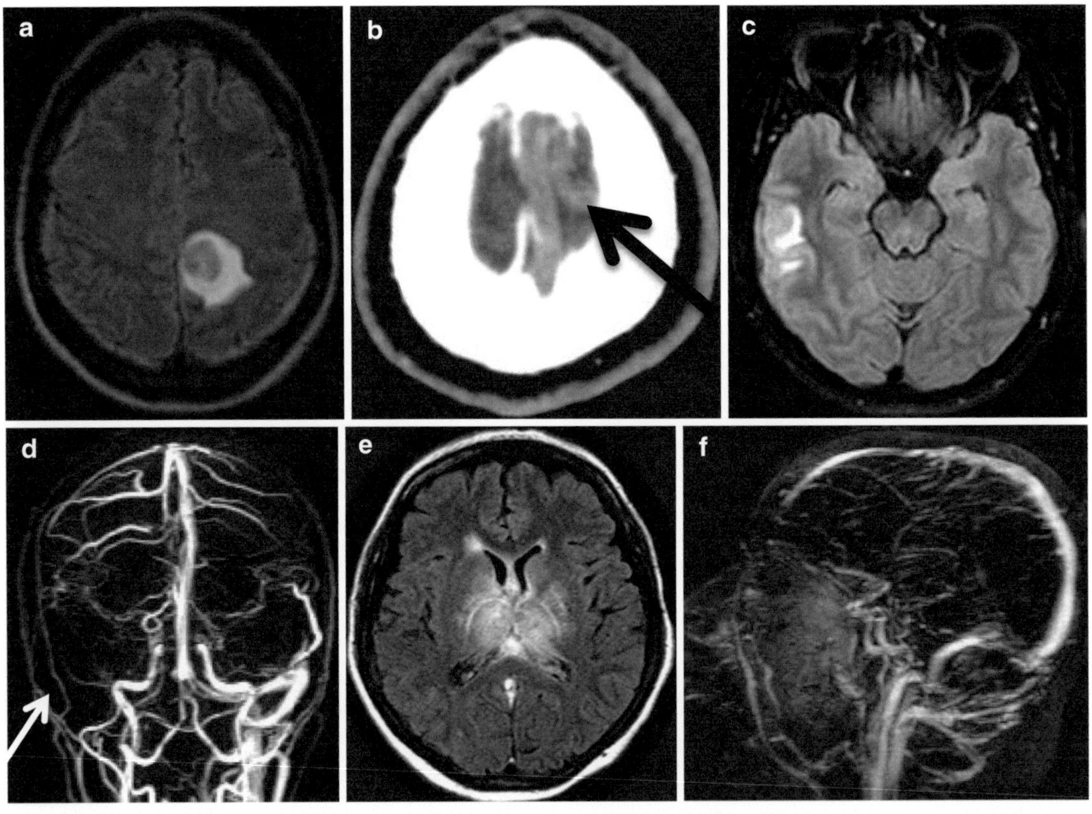

Fig. 10.1 Cerebral venous thrombosis and focal brain lesions. A parasagittal intraparenchymal hematoma shown on axial FLAIR image (**a**) suggests superior sagittal sinus and Trolard vein thrombosis as shown on contrast-enhanced CT in which these structures are not filled (*arrow* on **b**). A temporo-occipital lesion (axial FLAIR image on **c**) can be found in transverse sinus and Labbé vein thrombosis (*arrow* in MRV 3D reconstruction on **d**). Bilateral thalamic lesions (axial FLAIR image on **e**) suggest deep cerebral venous thrombosis, and 3D MRV reconstruction (**f**) shows absence of visualization of the deep venous system

They usually present with seizures, lethargy, irritability, poor feeding, apnea, jitteriness, or changes in muscle tone, whereas in older children, headache, papilledema, and focal neurological deficits are the main clinical manifestations [8]. Nevertheless, most of these clinical scenarios occur in all age groups [9].

Key Points

Etiology

There is a wide range of causes and risk factors associated with CVT. They include genetic and acquired prothrombotic states, dehydration, inflammatory, and hematologic diseases and drugs. Most commonly, the etiology cannot be determined by imaging, as the resulting appearance of CVT is similar regardless of its cause. Nevertheless, in some situations, imaging can show central nervous system (CNS) infections or adjacent infections, such as complicated mastoiditis. Intracranial hypotension related to lumbar puncture trauma, and neurosurgical interventions may cause CVT [2].

Among children, neonates are known to have a higher risk of thrombotic events compared with children of older age groups due to a developing hemostatic system and perinatal and maternal risk factors that are unique during this period of life including fetal distress and birth asphyxia, forceps delivery, meconium aspiration, dehydration, sepsis, cardiac defects, and meningitis [8, 9]. In addition, the normal process of molding and overlapping of the cranial bones during vaginal birth also causes injuries to the underlying dural sinuses thereby increasing the propensity for clot formation [8]. Maternal preeclampsia which is in itself a hypercoagulable state and chorioamnionitis are well-established maternal risk factors for neonatal CVT [8, 10]. CVT in older children is often associated with ear infections, meningitis, anemia, diabetes, head injury, dehydration, nephrotic syndrome, cancer, and hematologic disorder, among other prothrombotic conditions also present in adults [6, 8, 9].

Best Imaging Modality

The imaging modality that best depicts the thrombus inside of a vein or a venous sinus is magnetic resonance imaging (MRI). It demonstrates the location and extension of the thrombus, as well as the temporal evolution of the thrombosis. Multiplanar images on T1-weighted imaging (T1WI), T2-weighted imaging (T2WI), fluid-attenuated inversion recovery (FLAIR), and susceptibility-weighted imaging (SWI) as well as T2* sequences are sensitive to characterize an intraluminal thrombus, but the current gold standard is the combination of conventional MRI with magnetic resonance venography (MRV). This combination confidently defines the extension of the thrombosis and the patent venous drainage pathways of the brain, making the use of invasive methods such as catheter angiography unusual in clinical practice [1].

MRV sequences alone are many times not sufficient to distinguish sinus occlusion from normal variants of the sinus anatomy such as narrowing and/or hypoplasia [2, 5]. Nevertheless, MRV is especially important on chronic thrombosis follow-up, when it delineates the sinus partial recanalization, demonstrating its characteristic irregularities in the sinus contour and helping to detect complications, such as dural arteriovenous fistulas (DAVFs). In neonates, MRV false-positive results are likely due to deformability of the skull resulting in the appearance of slow flow in the sinuses. Consequently, contrast-enhanced MRV, which is less susceptible to alterations in flow, is recommended in neonates [1, 8, 10].

During the acute stage, thrombosed sinuses or veins are isointense on T1WI and hypointense on T2WI, and therefore, hardly distinguishable from normal veins. In this situation, intravenous gadolinium injection is helpful. Adding T2* or SWI images is important because patent veins and sinuses appear bright and the thrombus appears dark in these sequences [1].

In cases when MRI is not readily available or cannot be obtained, computed tomography (CT) is useful. Non-enhanced CT is often unremarkable, but venous or sinus hyperdensity is observed in about one-third of acute CVT patients. Contrast-enhanced CT is recommended to depict enhancement of the dural linings of a vein or sinus as well as filling defects within them. Reformatted images are also important to assess these filling defects on different planes [5, 11].

In neonates, ultrasonography commonly the preliminary screening test for hemorrhage in the neonatal period, may detect intraventricular bleeding, centrally located venous infarcts, or hemorrhages, as well as ventricular dilatation and leukomalacia secondary to CVT infarction and ischemia [8]. Doppler ultrasound can detect absent or reduced flow in the superficial sinovenous channels. Nonetheless, ultrasound has poor sensitivity and should not be used primarily for detection of CVT [8].

Major Findings

The imaging findings of CVT are not only the actual intraluminal thrombosis, but also the consequences of the obstructed venous drainage, such as parenchymal alterations, venous congestion, and parenchymal and/or subarachnoid hemorrhage [1].

The "dense triangle sign" and the "cord sign" have been described on unenhanced CT as a result of acute hyperdense thrombus within a dural sinus or a vein, respectively. These signs are reported on 20 % of patients in the first 1–2 weeks of CVT. Also, the thrombosed sinus and cortical vein are often enlarged and irregular in contour. Higher accuracy is achieved with contrast-enhanced CT which is able to demonstrate a filling defect in a sinus caused by the thrombus ("empty delta sign") in about 25–75 % of patients. All these imaging signs depend on the imaging plane used to visualize the involved venous structures. Since the sinuses and veins are often curved, reformatted CT images are very useful (Fig. 10.2) [11, 12].

On MRI, it is of importance to recognize a normal patent vein or sinus and the *time-related changes* in characteristics of intraluminal thrombus (Fig. 10.3):

Acute stage: Signal void which appears dark on T1WI and T2WI indicates presence of flow and is more conspicuous for higher speed flow and when the acquired imaging plane is perpendicular to the flow direction [12]. Clot during the acute CVT stage (1–5 days) contains intracellular deoxyhemoglobin typically showing isointensity to mild hyperintensity on T1WI and hypointensity on T2WI [1, 12]. The use of T2* and especially SWI images helps to depict thrombosed blood vessels (Fig. 10.4). A combination of marked intravascular hypointensity coupled with enlargement of a venous structure on these sequences is sensitive for the identification of CVT especially during the acute stage. Sometimes it is also possible to depict small congested vessels surrounding the dural layers of a sinus [1, 13].

Subacute stage: The subacute stage (5–15 days) has an early phase in which intracellular methemoglobin is markedly hyperintense on T1WI but still hypointense on T2WI. Only in the late subacute stage after red blood cell lysis does methemoglobin become extracellular and the thrombus appear hyperintense on both T1WI and T2WI [12].

Chronic stage: The major importance of MRV relies on the capacity to evaluate the chronic CVT phase (over 15 days). It also shows recanalization which characteristically presents irregular and thin flow in a venous sinus [14].

Evaluation of brain parenchyma is crucial when CVT is suspected. Supporting findings include that focal brain lesions are located in territories drained by corresponding specific veins and sinus and in non-arterial territories (Fig. 10.1) [11]. Increased cerebral venous pressure due to cerebral venous occlusion can result in a dilated venous and capillary bed, promoting interstitial edema and rupture of venous structures [15]. Focal vasogenic edema is demonstrated in 50–60 % of CVT patients, while brain hematoma occurs in 35–40 % of patients [16]. Brain lesions

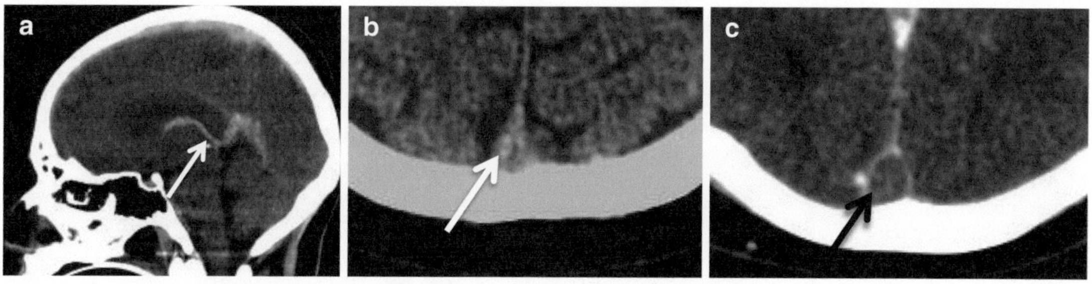

Fig. 10.2 Cord sign and dense triangle sign. (**a**) Sagittal non-enhanced CT image shows an acute hyperdense thrombus inside an internal cerebral vein and vein of Galen resulting in the "cord sign" (*arrow*). (**b**) Axial non-enhanced CT image reveals that the acute hyperdense thrombus inside the superior sagittal sinus results in the "dense triangle sign" (*arrow*). (**c**) Corresponding postcontrast CT image demonstrates a filling defect (clot) resulting in the "empty delta sign" (*arrow*)

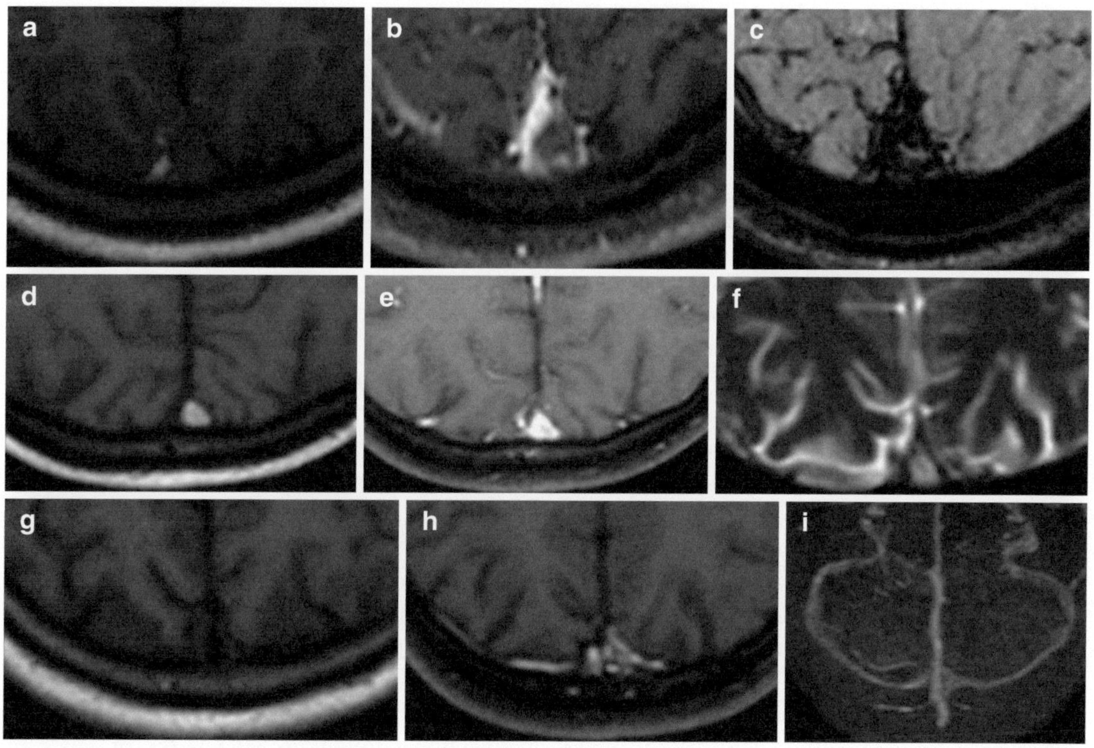

Fig. 10.3 Sinus thrombosis in different phases of evolution. (**a–c**) Axial non-enhanced T1WI, postcontrast T1WI, and SWI images demonstrate acute superior sagittal sinus thrombosis. (**d–f**) Axial non-enhanced T1WI, postcontrast T1WI, and T2WI images reveal subacute superior sagittal sinus thrombosis. Note the T1 bright clot (**d**) before contrast which is indistinguishable from surrounding contrast-enhanced blood in (**e–i**). Axial non-enhanced T1WI, postcontrast T1WI, and 3D MRV reconstruction images show signs of recanalization of the superior sagittal sinus, characterized by an irregular and thin flow inside it

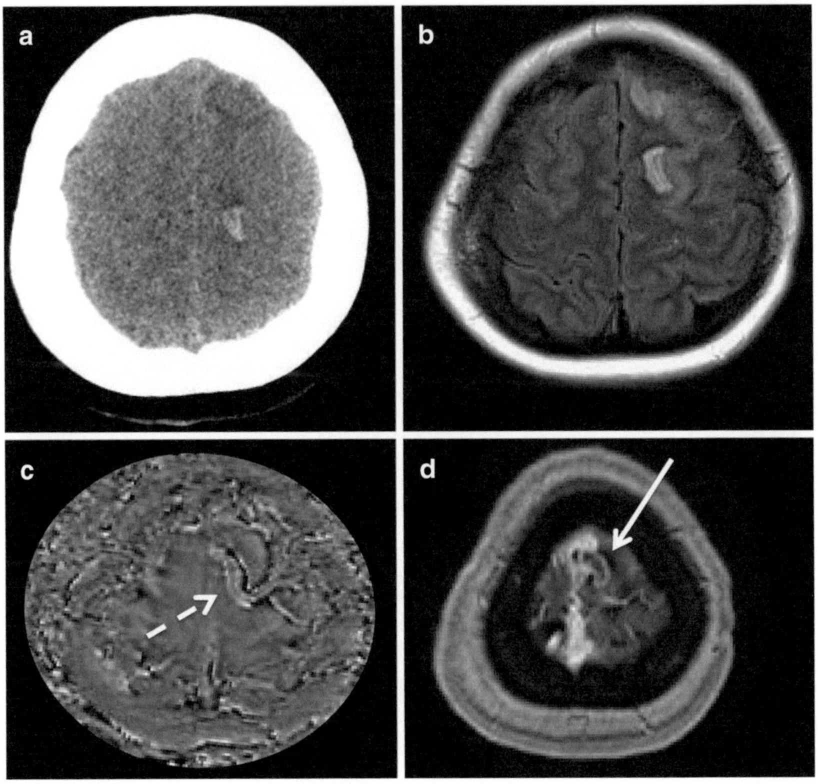

Fig. 10.4 Cortical vein thrombosis. (**a**) Axial CT image demonstrates a left parasagittal frontal small intraparenchymal hemorrhage. (**b**) Axial FLAIR image reveals a corticosubcortical hyperintense lesion with adjacent cortex swelling in the left frontal lobe. (**c**) Axial SWI phase image depicts a bright (blood products) curvilinear structure (*arrow*) in the left frontal lobe near the convexity. (**d**) Axial postcontrast T1WI confirms that the bright structure on SWI is a thrombosed cortical vein containing a filling defect (*arrow*)

related to CVT seem to be reversible even when presenting restricted diffusion, different from those due to arterial strokes (Fig. 10.5) [16–18]. Because cortical veins can rupture and bleed into the subarachnoid space, subarachnoid hemorrhage can be an initial finding of CVT (6%) [19]. Other imaging findings associated to CVT are brain edema, especially in sinus thrombosis, and enhancement of the falx and/or tentorium due to collateral circulation [5, 12, 20].

Cavernous sinus thrombosis (CST) takes place in a different setting. While CVT occurs due to prothrombotic states, CST is usually related to face or paranasal sinus infections. Unlike with other venous sinuses, contrast-enhanced CT is the primary imaging technique to detect CST demonstrating enlargement of the affected sinus, convexity of its lateral wall, and filling defects. The cavernous segment of the internal carotid artery and the dural wall of the cavernous sinus may demonstrate contrast enhancement, and these findings may be better seen on MRI than CT [21].

Imaging Follow-Up

On imaging follow-up, recanalization might be appreciated, as well as resolution of brain lesions. Large parenchymal changes can resolve independent from recanalization of underlying thrombosed veins and sinuses [17] even in the presence of previous restricted diffusion [16]. If the first examination showed parenchymal hemorrhage, gliosis and superficial siderosis may be observed on follow-up. Presence of large hematomas is a prognostic factor for death or disability [22].

A critical finding that should be sought out on conventional follow-up MRI is the presence of numerous and dilated cortical veins in the surrounding affected brain parenchyma. This finding may be related to venous hypertension/collaterals, but when focal, it may indicate the presence of an underlying DAVF (Fig. 10.6). The involved dural sinus receives arterialized blood flow leading to retrograde flow into dilated cortical veins predisposing to brain dysfunction with eventual dementia and intracranial hemorrhages [14, 23].

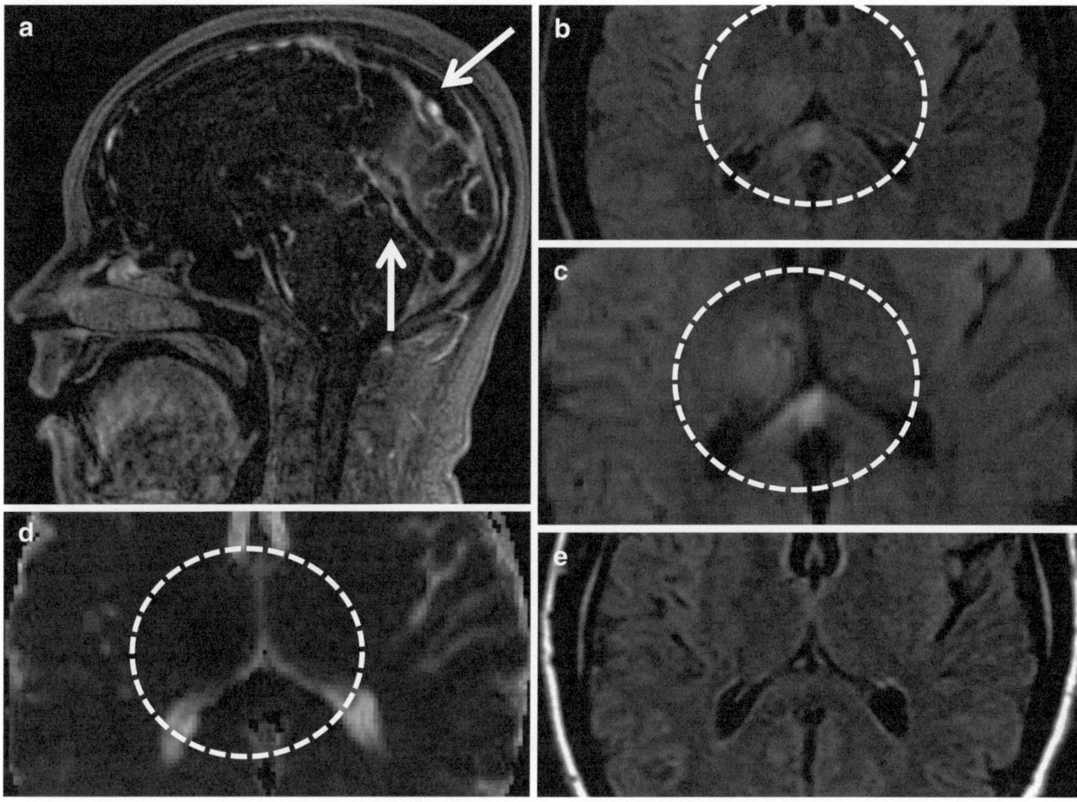

Fig. 10.5 (**a**) Sagittal post-gadolinium T1WI (**a**) shows filling defects in the superior sagittal and straight sinuses (*arrows*), as well as in the vein of Galen. (**b–d**) Axial FLAIR image reveals a hyperintense lesion in the right thalamus and splenium (*circle*) in part of the territory drained by the deep venous system. (**c, d**) Axial diffusion-weighted imaging and apparent diffusion coefficient map images depict areas of restricted diffusion within the lesion (*circles*). (**e**) Axial FLAIR image demonstrates a normal brain parenchyma on follow-up scan 4 months after clinical treatment

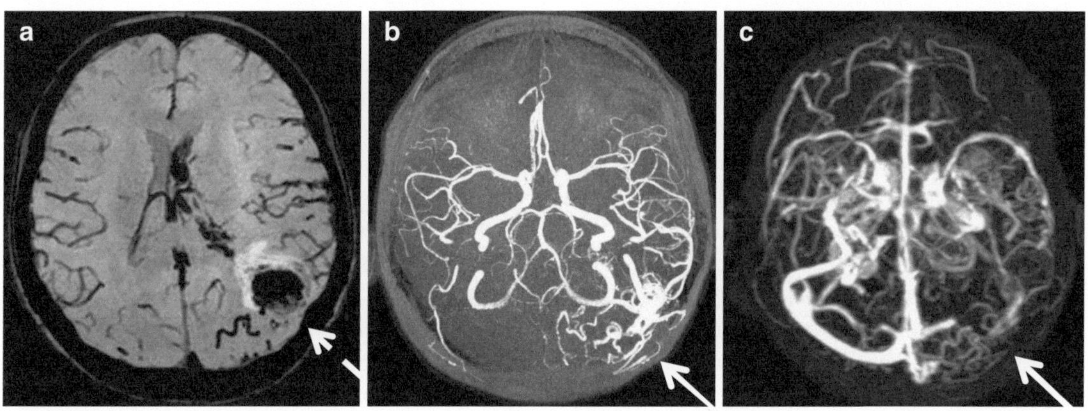

Fig. 10.6 Dural arteriovenous fistula. (**a–c**) SWI, 3D time-of-flight MIP, and 3D MRV MIP images show findings suggestive of a dural arteriovenous fistula with numerous small and tortuous vessels (*arrows*) on the parenchyma superior to a previously thrombosed left transverse sinus. This dural arteriovenous fistula is complicated by an intraparenchymal hematoma seen on SWI (*dashed arrow* on **a**)

Main Differential Diagnosis

Anatomic variations: One frequent anatomic variation is sinus asymmetry mainly observed in transverse sinuses. If the corresponding jugular foramen is also small, the size of the sinus may be considered as a normal variant. Sinus fenestrations, presence of arachnoid granulations, septa, and partial sinus absence may also be sources of misdiagnosis [24].

Intrasinus arachnoid granulation: They are common projections of the subarachnoid space into a sinus through which cerebrospinal fluid presumably reenters the venous system. They usually do not occupy the entire sinus like CVT does and are referred to as "giant" when they are of sufficient size to fill the lumen of a dural sinus and cause local dilation and/or filling defects which are incidental and commonly seen in the transverse and posterior superior sagittal sinuses [25].

Increased hematocrit levels: In situations like dehydration and polycythemia, the sinuses and veins may appear relatively hyperdense on non-enhanced CT (Fig. 10.7). However, arteries will have a similar appearance confirming that the blood is diffusively hyperdense and not attributable to thrombosis [12, 24].

Unmyelinated brain: Physiologic polycythemia and the relative hypodense unmyelinated brain of neonates can also make the sinuses appear hyperdense on CT (Fig. 10.7) [8, 12].

Diffuse brain edema: Parenchymal hypodensity may also make the venous structures appear relatively hyperdense on CT.

Subdural and subarachnoid hemorrhages on CT: Acute blood along a dural surface may mimic the empty delta sign ("pseudo-delta sign"). This sign is restricted to non-enhanced CT while the classically described "empty delta sign" is seen on postcontrast scans [12, 24].

T2WI hypointensity of acute CVT: Intracellular deoxyhemoglobin which is isointense on T1WI and low on T2WI may mimic a flow void and thus be missed. Intravenous gadolinium administration shows a filling defect within a vein or sinus [1, 12].

T1WI hyperintensity of subacute CVT: CVT may exhibit hyperintense signal on T1WI that may mimic a normal contrast filled and patent sinus on postcontrast studies since the thrombus is already hyperintense on non-enhanced images due to intracellular methemoglobin. Careful comparison between the pre- and post-gadolinium images avoids this potential false-negative finding (Fig. 10.3) [1, 12].

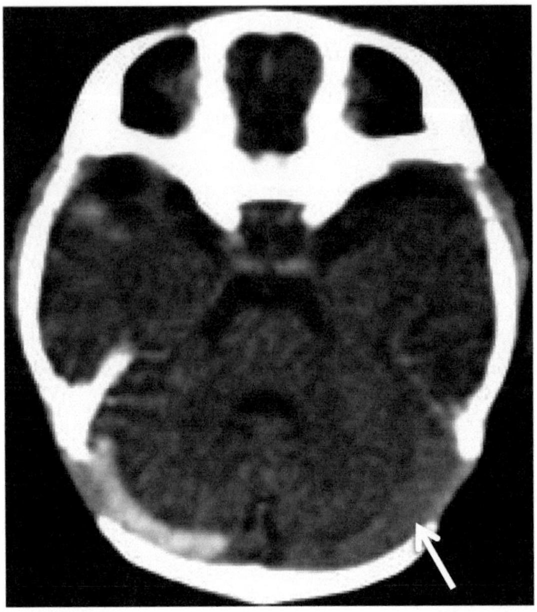

Fig. 10.7 Acute sinus thrombosis in a newborn. Axial non-enhanced CT image demonstrates right transverse sinus thrombosis. Note that the left transverse sinus is also mild hyperdense (*arrow*), a finding that may be due to physiologic polycythemia and the relative hypodense unmyelinated surrounding brain of this newborn as well as the thin skull

Enhancing chronic thrombus: Chronic clots have a propensity to enhance due to their replacement by vascularized connective tissues mimicking thus sinus patency. Comparison between the pre and post-gadolinium images and MRV findings avoids this misinterpretation [1, 12].

Flow artifacts on MRI: Slow flow leads to inconsistent flow void [24]. In the elderly, slow flow may be observed on the left jugular vein and the left sigmoid and transverse sinuses due to brachiocephalic vein compression between the sternum and an ectatic aortic arch. The blood flow of the internal jugular veins and intracranial venous sinuses may also be affected by respiration [26]. Another flow pitfall is the "entry section phenomenon" which is a flow-related enhancement artifact dependent on flow direction. Postcontrast studies clarify the diagnosis [11].

Tips

- Always evaluate reformatted pre- and postcontrast CT images to detect hyperdense veins or dural sinuses in different planes. Maximum intensity projection (MIP) and volume rendering reconstructions may be useful to delineate normal anatomy and variants.
- Analyze all acquired MRI planes and all available sequences. This will avoid interpretation errors particularly in the presence of flow-related artifacts and underlying T1 bright clots. Use the imaging plane acquired perpendicularly to the main flow direction of each evaluated venous segment to prevent misinterpretation as the signal intensity within these curved structures may occasionally simulate clots.
- When analyzing post-gadolinium images, remember to compare them, side-by-side, to non-enhanced images to avoid incorrect interpretation in the presence of subacute CVT as bright T1 clots may be indistinguishable from a contrast filled vessel.
- SWI increases sensitivity in the diagnosis of CVT especially in cortical vein thrombosis because it depicts them as very dark vascular structures. Careful scrutiny is recommended as susceptibility effects do not always indicate intravascular thrombosis since arterial flow voids and calcifications may also determine susceptibility artifacts [11, 13].
- Mention if a brain lesion can possibly be a consequence of a still non-depicted CVT based mainly on its location. And remember that those lesions tend to be temporary, mainly in the absence of hemorrhage but even in the presence of restricted diffusion.
- On follow-up studies, MRV is mandatory to grade the degree of sinus recanalization.
- On conventional MRI, search for dilated vessels in the brain parenchyma that surrounds the previously thrombosed venous sinus. Dilated veins may indicate high venous pressure and a DAVF should be suspected.

References

1. Bousser MG, Ferro JM. Cerebral venous thrombosis: an update. Lancet Neurol. 2007;6(2):162–70.
2. Stam J. Thrombosis of the cerebral veins and sinuses. N Engl J Med. 2005;352(17):1791–8.
3. Linn J, Bruckmann H. Cerebral venous and dural sinus thrombosis*: state-of-the-art imaging. Clin Neuroradiol. 2010;20(1):25–37.
4. Sheerin F. The imaging of the cerebral venous sinuses. Semin Ultrasound CT MR. 2009;30(6):525–58.
5. Saposnik G, Barinagarrementeria F, Brown Jr RD, Bushnell CD, Cucchiara B, Cushman M, et al. Diagnosis and management of cerebral venous thrombosis: a statement for healthcare professionals from the American Heart Association/American Stroke Association. Stroke J Cereb Circ. 2011;42(4):1158–92.
6. Wagner MW, Bosemani T, Oshmyansky A, Poretti A, Huisman TA. Neuroimaging findings in pediatric cerebral sinovenous thrombosis. Childs Nerv Syst ChNS Off J Int Soc Pediatr Neurosurg. 2015; 31(5):705–12.
7. Kersbergen KJ, Groenendaal F, Benders MJ, de Vries LS. Neonatal cerebral sinovenous thrombosis: neuroimaging and long-term follow-up. J Child Neurol. 2011;26(9):1111–20.
8. Yang JY, Chan AK, Callen DJ, Paes BA. Neonatal cerebral sinovenous thrombosis: sifting the evidence for a diagnostic plan and treatment strategy. Pediatrics. 2010;126(3):e693–700.
9. Sebire G, Tabarki B, Saunders DE, Leroy I, Liesner R, Saint-Martin C, et al. Cerebral venous sinus thrombosis in children: risk factors, presentation, diagnosis and outcome. Brain J Neurol. 2005;128(Pt 3): 477–89.
10. Wu YW, Miller SP, Chin K, Collins AE, Lomeli SC, Chuang NA, et al. Multiple risk factors in neonatal sinovenous thrombosis. Neurology. 2002;59(3): 438–40.
11. Rodallec MH, Krainik A, Feydy A, Helias A, Colombani JM, Julles MC, et al. Cerebral venous thrombosis and multidetector CT angiography: tips and tricks. Radiogr Rev Publ Radiol Soc N Am Inc. 2006;26 Suppl 1:S5–18; discussion S42–3.
12. Naidich TP, Castillo M, Cha S, Smirniotopoulos JG. Imaging brain. Available from: http://www.clinicalkey.com/dura/browse/bookChapter/3-s2.0-C20090368506 (n.d.).
13. Leach JL, Strub WM, Gaskill-Shipley MF. Cerebral venous thrombus signal intensity and susceptibility effects on gradient recalled-echo MR imaging. AJNR Am J Neuroradiol. 2007;28(5):940–5.
14. Leach JL, Wolujewicz M, Strub WM. Partially recanalized chronic dural sinus thrombosis: findings on MR imaging, time-of-flight MR venography, and contrast-enhanced MR venography. AJNR Am J Neuroradiol. 2007;28(4):782–9.
15. Schaller B, Graf R. Cerebral venous infarction: the pathophysiological concept. Cerebrovasc Dis. 2004;18(3):179–88.

16. Mullins ME, Grant PE, Wang B, Gonzalez RG, Schaefer PW. Parenchymal abnormalities associated with cerebral venous sinus thrombosis: assessment with diffusion-weighted MR imaging. AJNR Am J Neuroradiol. 2004;25(10):1666–75.
17. Rottger C, Trittmacher S, Gerriets T, Blaes F, Kaps M, Stolz E. Reversible MR imaging abnormalities following cerebral venous thrombosis. AJNR Am J Neuroradiol. 2005;26(3):607–13.
18. Ducreux D, Oppenheim C, Vandamme X, Dormont D, Samson Y, Rancurel G, et al. Diffusion-weighted imaging patterns of brain damage associated with cerebral venous thrombosis. AJNR Am J Neuroradiol. 2001;22(2):261–8.
19. Oppenheim C, Domigo V, Gauvrit JY, Lamy C, Mackowiak-Cordoliani MA, Pruvo JP, et al. Subarachnoid hemorrhage as the initial presentation of dural sinus thrombosis. AJNR Am J Neuroradiol. 2005;26(3):614–7.
20. Qu H, Yang M. Early imaging characteristics of 62 cases of cerebral venous sinus thrombosis. Exp Ther Med. 2013;5(1):233–6.
21. Schuknecht B, Simmen D, Yuksel C, Valavanis A. Tributary venosinus occlusion and septic cavernous sinus thrombosis: CT and MR findings. AJNR Am J Neuroradiol. 1998;19(4):617–26.
22. Ferro JM, Canhao P, Stam J, Bousser MG, Barinagarrementeria F, Investigators I. Prognosis of cerebral vein and dural sinus thrombosis: results of the International Study on Cerebral Vein and Dural Sinus Thrombosis (ISCVT). Stroke J Cereb Circ. 2004;35(3):664–70.
23. Gupta A, Periakaruppan A. Intracranial dural arterio-venous fistulas: a review. Indian J Radiol Imaging. 2009;19(1):43–8.
24. Poon CS, Chang JK, Swarnkar A, Johnson MH, Wasenko J. Radiologic diagnosis of cerebral venous thrombosis: pictorial review. AJR Am J Roentgenol. 2007;189(6 Suppl):S64–75.
25. Kan P, Stevens EA, Couldwell WT. Incidental giant arachnoid granulation. AJNR Am J Neuroradiol. 2006;27(7):1491–2.
26. Kudo K, Terae S, Ishii A, Omatsu T, Asano T, Tha KK, et al. Physiologic change in flow velocity and direction of dural venous sinuses with respiration: MR venography and flow analysis. AJNR Am J Neuroradiol. 2004;25(4):551–7.

Dural Arteriovenous Fistulas

11

Carlos Eduardo Baccin, Antônio José da Rocha, and Renato Hoffmann Nunes

Abstract

Dural arteriovenous fistulas are abnormal connections between meningeal arteries and dural venous sinuses, meningeal veins, or cortical veins that result in direct arteriovenous shunting. They represent 10–15 % of cerebrovascular malformations with arteriovenous shunting. Their dural arterial supply and lack of a parenchymal nidus differentiate them from pial arteriovenous malformations. Dural arteriovenous fistulas generally are acquired lesions that are frequently associated with prior dural venous sinus thrombosis. Patterns of venous drainage are paramount in determining lesion severity and in guiding treatment. Diagnosis at their early stage may be difficult because of nonspecific clinical and imaging findings. Although the diagnosis has traditionally been by catheter angiography, many of these lesions are now first detected or suspected on cross-sectional imaging.

C.E. Baccin, MD (✉)
Division of Interventional Neuroradiology, Hospital Beneficência Portuguesa de São Paulo, Rua Maestro Cardim, 769. Bela Vista, Sao Paulo, SP 01323-001, Brazil

Division of Interventional Neuroradiology, Hospital Israelita Albert Einstein, Sao Paulo, SP, Brazil
e-mail: cebaccin@gmail.com

A.J. da Rocha, MD, PhD
Division of Neuroradiology, Hospital Santa Casa de Misericórdia de São Paulo, Rua Dr. Cesário Motta Junior 112, Vila Buarque, Sao Paulo, SP 01221-020, Brazil

Division of Neuroradiology, Grupo Fleury, Sao Paulo, SP, Brazil
e-mail: antonio.rocha@grupofleury.com.br

R. Hoffmann Nunes, MD
Division of Neuroradiology, Santa Casa de São Paulo, São Paulo, Brazil
e-mail: renatohn@hotmail.com

Background

Dural arteriovenous fistulas (DAVFs) are abnormal connections between meningeal arteries and dural venous sinuses, meningeal veins, or cortical veins that result in direct arteriovenous shunting repre senting 10–15 % of cerebrovascular malformations with arteriovenous shunting. Their dural arterial supply and lack of a parenchymal nidus differentiate them from the more common pial arteriovenous malformations. DAVFs are generally acquired lesions and are frequently associated with prior dural venous sinus thrombosis [1, 2].

Adult DAVFs constitute the majority of these lesions and are most common at the transverse, sigmoid, and cavernous sinuses [3]. There is also a subset of pediatric lesions that often involve

R. Hoffmann Nunes et al. (eds.), *Critical Findings in Neuroradiology*,
DOI 10.1007/978-3-319-27987-9_11

the torcula, superior sagittal sinus, and venous lakes [4].

Dural fistulas of the cavernous sinus, also called cavernous carotid fistulas (CCFs), are the second most common type and are classified as either direct (a direct connection between the cavernous internal carotid artery and the cavernous sinus) or indirect (connection between multiple external carotid artery branches or dural branches of the internal carotid artery and the cavernous sinus) [1, 2, 5]. Direct CCFs are high-flow and often devastating lesions that result from rupture of the cavernous carotid artery typically in the setting of skull base fractures. Indirect CCFs are slow-flow, low-pressure lesions thought to be degenerative in etiology, and their symptoms are often insidious. Unlike other DAVFs, indirect CCFs are rarely associated with dural sinus thrombosis [5].

Patterns of venous drainage are paramount in determining lesion severity and are graded using the Cognard classification system (Table 11.1) [6]. Low-grade lesions (types I and IIa) lack cortical venous drainage and rarely, if ever, cause intracranial hemorrhage. High-grade lesions (type IIb and above) demonstrate absent venous sinus drainage and retrograde flow through cortical veins which may become ectatic (type IV) under arterial pressure. Increased hemodynamic stress makes these fragile cortical veins prone to rupture. Lesions which demonstrate cortical venous drainage are associated with an 8.1 % annual risk of intracranial hemorrhage and an annual mortality risk of 10.4 % [2].

Most DAVFs present most in the fifth and sixth decades of life with symptoms that vary with lesion location and venous drainage pattern. Low-grade DAVFs at the junction of the transverse and sigmoid sinuses often present with pulsatile tinnitus. High-grade lesions present with severe headaches and stroke-like symptoms from lobar hemorrhage or venous infarctions as well as seizures and/or cerebellar symptoms. CCFs can initially present with sudden palsies of cranial nerves traversing the cavernous sinus. Eventually, varying degrees of proptosis, altered vision, and periorbital edema develop depending on lesion severity [1, 2, 5, 7].

Treatment options vary with lesion grade and clinical presentation. In general, clinical observation is indicated in asymptomatic, low-grade lesions without cortical venous drainage (Cognard type I and IIa). Symptomatic low-grade lesions (i.e., tinnitus and impaired vision) or high-grade lesions may require endovascular embolization which is currently considered the first line of treatment in the majority patients. Surgery is generally reserved for patients where endovascular approaches have previously failed or are technically difficult [2].

Table 11.1 Cognard classification of dural arteriovenous fistulas

Type I	Venous drainage into dural sinus with anterograde flow
Type IIa	Venous drainage into dural sinus with retrograde flow
Type IIb	Venous drainage into dural sinus with anterograde flow and cortical vein drainage
Type IIc	Venous drainage into dural sinus with retrograde flow and cortical vein drainage
Type III	Venous drainage into cortical veins
Type IV	Venous drainage into cortical veins with associated venous ectasia(s)
Type V	Venous drainage into spinal perimedullary veins

Key Points

Etiology

DAVFs are usually acquired lesions associated with history of trauma, previous craniotomy, and/or dural venous sinus thrombosis. Prevailing etiologic theories focus on venous hypertension and neoangiogenesis in response to local thrombosis and hypoperfusion resulting in proliferation of microvascular fistulous networks within the walls of a dural venous sinus [1, 2]. This correlates with findings on gross pathology which demonstrate numerous tiny, hair-like vessels in the sinus wall. Pediatric DAVFs are thought to be congenital or related to birth trauma, infection, or in utero venous thrombosis [7].

Best Imaging Modality

The early diagnosis of DAVFs may be difficult because of their nonspecific clinical and imaging findings. Although the diagnosis of DAVFs has traditionally been by digital subtraction (catheter) angiography (DSA), many of these lesions are now first detected or suspected on cross-sectional imaging [1, 2].

Computed tomography (CT) is often used as an initial screening tool to determine presence of hemorrhage or edema from venous congestion [1, 2].

Magnetic resonance imaging (MRI) is more sensitive for the diagnosis as it readily demonstrates the intracranial vasculature and signs of venous hypertension. Multiplanar images on T1-weighted imaging (T1WI), T2-weighted imaging (T2WI), fluid-attenuated inversion recovery (FLAIR), and susceptibility-weighted imaging (SWI) or gradient-echo T2* sequences are recommended in order to detect the presence of hemorrhage, edema from venous congestion, or signs of venous infarct. Postcontrast imaging is also important to depict engorged vessels, enhancing dural linings of a vein or sinus, as well as filling defects within them [1, 2].

3D time-of-flight (3D TOF) MR angiography (MRA) is limited in the evaluation of DAVFs but can suggest the presence of a lesion, demonstrating abnormal high flow in arteries close to venous structures [8].

Dynamic MRA using time-resolved imaging of contrast kinetics (TRICKS) has an increasing role in DAVF imaging. The dynamic resolution of this modality is adequate for separating early arterial, arterial, parenchymal, and venous phases. However, limitations in spatial resolution hinder its ability to fully characterize lesions for therapeutic purposes [9].

Dynamic-susceptibility contrast MRI perfusion can be a very sensitive for evaluation of impaired venous drainage in the setting of cerebral DAVF and permits quantitative evaluation of multiple perfusion parameters. In patients with high-grade DAVFs, there are increased cerebral brain blood volume values involving the affected cerebral hemisphere secondary to impaired venous drainage. However, the correlation of increased parenchymal perfusion to retrograde cortical venous drainage is controversial [10].

Arterial spin labeling (ASL) is a promising technique for selecting candidates for DSA. It has been reported that the presence of focal high signal on ASL is concerning for a shunt-type lesion. Lesions may be quite small and not appreciated on other imaging sequences, particularly if there is intracranial hemorrhage but they may be clearly identified by ASL [11].

CTA may provide a useful adjunct for treatment planning by defining the location of the arteriovenous shunt relative to the surrounding brain and skull. DAVFs, however, may be obscured by overlapping osseous structures on conventional CTA [12].

The goal of imaging is not only to determine the presence or absence of a DAVF but also to clarify its pattern of venous drainage. Once the morphology and hemodynamics of the lesion are delineated, the need to pursue aggressive therapies can be determined. DSA is the most accurate method for characterization of DAVFs and is generally required to identify the exact fistula site, feeding arteries, and venous outflow pathways. The temporal resolution of DSA and the ability to perform selective injections allow precise identification of early dural venous sinus filling or cortical venous reflux. DSA also provides critical information before endovascular embolization which is the first line of therapy for DAVFs [1, 2, 7].

Major Findings

Parenchymal imaging findings of DAVFs are generally a consequence of venous hypertension, venous congestion and/or infarction, and parenchymal and/or subarachnoid hemorrhage [1, 2].

Edema may be demonstrated on CT, but it is better depicted on MRI (Figs. 11.1 and 11.2). Areas of T2 and FLAIR white matter hyperintensity

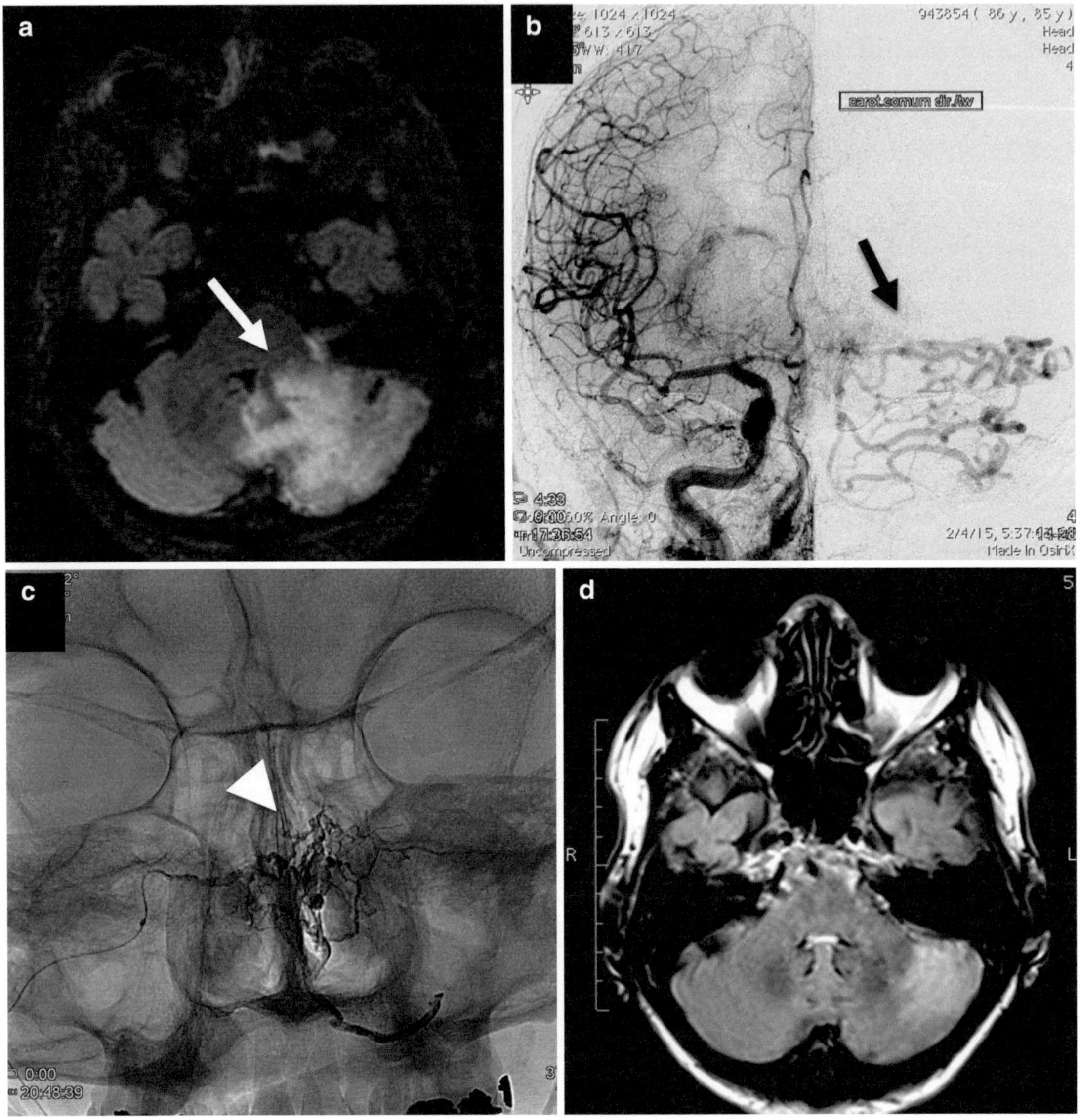

Fig. 11.1 Posterior fossa DAVF. (**a**) Axial FLAIR image shows hyperintenisty in the left cerebellar hemisphere (*white arrow*) with mass effect on the fourth ventricle, due to venous congestion. (**b**) Right common carotid artery DSA reveals enlarged veins (*black arrow*) in the left cerebellar hemisphere consistent with cortical venous reflux. (**c**) Radiograph during embolization of the arteriovenous shunt demonstrates embolic material occluding the vessels to the shunt (*arrowhead*). (**d**) Follow-up axial FLAIR image shows improvement of left cerebellar hemisphere edema after endovascular treatment (Courtesy of Ronie L. Piske, MD, PhD, Hospital Beneficência Portuguesa de São Paulo, Brazil)

with or without restricted diffusion are seen in the setting of venous hypertension and may reverse following treatment [1, 2].

Venous congestion in high-grade lesions may lead to *parenchymal and/or subarachnoid hemorrhage* due to venous rupture and are depicted on CT or MRI (Fig. 11.3). Hemorrhage has variable signal depending on the stage but usually demonstrates "blooming" on SWI and T2* sequences [1, 2, 7].

Engorged vessels close to the meninges or dural sinus walls and dilated venous pouches are

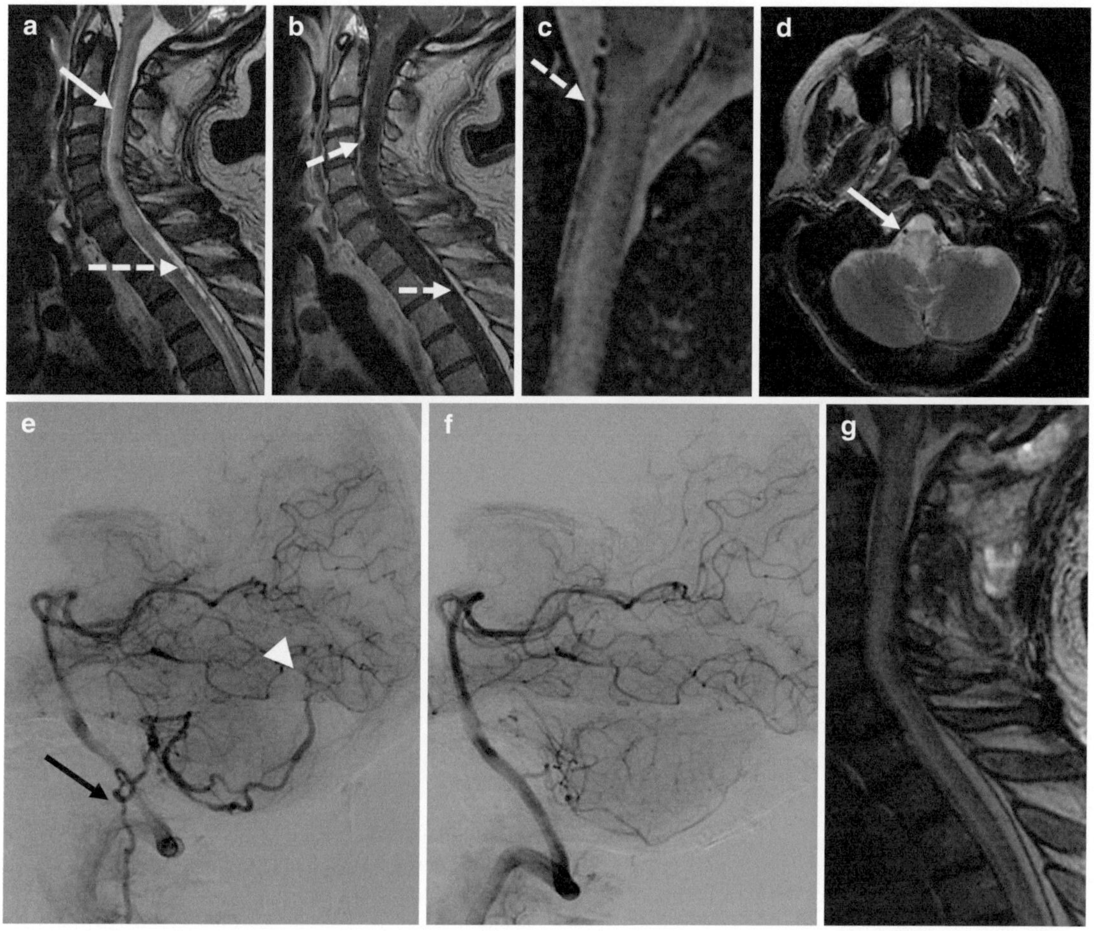

Fig. 11.2 Intracranial dural arteriovenous shunt with spinal cord edema due to venous drainage. Sagittal T2WI (**a**) and postcontrast T1WI (**b**) images of the cervical spine show extensive hyperintensity of the cervical cord consistent with spinal cord edema (*solid arrow* on **a**) and perimedullary venous ectasia (*dashed arrows* on **a** and **b**). Proton density sagittal image (**c**) of the cervical spinal reveals perimedullary venous ectasia (*dashed arrow*). Axial T2WI (**d**) demonstrates that the spinal cord edema extends to the medulla oblongata (*arrow*). Lateral DSA view (**e**) of the left vertebral artery injection before treatment shows an arteriovenous shunt in the posterior fossa (*arrowhead*) draining into perimedullary cervical veins (*arrow*). After surgical treatment, lateral DSA view (**f**) of the left vertebral artery injection reveals complete occlusion of the shunt. Sagittal T2WI image (**g**) of the cervical spine after surgical treatment shows resolution of the perimedullary cervical vein ectasia and near-complete resolution of cord edema (Courtesy of Christopher Ogilvy, MD, Massachusetts General Hospital, Harvard Medical School, Boston)

a result of venous congestion and can be identified as the presence of flow-void clusters on MRI next to the dural sinuses and meninges (Figs. 11.2 and 11.4) and on postcontrast CT and MRI as abnormally prominent vascular enhancement within suspect areas (Fig. 11.3) [1, 2]. There is a significant association between dilated vessels and prominent vascular enhancement with the presence of retrograde cortical vein drainage in DAVFs [13]. CTA and MRA may better depict enlarged veins and feeding arteries as well as a shaggy appearance to the venous sinuses and/or tentorium (Figs. 11.3 and 11.5) [1, 2, 12].

Abnormal signal within veins may be demonstrated on SWI and seen as hyperintense venous signal related to rapid wash-in of oxygenated blood in the setting of arteriovenous shunting [14]. Impaired venous drainage and increased venous

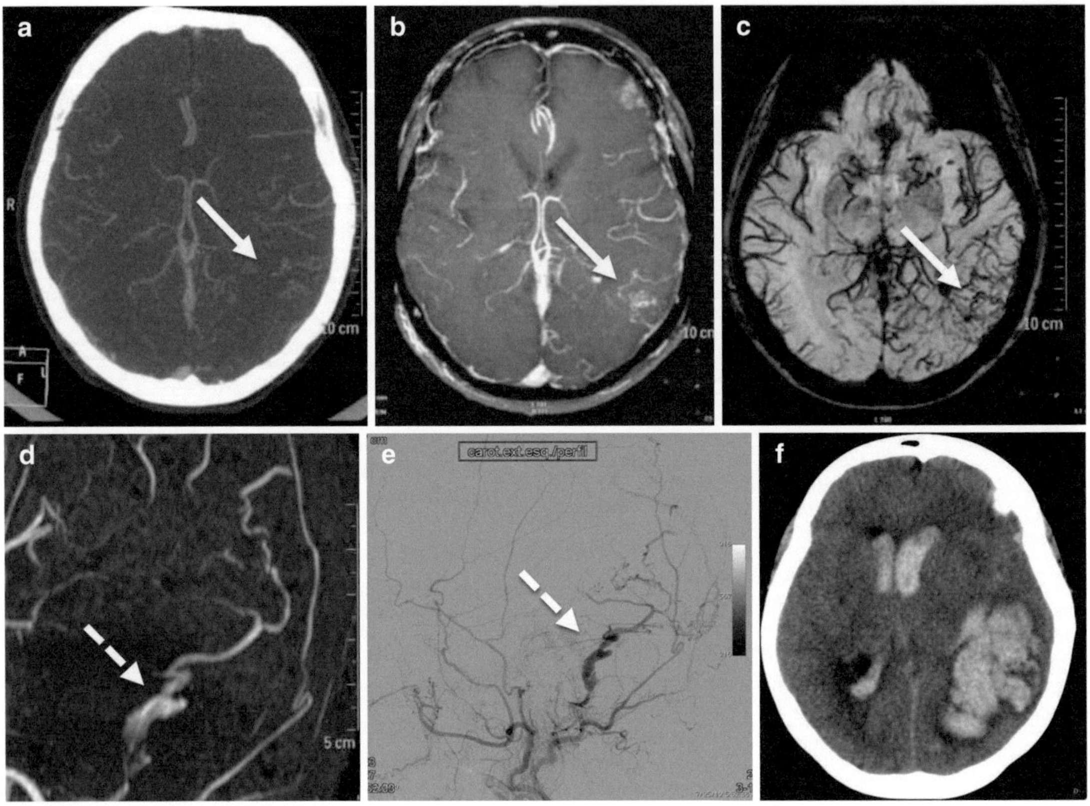

Fig. 11.3 Sigmoid sinus dural arteriovenous shunt. Axial venous phase head CTA (**a**) shows a tangle of vessels in the left temporal lobe (*arrow*). Axial postcontrast T1WI (**b**) and (**c**) SWI images confirm anomalous enlarged cortical vessels (*arrows*). Sagittal magnified TRICKS angiographic image (**d**) reveals the arteriovenous dural shunt (*dashed arrow*) from a branch of the external carotid artery into the sigmoid sinus and cortical venous drainage. Lateral DSA view (**e**) of the left external carotid artery injection shows the arteriovenous shunt between the occipital artery and the sigmoid sinus (*dashed arrow*) with reflux into cortical veins of the temporal and occipital lobes. Follow-up axial CT (**f**) shows intraparenchymal and intraventricular hemorrhage

pressure result in cortical venous engorgement as well as prolonged venous stagnation leading to increased venous oxygen extraction. These factors are thought to result in increased prominence of cortical veins on SWI in the setting of retrograde cortical vein drainage with DAVFs [15]. ASL is also considered very useful for this purpose. The abnormal venous signal on ASL observed in the draining veins of an arteriovenous shunt is related to the blood that bypasses the capillary bed and is shunted directly into veins [11].

Asymmetric contrast opacification of the jugular veins depicted on CTA when associated with other findings described in this chapter has high sensitivity and specificity for the diagnosis of DAVFs in patients with pulsatile tinnitus [12].

DSA defines dural and trans-osseous feeders as well as the venous drainage of DAVFs. Anterograde or retrograde drainage of DAVF (to dural sinuses or cortical veins) can be easily identified in DSA and is important in treatment decision and prognosis (Figs. 11.1, 11.2, 11.3, and 11.4) [1, 2].

CCF imaging findings are also related to the degree of venous congestion, including proptosis, retro-orbital edema, cavernous sinus enlargement, prominent flow voids with strong contrast enhancement, and enlargement of the cavernous sinus(es) and superior ophthalmic vein. Retrograde flow from the cavernous sinus is most commonly into the ophthalmic veins (Figs. 11.5 and 11.6). A direct CCF shows rapid flow with

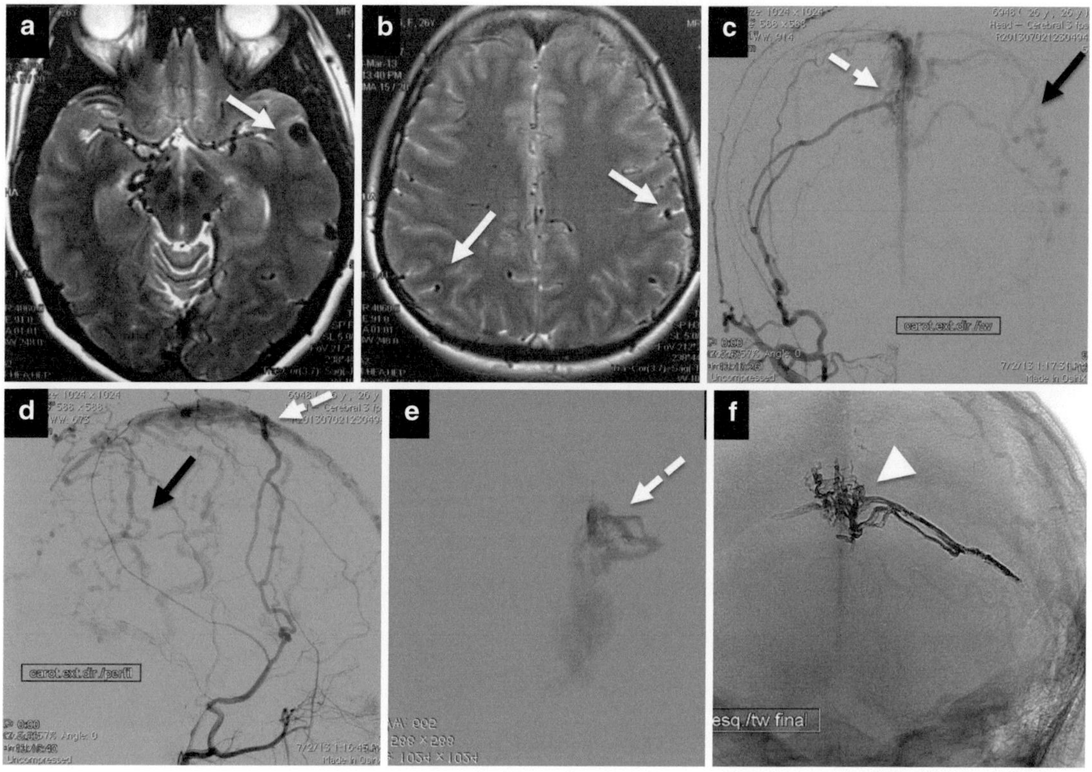

Fig. 11.4 Superior sagittal sinus dural arteriovenous shunt. Brain axial T2WI images (**a**, **b**) show bilateral dilated cortical veins (*arrows*). DSA views of the right external carotid artery injections in anteroposterior (**c**) and lateral (**d**) planes demonstrate the arteriovenous superior sagittal sinus shunt supplied by the right middle meningeal artery (*dashed white arrows*) which drains via the superior sagittal sinus with reflux into cortical veins (*black arrows*) in the opposite cerebral hemisphere due to thrombosis of the superior sagittal sinus. Superselective DSA (**e**) with injection of contrast into a left frontal branch of the middle meningeal artery depicts the shunt (*dashed arrow*). Frontal radiograph of the head (**f**) after injection of the embolic material reveals its cast (*arrowhead*) occluding the arterial and venous connections from the right and left middle meningeal arteries into the superior sagittal sinus resulting in the cure of the fistula

early opacification of cavernous sinus. An indirect CCF typically has multiple feeders from internal carotid artery and dural branches of external carotid artery and shows less prominent findings than a direct fistula [5, 7].

Imaging Follow-Up

In patients with a diagnosis of venous thrombosis, the presence of numerous and dilated cortical veins in the surrounding brain parenchyma should rise the suspicion of venous hypertension/collaterals and may indicate the presence of an underlying DAVF [16, 17].

DAVFs have a poorly understood natural history. Some progress over time and others remain stable for unknown reasons. Hemorrhagic risk is associated with their location and venous drainage pattern. In the presence of cortical venous drainage, the risk of hemorrhage is about 8.1 %/year for symptomatic patients and 1.5 %/year for asymptomatic ones. Without cortical venous drainage, the risk of hemorrhage is extremely low. DSA is the gold standard method for post-treatment follow-up; however, noninvasive methods such as ASL may suffice [1, 11].

On imaging follow-up, resolution of associated brain abnormalities may be appreciated after treatment even in the presence of previously

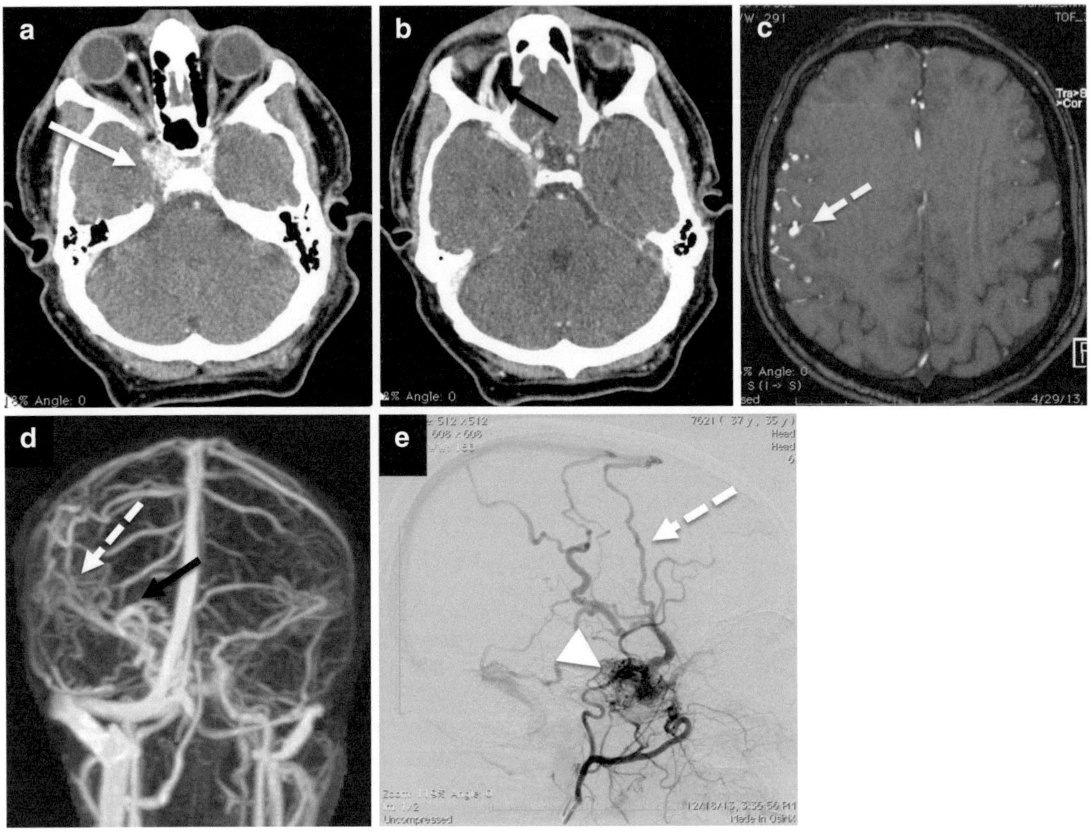

Fig. 11.5 Cavernous sinus dural shunt. Axial postcontrast head CT images (**a**, **b**) show an enlarged right cavernous sinus (*white arrow*) and an enlarged right superior ophthalmic vein (*black arrow*). Axial TOF MRA image (**c**) reveals enlarged cortical veins on the convexity of the right hemisphere (*dashed arrow*). Coronal 3D MRV (**d**) image demonstrates an enlarged right superior ophthalmic vein (*black arrow*) and dilated cortical veins in the right hemisphere (*dashed white arrow*). Lateral DSA view (**e**) of the external carotid artery injection reveals the cavernous sinus arteriovenous shunt (*arrowhead*) draining into the cortical veins (*dashed arrow*)

restricted diffusion [18]. If the first examination showed parenchymal hemorrhage, gliosis and superficial siderosis may be observed on follow-up studies. The presence of large hematomas is a prognostic factor for death or disability [19].

Main Differential Diagnosis

Sinus thrombosis: An isolated thrombosed dural sinus with prominent collateral veins is the major differential diagnosis of a DAVF; however, arterial feeders are absent in isolated venous thrombosis [1].

Other vascular malformations: Prominent vessels may also be seen in arteriovenous malformations (AVMs) and developmental venous anomalies (DVAs). However, AVMs typically present with a nidus which is not seen in DAVFs. A "medusa head" or caput medusa, seen on the venous phase of angiographic studies, is a typical sign of a DVA [1, 7].

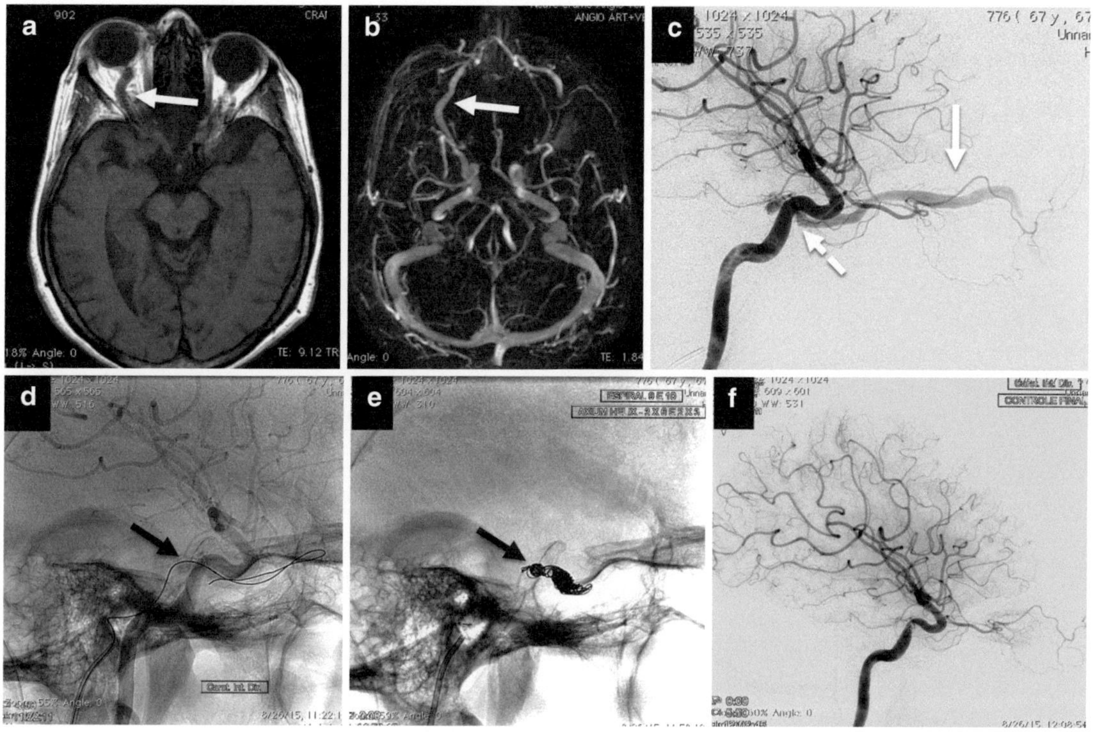

Fig. 11.6 Cavernous sinus dural arteriovenous shunt. Axial T1WI (**a**) and time-resolved contrast-enhanced MRA (**b**) show right proptosis and enlargement of the superior ophthalmic vein (*arrows*). Lateral DSA image (**c**) of the right internal carotid artery injection reveals the arteriovenous shunt adjacent to the cavernous internal carotid artery (*dashed arrow*) and enlargement of the superior ophthalmic vein (*solid arrow*). Non-subtracted DSA lateral images (**d**, **e**) obtained during the neurointerventional procedure performed through the inferior petrous sinus show microcatheterization of the proximal segment of a vein at the site of the arteriovenous shunt (*arrow* on **d**) and coils deployed to occlude the shunt (*arrow* on **e**). DSA lateral image (**f**) of the right internal carotid artery injection confirms complete occlusion of the arteriovenous shunt

Tips

- Patterns of venous drainage are paramount in determining lesion severity and frequently classified using the Cognard system. The direction of dural sinus drainage (antegrade vs. retrograde), presence of cortical venous drainage, and venous outflow architecture all contribute to lesion grading.
- In patients with a diagnosis of venous thrombosis, the presence of numerous and dilated cortical veins in the surrounding brain parenchyma may be related to venous hypertension/collaterals, but when focal, they may indicate the presence of an underlying DAVF.
- Direct CCFs are high-flow lesions which are often devastating lesions that

result from rupture of the cavernous carotid artery typically in the setting of a skull base fractures. They show rapid flow with early opacification of cavernous sinus. A single-hole arterial fistula is often present.

- Indirect CCFs are slow-flow, low-pressure lesions thought to be degenerative in etiology, and their symptoms are often insidious. They typically have multiple feeders from internal carotid artery and dural branches of external carotid artery.
- The diagnosis of DAVFs at an early stage may be difficult because of nonspecific clinical and imaging findings. The presence of venous thrombosis, engorged vessels and dilated venous pouches, abnormal signal within the veins, and asymmetric contrast opacification of the jugular veins should raise suspicion.
- In patients who have equivocal findings for a vascular malformation and who may be poor candidates for DSA, a negative ASL study generally excludes a fistula.

References

1. Gandhi D, Chen J, Pearl M, Huang J, Gemmete JJ, Kathuria S. Intracranial dural arteriovenous fistulas: classification, imaging findings, and treatment. AJNR Am J Neuroradiol. 2012;33(6):1007–13.
2. Miller TR, Gandhi D. Intracranial dural arteriovenous fistulae: clinical presentation and management strategies. Stroke. 2015;46(7):2017–25.
3. Kirsch M, Liebig T, Kuhne D, Henkes H. Endovascular management of dural arteriovenous fistulas of the transverse and sigmoid sinus in 150 patients. Neuroradiology. 2009;51(7):477–83.
4. Morita A, Meyer FB, Nichols DA, Patterson MC. Childhood dural arteriovenous fistulae of the posterior dural sinuses: three case reports and literature review. Neurosurgery. 1995;37(6):1193–9; discussion 9–200.
5. Miller NR. Dural carotid-cavernous fistulas: epidemiology, clinical presentation, and management. Neurosurg Clin N Am. 2012;23(1):179–92.
6. Cognard C, Gobin YP, Pierot L, Bailly AL, Houdart E, Casasco A, et al. Cerebral dural arteriovenous fistulas: clinical and angiographic correlation with a revised classification of venous drainage. Radiology. 1995;194(3):671–80.
7. Mossa-Basha M, Chen J, Gandhi D. Imaging of cerebral arteriovenous malformations and dural arteriovenous fistulas. Neurosurg Clin N Am. 2012;23(1):27–42.
8. Noguchi K, Melhem ER, Kanazawa T, Kubo M, Kuwayama N, Seto H. Intracranial dural arteriovenous fistulas: evaluation with combined 3D time-of-flight MR angiography and MR digital subtraction angiography. AJR Am J Roentgenol. 2004;182(1):183–90.
9. Akiba H, Tamakawa M, Hyodoh H, Hyodoh K, Yama N, Nonaka T, et al. Assessment of dural arteriovenous fistulas of the cavernous sinuses on 3D dynamic MR angiography. AJNR Am J Neuroradiol. 2008;29(9):1652–7.
10. Noguchi K, Kuwayama N, Kubo M, Kamisaki Y, Kameda K, Tomizawa G, et al. Intracranial dural arteriovenous fistula with retrograde cortical venous drainage: use of susceptibility-weighted imaging in combination with dynamic susceptibility contrast imaging. AJNR Am J Neuroradiol. 2010;31(10):1903–10.
11. Alexander M, McTaggart R, Santarelli J, Fischbein N, Marks M, Zaharchuk G, et al. Multimodality evaluation of dural arteriovenous fistula with CT angiography, MR with arterial spin labeling, and digital subtraction angiography: case report. J Neuroimaging. 2014;24(5):520–3.
12. Lee CW, Huang A, Wang YH, Yang CY, Chen YF, Liu HM. Intracranial dural arteriovenous fistulas: diagnosis and evaluation with 64-detector row CT angiography. Radiology. 2010;256(1):219–28.
13. Kwon BJ, Han MH, Kang HS, Chang KH. MR imaging findings of intracranial dural arteriovenous fistulas: relations with venous drainage patterns. AJNR Am J Neuroradiol. 2005;26(10):2500–7.
14. Jagadeesan BD, Delgado Almandoz JE, Moran CJ, Benzinger TL. Accuracy of susceptibility-weighted imaging for the detection of arteriovenous shunting in vascular malformations of the brain. Stroke. 2011;42(1):87–92.
15. Saini J, Thomas B, Bodhey NK, Periakaruppan A, Babulal JM. Susceptibility-weighted imaging in cranial dural arteriovenous fistulas. AJNR Am J Neuroradiol. 2009;30(1):E6.
16. Leach JL, Wolujewicz M, Strub WM. Partially recanalized chronic dural sinus thrombosis: findings on MR imaging, time-of-flight MR venography, and contrast-enhanced MR venography. AJNR Am J Neuroradiol. 2007;28(4):782–9.
17. Gupta A, Periakaruppan A. Intracranial dural arteriovenous fistulas: a review. Indian J Radiol Imaging. 2009;19(1):43–8.
18. Mullins ME, Grant PE, Wang B, Gonzalez RG, Schaefer PW. Parenchymal abnormalities associated with cerebral venous sinus thrombosis: assessment with diffusion-weighted MR imaging. AJNR Am J Neuroradiol. 2004;25(10):1666–75.
19. Ferro JM, Canhao P, Stam J, Bousser MG, Barinagarrementeria F, Investigators I. Prognosis of cerebral vein and dural sinus thrombosis: results of the International Study on Cerebral Vein and Dural Sinus Thrombosis (ISCVT). Stroke J Cereb Circ. 2004;35(3):664–70.

Subarachnoid Hemorrhage

12

Ana Lorena Abello and Renato Hoffmann Nunes

Abstract

Subarachnoid hemorrhage is a condition defined by extravasation of blood into the subarachnoid space. In patients with nontraumatic subarachnoid hemorrhage, the most frequent cause is the rupture of a saccular aneurysm. Non-contrast head computed tomography is the first choice for the diagnosis.

Background

Subarachnoid hemorrhage (SAH) (Fig. 12.1) is a condition defined by extravasation of blood into the subarachnoid space. In patients with nontraumatic SAH, the most frequent cause is the rupture of a saccular aneurysm (aSAH). The incidence of aSAH ranges from 2 to 16 per 100,000 and is highest in Japan and Finland (about 3–5: 100,000 in the United States). It occurs more often in middle-age women, with a 3:2 female-to-male ratio and a peak incidence in the sixth decade of life. The only consistently reported risk factors for SAH are hypertension, smoking, and alcoholism.

The typical presentation of a patient who has aSAH is the paroxysmal onset of a severe diffuse headache accompanied by vomiting and occasionally variable periods of loss of consciousness. The headache often is described as "the worst headache of my life" (thunderclap headache). Patients may develop meningismus, retinal hemorrhages, or focal neurologic signs [1–6].

A.L. Abello, MD (✉)
Department of Radiology, University of North Carolina, Chapel Hill, NC, USA
e-mail: anaabellop@hotmail.com

R. Hoffmann Nunes, MD
Division of Neuroradiology, Santa Casa de São Paulo, São Paulo, Brazil
e-mail: renatohn@hotmail.com

Key Points

Etiology

Aneurysmal subarachnoid hemorrhage: The most frequent type of aneurysms is the saccular aneurysms, which arise at sites of arterial branching, usually at the base of the brain, either in the circle of Willis itself or at a nearby branching point (Fig. 12.2). The formation of aneurysms at

R. Hoffmann Nunes et al. (eds.), *Critical Findings in Neuroradiology*,
DOI 10.1007/978-3-319-27987-9_12

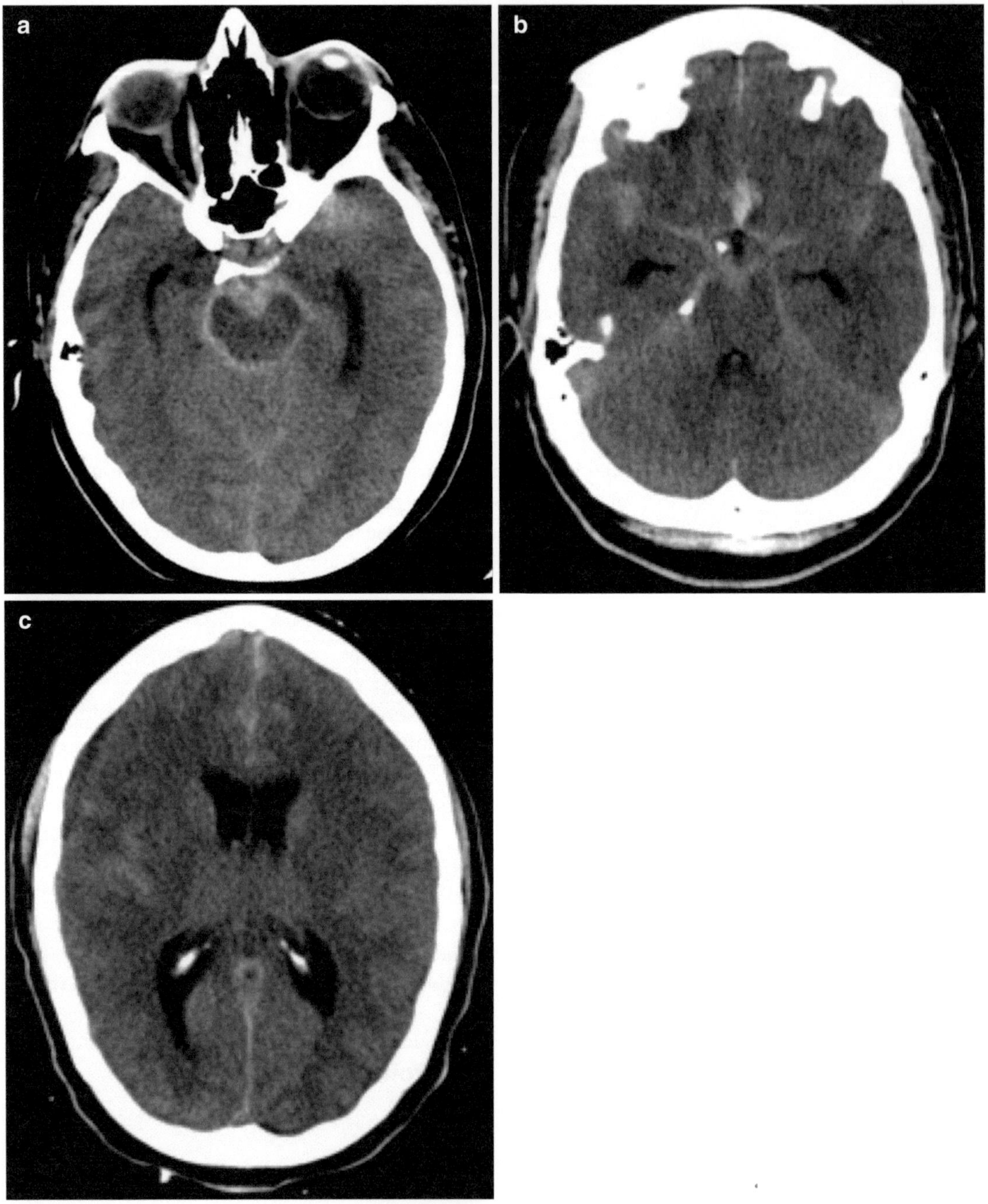

Fig. 12.1 Subarachnoid hemorrhage with hydrocephalus (Fisher-3). (**a**–**c**) Axial non-contrast head CT images reveal hyperdensity along the basal cisterns and fissures with sulci effacement. Hemorrhage is also observed in enlarged ventricles due to hydrocephalus

characteristic locations is the result of the turbulent flow patterns at these locations and possible differences in gene expressions at different arterial sites. Blood blister-like aneurysms are thin-walled hemispheric bulges that, as their name suggests, resemble cutaneous blood blisters in appearance. Fusiform aneurysms are focal dilatations that involve the entire circumference of a vessel, extend for relatively limited distances, and do not arise at branch points.

Perimesencephalic non-aneurysmal subarachnoid hemorrhage: It is much more limited in extent than aSAH and is localized to the interpeduncular, ambiens, and prepontine cisterns (Fig. 12.3). It eventually spreads into the posterior aspect of the suprasellar cistern. It rarely extends into the Sylvian fissures. In nearly, all cases, no cause is found.

Convexity subarachnoid hemorrhage: Convexity subarachnoid hemorrhages (Fig. 12.4) are usually non-aneurysmal, usually mild, and unilateral. The importance of this condition is the lack of sensibility of the CT to detect it. It is estimated that 52 % of cases are missed by CT. Some related causes are amyloid angiopathy, vasculitis, venous thrombosis, and reversible cerebral vasoconstriction syndrome [6–11].

Best Imaging Modality

Non-contrast head computed tomography (CT): Non-contrast head CT is the first choice for the diagnosis (Fig. 12.1). The sensitivity of CT in the first 3 days for SAH is very high (close to 100 %), after which it decreases moderately during the

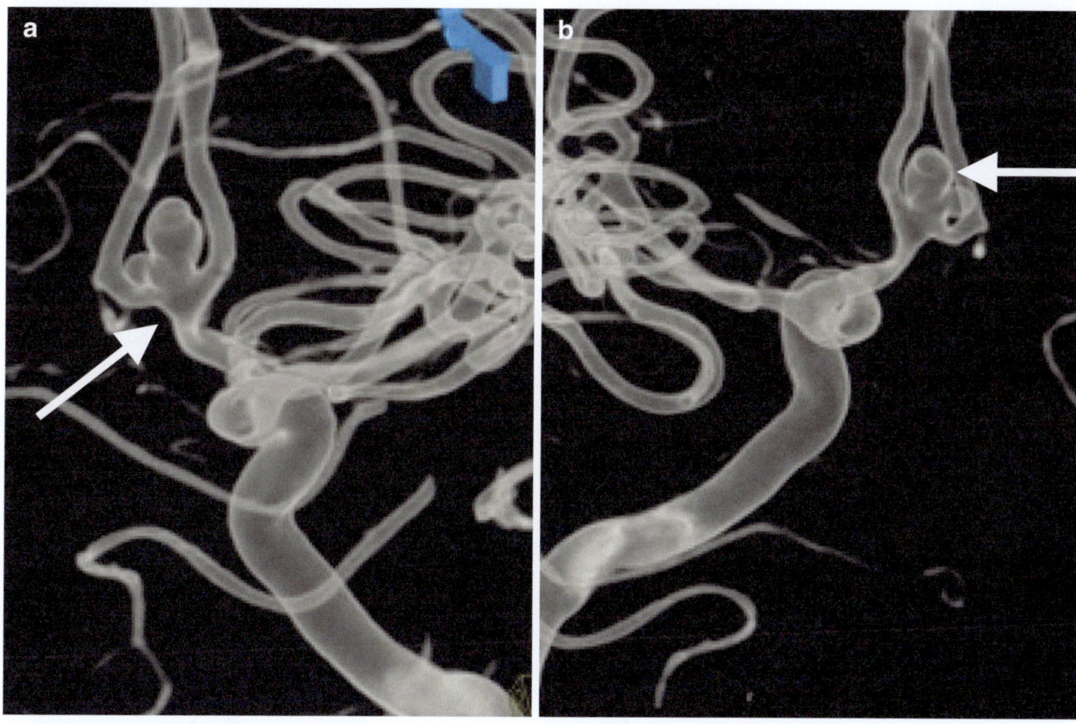

Fig. 12.2 Saccular aneurysm. (**a**, **b**) Reformatted 3D DSA images demonstrate a saccular dilatation in the anterior communicating artery (*arrows*)

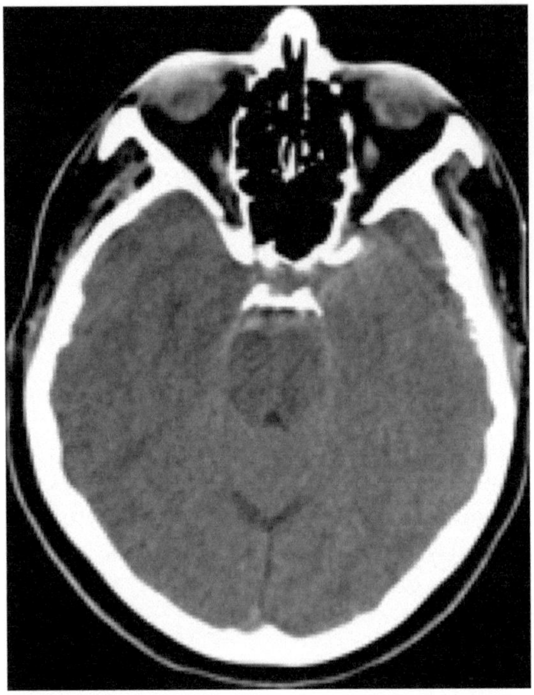

Fig. 12.3 Perimesencephalic non-aneurysmal subarachnoid hemorrhage. Axial non-contrast head CT image reveals hyperdensity restricted to the perimesencephalic cisterns

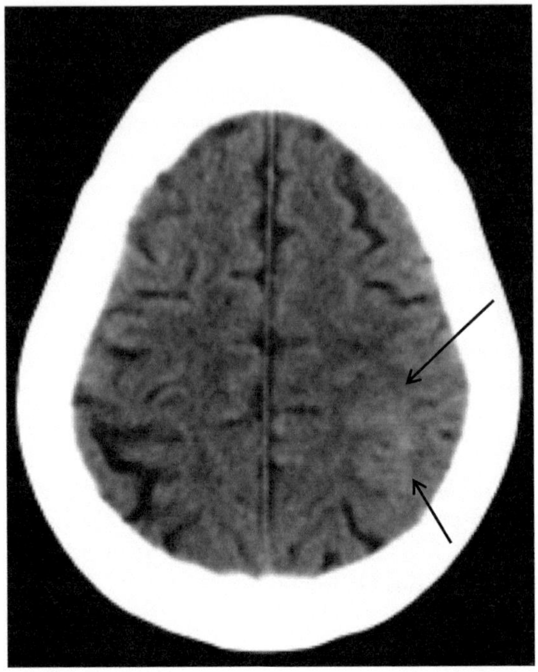

Fig. 12.4 Convexity subarachnoid hemorrhage in a 34 year old female with reversible cerebral vasoconstriction syndrome. Axial non-contrast head CT image demonstrates a hyperdensity (*arrows*) in left fronto-parietal sulci as well as effacement of cortical sulci

next few days. After 5–7 days, the rate of negative CT increases sharply (Fig. 12.4).

Head computed tomography angiography (*CTA*): CTA is recommended for the investigation of the cause and treatment planning (Fig. 12.2).

Magnetic resonance imaging (*MRI*): MRI may be considered in cases when CT is equivocal or in patients with high clinical suspicion of a late-onset SAH (Fig. 12.5) [6–9, 12].

Major Findings

- Hyperdensity within the cisterns at the base of the brain (Figs. 12.1 and 12.3).
- Hyperdensity in the Sylvian fissures and in the superficial sulci overlying more superior aspects of the brain (Figs. 12.1 and 12.4).
- Hydrocephalus is present in many patients (Fig. 12.1).
- The hemorrhage from an intracranial aneurysm may not be confined to the subarachnoid cisterns but can extend into the brain, to the ventricular system, or sometimes to the subdural space, leading to an intraparenchymal or a subdural hematoma that nearly always is accompanied by SAH (Fig. 12.6).
- On MRI, FLAIR is the best sequence to depict aSAH. The change in T1 induced by red cells and by blood serum protein is sufficient to prevent fluid signal suppression. Hyperintense CSF is present in sulci and cisterns in FLAIR (Fig. 12.5). SWI is probably as good as FLAIR, but it is relatively long acquisition time results in motion artifacts in unstable SAH patients [6–9].

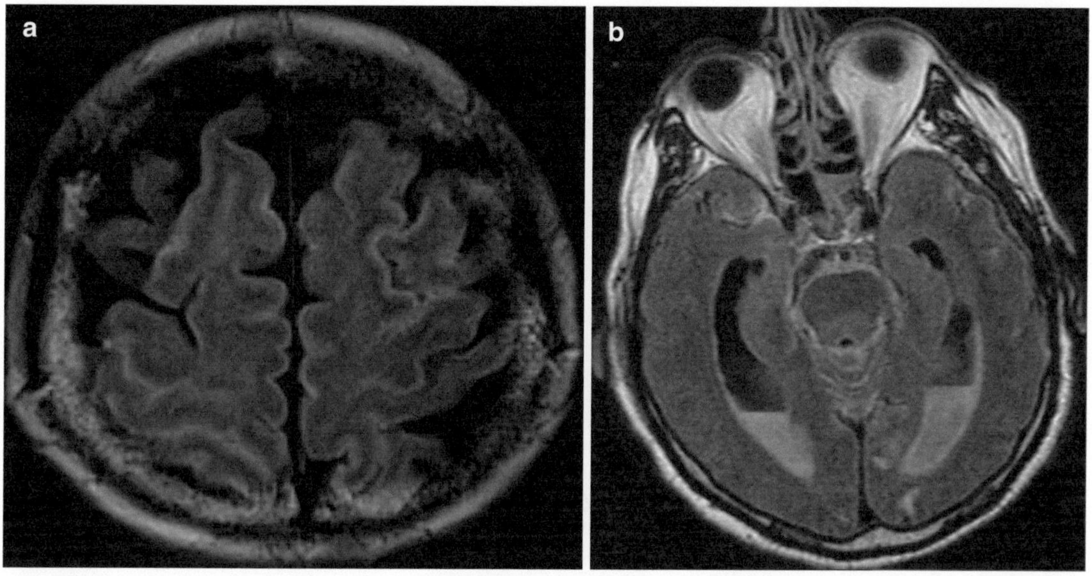

Fig. 12.5 Subarachnoid hemorrhage. (**a**) Axial FLAIR MRI shows hyperintense signal in the frontal and parietal convexity sulci. (**b**) Axial FLAIR MRI reveals hyperintense signal along the cerebellar fissures and in prepontine cisterns. Also note that a fluid–fluid level is demonstrated inside the lateral ventricles, corresponding to intraventricular hemorrhage

Imaging Follow-Up

CT: First choice modality.

- CTA should be the second step investigation of nontraumatic SAH.
  - Positive CTA: aneurysmal subarachnoid hemorrhage
    Consider treatment (endovascular or surgical).
  - Negative CTA:
    DSA is recommended for the diagnosis and, if negative, it should be repeated after 1 and/or 6 weeks.

Special conditions:

- When the hemorrhage is peripherally located (Fig. 12.4), CTA should be carefully scrutinized for vasculitis and DSA is recommended for confirmation.
- In cases when the hemorrhage is confined to the perimesencephalic region and the CTA is negative (Fig. 12.3), DSA may not be needed [12, 13].

Main Differential Diagnosis

- *Pseudo-subarachnoid hemorrhage* is caused by severe cerebral edema. The hypodensity of the brain makes blood in the cerebral arteries and veins to appear dense, mimicking the appearance of SAH.
- *Meningitis* may mimic SAH on FLAIR sequences. SWI may provide information helpful to make this differentiation demonstrating that blood is strikingly hypointense.

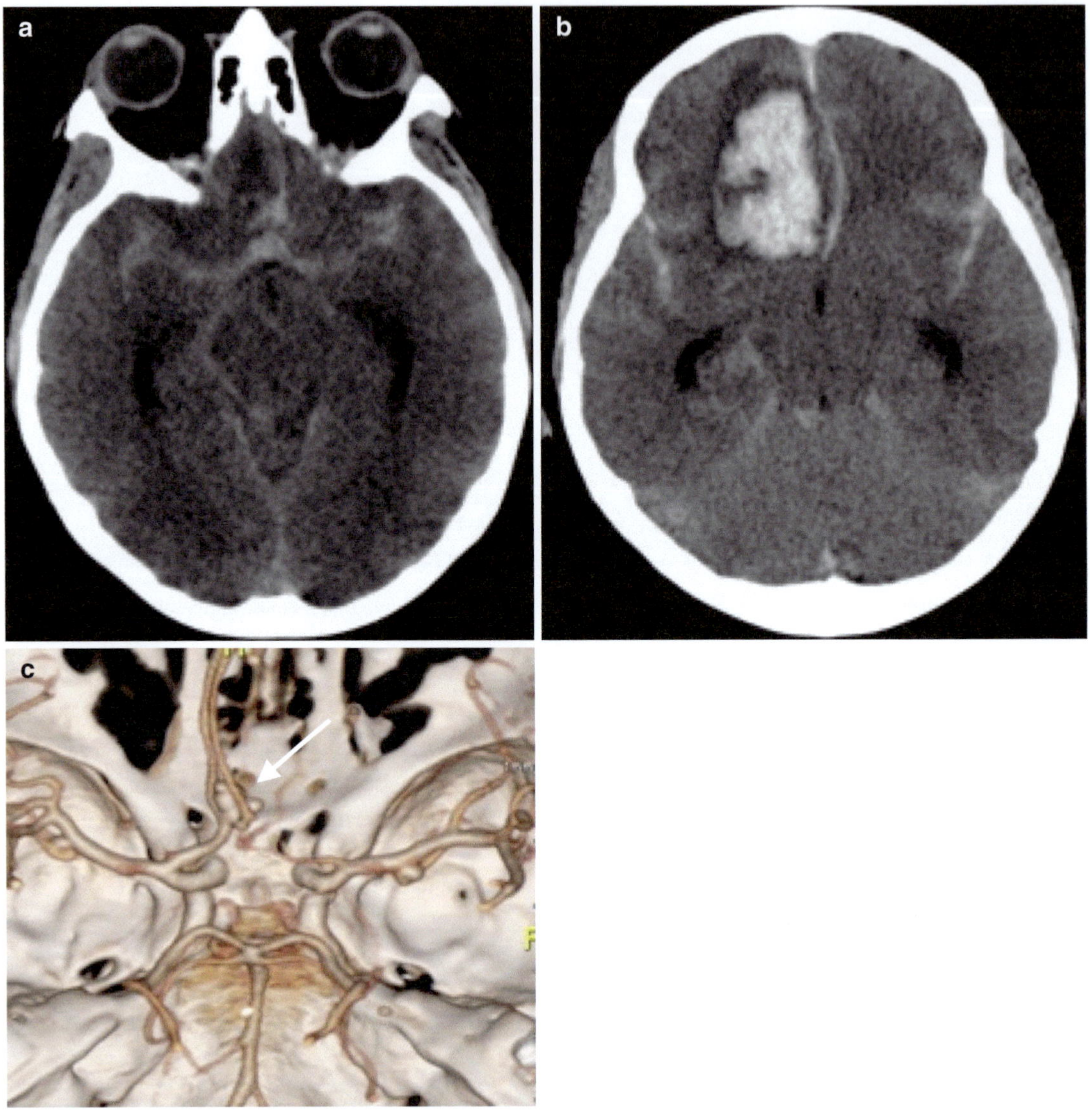

Fig. 12.6 Intraparenchymal hematoma and subarachnoid hemorrhage (Fisher-4). (**a**, **b**) Axial non-contrast head CT reveals a right frontal intraparenchymal hematoma and hyperdensity in the basal cisterns and fissures with sulci effacement. Also note enlarged temporal horns due to hydrocephalus. (**c**) Reformatted 3D CTA demonstrates a saccular dilatation (*arrow*) in the anterior communicating artery

Tips

- *Always mention the amount of blood and its location* (cisterns and fissures involved). The amount of blood seen on the initial head CT is one of the best predictors for vasospasm in SAH. In order to predict prognosis, information must be provided in the report using the Fisher classification, which mainly takes into account the amount of blood and the Hijdra classification, which also considers the number of cisterns and fissures involved.
- *The best well-known classification is the Fisher*: (1) no blood detected on the CT, (2) thin (<1 mm) SAH, (3) thick (>1 mm) SAH or clots, (4) intraparenchymal or intraventricular blood.

- Tips for localizing an aneurysm on the CTA:
  - Look for the most common locations: AComA, MCA, PComA, and the tip of the basilar artery.
  - Pay attention to the vessels that are close to the areas which contain the greater amount of blood.
- In a patient with a posterior fossa nonaneurysmal SAH, it is important to consider vertebral artery dissection as one of the possible causes.
- During the follow-up, look for ischemic areas, related to vasospasm.

References

1. Kwiatkowski T, Alagappan K. Headache. In: Marx J et al., editors. Rosen's emergency medicine: concepts and clinical practice. Philadelphia: Mosby-Elsevier; 2005. p. 1635–7.
2. Feigin VL, Lawes CM, Bennett DA, Barker-Collo SL, Parag V. Worldwide stroke incidence and early case fatality reported in 56 population-based studies: a systematic review. Lancet Neurol. 2009;8:355–69.
3. Linn FHH, Rinkel GJE, Algra A, van Gijn J. Incidence of subarachnoid hemorrhage: role of region, year, and rate of computed tomography: a meta-analysis. Stroke. 1996;27:625–9.
4. Ingall TJ, Wiebers DO. Natural history of subarachnoid hemorrhage. In: Whistnat JP, editor. Stroke: population cohorts and clinical trials. Boston: Butterworth-Heinmann; 1993.
5. Teunissen LL, Rinkel GJE, Algra A, van Gijn J. Risk factors for subarachnoid hemorrhage a systematic review. Stroke. 1996;27:544–9.
6. Edlow JA, Caplan LR. Avoiding pitfalls in the diagnosis of subarachnoid hemorrhage. N Engl J Med. 2000;342:29–36.
7. van Gijn J, Kerr RS, Rinkel GJE. Subarachnoid haemorrhage. Lancet. 2007;369:306–18.
8. Naidich T, Castillo M, Cha S, Smirniotopoulos J. Imaging of the brain. 1st ed. Philadelphia. Saunders an imprint of Elsevier Inc. 2013.
9. Osborn A. Brain: Imaging, pathology, and anatomy. 1st ed. Salt Lake City: Amirsys; 2013.
10. Ducros A. Reversible cerebral vasoconstriction syndrome. Lancet Neurol. 2012;11:906–17.
11. Ducros A, Fiedler U, Porcher R, Boukobza M, Stapf C, Bousser MG. Hemorrhagic manifestations of reversible cerebral vasoconstriction syndrome: frequency, features, and risk factors. Stroke. 2010; 41:2505–11.
12. Cortnum S, Sørensen P, Jorgensen J. Determining the sensitivity of computed tomography scanning in early detection of subarachnoid hemorrhage. Neurosurgery. 2010;66:900–2. 101.
13. Agid R, Andersson T, Almqvist H, Willinsky RA, Lee S-K, TerBrugge KG, Farb RI, Söderman M. Negative CT angiography findings in patients with spontaneous subarachnoid hemorrhage: when is digital subtraction angiography still needed? AJNR Am J Neuroradiol. 2010;31:696–705.

Incorrectly Clipped/Coiled Aneurysms 13

João Maia Jacinto and Isabel Ribeiro Fragata

Abstract

Incorrectly clipped/coiled aneurysms may grow over time and be prone to re-rupture. Aneurysm remnant rupture may cause the same clinical manifestations as untreated lesions and have serious clinical consequences. The most common presentation is also a "thunderclap" headache due to acute subarachnoid hemorrhage.

Imaging follow-up is crucial after surgical or endovascular procedures to confirm aneurysm exclusion. Digital subtraction angiography remains the standard modality for evaluation of both coiled and clipped aneurysms. However, it is increasingly being replaced by noninvasive techniques such as CTA/MRA.

Background

Surgical clipping and endovascular coiling are the two alternatives for treatment of ruptured and unruptured intracranial aneurysms. Follow-up imaging is essential after both treatments. Regarding surgical treatment, incorrectly clipped aneurysms and postoperative remnants occur in about 4–8 % of patients [1], and these may grow over time resulting in rupture and bleeding with a mortality rate of approximately 50 % [2]. Also, endovascular treatment can leave aneurysm remnants in about 20 % [3] of patients leading to retreatment in 10 % of them. Postoperative imaging follow-up is important to confirm aneurysm exclusion and can be important to evaluate complications related to treatment.

Surgical re-intervention and endovascular procedures are valid options to treat incompletely excluded aneurysms. Incompletely clipped or coiled aneurysms may cause the same symptoms as non-treated lesions. Unruptured lesions may be asymptomatic or cause headache and focal neurological deficits, depending on their location. Surgical or endovascular treatment may cause parent vessel occlusion or stenosis and consequently stroke.

The most common presentation of aneurysm re-rupture is severe headache ("thunderclap") with subarachnoid hemorrhage (SAH) [4].

J.M. Jacinto, MD (✉) • I.R. Fragata, MD
Department of Neuroradiology, Centro Hospitalar Lisboa Central, Rua José António Serrano, Lisbon 1150-199, Portugal
e-mail: jnmjacinto@gmail.com; isabelfragata@gmail.com

R. Hoffmann Nunes et al. (eds.), *Critical Findings in Neuroradiology*,
DOI 10.1007/978-3-319-27987-9_13

Key Points

Etiology

Difficult anatomical access and/or surgical approach may lead to suboptimal aneurysm clipping including incomplete neck clipping, wrong positioning of the clip blades (above the neck or involving parent vessels or other adjacent structures), and, if multiple aneurysms exist, clipping of the incorrect one.

Incomplete aneurysm coiling can also occur, leaving a permeable neck or even a dome with residual filling within coil interstices (due to loose packing) or along aneurysm wall. Although rare in small neck aneurysms, a coil loop may externalize into the parent vessel a finding that is generally of no long-term significance for the patient. In ruptured aneurysms with a wide neck, a stent can be used as an adjuvant to coiling, and, in this circumstance, malpositioning or dislocation of the stent may occur.

Best Imaging Modality

Computed tomography (CT) and CT angiography (CTA). Generally performed as the first imaging study on both elective and urgent clinical contexts. In the early perioperative period, both techniques are generally used to determine the cause of acute SAH and assess ischemic lesions, hydrocephalus, and mass effect. For initial diagnosis and evaluation of acute SAH, modern CT scanners have a 100 % accuracy [2]. CTA, with multiplanar reformatted images and 3D volume rendering, has specificity rates of 96–98 % for aneurysms smaller than 3 mm and of 100 % for those larger than 4 mm [2] and may provide effective assessment of surgically treated aneurysms, aneurysmal remnants, and the remainder arterial vasculature. However, very small remnants may be undetectable with this technique. Additionally, metal artifacts may make assessment of adjacent tissues and small residues difficult. Titanium clips produce lesser artifacts than cobalt and stainless steel clips. A clip positioned perpendicular or oblique to the scanning plane produces less artifacts than in-plane clips [5]. Adjusting the window settings may be required to optimize vascular clip visualization. CT and CTA are not useful for follow-up of coiled aneurysms [6]. In fact, the artifact caused by the platinum coils inside the aneurysm renders interpretation of adjacent parenchymal densities almost impossible, and MRI is a preferable technique in this situation.

Magnetic resonance imaging (MRI) and MR angiography (MRA). Both are less useful than CT/CTA since the metal clips (if compatible with MRI) can cause substantial artifacts in the peri-aneurysmal regions. In addition, T1 shortening artifacts caused by spin saturation in associated hematomas (due to presence of methemoglobin) can contaminate time-of-flight (TOF) MRA mimicking the signal intensity of aneurysm remnants [2]. Despite these limitations, MRI is useful to evaluate clinical abnormalities not explained on CT (e.g., diffusion-weighted imaging (DWI) for diagnosis of acute stroke after surgery or endovascular treatment).

Three-dimensional TOF is the most used sequence to detect aneurysms since it provides good spatial resolution (1 mm at 1.5 T and 0.6 mm at 3.0 T MRI) [2, 7]. However, contrast-enhanced MRA may have higher sensitivity than non-contrast time-of-flight MRA especially in partially thrombosed aneurysms where the hyperintensity of thrombus (due to presence of methemoglobin and T1 shortening) may mimic flow [2]. MRI can be safely performed immediately after surgery because most skin sutures and staples are MRI compatible. MRA is preferred to CTA for follow-up imaging of coiled aneurysms. All current coils are compatible with MRI, as well as intracranial stents. TOF MRA is usually good enough for follow-up studies of coiled aneurysms, but if a stent was used, contrast MRA is preferred to compensate for the loss of signal caused by the stent metal struts.

Digital subtraction angiography (DSA). DSA is the gold standard for the evaluation of treated aneurysms both coiled and clipped. Although high-resolution CTA is very sensitive as previously mentioned, it can potentially miss small aneurysm remnants which may be easily seen by DSA [2]. However, DSA is increasingly being replaced by noninvasive techniques in the follow-up of aneurysms and now performed only after diagnosis of a residual/recurrent aneurysm by a noninvasive technique since it carries a small but non-negligible risk of complications such as groin hematoma and even stroke.

Major Findings

Exclusion of an aneurysm from the cerebral circulation is the main goal of both surgical clipping and endovascular treatments. The surgical technique consists of exposing the aneurysm neck and occluding it with a clip. Postsurgical imaging may reveal incorrect positioning of clips. Direct findings include incomplete clipping with the clip blades only partially occluding the neck or the blades positioned above the aneurysmal neck (Fig. 13.1) and/or involving parent vessels or other structures and even clipping of the wrong aneurysm in patients with multiple aneurysms.

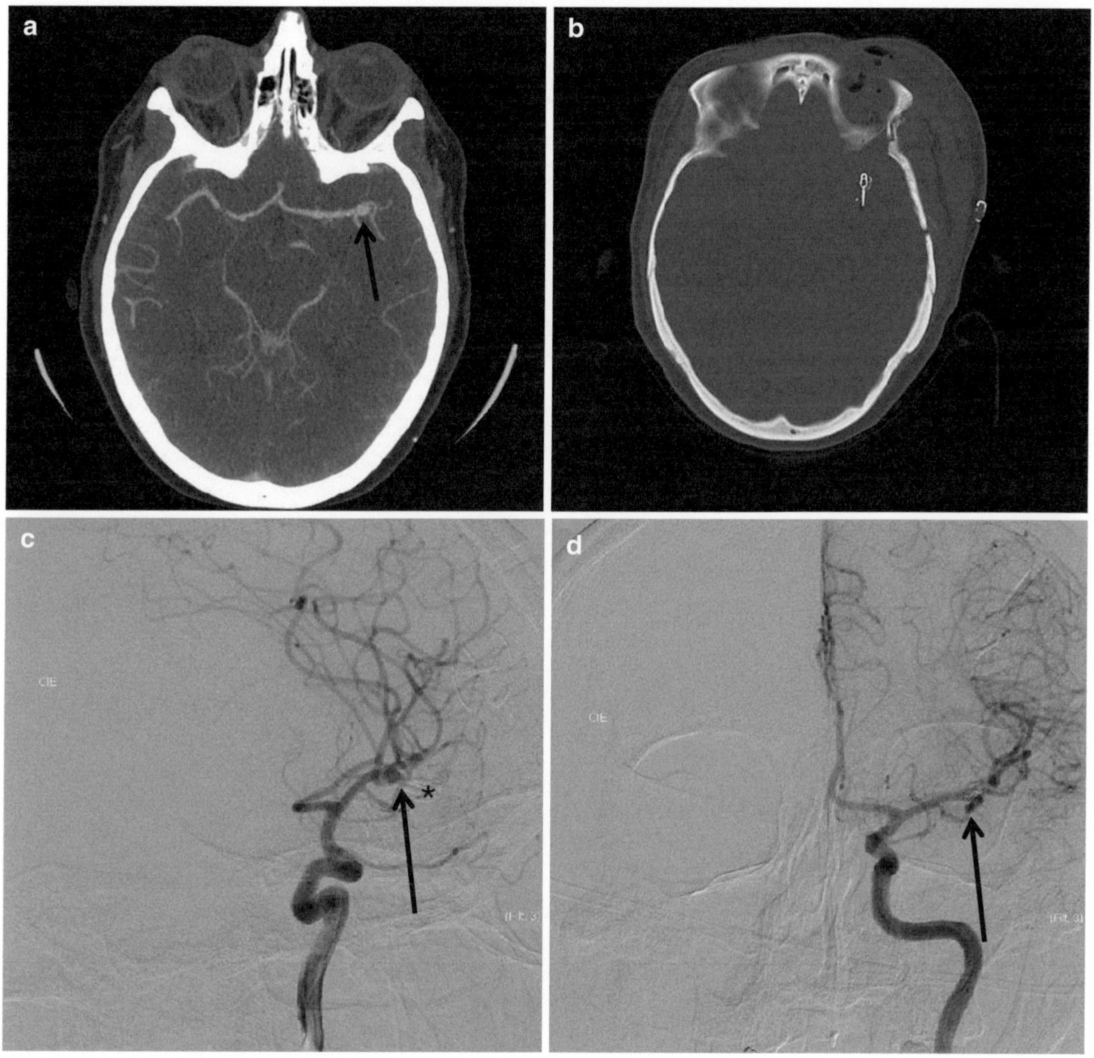

Fig. 13.1 Residual aneurysmal neck. (**a**) Head CTA shows a saccular aneurysm on left middle cerebral artery bifurcation (*arrow*). (**b**) Head CT using bone window settings shows the clip position. (**c**, **d**) Postsurgery DSA (right oblique and AP views) detect a residual neck (*arrows*). The clip position (*) is also appreciated on this study

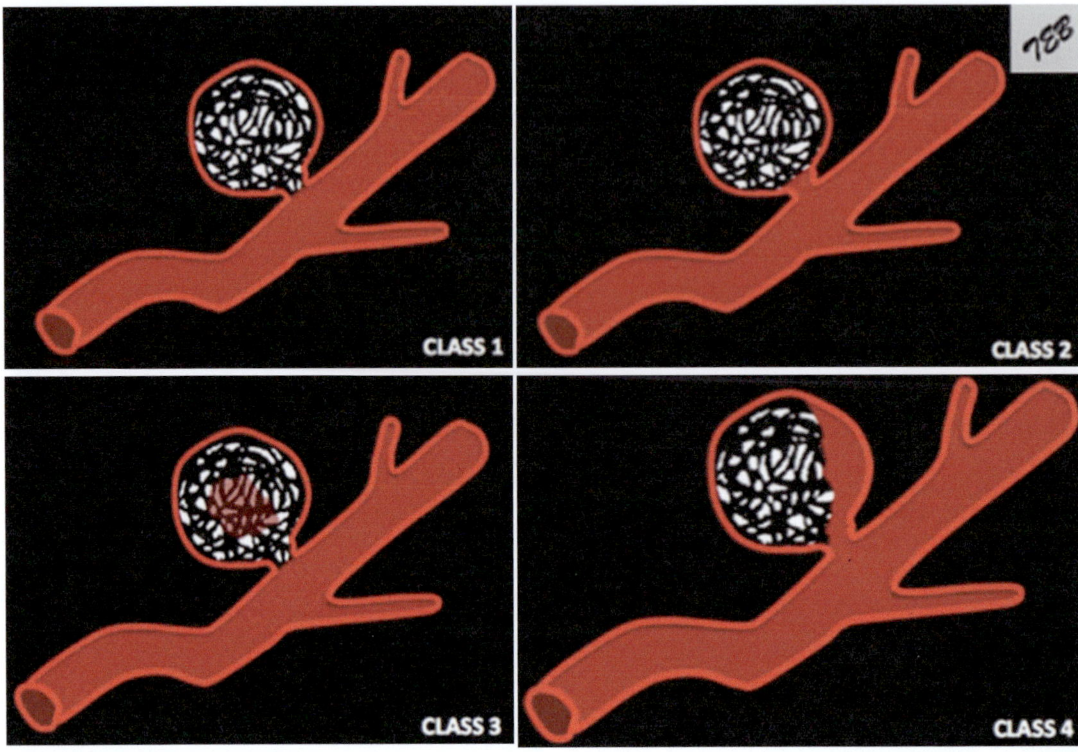

Fig 13.2 Modified Raymond–Roy classification of intracranial aneurysms treated with coil embolization. *Class 1* complete obliteration, *class 2* residual neck, *class 3* residual aneurysm with contrast within coil interstices, *class 4* residual aneurysm with contrast along aneurysm wall (Modified from Mascitelli et al. [9])

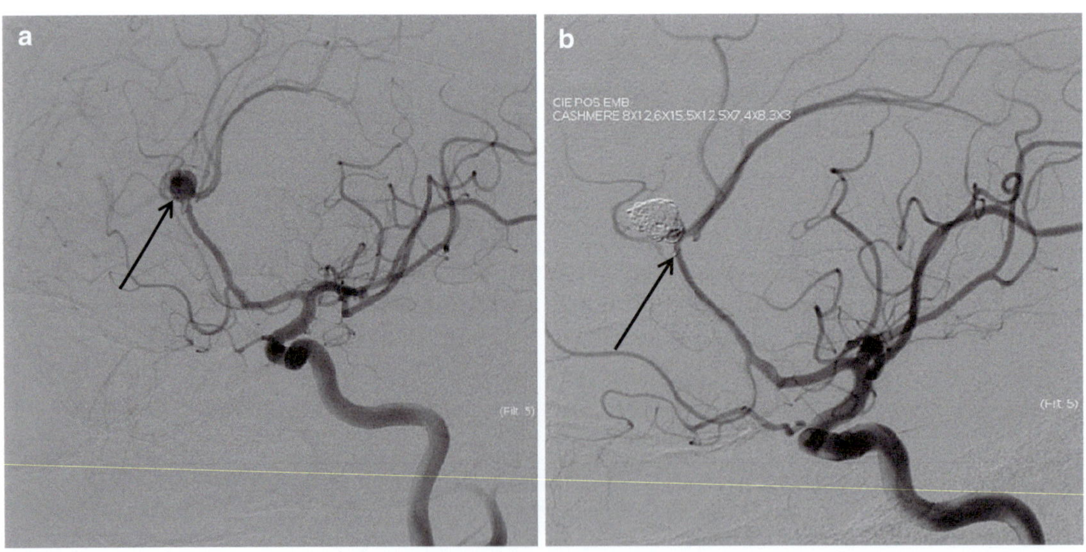

Fig. 13.3 Coil loop outside the aneurysmal sac. (**a**) DSA left oblique view shows a saccular aneurysm which had rupture located at the left anterior cerebral artery (*arrow*). (**b**) The aneurysm was treated with endovascular coils, and a small coil loop is visible outside the aneurysmal sac and inside the parent vessel lumen (*arrow*)

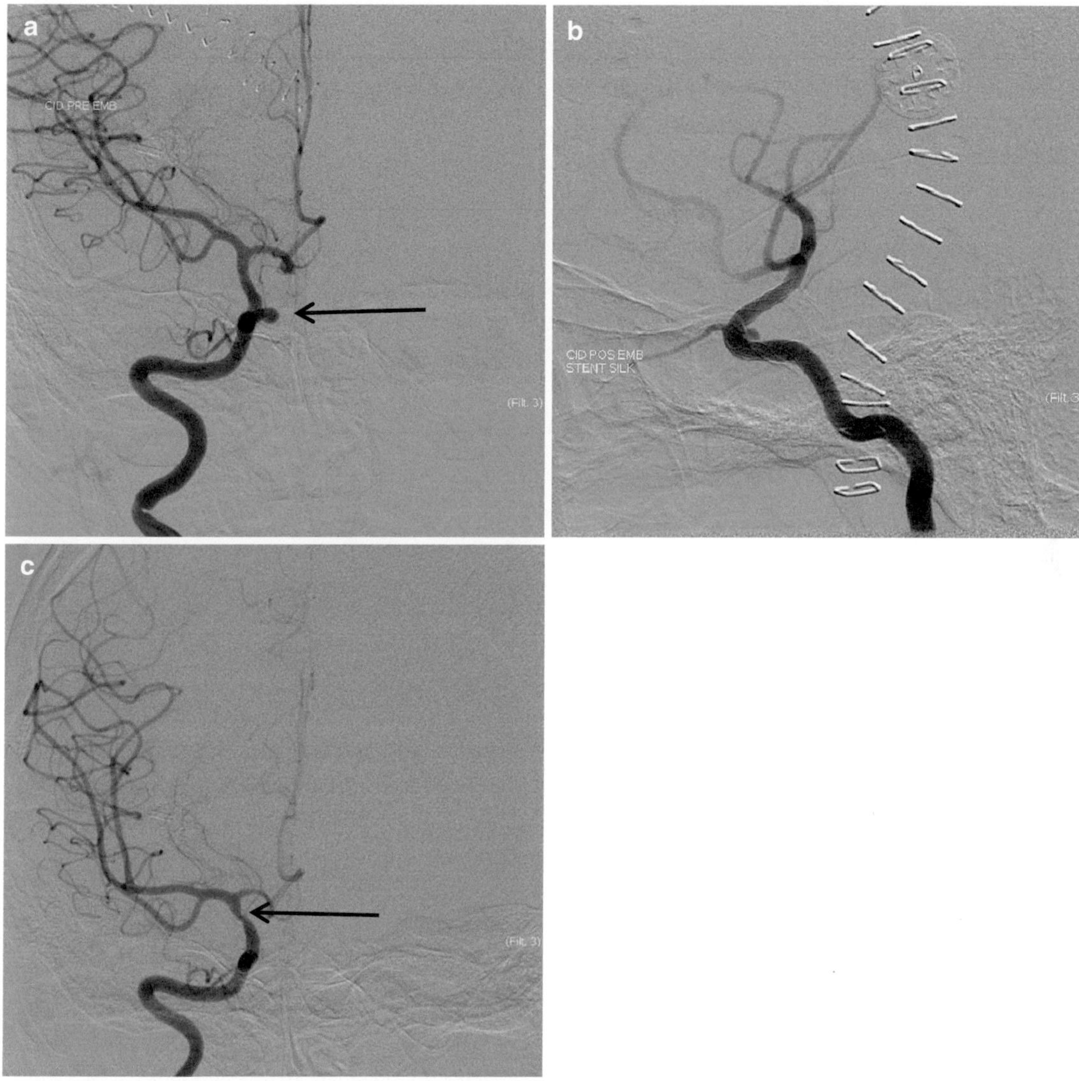

Fig. 13.4 Intimal hyperplasia and stenosis after treatment with stent. (**a**) DSA displays an unruptured paraophtalmic aneurysm (*arrow*). (**b**) DSA after treatment shows a flow diverter stent placed across the neck of the aneurysm in the right internal carotid artery. (**c**) A follow-up DSA was performed 3 months later and shows total obliteration of the aneurysm. Intra-stent stenosis due to intimal hyperplasia (*arrow*) is also visible

The endovascular technique for aneurysm treatment consists, in the majority of patients, in filling the aneurysm sac with platinum coils and obtaining a high metal filling density inside the aneurysm to occlude its lumen. Contrast filling of a part of the previously embolized aneurysm is considered as "partial coiling" and should be mentioned and described in the imaging report. There are a few classifications available, but the Raymond–Roy classification is probably the mostly used version (Fig. 13.2) [8, 9]. In some wide neck aneurysms, a stent covering the neck of the aneurysm is used to secure the coils inside the sac and avoid their extrusion into the vessel lumen (Fig. 13.3). Other posttreatment findings may be seen such as malpositioning/dislocation of the stent and in-stent intimal hyperplasia with parent vessel stenosis (Fig. 13.4).

Imaging Follow-Up

Intraoperative or immediate postoperative imaging is required for clipped aneurysms in order to evaluate the success of the procedure, aneurysm remnants, and patency of the parent vessel.

If complete exclusion of a clipped aneurysm is confirmed in the early postoperative period, recurrence is close to 0 % [10] and usually no further follow-up imaging is required. In case of MRI follow-up, it should not be forgotten that only titanium and titanium alloy clips are entirely safe, due to their total lack of interactions with the magnetic field.

After a successful endovascular procedure, there is a low recurrence rate of aneurysm recanalization and de novo lesions, but contrary to the case of clipped aneurysms, long-term follow-up is usually recommended. At present, TOF MRA and contrast-enhanced MRA are recommended for follow-up of coiled aneurysms. Timing and duration of follow-ups are variable in different centers, but usually at least a 3–6 month, a 12–15-month, and a 24–36-month follow-up are performed [6].

Main Differential Diagnosis

There is no differential diagnosis. Nevertheless, there are some challenging cases, such as patients with multiple intracranial aneurysms in the context of SAH, where it can be difficult to decide which aneurysm ruptured. Additionally, some clips may be positioned close to bone, and evaluation of aneurysm recurrences may be difficult, particularly on CT.

Tips

- It is important to contact the patient's surgeon if one suspects possible incorrect aneurysm clipping with or without associated clinical symptoms since it might need treatment.
- Mention and measure all aneurysm remnants; try to describe the clip position and its relation with parent vessels and other neighboring intracranial structures.
- In case of endovascular coiling, look for aneurysm remnants, use scales such as the modified Raymond–Roy scale to quantify these remnants, and also report malpositioned coils or vessel stenosis.
- If a stent was used, look for stenosis of the parent vessel, sometimes due to intimal hyperplasia. CTA can show malpositioning of the stent struts and kinking/non-apposition of the stent to the vessel walls.
- Characterize other aneurysms, known or de novo, and compare them to previous imaging studies to assess any change especially growth.

References

1. Mangiafico S, Cellerini M, Villa G, et al. Endovascular coiling of aneurysm remnants after clipping in patients with follow-up – a single center experience. Interv Neuroradiol. 2005;11:41–8.
2. Hacein-Bey L, Provenzale J. Current imaging assessment and treatment of intracranial aneurysms. Am J Roentgenol. 2011;196:32–44.
3. Ferns SP, Sprengers ME, van Rooij WJ, et al. Coiling of intracranial aneurysms: a systematic review on initial occlusion and reopening and retreatment rates. Stroke. 2009;40:e523–9.
4. Osborn AG. Osborn's brain: imaging, pathology, and anatomy. 1st ed. Salt Lake City: Amirsys; 2013. p. XI. 1272 p.
5. Wallace R, Karis JP, Partovi S, et al. Noninvasive imaging of treated cerebral aneuryms, part II: CT angiographic follow-up of surgically clipped aneurysms. AJNR. 2007;28:1207–12.
6. Wallace R, Karis JP, Partovi S, et al. Noninvasive imaging of treated cerebral aneuryms, part I: MR angiographic follow-up of coiled aneurysms. AJNR. 2007;28:1001–8.
7. Shellock FG, Tkach JA, Ruggieri PM, et al. Aneurysm clips: evaluation of magnetic field interactions and translational attraction by use of 'Long-Bore' and 'Short-Bore' 3.0T MR imaging systems. AJNR. 2003;24:463–71.

8. Roy D, Milot G, Raymond J. Endovascular treatment of unruptured aneurysms. Stroke. 2001;32: 1998–2004.
9. Mascitelli JR, Moyle H, Oermann EK, et al. An update to the Raymond-Roy occlusion classification of intracranial aneurysms treated with coil embolization. J Neurointerv Surg. 2015;7(7):496–502.
10. Tsutsumi K, et al. Risk of aneurysm recurrence in patients with clipped cerebral aneurysms. Stroke. 2011;32:1191–4.

Brain Death

14

Jaime Leal Pamplona, Ana Maria Braz, and Renato Hoffmann Nunes

Abstract

Brain death refers to the irreversible cessation of brain function and is usually clinically determined. Brain death is a legal definition that incorporates different medical parameters in different locations. The three essential findings are coma, absence of brainstem reflexes, and apnea. However, diagnostic criteria of brain death vary widely among countries. In some countries, imaging studies are exclusively used as ancillary tools, while in other countries they must be obtained to determine the diagnosis of brain death.

Background

Brain death is a clinical expression of a generalized irreparable brain damage characterized by irreversible coma, absent brainstem reflexes, and apnea [1–3]. The etiologies of brain death differ between adults and children, but overall traumatic brain injury is the main cause [3]. There is a clear difference between severe brain damage and brain death. Brain death means that life support is futile and represents the principal prerequisite for the donation of organs for transplantation [4]. Since the 1950s, there has been a constant refinement of guidelines to achieve the correct diagnosis of brain death, and today with the increasing demand for organs for transplantation, a rapid and accurate diagnosis of brain death is more important than ever [3, 4]. In some countries (e.g., USA, England, Canada) the diagnosis of brain death is based on clinical criteria and an apnea test, but ancillary or confirmatory tests may be used when uncertainty exists about the reliability of the neurologic examination or when the apnea test cannot be correctly performed [4]. Conversely, in other countries, at least one of these ancillary tests is mandatory for the diagnosis of brain death. Despite the brain death criteria used, a patient properly determined to be brain dead is legally and clinically dead [1, 3, 4].

Determination of brain death relies first on clinical evaluation, neurologic examination, apnea test, and, if indicated, ancillary tests [1] as follows:

J.L. Pamplona, MSc, MD (✉) • A.M. Braz, MD
Centro Hospitalar Lisboa Central, Lisbon, Portugal
e-mail: jaime.rlpamplona@gmail.com; amfbraz@gmail.com

R. Hoffmann Nunes, MD
Division of Neuroradiology,
Santa Casa de São Paulo, São Paulo, Brazil
e-mail: renatohn@hotmail.com

R. Hoffmann Nunes et al. (eds.), *Critical Findings in Neuroradiology*,
DOI 10.1007/978-3-319-27987-9_14

Clinical evaluation:

- The first step in clinical evaluation is to establish and document the irreversibility of the brain injury. Potentially reversible causes of apparent marked depression of consciousness, such as drugs or any pathologic disturbances that may mimic brain death must be ruled out [1, 3, 4].

Neurologic exam:

- Establish coma – Lack of consciousness and unresponsiveness to noxious stimuli reflect severe brain dysfunction above the brainstem. Assessment of consciousness or responsiveness may be done initially by using the Glasgow Coma Scale (GCS). A score of 3 (no eye opening, no verbal response, or movement either spontaneously or in response to stimulation thus, the lowest possible) indicates complete loss of consciousness or responsiveness [1, 5].
- Establish absence of brainstem reflexes – Brainstem function is determined by assessing pupil size, reactivity, and other reflexes mediated by the brainstem including oculocephalic, oculovestibular, corneal, cough, and gag reflexes [1, 5]. Facial trauma and/or drugs may compromise the ability to perform an optimal cranial nerve examination [4, 5].
- Establish absence of any motor response – Patients' movements in brain death may be confounding factors in clinical evaluation. Movements in the brain dead may be due to complex spinal reflexes or ventilator auto triggering [5].

Apnea test: The apnea test is usually performed after a second examination of brainstem reflexes [1, 6]. It demonstrates absence of respiratory drive in the presence of hypercapnia. Patient body temperature has to be above 36 °C and systolic blood pressure above 100 mmHg to perform the apnea test.

Ancillary tests: If the apnea test is not tolerated, the results are inconclusive, or shorter intervals are required between initiation and completion of a brain death protocol; ancillary tests may be appropriate. Ancillary tests include cerebral catheter angiography, transcranial Doppler ultrasonography, computed tomography angiography (CTA), magnetic resonance angiography (MRA), electroencephalography, and cerebral scintigraphy [1–3].

Key Points

Etiology

In adults, the main causes of brain death include traumatic brain injury, subarachnoid hemorrhage, and cardiac arrest. In children, non-accidental trauma, motor vehicle accidents, and asphyxia (especially drowning) account for the major causes [3].

Terminal brainstem herniation is often the final stage in refractory brain injury caused by trauma, ischemia or infarction, hemorrhage, intracranial tumors, or infectious processes. Terminal brainstem dysfunction can also be caused by neuronal death induced by anoxic or ischemic injury after cardiopulmonary arrest [5]. Rapid progression of brain edema with associated increased intracranial pressure leads to cerebral cortex compression and microvascular blood flow impairment with consequent cortical dysfunction as evidenced by progressive loss of consciousness. Further progression of the process may lead to pathological posturing and/or seizure activity and finally transtentorial herniation with distortion of the posterior fossa and brainstem displacement through the foramen magnum [5]. Brainstem distortion results in a hypertensive state that reflects a reflex response to maintain brain perfusion. Finally, brainstem dysfunction, with total loss of catecholamine regulation, causes loss of sympathetic control ending with hypotension and loss of vasomotor tone [5].

Best Imaging Modality

The diagnosis of brain death is a clinical diagnosis, which means that ancillary tests should be used when the apnea test cannot be performed or when it is impossible to rely on the neurologic

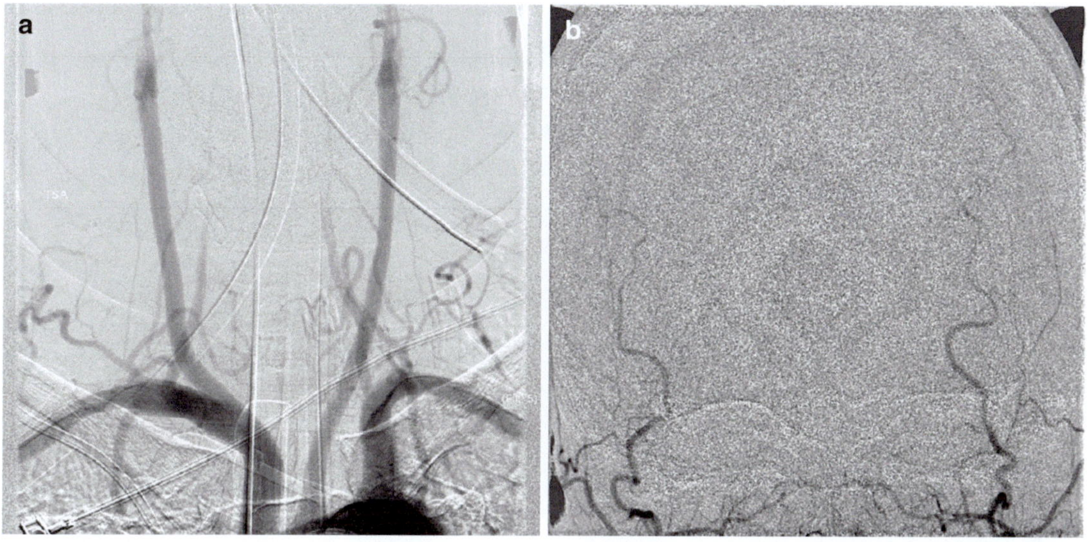

Fig. 14.1 Brain death demonstrated on digital subtraction catheter angiography. (**a**) AP view angiogram of supra-aortic vessels show bilateral filling of the common and external carotid arteries, vertebral arteries, and proximal cervical segment of the internal carotid arteries. (**b**) AP view the head reveals no filling of the intracranial arteries (anterior and posterior circulation) but patency of both external carotid arteries

examination [2]. There is a worldwide controversy about the newer ancillary tests, and there is still insufficient evidence on some emerging tests that can be used to confirm the diagnosis of brain death.

Ancillary Tests

Ancillary tests can be divided into those that demonstrate loss of bioelectrical activity and those that show absence of cerebral blood flow (CBF). To demonstrate loss of bioelectrical activity, electroencephalography is the most used test. To confirm absence of CBF, cerebral catheter angiography, CTA, MRA, MRI perfusion, and nuclear medicine are the most reliable methods [7].

Cerebral catheter angiography or digital subtraction angiography is an imaging modality that has traditionally been used to diagnose brain death (Fig. 14.1) [2, 8]. Anterior and posterior circulations should be accessed by performing separate contrast injections in both common carotid and both vertebral arteries not in the aortic arch [8]. A delayed venous phase should be assessed to assure that there is no delay filling of intradural segments of internal carotid and vertebral arteries. Similar

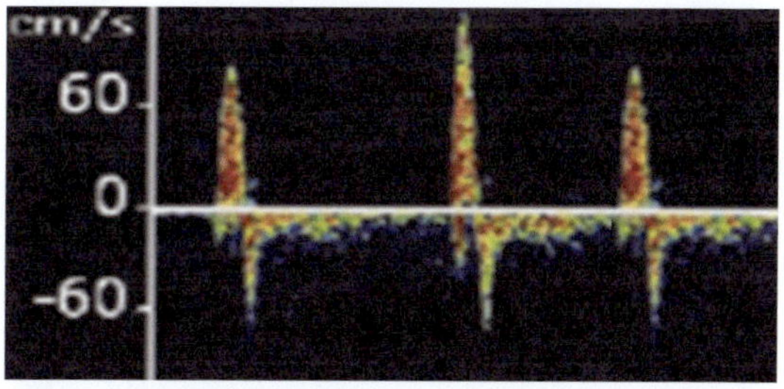

Fig. 14.2 Brain death signs demonstrated on transcranial Doppler ultrasound: insonation via trans-temporal window for the middle cerebral artery. Figure (**a**) depicts reverberating flow, anterograde in systole and retrograde in diastole characteristic of brain death

findings can be expected using CTA, MRA, and even CT or MRI perfusion-based techniques [2, 8].

Transcranial Doppler ultrasonography is a simple but limited method to assess intracranial vascularization. Bilateral insonation should always be done via temporal bone windows and the suboccipital transcranial window to assess anterior and posterior circulations respectively. In absence of signal, insonation through the orbital window should be considered (Fig. 14.2) [9].

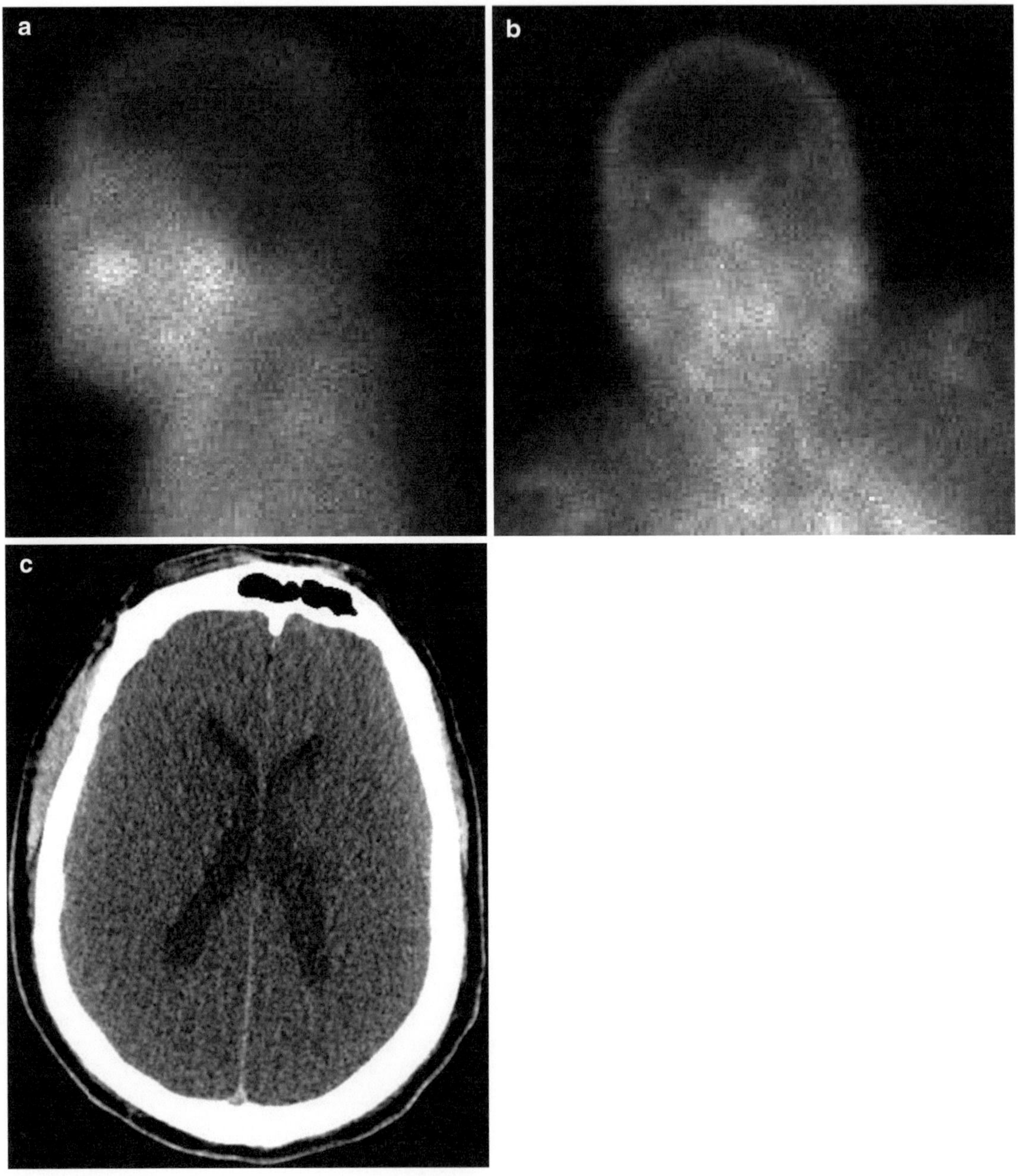

Fig. 14.3 Brain death signs demonstrated on cerebral scintigraphy and CT. (**a**) Anteroposterior and (**b**) lateral views reveal the characteristic empty skull phenomenon that represents absence of radionuclide in all cerebral vascular territories. (**c**) The axial non-contrast enhancement brain CT in the same patient shows diffuse brain edema and swelling with sulci effacement and loss of the normal differentiation between gray and white matter

Cerebral scintigraphy is less invasive than catheter angiography and more accurate than ultrasound. Several 99mTc-labeled agents may be used, brain-specific agents as 99mTc-HMPAO and 99mTc-ECD and non-brain-binding agent such as 99mTc-DTPA (Fig. 14.3) [10]. The isotope should be injected, and images of the head should be obtained in three different time points: immediately, at 30–60 min and after 2 h [10].

Electroencephalography is used in most countries; it remains the most well-validated ancillary test. It is noninvasive, easily performed at bedside, and with quickly available results [11]. Full diagnostic EEG with a minimum of eight scalp electrodes should be used [1]. The device sensitivity should be ≥2 μV and tracing ≥30 min. Tracing is evaluated in response to visual/auditory stimulation [11].

Emerging ancillary test (currently there are insufficient levels of evidence for these techniques):

Magnetic resonance imaging and magnetic resonance angiography (*MRI/MRA*) are used to document the lack of intracerebral blood flow and also to assess parenchymal lesions (Figs. 14.4, 14.5, 14.6, and 14.7) [12]. To study brain lesions and the related mass effect, a standard brain protocol is performed, including T1-weighted and T2-weighted sequences in the axial plane. Advanced magnetic resonance imaging techniques, including diffusion (DWI), spectroscopy (MRS), and perfusion, may also be performed. To access the blood flow, an MRA must be performed using phase-contrast angiography, contrast-enhanced angiography, or time-of-flight (TOF) angiography. The latter is the most commonly used [12].

CTA is a widely available technique that is less invasive and faster than catheter angiography in accessing intracranial blood flow. Three different acquisitions may be obtained, starting at the C1–C2 level and extending to the convexities. A nonionic contrast medium should be injected through a peripheral vein using a power injector, and early arterial and delayed venous phases need to be acquired [13].

Somatosensory evoked potentials (*EPs*) and *bispectral index* are also used, but a description of them is beyond the scope of this text.

Major Findings

Cerebral catheter angiography shows absence of intracerebral filling at the level of skull entry of the internal carotid and vertebral arteries. The internal carotid and vertebral arteries should fill until they pierce the dura without any filling thereafter. The external carotid arteries should be patent. Delay filling of the superior longitudinal sinus may be seen [2, 8].

Transcranial Doppler ultrasonography may show: (1) brief systolic forward flow or systolic spikes and diastolic reverse flow, (2) brief systolic forward flow or systolic spikes and no diastolic flow, (3) or no demonstrable flow in a patient in whom flow was previously evident on Doppler images [3].

Cerebral scintigraphy shows the characteristic empty skull phenomenon defined as no uptake of radionuclide in all cerebral artery territories (basilar artery, middle, anterior, and posterior cerebral arteries) [10].

Electroencephalography shows no electrical activity during at least 30 min after intense somatosensory or audiovisual stimuli [11].

MRA demonstrates absence of intracranial (anterior and posterior) circulation perfusion with preservation of external carotid artery perfusion [1, 12].

Pitfalls

- On TOF imaging, slow flow, in-plane flow, and non-laminar flow may be incorrectly interpreted as absence of flow [1, 12].
- There are not enough studies in the literature using contrast-enhanced MRA to confirm its utility [1, 12].

CTA shows a strong correlation with results of four-vessel angiography with absence of contrast filling of intracranial anterior and posterior circulation arteries and patency of the external carotid arteries (Fig. 14.8) [1].

Pitfalls

- There are studies that show intracranial opacification of blood vessels in CTA in patients who fulfill the EEG and cerebral catheter angiography criteria for brain death [1].
- This delayed, weak, and persistent opacification of the proximal segments of the cerebral

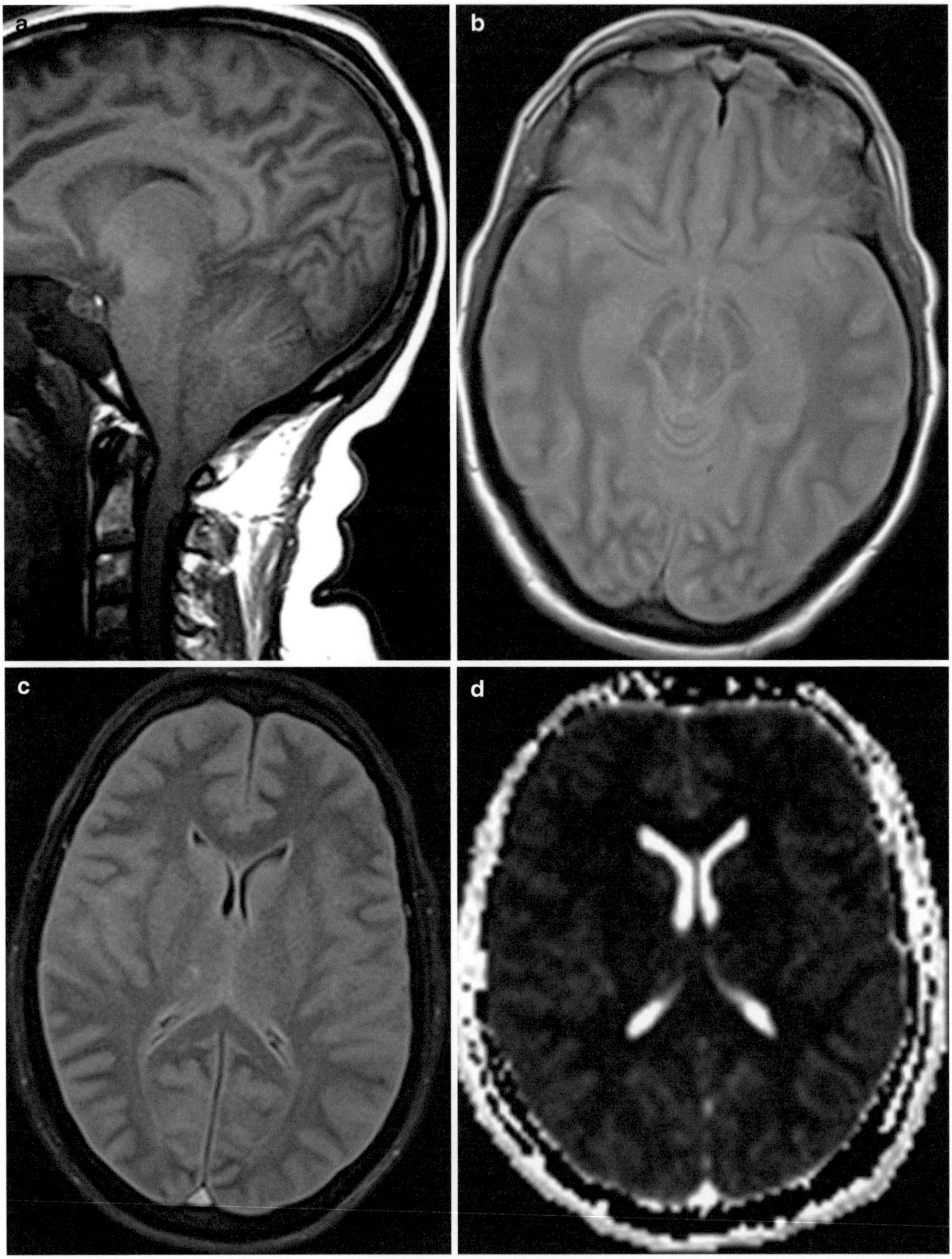

Fig. 14.4 Brain death signs demonstrated on MRI. (**a**) Sagittal T1WI shows downward displacement of diencephalon, brainstem, and cerebellum; lack of cortical sulci and cerebellar fissures; and obliteration of all basal cisterns and of the infratentorial ventricular system. (**b**) Axial proton density image depicts absence of flow voids in the middle, anterior, and posterior cerebral arteries. (**c**) Axial FLAIR reveals diffuse brain swelling, gyral swelling, and diffuse gray matter high signal intensity. (**d**) Axial apparent diffusion coefficient (*ADC*) map shows severe drop in the values of ADC more pronounced in the white matter compatible with early subacute diffuse ischemia

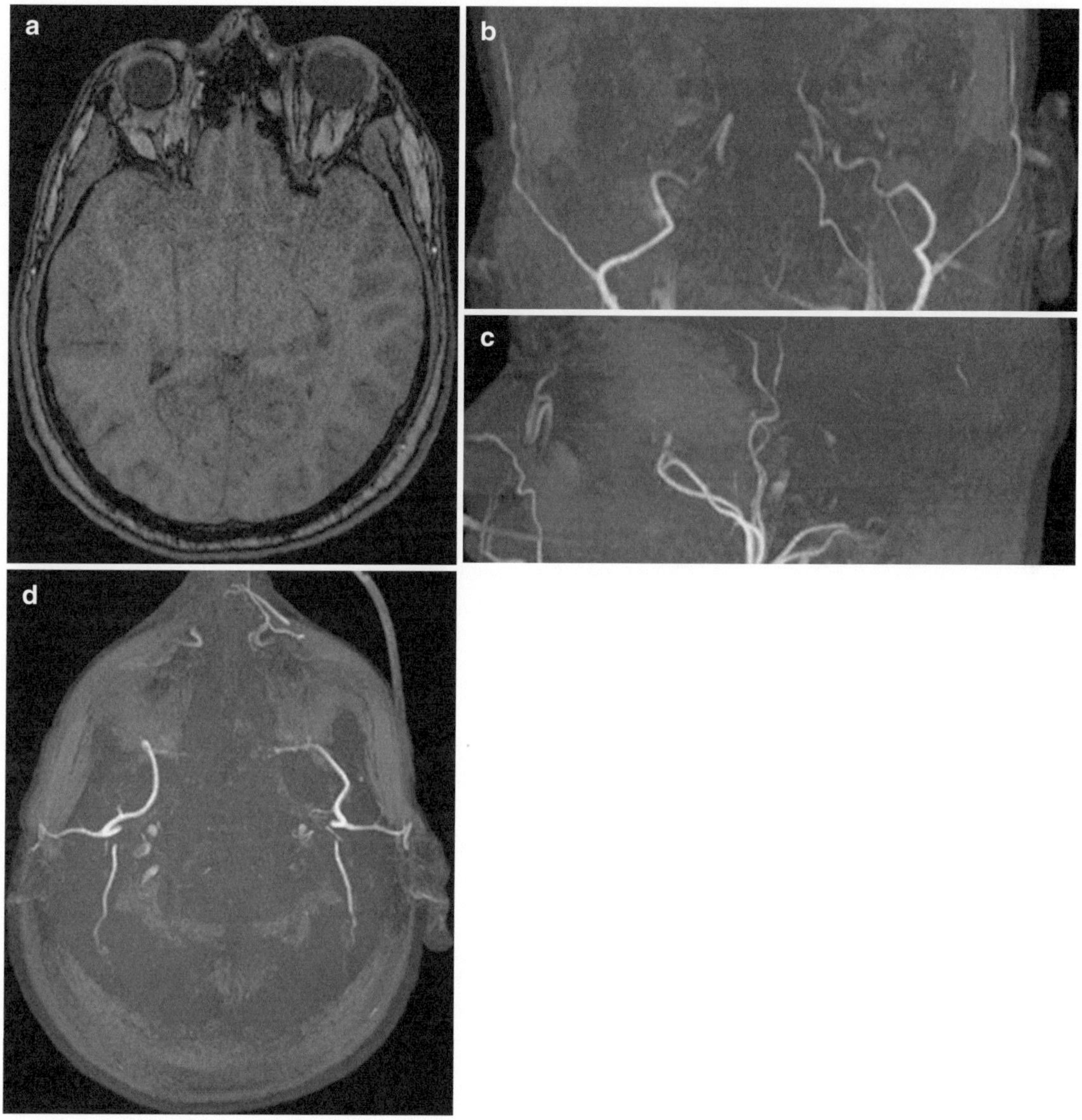

Fig. 14.5 Brain death signs on MRA. (**a**) Axial time-of-flight source image (**b–d**) and 3D reconstructions (**b**) coronal, (**c**) sagittal, and (**d**) axial show absence of the normal flow-related signal in the intracranial arteries. Note that both external carotid arteries and branches are normally seen

arteries, termed "stasis filling," indicates inadequate brain perfusion and should be recognized as an important pitfall when CTA is used [14].

Somatosensory evoked potentials (*EPs*) demonstrate bilateral absence of N20-P22 response with median nerve stimulation and disappearance of P14 nasopharyngeal electrode [1].

Pitfalls

- All types of evoked potentials can be absent in patients who have lost brainstem reflexes but are not clinically brain death [1].
- EPs do not test the functional integrity of all CNS structures.

Bi-spectral index may show gradual decline in bi-spectral index values to 0 [1].

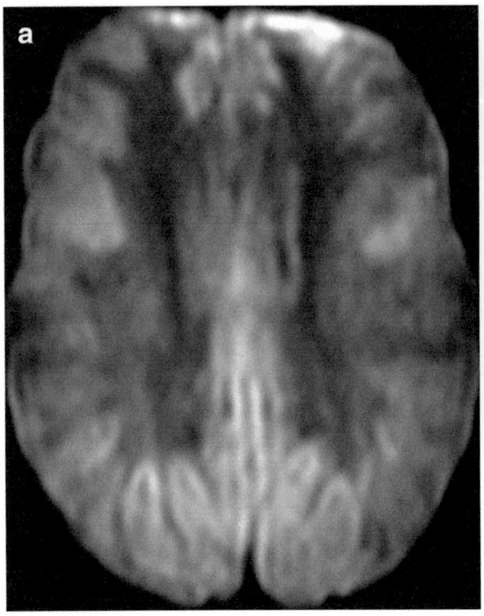

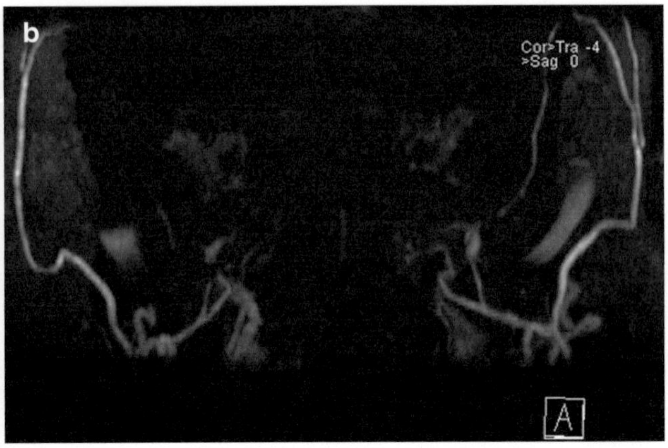

Fig. 14.6 Brain death signs demonstrated on MRI. (**a**) DWI reveals diffuse cortical high signal intensity which corresponded to low ADC values, and (**b**) 3D coronal reformation of MRA studies shows absence of visible intracerebral arteries which the external carotid arteries are seen

Pitfalls

- This technology is rarely used in intensive care units and has not been compared to flow studies [1].

Imaging Follow-Up

As stated before, the diagnosis of brain death is mainly clinical. Assessment of absence of brainstem reflexes should be performed at least on two different occasions, and the apnea test is usually done after the second examination. Ancillary tests may be repeated according with the institutional policies until definitive proof of brain death is obtained [1, 2, 5].

Main Differential Diagnosis

Clinically, the main differential diagnosis includes fulminant Guillain–Barré syndrome, organophosphate intoxication, high cervical spinal cord injury, drugs toxicity, severe hypothermia, *locked-in* syndrome, and post-cardiac arrest syndrome [1, 2, 5].

The main imaging differential diagnosis includes:

Severe intracranial hypertension: may delay filling of intracranial vessels due to cerebral circulation arrest.

Extradural origin of the ophthalmic artery: in 6–10 % of patients, the ophthalmic artery emerges proximal to the distal dural ring. In these patients, its filling does not indicate patency of intracranial flow.

Extradural origin of the posterior inferior cerebellar artery (*PICA*): in some patients, the PICA emerges from V3 segment (extradural) of vertebral artery or even from occipital artery and may fill even when a patient is brain dead.

Tips

Cerebral catheter angiography, MRA, and CTA:

- The origin of the ophthalmic artery is commonly used as the angiographic limit between the extradural and intradural ICA (Fig. 14.9). A positive

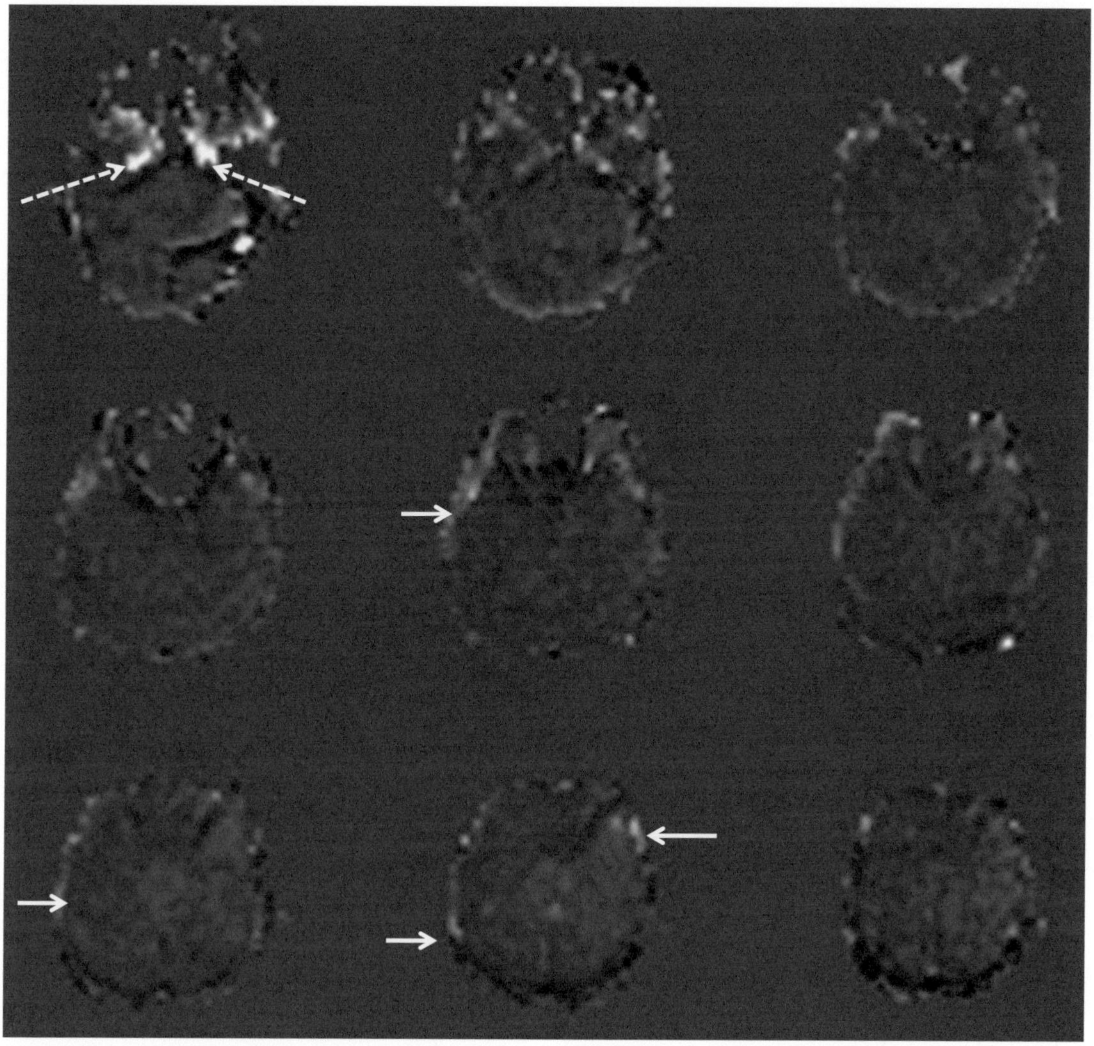

Fig. 14.7 Brain death signs demonstrated on arterial spin labeling (*ASL*). The CBF map shows ASL criteria supporting brain death: extremely diffuse decreased perfusion, bright signal intensity in the ICAs (*dashed arrows*) at their entry into the skull base that suggests flow stagnation, and patent external carotid circulation (*arrows*)

study shows no visualization of anterior circulation beyond level of supraclinoid ICAs and no posterior circulation filling beyond dural penetration of vertebral arteries.

- External carotid arteries and their branches should be patent without retrograde flow at the supraclinoid segment of ICA via the ophthalmic artery (Fig. 14.1).
- Sometimes the sagittal superior sinus can be seen due to meningeal artery perfusion or trans-diploic emissary veins draining the scalp tissues. However, no filling is seen in most brain dead patients.

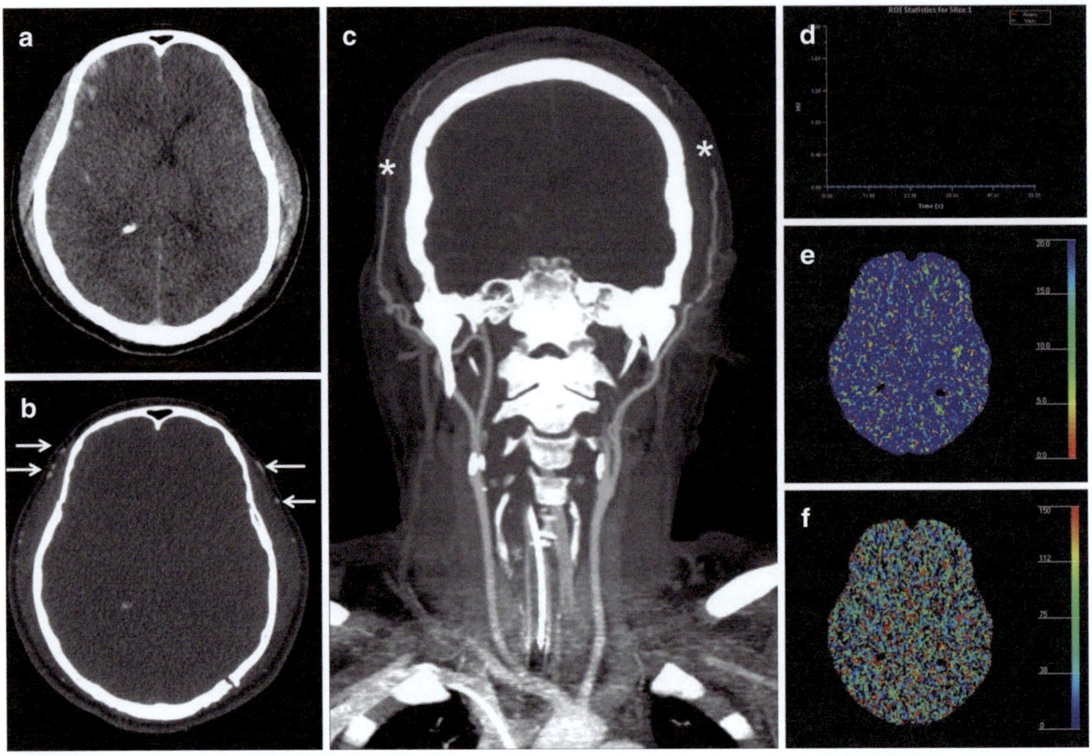

Fig. 14.8 Brain death signs demonstrated on CTA and CT perfusion. (**a**) Non-contrast CT in a patient with severe head trauma. (**b**) Axial CTA and (**c**) coronal MIP CTA image depict complete absence of intracranial vascular enhancement. Note patent external carotid arteries (*arrows* on **b** and * on **c**). CT perfusion study including (**d**) perfusion curve, (**e**) mean transit time, and (**f**) cerebral blood flow maps demonstrate absence of brain perfusion (Courtesy of Dr. Antônio Rocha, MD, PhD – Sao Paulo, Brazil)

- Absence of internal cerebral veins filling should also be present.

Head CT:

- Diffuse cerebral edema, loss of differentiation between the gray and white matter, and different types of herniations are usually seen (Fig. 14.3).
- After a global brain injury, the use of CT perfusion could potentially be an issue since it relies on comparisons to the contralateral "normal" side.

MRI:

- Loss of flow voids in the intracranial ICAs and any distal cerebral vessels, central and tonsillar herniations, diffuse brain swelling, obliteration of the CSF spaces, and compression of the ventricules are typical findings (Fig. 14.4).
- Significant drop in the apparent diffusion coefficient (ADC) values (white matter may demonstrate greater ADC reduction than the gray matter) may be seen (Fig. 14.4).
- MRS findings vary; there no characteristic pattern typical of brain death. The most common findings are an increase of the lactate peak and reduction of all other metabolites.
- In perfusion studies, there should be absence of CBF, but in certain cases (i.e., craniectomies), CBF can be maintained despite documented brain death.

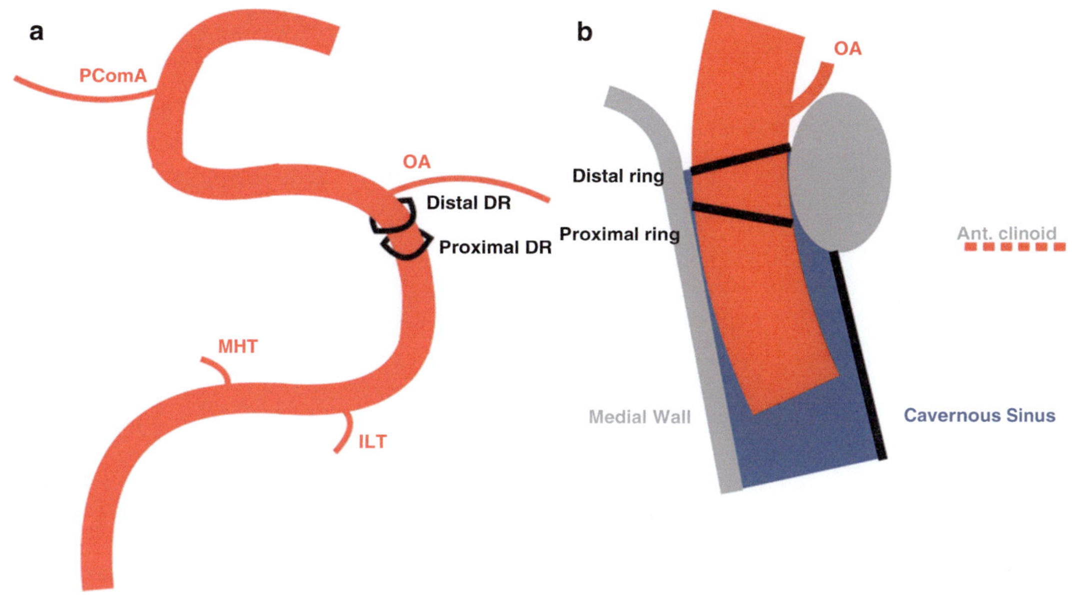

Fig. 14.9 Anatomy of the internal carotid artery (*ICA*). Simplified anatomic drawing of the ICA showing the origin of the ophthalmic artery (*OA*) which is the angiographic limit between extradural and intradural ICA. Lateral view (**a**) and posteroanterior view (**b**) of the ICA show that the emergence of ophthalmic artery is distal to the distal dural ring. *ILT* inferolateral trunk, *MHT* meningo-hypophyseal trunk, *PComA* posterior communicating artery, *DR* dural ring, *Ant. clinoid* anterior clinoid process

- Arterial spin labeling (ASL) MRI perfusion has been studied as a potential noninvasive and reliable confirmatory test for diagnosing brain death (Fig. 14.7) [7].

Further investigation is needed to validate these techniques. Non-enhanced CT and conventional/advance MRI still lack sensitivity and specificity for brain death.

References

1. Wijdicks EF, Varelas PN, Gronseth GS, et al. Evidence-based guideline update: determining brain death in adults: report of the Quality Standards Subcommittee of the American Academy of Neurology. Neurology. 2010;74:1911.
2. Heran M, Heran N. Potential ancillary tests in the evaluation of brain death: the value of cerebral blood flow assessment. Can J Neurol Sci. 2008;35:409–19.
3. Wijdicks EF. The diagnosis of brain death. N Engl J Med. 2001;344:1215–21.
4. Hwang DY, Gilmore EJ, Greer DM. Assessment of brain death in the neurocritical care unit. Neurosurg Clin N Am. 2013;24:469–82.
5. Arbour RB. Brain death: assessment, controversy, and confounding factors. Crit Care Nurse. 2013;33(6):27–46.
6. Goila AK, Pawer M. The diagnosis of brain death. Indian J Crit Care Med. 2009;13(1):7–11.
7. Kang KM, Han MH, et al. Clinical utility of arterial spin-labeling as a confirmatory test for suspected brain death. Am J Neuroradiol. 2015;36:909–14.
8. Busl KM, Greer DM. Pitfalls in the diagnosis of brain death. Neurocrit Care. 2009;11(2):276–87.
9. Lamp Y, Sadeh M, et al. Diagnosis of brain death using the transcranial doppler with a transorbital approach. Arch Neurol. 2002;59:58–60.
10. Donohoe KJ, Stokes MK, et al. DSNM practice guideline for brain death scintigraphy 2.0. J Nucl Med Technol. 2012;40(3):198–203.
11. Chen Z, Cichocki A, et al. An empirical EEG analysis in brain death diagnosis for adults. Cogn Neurodyn. 2008;2:257–71.
12. Karantanas AH, Komnos A, et al. Contribution of MRI and MR angiography in early diagnosis of brain death. Eur Radiol. 2002;12:2710–6.
13. Frumps E, Dupas B, et al. CT angiography for brain death diagnosis. Am J Neuroradiol. 2009;30:1566–70.
14. Nunes D, Rocha AJ, Boni RC. Pitfalls in vascular imaging when brain death is suspected: multiparametric multidetector computed tomography as a complementary diagnostic tool. Arq Neuropsiquiatr. 2014;72(6):473–4.

Meningitis, Empyema, and Brain Abscess in Adults

15

Thiago Luiz Pereira Donoso Scoppetta, Antônio José da Rocha, and Renato Hoffmann Nunes

Abstract

Central nervous system infections remain an important cause of morbidity and mortality worldwide. Meningitis is the most common manifestation. Pathogens vary based on the location of the infection, geography, vaccination status, age, surgical intervention, and immune status. They are considered medical emergencies requiring immediate diagnosis and therapy, and crucial steps are needed to achieve a good clinical outcome. Lumbar puncture is the first step in their evaluation, and imaging of the brain is often indicated in patients with neurologic deficits, altered immunity, or decreased level of consciousness.

T.L.P.D. Scoppetta, MD (✉)
Division of Neuroradiology,
Hospital Santa Casa de Misericórdia de São Paulo,
Rua Dr. Cesário Motta Junior 112, Vila Buarque,
Sao Paulo, SP 01221-020, Brazil

Division of Neuroradiology,
Hospital São Camilo Pompéia,
Sao Paulo, Brazil

Division of Neuroradiology,
Clinica de Diagnósticos Dr. Luiz Scoppetta,
Sao Paulo, Brazil

Division of Neuroradiology,
Grupo Fleury, Sao Paulo, SP, Brazil
e-mail: thiagoscoppetta@hotmail.com

A.J. da Rocha, MD, PhD
Division of Neuroradiology,
Hospital Santa Casa de Misericórdia de São Paulo,
Rua Dr. Cesário Motta Junior 112, Vila Buarque,
Sao Paulo, SP 01221-020, Brazil

Division of Neuroradiology, Grupo Fleury,
Sao Paulo, SP, Brazil
e-mail: antonio.rocha@grupofleury.com.br

R. Hoffmann Nunes, MD
Division of Neuroradiology,
Santa Casa de São Paulo, São Paulo, Brazil
e-mail: renatohn@hotmail.com

R. Hoffmann Nunes et al. (eds.), *Critical Findings in Neuroradiology*,
DOI 10.1007/978-3-319-27987-9_15

Background

Central nervous system (CNS) infections remain an important cause of morbidity and mortality worldwide, resulting in an estimated 340,000 deaths caused by meningitis [1]. Meningitis is a common form of CNS involvement characterized by infection of cerebrospinal fluid (CSF) and the meningeal layers surrounding the brain. Bacteria as well as other agents, such as mycobacteria, viruses, fungi, parasites, and noninfectious causes, can induce meningeal inflammation. Organisms may reach the brain parenchyma and meninges by different routes from contiguous or distant foci [2].

Pathogens vary based on the location of infection within the CNS, patient's origin, vaccination status, age, surgical intervention, and immune suppression. Knowledge of the epidemiology is crucial in the selection of appropriate empiric antimicrobial therapy [2].

The classic clinical features of meningitis include headache, nuchal rigidity, fever, and vomiting, followed by mental status changes. The clinical features of an empyema or a cerebral abscess depend on lesion size, location, virulence of the organism, and the patient's underlying condition. Usually both present with seizures, focal deficits, and progressive neurologic deterioration. Typically, a subdural empyema has a faster clinical course compared to an epidural empyema. Cerebral abscesses usually manifest as focal neurological deficits and fever is only present in 50 % of patients [2].

CNS infections are a medical emergency requiring immediate diagnosis and subsequent therapies, crucial steps to achieve favorable clinical outcomes. The lumbar puncture is the first step in the evaluation of any patient suspected of CNS infection. Imaging of the brain is often indicated in patients with neurologic deficits, immunocompromising conditions, or decreased level of consciousness [3, 4]. Subdural empyema also requires prompt surgical decompression. Brain abscess can be managed without neurosurgical procedure. However, stereotactic biopsy and drainage are required when there is significant mass effect, no primary sites identified for culture, neurological deterioration, or poor response to antibiotic treatment [5].

A lengthy description of the neuroimaging and clinical manifestations of all infections is beyond the scope of this chapter; therefore, herein, we present the most common causes of intracranial infections, particularly pyogenic.

Key Points

Etiology

Pathogens differ based on a wide variety of clinical and socio-geographic conditions. Even though meningitis usually results from viral or bacterial infections, bacterial infections result in more complications such as empyemas and brain abscesses [4].

Age: Incidence is age dependent. *S. pneumoniae* and *N. meningitidis* are the most common bacteria in young adults. *Listeria* is more likely to be observed in elderly patients [6].

Surgical intervention: Iatrogenic CNS infections are usually caused by *S. aureus*, coagulase-negative staphylococci, streptococci, *Enterobacteriaceae*, and *P. aeruginosa* [7].

Vaccination status: The epidemiology of CNS infections has markedly changed by virtue of vaccination. Currently, *S. pneumoniae* and *N. meningitidis* are the most common and aggressive bacteria-causing meningitis. The most common viruses are enteroviruses, herpes simplex virus (HSV) 1 and 2, and varicella-zoster virus (VZV) [6, 8, 9].

Immune status: Immunocompromised patients are prone to *E. coli*, *Klebsiella*, and *Listeria* meningitis. *Nocardia asteroides* is also an important cause of abscesses in this population.

Location: The two most common bacteria-causing ventriculitis are *Staphylococcus* and *Enterobacter* [4]. Empyema is most frequently caused by *Streptococcus milleri*, enterococci, and gram-negative bacilli [2]; brain abscess are usually secondary to hematogenous dissemination of anaerobic and gram-negative bacteria or both [10].

Pathophysiology

Meningitis: The organism may reach the meninges hematogenously, by direct spread from the paranasal sinuses or middle ears or by direct inoculation after a penetrating head trauma or neurosurgery. Meningitis is the most common expression of CNS infection after intracranial, otolaryngology, and sinus surgeries [6].

Ventriculitis: A pathogen may reach the ventricular system by direct implantation secondary to trauma or neurosurgical procedures; contiguous extension, such as a brain abscess rupture; and hematogenous spread. Subarachnoid extension from extraventricular sites into the ventricles is another possible route [4].

Empyema: Usually occurs secondary to retrograde thrombophlebitis via the calvarial emissary veins from a parameningeal focus. Seventy-five percent of patients with empyema have an adjacent aerated cavity (paranasal sinuses, middle ear, mastoid) infection. Empyema may also arise from concurrent meningitis or from rupture of a brain abscess into the subdural space [11].

Cerebritis and abscess: The most commonly identified sources are otomastoiditis, sinusitis, odontogenic abscess, and hematogenous spread. Abscess may also be observed as a complication of meningitis. However, in 20–30 %, no clear source of infection is identified [12]. Abscess formation follows a predictable path that can be divided into four sequential stages: early cerebritis (1–3 days), late cerebritis (4–9 days), early capsule (10–14 days), and late capsule (beyond the 14th day) [12].

Best Imaging Modality

Computed tomography (CT) is useful as a first-line study in view of its wide availability and speed especially in individuals with mental status changes or other systemic complications before performing a lumbar puncture. CT is critical in ruling out meningitis mimics such as acute subarachnoid hemorrhage and in depicting parameningeal foci [11]. However, it has several limitations. Besides the low sensibility to depict meningeal enhancement, CT does not provide enough information about the abscess cavity, and its depiction of small collections located close to bones is limited [4, 13, 14].

Magnetic resonance imaging (MRI) is the imaging method of choice because of its higher contrast resolution and sensitivity to contrast enhancement. Postcontrast images should be included in any imaging protocol, postcontrast fluid-attenuated inversion recovery (FLAIR) are helpful. Diffusion-weighted imaging (DWI) is also important for diagnostic and follow-up purposes. Furthermore, newer MRI techniques including susceptibility-weighted imaging (SWI), MR perfusion, MR spectroscopy, and diffusion tensor imaging (DTI) can support the diagnosis, help to plan surgery or biopsy, and even predict the infective agent [14–20].

Major Findings

Meningitis: It is characterized by hyperintense material filling the subarachnoid spaces, better demonstrated on FLAIR. DWI characteristically shows restricted diffusion when a purulent meningitis is present [21]. Leptomeningeal and subarachnoid space contrast enhancement is depicted on postcontrast T1-weighted images (T1WI) and postcontrast FLAIR; the latter is considered more sensitive for this purpose (Fig. 15.1) [22, 23]. These findings are not specific for bacterial infections and a wide variety of conditions may result in a similar imaging appearance (Fig. 15.2). Although nonbacterial meningitis may display the same imaging findings, it does not result in areas of restricted diffusion. Hydrocephalus, venous thrombosis, artery vasculopathy, and ischemic infarcts are complications that should be promptly diagnosed [4].

Ventriculitis: Thickening and abnormal ependymal contrast enhancement are the findings of ventriculitis (Fig. 15.3). The degree of thickness and morphology of the contrast enhancement should be evaluated, and in bacterial and viral infections, it is thin and smooth. The ventricles themselves may be dilated, and debris may be seen in their dependent portions. Pyogenic intraventricular empyema is most often caused by brain abscess rupture to inside the ventricles. DWI is crucial for diagnosis, demonstrating restricted diffusion in the dependent portions [4].

Empyema: CT demonstrates extra-axial collections, single, multiple, or bilateral, with variable attenuation that is usually higher than

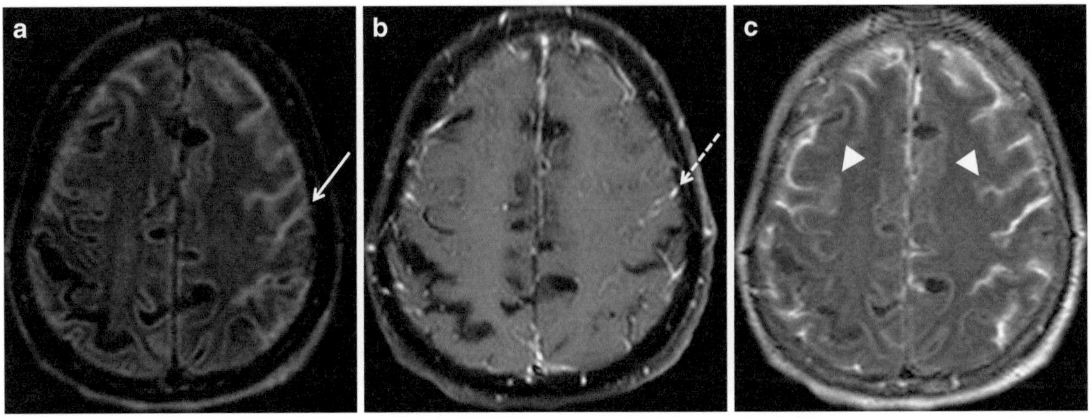

Fig. 15.1 Bacterial meningitis. (**a**) Axial FLAIR image shows high signal intensity along the bilateral frontal and left parietal sulci (*arrow*). (**b**) Corresponding axial postcontrast T1WI image demonstrates minimal leptomeningeal enhancement over the convexities (*dashed arrow*). (**c**). Axial FLAIR postcontrast image better depicts the bilateral leptomeningeal enhancement (*arrowheads*)

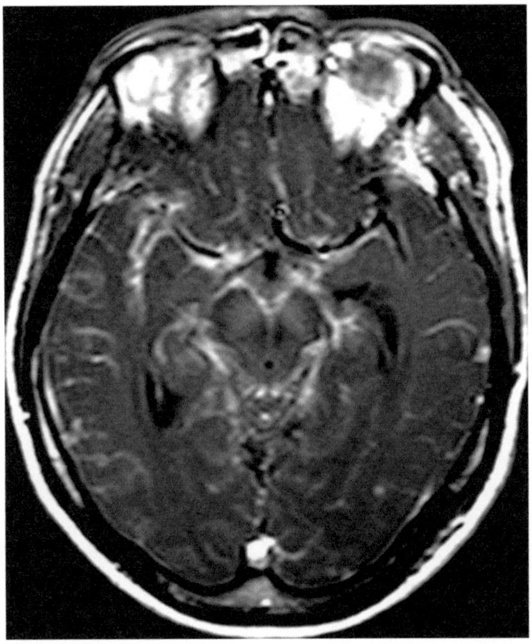

Fig. 15.2 Tuberculous meningitis. Postcontrast axial T1WI shows leptomeningeal thickening and enhancement centered within the basilar cisterns around anterior and middle cerebral arteries

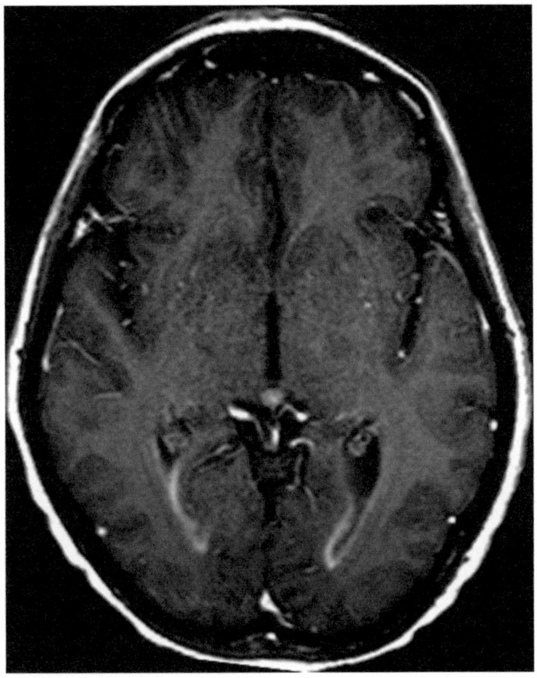

Fig. 15.3 CMV ventriculitis. Postcontrast axial T1WI shows ependymal enhancement along the occipital horns of the lateral ventricles

that of CSF and peripheral contrast enhancement. The morphology of the collection is usually concave, as the subdural space is far more affected than the epidural space. Similar findings are observed on MRI and are characterized by extra-axial collections that are hyperintense on FLAIR with peripheral contrast enhancement. DWI is crucial for the diagnosis showing restricted diffusion in the empyemas (Fig. 15.4). MRI also better depicts findings related to paranasal sinus and mastoid infections, which may be associated with intracranial extension [4].

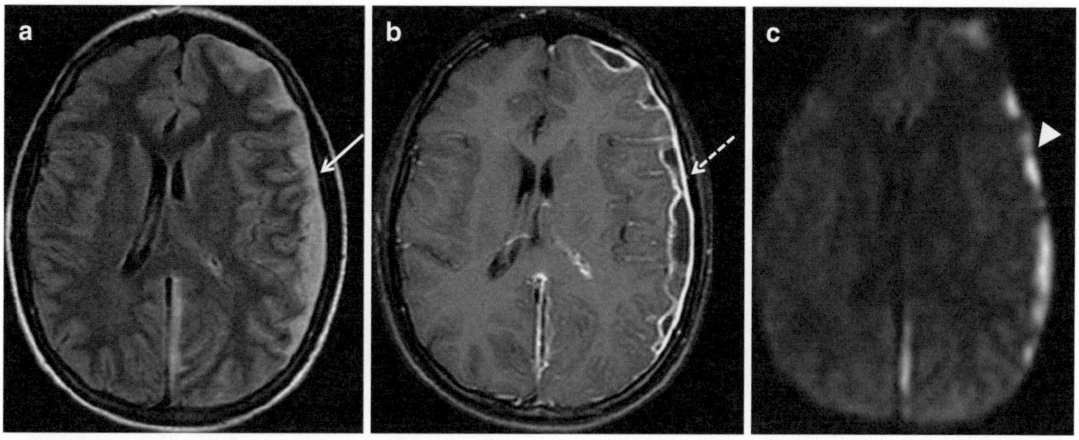

Fig. 15.4 Left subdural empyema secondary to otomastoiditis (not shown). (**a**) Axial FLAIR image shows a subdural collection with high signal intensity extending over the cerebral convexity (*arrow*) and along the left posterior falx cerebri. (**b**) Axial postcontrast T1WI reveals peripheral enhancement of the subdural collection (*dashed arrow*). (**c**) Axial DWI shows restricted diffusion within the subdural empyema (*arrowhead*), which was confirmed on the ADC map (not shown)

Cerebritis: It is the earliest manifestation of a cerebral infection, occurring about 2–3 days after pathogen inoculation and may progress to abscess formation. Initially, CT shows an ill-defined area of low attenuation with subtle mass effect. MRI shows increased T2/FLAIR signal and little or absent contrast enhancement. DWI signal is variable; however, the presence of restricted diffusion supports the diagnosis [21]. A capsule is formed as an attempt to contain the infection while the central portion undergoes liquefactive necrosis [21].

Abscess: Typically appears as a ring-enhancing lesion. The capsule of the abscess is thinner on its ventricular side than on its cortical side. The abscess cavity demonstrates high signal intensity on T2-weighted imaging (T2WI) and low or intermediate signal intensity on T1WI. The capsule may present with high signal intensity on T1WI and low signal intensity on T2WI. DWI characteristically demonstrates restricted diffusion within the cavity, often helping to differentiate it from other lesions (Fig. 15.5) [15, 18]. One should consider that restricted diffusion may vary with the concentration of purulent material in the cavity, and partially treated abscess may not show diffusion restriction [24–26]. MR spectroscopy (MRS) can be useful for characterization of some metabolites typically found in pyogenic abscess, especially certain amino acids such as valine, leucine, and isoleucine (0.9 ppm), which are final products of the action of proteolytic enzymes in liquefactive necrosis. Other metabolites have also been described, including lactate (1.3 ppm), alanine (1,5 ppm), acetate (1.92 ppm), and succinate (2.4 ppm), derived from tissue necrosis and different fermentation and glycolysis pathways (Table 15.1) [14, 16, 17]. SWI typically depicts in late abscesses two concentric rims, with the outer one being hypointense and the inner one hyperintense relative to the cavity content, characterizing the "dual rim sign" [27].

Imaging Follow-Up

CT should be performed if patients fail to improve within 48 h of antibiotic treatment or if a new focal neurological deficit appears. DWI is useful to follow-up treatment response in pyogenic abscesses. A decrease of restricted diffusion in the abscess cavity is correlated with treatment response and good outcome (Fig. 15.6). Conversely, persisting or reappearing restricted diffusion indicates treatment failure [26]. MRS can also be used to follow-up, and it is assumed that reduction or disappearance of abnormal metabolites despite persistence of isolated lactate peak reflect good therapeutic response [28]

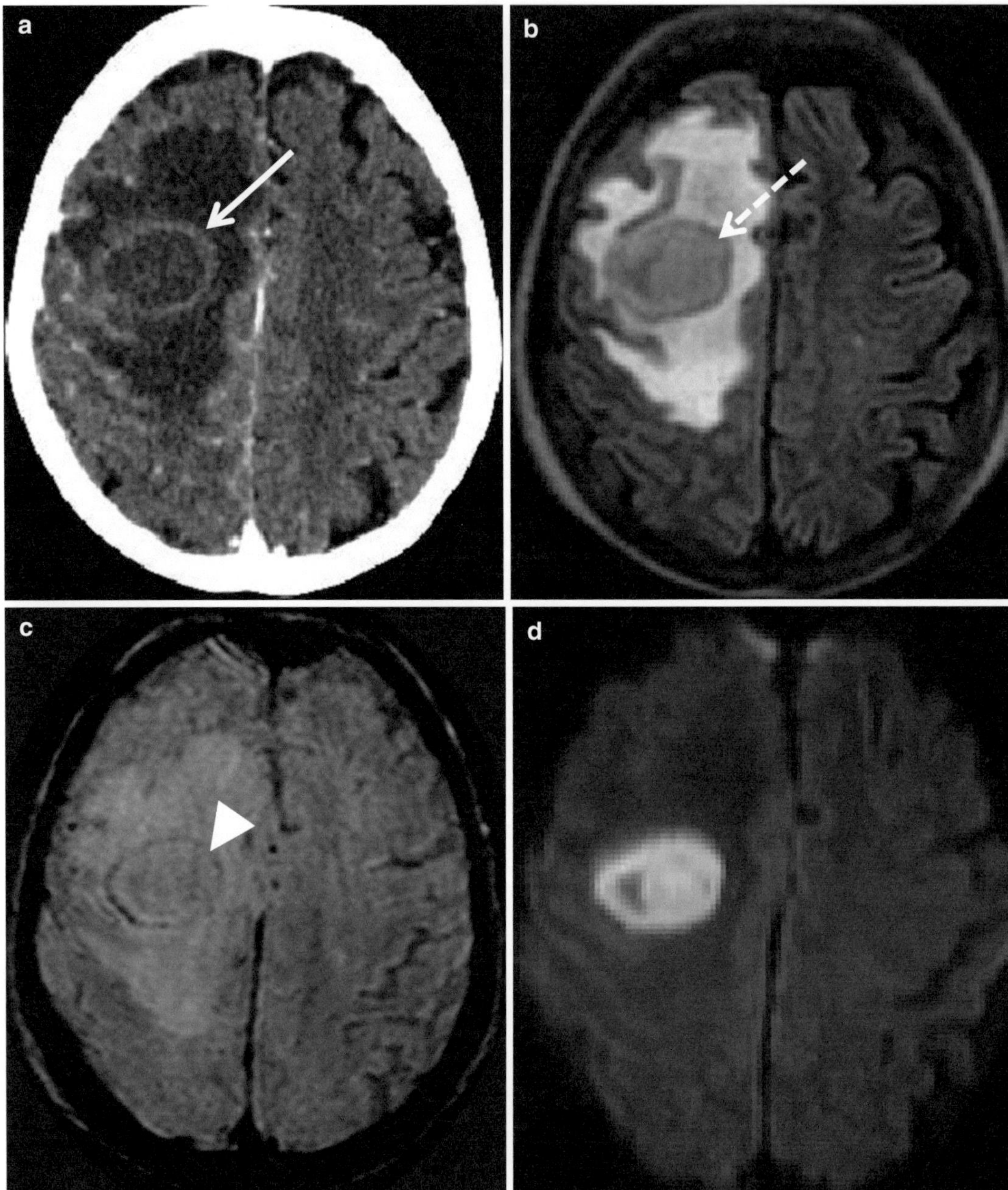

Fig. 15.5 Right frontal lobe pyogenic brain abscess. (**a**) Contrast-enhanced CT demonstrates ring-enhancing mass in the right frontal lobe (*arrow*) with surrounding extensive vasogenic edema. (**b**) Axial FLAIR image depicts the surrounding T2 hypointense signal of the abscess capsule (*dashed arrow*). (**c**) On axial SWI, the abscesses are bordered by two concentric rims, with the outer one being hypointense and the inner one hyperintense relative to cavity content, forming the "dual rim sign" (*arrowhead*). (**d**) Axial DWI reveals high signal, which corresponded with restricted water diffusion on the ADC map (not shown) within the abscess cavity. (**e**) Sagittal postcontrast T1WI shows the regular rim enhancement and a posterosuperior satellite lesion (*dashed arrow*, "daughter abscess"). (**f**) Perfusion MR image (relative CBV map) demonstrates minimal increased values corresponding to the ring-enhancing area. (**g**) 1H-MR spectroscopy using SE sequence (TR/TE/NEX – 3000 ms/144 ms/128) from the center of the lesion shows resonances of AAs, 0.9 ppm; Lip/Lac, 1.3 ppm; Ac, 1.9 ppm; and Suc, 2.4 ppm (*arrows*)

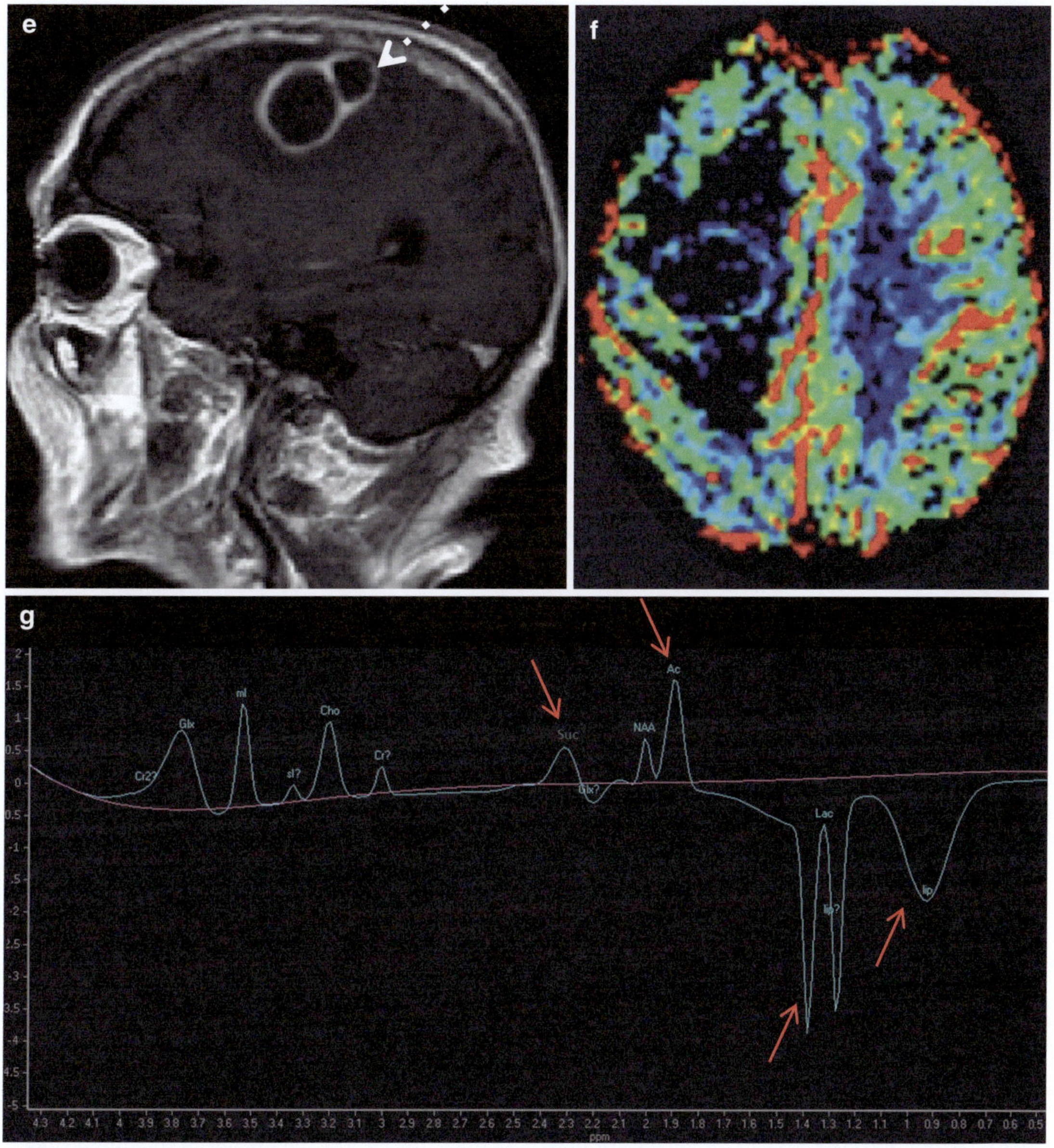

Fig. 15.5 (continued)

Main Differential Diagnosis

Meningitis: Subarachnoid FLAIR hyperintensity can be caused by a wide range of conditions, pathologic and artifactual. Meningitis, subarachnoid hemorrhage, leptomeningeal spread of malignant disease, and supplemental oxygen are the most important ones (Table 15.2) [29]. The differential diagnosis of meningeal enhancement is extensive and includes neoplastic (primary or secondary tumors), granulomatous, infectious, and inflammatory conditions. Imaging helps in differentiation of infective from the noninfective conditions since carcinomatous meningitis typically presents with dural enhancement and produces a thicker and/or nodular contrast enhancement. Cancer history and systemic disease may guide the diagnosis. However, CSF

Table 15.1 Abscess imaging findings

Etiologic agent	Conventional MRI	Advanced MRI techniques
Pyogenic	Capsule: high signal on T1WI and low signal on T2WI. Thin and smooth rim enhancement Cavity: low signal on T1WI and high signal on T2WI, restricted diffusion Associated findings: satellite lesions, parameningeal focus, pyogenic leptomeningitis, pyogenic intraventricular empyema, or subdural empyema	MR perfusion: low cerebral blood volume (rCBV) on dynamic susceptibility contrast (DSC-MRI) MRS: AAs, alanine, acetate, and succinate. The presence of acetate and succinate has been attributed to anaerobic bacteria SWI: dual rim sign
Tuberculous	Variable imaging presentation Low signal on T2WI within the cavity suggests a granulomatous process Smooth, lobulated, or crenated wall contrast enhancement May present restricted diffusion Associated findings: thick basal leptomeningeal enhancement, basal ganglia infarcts, and hydrocephalus	MR perfusion: low rCBV on DSC-MRI MRS: increased lipids and lactate
Fungal	May present low signal on T2WI Lobulated or crenated wall contrast enhancement Intracavitary projections (specific finding) Restricted diffusion (including the walls)	MR perfusion: low rCBV on DSC-MRI MRS: AAs, lipids, lactate, and trehalose (3,6-3,8 ppm)

cytology is regarded as the cornerstone of diagnosis. Sometimes biopsy of the affected leptomeningeal areas may help to reach the etiologic diagnosis [4].

Ventriculitis: It can be caused by a wide variety of infectious agents. Thin and linear ependymal contrast enhancements are characteristics that suggest underlying infectious disease (Fig. 15.3). Chorioretinitis and ependymal enhancement when present are suspicious for CMV ventriculitis, particularly in the setting of AIDS. Lymphoproliferative malignancies or neoplastic spread typically produce thicker, lumpy, or nodular contrast enhancement [4].

Empyema: Subdural empyemas typically resemble subdural hematomas in their shape and relationship to sutures and dural reflections. It is also important to consider that blood products may cause high signal intensity on DWI due to susceptibility artifacts. However, CT scan or SWI is able to confirm blood products in cases of subdural hematomas. Subdural hygroma is another differential diagnosis. It is a common complication and is seen in up to one-third of patients with meningitis. Typically, it presents with signal intensity similar to the CSF in all sequences, including DWI [4].

Cerebritis: a wide range of conditions can cause parenchymal areas of signal intensity on T2WI/FLAIR. Acute ischemic stroke should be considered when a vascular territory is affected. Neoplasms usually present with a more infiltrative pattern, and advanced MR techniques may depict increased perfusion and high choline in high-grade neoplasms. HSV-1 may result in meningitis and a cerebritis; however, it characteristically has a predilection for the limbic system [10, 21].

Abscess: The presence of a *ring-enhancing lesion* in the brain is not diagnostic of an abscess and must be distinguished from necrotic neoplasms and other cystic lesions. The differential diagnosis can be accessed by the mnemonics *MAGICAL DR*, where "M" stands for metastasis, "A" for abscess, "G" for gliomas (in adults, particularly glioblastoma), "I" for infarction (subacute), "C" for contusion (resolving hema-

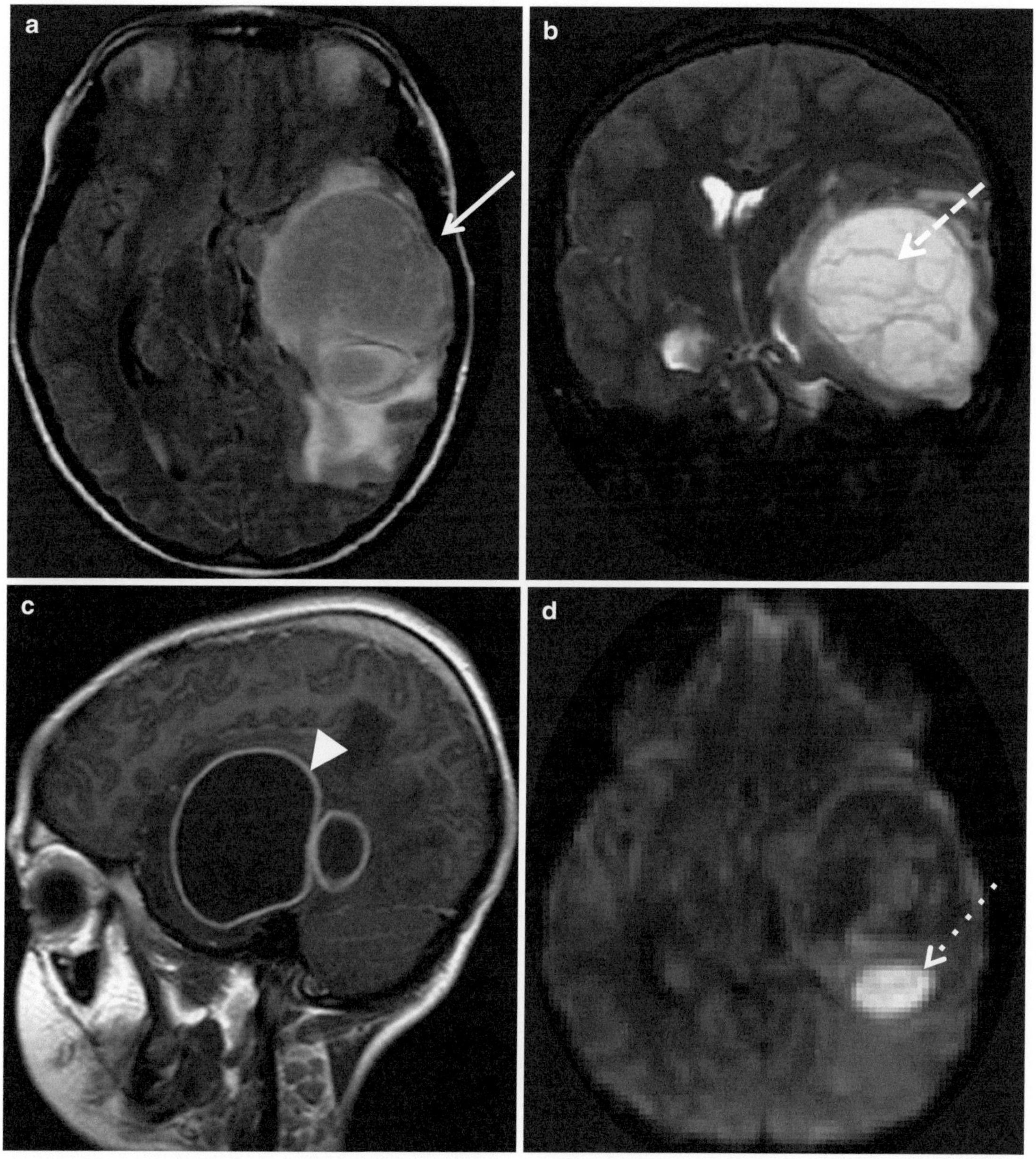

Fig. 15.6 Left temporal pyogenic brain abscess after antibiotic treatment. (**a**) Axial FLAIR image depicts a complex mass in the left temporal lobe with the surrounding T2 hypointense signal of the abscess capsule (*arrow*) and surrounding vasogenic edema. (**b**) Coronal T2WI shows a multiloculated cystic mass (*dashed arrow*). (**c**) Sagittal postcontrast T1WI demonstrates the two ring-enhancing masses with regular rim enhancement (*arrowhead*). (**d**) Axial DWI reveals restricted water diffusion within the smaller posterior cavity corresponding to an abscess (*dashed arrow*). Note the decreased signal intensity within the large abscess cavity after antibiotic treatment (better response than the posterior one)

toma), "A" for AIDS (opportunistic infections), "L" for lymphoma (especially in immunocompromised patients), "D" for demyelination, and "R" for radiation necrosis. Besides, one should consider that patients from endemic regions are prone to cysticercosis and its diagnostic criteria are based on clinical, imaging, immunologic, and epidemiologic data [30]. The term "abscess" is

Table 15.2 Causes of sulcal hyperintensity on FLAIR images

Pathologic	Meningitis
	Leptomeningeal spread of malignant disease
	Leptomeningeal melanosis
	Primary meningeal tumors
	Subarachnoid hemorrhage
	Fat-containing tumors
	Contrast media
	Vascular hyperintensity (moyamoya disease, acute stroke)
Artifacts	Supplemental oxygen
	CSF pulsation
	Vascular pulsation
	Magnetic susceptibility artifact
	Motion artifact

not restricted to pyogenic lesions, as tuberculosis and fungus may also cause similar lesions. Clinical history and advanced MRI techniques may help in the diagnostic workflow (Table 15.3) [15, 18–20].

Tips

- Subarachnoid FLAIR hyperintensity can be caused by many conditions, either pathologic or artifactual (Table 15.2). Sagittal MR imaging can easily depict oropharyngeal aperture helping identify patients receiving supplemental oxygen. The concentration of administered supplemental oxygen is crucial in producing hyperintensity on FLAIR images.
- Meningeal contrast enhancement is nonspecific and can be seen in meningitis of any cause, including noninfectious processes.
- Leptomeningeal thickening and contrast enhancement that is centered within the basal cisterns are characteristic findings of tuberculous meningitis.
- Restricted diffusion on DWI within a centrally T2 hyperintense ring-enhancing mass is characteristic but not pathognomonic of a pyogenic abscess.
- "Thinking outside the box" – literally. The most common identified sources of empyema, cerebritis, and brain abscess are parameningeal foci.
- Restricted diffusion within the pyogenic abscess cavity may vary with the concentration of purulent material. A partially treated abscess may not present with diffusion restriction.
- Keep in mind the mnemonics *MAGICAL DR* to remember the potential causes of a cerebral ring-enhancing lesion (see above). Clinical history and advanced imaging techniques may help narrowing the differential diagnosis list.
- Always remember to consider toxoplasmosis, cryptococcosis, neurosyphilis, and fungal infections in immunocompromised patients, particularly in the setting of AIDS.

Table 15.3 Differential diagnosis of ring-enhancing lesions

Mnemonics	Clinical history	Image findings	Examples
Metastasis	Primary neoplasm known Malignant cells in CSF analysis	Thicker rim of enhancement and DWI hyperintensity within solid component High rCBV with poor baseline return in DSC-MRI, high choline, lactate and lipids on ^{1}H MR spectroscopy	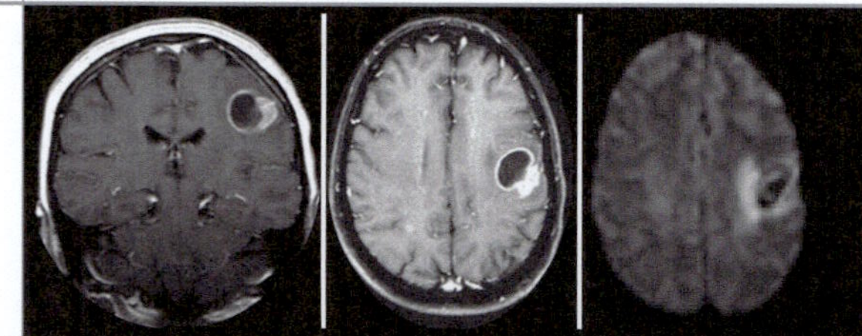
Abscess	Fever in 50 % Primary infectious focus known Infectious CSF findings	Varies according to the agent (see Table 15.1)	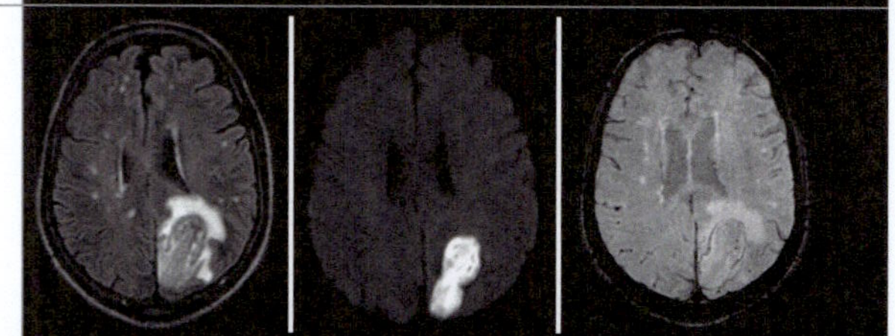
Glioma	No signs of clinical and laboratory infection	GBM usually shows thicker rim of contrast enhancement and DWI hyperintensity within solid component (hypercellularity and high nuclear to cytoplasmic ratio) High CBV with moderate baseline return on DSC-MRI High choline, Lactate and lipid on MRS	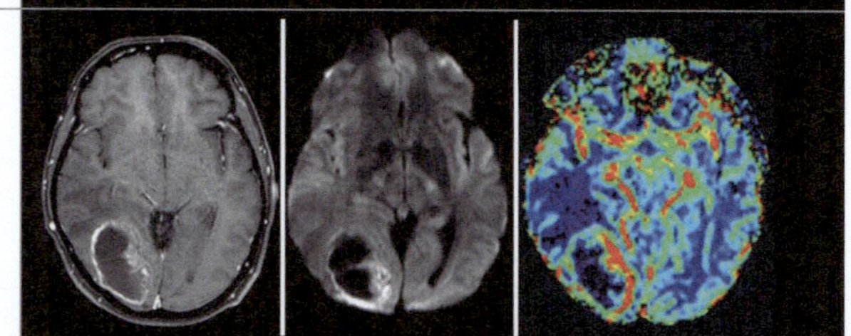
Infarct (subacute)	The presence of cardiovascular risks Previous images available No signs of clinical and laboratory infection	Lesion respecting a specific arterial territory, characteristic gyriform enhancement in subacute stage Predictable imaging course Vascular study may add information	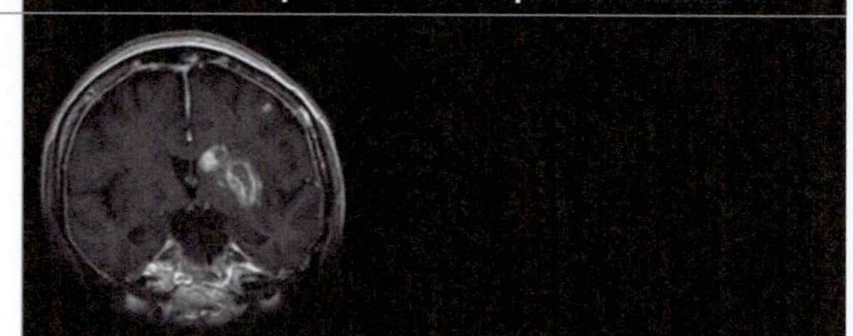

(continued)

Table 15.3 (continued)

Mnemonics	Clinical history	Image findings	Examples
Contusion	History of trauma Previous images available No signs of clinical and laboratory infection	Characteristic location (frontal and temporal poles), skull fracture Blood products depicted on GRE or SWI. DWI may show susceptibility artifacts inside hematoma	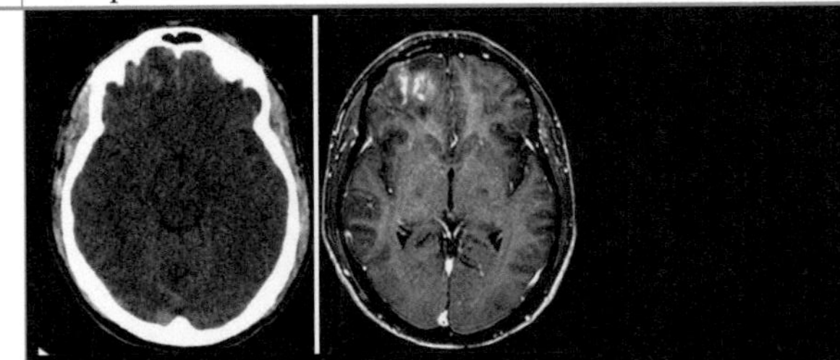
AIDS (opportunistic infections)	Immunocompromised patients Signs of systemic disease	*Toxoplasmosis*: Iso to low T2 signal within the lesion surrounded by vasogenic edema. "Eccentric target sign" *Cryptococcosis*: usually presents as meningitis. Gelatinous pseudocysts and cryptococcomas are other forms of presentation	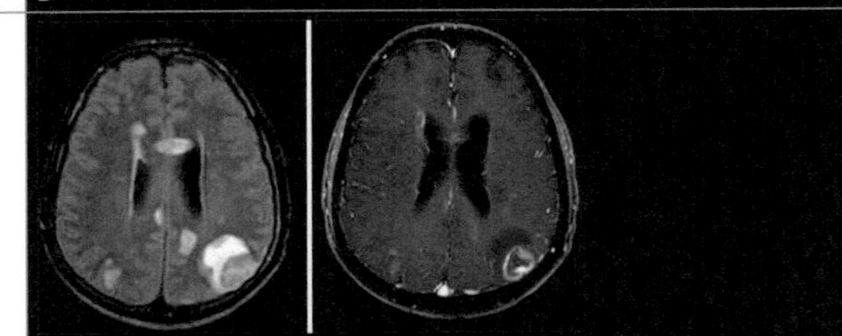
Lymphoma	Immunocompromised patients, particularly in AIDS or posttransplantation	Usually centered in basal ganglia and periventricular region, usually show low signal on T2WI and hyperintensity on DWI within solid component, higher vascular permeability on DCE-MRI High rCBV on DSC-MRI	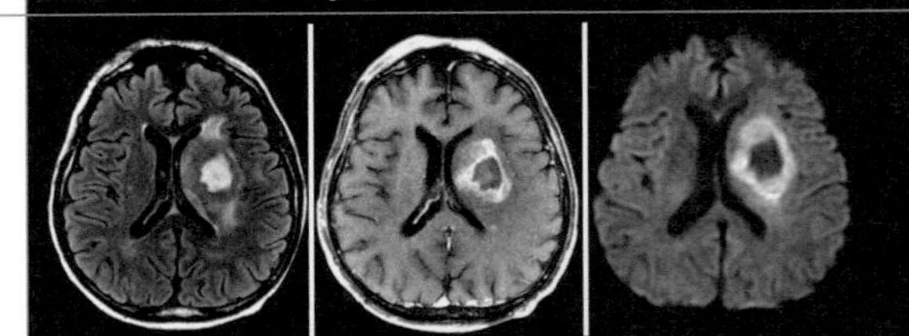
Demyelination	Clinical history of focal neurologic deficits or optic neuritis Diagnosis of multiple sclerosis (MS) on clinical basis No signs of clinical and laboratory infection	Incomplete peripheral enhancement (open-ring enhancement) Characteristic lesion distribution and callosal–septal interface involvement in MS patients	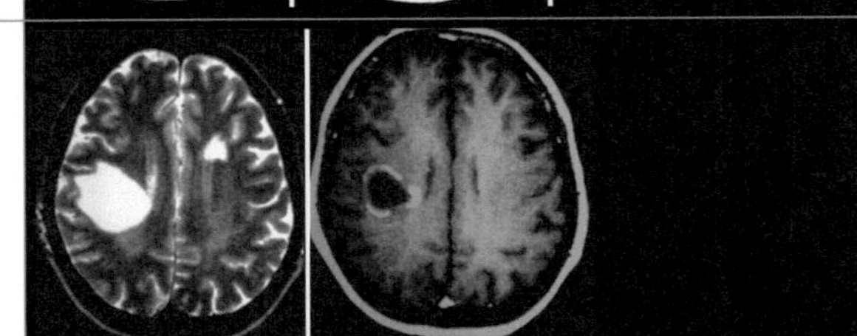

Radiation necrosis	History of radiation therapy is crucial No signs of clinical and laboratory infection	White matter T2/FLAIR hyperintensity Lesion within the field of radiation Contrast enhancement Low perfusion MRS shows no viable metabolites	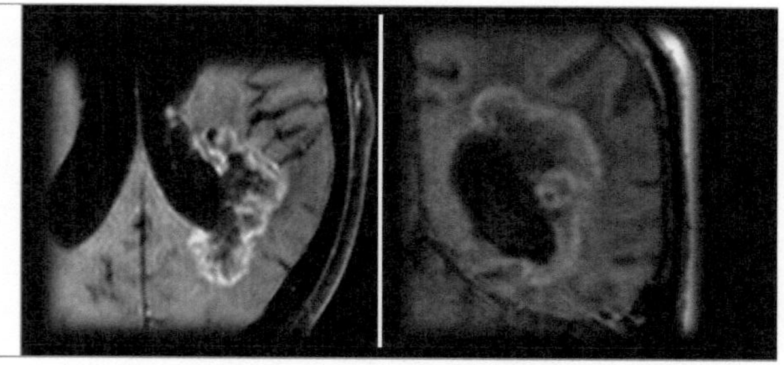
Might consider the following differential diagnosis in special epidemiological conditions			
Cysticercosis	Patients from endemic regions	Parenchymal lesions can be divided into four stages with unique imaging and clinical features: Vesicular, colloidal vesicular, granular nodular, and nodular calcified Scolex seen inside the cyst is an absolute feature according to the proposed diagnostic criteria	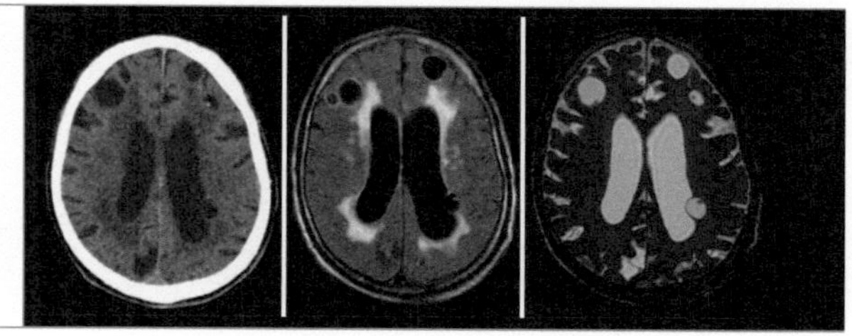

References

1. Mathers C, Fat DM, Boerma JT, World Health Organization. The global burden of disease: 2004 update. Geneva: World Health Organization; 2008.
2. Naidich TP. Imaging of the brain. Philadelphia: Saunders/Elsevier; 2013.
3. van de Beek D, de Gans J, Spanjaard L, Weisfelt M, Reitsma JB, Vermeulen M. Clinical features and prognostic factors in adults with bacterial meningitis. N Engl J Med. 2004;351(18):1849–59.
4. Mohan S, Jain KK, Arabi M, Shah GV. Imaging of meningitis and ventriculitis. Neuroimaging Clin N Am. 2012;22(4):557–83.
5. Heth JA. Neurosurgical aspects of central nervous system infections. Neuroimaging Clin N Am. 2012; 22(4):791–9.
6. Riddell J, Shuman EK. Epidemiology of central nervous system infection. Neuroimaging Clin N Am. 2012;22(4):543–56.
7. Korinek AM. Risk factors for neurosurgical site infections after craniotomy: a prospective multicenter study of 2944 patients. The French Study Group of Neurosurgical Infections, the SEHP, and the C-CLIN Paris-Nord. Service Epidémiologie Hygiène et Prévention. Neurosurgery. 1997;41(5):1073–9; discussion1079–81.
8. Thigpen MC, Whitney CG, Messonnier NE, Zell ER, Lynfield R, Hadler JL, et al. Bacterial meningitis in the United States, 1998–2007. N Engl J Med. 2011;364(21):2016–25.
9. van de Beek D, de Gans J, Tunkel AR, Wijdicks EFM. Community-acquired bacterial meningitis in adults. N Engl J Med. 2006;354(1):44–53. Massachusetts Medical Society.
10. Rath TJ, Hughes M, Arabi M, Shah GV. Imaging of cerebritis, encephalitis, and brain abscess. Neuroimaging Clin N Am. 2012;22(4):585–607.
11. da Rocha AJ, Vedolin L, Mendonça RA. Encéfalo. Brasil: Elsevier; 2012. 1 p.
12. Mathisen GE, Johnson JP. Brain abscess. Clin Infect Dis. 1997;25(4):763–79. Oxford University Press.
13. Chang KH, Han MH, Roh JK, Kim IO, Han MC, Kim CW. Gd-DTPA-enhanced MR imaging of the brain in patients with meningitis: comparison with CT. Am J Roentgenol. 1990;154(4):809–16.
14. Lai PH, Li KT, Hsu SS, Hsiao CC, Yip CW, Ding S, et al. Pyogenic brain abscess: findings from in vivo 1.5-T and 11.7-T in vitro proton MR spectroscopy. Am J Neuroradiol. 2005;26(2):279–88.
15. Kim YJ, Chang KH, Song IC, Kim HD, Seong SO, Kim YH, et al. Brain abscess and necrotic or cystic brain tumor: discrimination with signal intensity on diffusion-weighted MR imaging. Am J Roentgenol. 1998;171(6):1487–90.
16. Luthra G, Parihar A, Nath K, Jaiswal S, Prasad KN, Husain N, et al. Comparative evaluation of fungal, tubercular, and pyogenic brain abscesses with conventional and diffusion MR imaging and proton MR spectroscopy. Am J Neuroradiol. 2007;28(7):1332–8.
17. Pal D, Bhattacharyya A, Husain M, Prasad KN, Pandey CM, Gupta RK. In vivo proton MR spectroscopy evaluation of pyogenic brain abscesses: a report of 194 cases. AJNR Am J Neuroradiol. 2010;31(2): 360–6.
18. Lai PH, Ho JT, Chen WL, Hsu SS, Wang JS, Pan HB, et al. Brain abscess and necrotic brain tumor: discrimination with proton MR spectroscopy and diffusion-weighted imaging. Am J Neuroradiol. 2002;23(8): 1369–77.
19. Öz G, Alger JR, Barker PB, Bartha R, Bizzi A, Boesch C, et al. Clinical proton MR spectroscopy in central nervous system disorders. Radiology. 2014;270(3):658–79.
20. Toh CH, Wei KC, Ng SH, Wan YL, Lin CP, Castillo M. Differentiation of brain abscesses from necrotic glioblastomas and cystic metastatic brain tumors with diffusion tensor imaging. Am J Neuroradiol. 2011; 32(9):1646–51.
21. Gasparetto EL, Cabral RF, da Cruz LCH, Domingues RC. Diffusion imaging in brain infections. Neuroimaging Clin N Am. 2011;21(1):89–113, vii.
22. Mathews VP, Caldemeyer KS, Lowe MJ, Greenspan SL, Weber DM, Ulmer JL. Brain: gadolinium-enhanced fast fluid-attenuated inversion-recovery MR imaging. Radiology. 1999;211(1):257–63.
23. Fukuoka H, Hirai T, Okuda T, Shigematsu Y, Sasao A, Kimura E, et al. Comparison of the added value of contrast-enhanced 3D fluid-attenuated inversion recovery and magnetization-prepared rapid acquisition of gradient echo sequences in relation to conventional postcontrast T1-weighted images for the evaluation of leptomeningeal diseases at 3T. AJNR Am J Neuroradiol. 2010;31(5):868–73.
24. Tomar V, Yadav A, Rathore RKS, Verma S, Awasthi R, Bharadwaj V, et al. Apparent diffusion coefficient with higher b-value correlates better with viable cell count quantified from the cavity of brain abscess. Am J Neuroradiol. 2011;32(11):2120–5.
25. Maia ACM Jr, Guedes BVS, Lucas A Jr, José da Rocha A. Diffusion MR imaging for monitoring treatment response. Neuroimaging Clin N Am. 2011; 21(1):153–78.
26. Cartes-Zumelzu FW, Stavrou I, Castillo M, Eisenhuber E, Knosp E, Thurnher MM. Diffusion-weighted imaging in the assessment of brain abscesses therapy. Am J Neuroradiol. 2004;25(8):1310–7.
27. Toh CH, Wei KC, Chang CN, Hsu PW, Wong HF, Ng SH, et al. Differentiation of pyogenic brain abscesses from necrotic glioblastomas with use of susceptibility-weighted imaging. Am J Neuroradiol. 2012;33(8):1534–8.
28. Burtscher IM, Holtås S. In vivo proton MR spectroscopy of untreated and treated brain abscesses. Am J Neuroradiol. 1999;20(6):1049–53.
29. Stuckey SL, Goh TD, Heffernan T, Rowan D. Hyperintensity in the subarachnoid space on FLAIR MRI. Am J Roentgenol. 2007;189(4):913–21.
30. Del Brutto OH, Rajshekhar V, White AC, Tsang VC, Nash TE, Takayanagui OM, et al. Proposed diagnostic criteria for neurocysticercosis. Am Acad Neurol. 2001;57(2):177–83.

Meningitis, Empyema, and Brain Abscess in Children

16

Thiago Luiz Pereira Donoso Scoppetta,
Antônio José da Rocha,
and Renato Hoffmann Nunes

Abstract

Central nervous system infection in children is an important condition for which early recognition is crucial to achieve a favorable clinical outcome. Infectious bacterial meningitis is the most common manifestation of CNS infections in this age group. Despite the fact that the imaging findings may be nonspecific, its clinical presentation has distinct peculiarities. The classical clinical features of infective meningitis in children include apathy, lethargy, stupor, poor feeding, and irritability. Clinical history and imaging techniques may help in the diagnostic workflow.

Background

Infectious bacterial meningitis is the most common presentation of central nervous system (CNS) infection in this age group and represents an inflammation of the meninges, in particular the arachnoid and the pia mater, associated with the invasion of bacteria to the subarachnoid space [1]. Besides bacteria, mycobacteria, viruses, fungi, parasites, and other noninfectious causes associated to systemic and neoplastic diseases as well as certain drugs can induce meningeal inflammation [2, 3].

T.L.P.D. Scoppetta, MD (✉)
Division of Neuroradiology,
Hospital Santa Casa de Misericórdia de São Paulo,
Rua Dr. Cesário Motta Junior 112, Vila Buarque,
Sao Paulo, SP 01221-020, Brazil

Division of Neuroradiology,
Hospital São Camilo Pompéia,
Sao Paulo, Brazil

Division of Neuroradiology,
Clinica de Diagnósticos Dr. Luiz Scoppetta,
Sao Paulo, Brazil

Division of Neuroradiology,
Grupo Fleury, Sao Paulo, SP, Brazil
e-mail: thiagoscoppetta@hotmail.com

A.J. da Rocha, MD, PhD
Division of Neuroradiology, Hospital Santa Casa de Misericóridia de São Paulo,
Rua Dr. Cesário Motta Junior 112, Vila Buarque,
Sao Paulo, SP 01221-020, Brazil

Division of Neuroradiology, Grupo Fleury,
Sao Paulo, SP, Brazil
e-mail: antonio.rocha@grupofleury.com.br

R. Hoffmann Nunes, MD
Division of Neuroradiology,
Santa Casa de São Paulo, São Paulo, Brazil
e-mail: renatohn@hotmail.com

R. Hoffmann Nunes et al. (eds.), *Critical Findings in Neuroradiology*,
DOI 10.1007/978-3-319-27987-9_16

Pathogens vary based on location of infection within the CNS, geographic exposure, vaccination status, age, surgical intervention, and immune suppression. Therefore, knowledge of the epidemiology of CNS infection is crucial in the selection of appropriate empiric antimicrobial therapy.

Despite the fact that imaging findings of CNS infection show similar features to those of adults, its clinical presentation is distinct and includes apathy, lethargy, stupor, poor feeding, and irritability. Seizures are present in 40 % of cases. Neonates and infants may present with a bulging fontanelle. The typical signs observed in adults such as headache, neck stiffness, and Kernig sign are less common, especially in younger children [1, 2].

Regardless of age, CNS infections are a medical emergency requiring immediate diagnosis and antimicrobial therapy. The diagnosis can be made by clinical, physical, and laboratory evaluations, especially cerebral spinal fluid (CSF) analysis. Generally, neuroimaging is performed in patients with complications [1, 3]. A special concern in the pediatric age group is radiation exposure [4].

Subdural effusions are commonly associated with meningitis and typically do not require neurosurgical drainage as they typically regress over time with antimicrobial treatment. However, when infected, result in subdural empyemas, requiring prompt surgical decompression. Brain abscesses can also be managed sometimes without neurosurgical procedure. However, stereotactic biopsy and drainage are required when there is significant mass effect, no primary sites identified for culture, and neurologically deterioration is observed or poor response to antibiotic treatment [5].

Key Points

Etiology

Successful vaccination against *Haemophilus influenzae* type B (Hib) and *Streptococcus pneumoniae* has changed the epidemiology of bacterial meningitis during the last 20 years, especially in children. The most common organisms vary based on the age group (Table 16.1) [3, 6]. Young malnourished children, in particular, are most susceptible to tuberculous meningitis which develops most often within 3 months of the primary infection, and the presence of concomitant deep parenchymal nodules is unusual [7].

Table 16.1 Most common bacteria according to age group

Age group	Most common bacteria
Newborns	Group B *streptococcus*, *Listeria monocytogenes*, *Citrobacter*, and gram-negative organisms such *Escherichia coli*
Children <7 years	*Streptococcus pneumoniae*, *Haemophilus influenzae* type B, *Neisseria meningitidis*, and *Citrobacter*
Children >7 years and adolescents	*Neisseria meningitides*

Meningitis: The organism may reach the meninges hematogeneously, by contiguous spread from infected adjacent aerated cavities (mastoid/middle ear or paranasal sinuses), via the choroid plexus, by abscess rupture to subarachnoid space, or by direct inoculation after penetrating head trauma or neurosurgery. A peculiarity in this age group is recurrent meningitis as a result of previous skull base trauma, cephaloceles, and dysraphic lesions such as dermal tracts, congenital cysts, and neuroenteric fistulae [1, 8]. Mollaret's meningitis is a particular entity in children which is characterized by a benign recurrent lymphocytic meningitis, recently attributed to herpes simplex viruses (HSV-2) [9].

Ventriculitis: The pathogen may reach the intraventricular system by direct implantation secondary to trauma or neurosurgical procedures; contiguous extension, such as brain abscess rupture; and hematogeneous spread [3]. In children, the main route is by subarachnoid extension from a meningeal focus into the ventricles. Ventriculitis occurs in almost 30 % of patients with bacterial meningitis, more commonly in neonates [10].

Empyema: Usually, it occurs secondary to retrograde thrombophlebitis via the calvarial emissary veins from a parameningeal focus. Empyema may also arise from concurrent meningitis, particularly in neonates.

Cerebritis and abscess: Most bacterial abscesses in children are caused by complications of bacterial meningitis. Once the infection is lodged in the meninges, it can spread via the leptomeningeal sheaths of the penetrating cortical vessels resulting in cerebritis and abscess formation. Other possible sources are otomastoiditis, sinusitis, odontogenic abscess, hematogeneous spread, and neurosurgical complications. Congenital cyanotic heart disease should be promptly investigated in cases of brain abscess in children, while recurrent brain abscess has been associated with congenital pulmonary arteriovenous fistula at any age.

Best Imaging Modality

Cranial sonography is a useful imaging modality in newborns for the evaluation of CNS infection complications, such as ventriculitis, extra-axial collections, and brain abscess. It is a wide available imaging modality and does not use radiation [1]. Because of its limited evaluation of the lateral brain surfaces, extra-axial fluid collections in the temporal lobes may be missed.

Computed tomography (CT) is useful before lumbar puncture when elevated intracranial pressure is suspected, and usually it does not require sedation. However, CT has low sensitivity to depict meningeal enhancement, does not provide enough data about the abscess cavity, and can miss small collections located close to the bone surface [11]. Another important limitation is its radiation [4, 12].

Magnetic resonance imaging (MRI) is the imaging modality of choice due to its higher contrast resolution, better sensitivity to contrast enhancement, and its ability to provide presumptive information about the type of infective agent. Nonetheless, it should be carefully used because it often requires sedation especially in younger children.

Postcontrast images are needed when there is no clinical contraindication to gadolinium-based agents. Recent evidence supporting the long-term deposition of gadolinium in certain regions of the brain calls for caution when used repeatedly and in children. Postcontrast fluid-attenuated inversion recovery (FLAIR) images are very helpful to detect meningeal enhancement. Diffusion weighted-imaging (DWI) must be added to the protocol for diagnosis and follow-up purposes as pus is depicted as zones of restricted diffusion regardless of its location.

There is high risk for venous thrombosis when subdural empyema is detected. Therefore, MR venography may be performed to evaluate the patency of dural venous sinuses.

MR perfusion and MR spectroscopy (MRS) should be included whenever there is a ring-enhancing mass present in absence of obvious signs of CNS infection and may help to differentiate an abscess from a tumor [13–16].

Major Findings

Meningitis: Mild ventriculomegaly and enlargement of the subarachnoid spaces are the earliest abnormalities that can be seen. Contrast-enhanced CT can also demonstrate effacement of the cerebral cortical sulci and leptomeningeal enhancement. However, a normal CT scan is the most common finding in children with acute bacterial meningitis [1].

FLAIR MR images usually show hyperintensity in the subarachnoid space over the cerebral convexities. Restricted diffusion on DWI can be observed in purulent meningitis [17]. Even though leptomeningeal enhancement is also depicted on postcontrast T1 weighted-images (T1WI), postcontrast FLAIR is the most sensitive sequence for this purpose (Fig. 16.1) [18].

Ventriculitis: Thickening and abnormal ependymal enhancement are classical findings for ventriculitis. The degree of thickness and morphology of the contrast enhancement should be evaluated to achieve the correct differential diagnosis as in bacterial and virus infections it is expected to be thin and smooth, while in neoplasia it tends to be thick and nodular. The ventricles themselves are nearly always dilated and debris can be seen in their dependent portions. Dependent pus, often a complication from bacterial meningitis in children, always shows restricted diffusion on DWI [3].

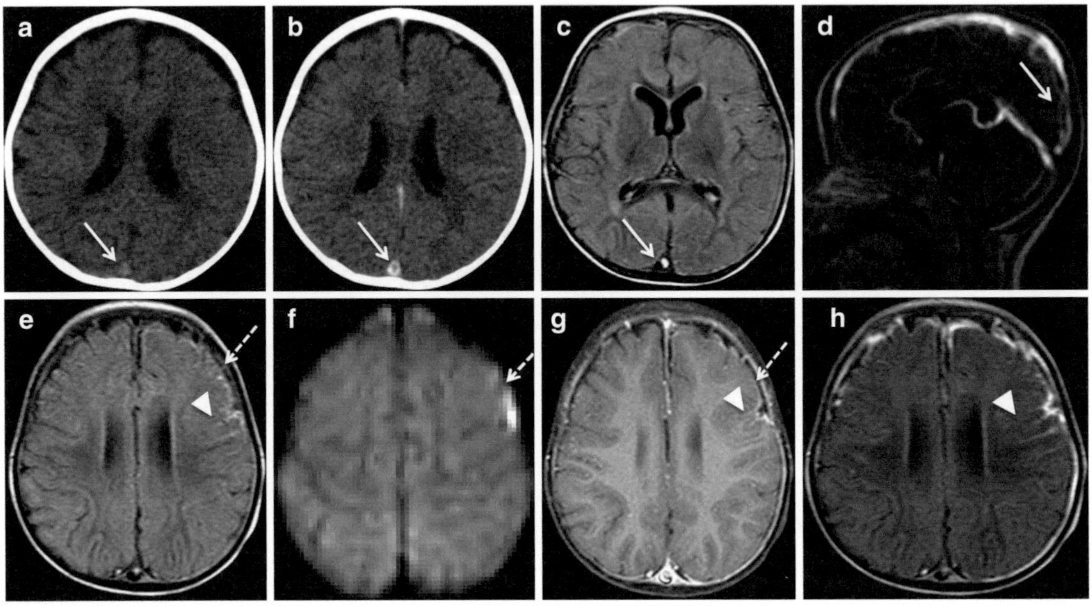

Fig. 16.1 Bacterial meningitis complicated with subdural empyema and superior sagittal sinus thrombosis. (**a**) Non-contrast CT depicts marked hyperattenuation of the superior sagittal sinus (*arrow*). (**b**) Corresponding postcontrast CT demonstrates the filling defect within it consistent with a thrombus (*arrow*). (**c**) Axial FLAIR image shows high signal intensity along the posterior part of superior sagittal sinus (*arrow*). (**d**) On phase contrast venography, there is incomplete filling of the superior sagittal sinus posteriorly (*arrow*). (**e**) Axial FLAIR image demonstrates a subdural collection with high signal intensity extending over the frontal convexity (*dashed arrow*). There is also increased signal in the underlying sulci (*arrowhead*). (**f**) Axial DWI reveals restricted diffusion within the subdural empyema (*dashed arrow*). (**g**) Axial postcontrast T1WI shows peripheral enhancement of the subdural collection (*dashed arrow*) and minimal leptomeningeal enhancement (*arrowhead*). (**h**) Axial FLAIR postcontrast image clearly depicts the leptomeningeal enhancement (*arrowhead*)

Empyema: CT scan and MRI demonstrate an extra-axial collection (concave or convex), uni- or bilateral, with different features from CSF. Peripheral contrast enhancement is virtually seen in all cases. Empyema characteristically displays restricted diffusion on DWI (Fig. 16.1). On T1-weighted images without contrast, its signal tends to be slightly higher than normal CSF. The underlying brain may show edema. Underlying infarcts due to venous thrombosis may be seen [3].

Cerebritis and abscess: Their formation follows a predictable path that can be divided into four sequential stages (Figs. 16.2 and 16.3). Imaging findings vary with the time (Table 16.2) [19, 20].

Hydrocephalus, venous thrombosis, artery vasculopathy, and ischemic stroke are complications that should be promptly addressed. Deep venous thrombosis is more commonly seen in children than in adults with meningitis (Fig. 16.1) [1].

Imaging Follow-Up

Neuroimaging should be performed when there is poor treatment response or complications are suspected [1]. The most common indication of complication in children is increasing head circumference. In such cases, CT or MRI is needed.

Congenital or acquired bone defects especially those communicating with sinonasal and middle ear cavities are an important cause of secondary recurrent meningitis in this age group [1, 8].

DWI and MRS are useful techniques in the pre- and posttreatment evaluation of brain abscesses. Decreased DWI signal intensity and increasing apparent diffusion coefficient (ADC) values in the abscess cavity correlated with successful treatment. The opposite is also true [19, 21]. The reduction or disappearance of the abnormal metabolite peaks by MRS or persistence of isolated peak lactate reflects the good therapeutic response [22].

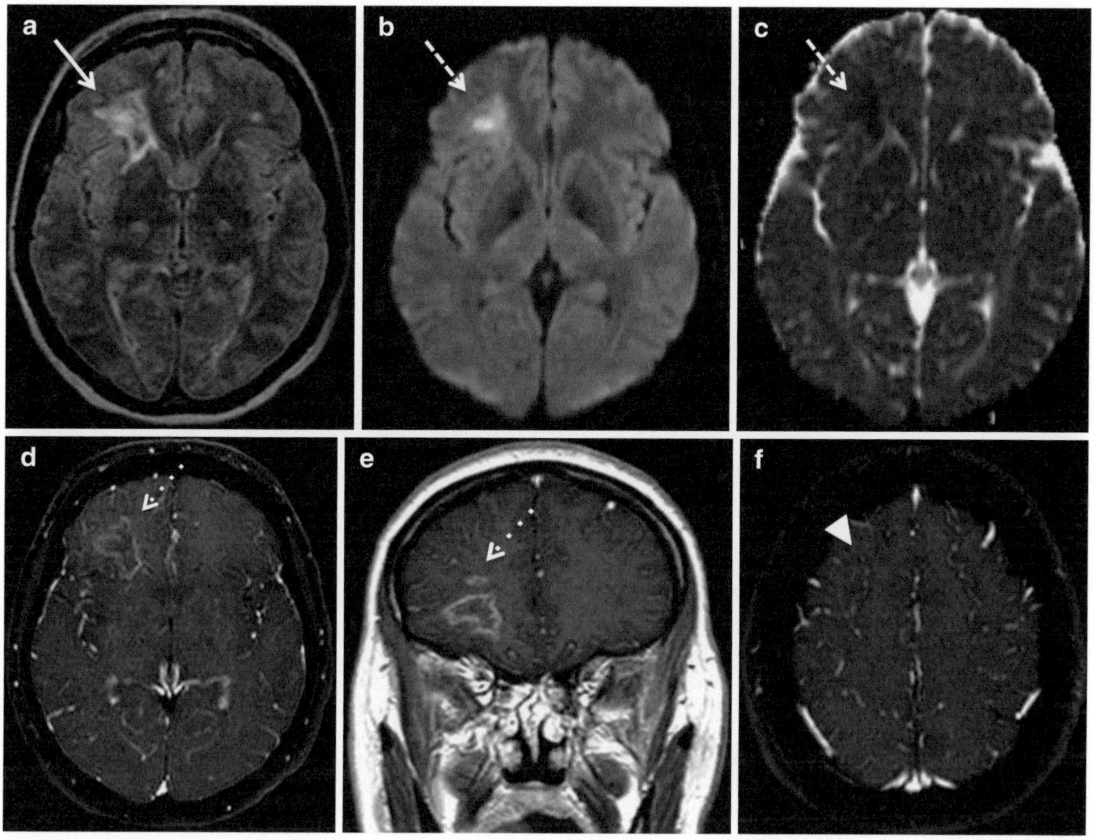

Fig. 16.2 Bacterial meningitis complicated with late cerebritis/early abscess in right frontal lobe. (**a**) Axial FLAIR image shows high signal intensity in the right frontal lobe (*arrow*). Axial DWI (**b**) and ADC (**c**) images demonstrate restricted diffusion (*dashed arrow*). (**d, e**) Corresponding axial and coronal postcontrast T1WI depict irregular peripheral enhancement (*dashed arrow*), consistent with late cerebritis/early abscess. (**f**) Axial postcontrast T1WI reveals leptomeningeal enhancement over the convexity (*arrow head*)

Main Differential Diagnosis

Subarachnoid FLAIR hyperintensity may be caused by a wide range of conditions, pathologic or artifactual. Meningitis, subarachnoid hemorrhage, leptomeningeal spread of malignant disease, and supplemental oxygen concentration are the most important ones [23].

The differential diagnosis of *meningeal enhancement* is extensive and includes neoplastic (primary or secondary tumors), granulomatous, infectious, and inflammatory conditions. Tuberculous meningitis is an important cause of meningitis in young children in endemic areas. Leptomeningeal thickening and enhancement, particularly in basal cisterns, leading to hydrocephalus are the major findings of tuberculous meningitis. Basal ganglia infarcts are also a well-known complication of tuberculosis [7]. Imaging helps in differentiation of infective from the non-infective conditions since carcinomatous meningitis typically presents with dural enhancement and produces thicker or nodular areas of contrast enhancement [3]. A cancer history and systemic disease may guide the differential diagnosis. However, CSF cytology is regarded as the cornerstone of diagnosis. Sometimes biopsy of the affected leptomeningeal areas may help to reach the final diagnosis [3].

Ventriculitis can be caused by a wide variety of infectious agents. Thickening degree and enhancement morphology should be evaluated to offer the correct differential diagnosis. Thereby, thin and linear ependymal enhancement is

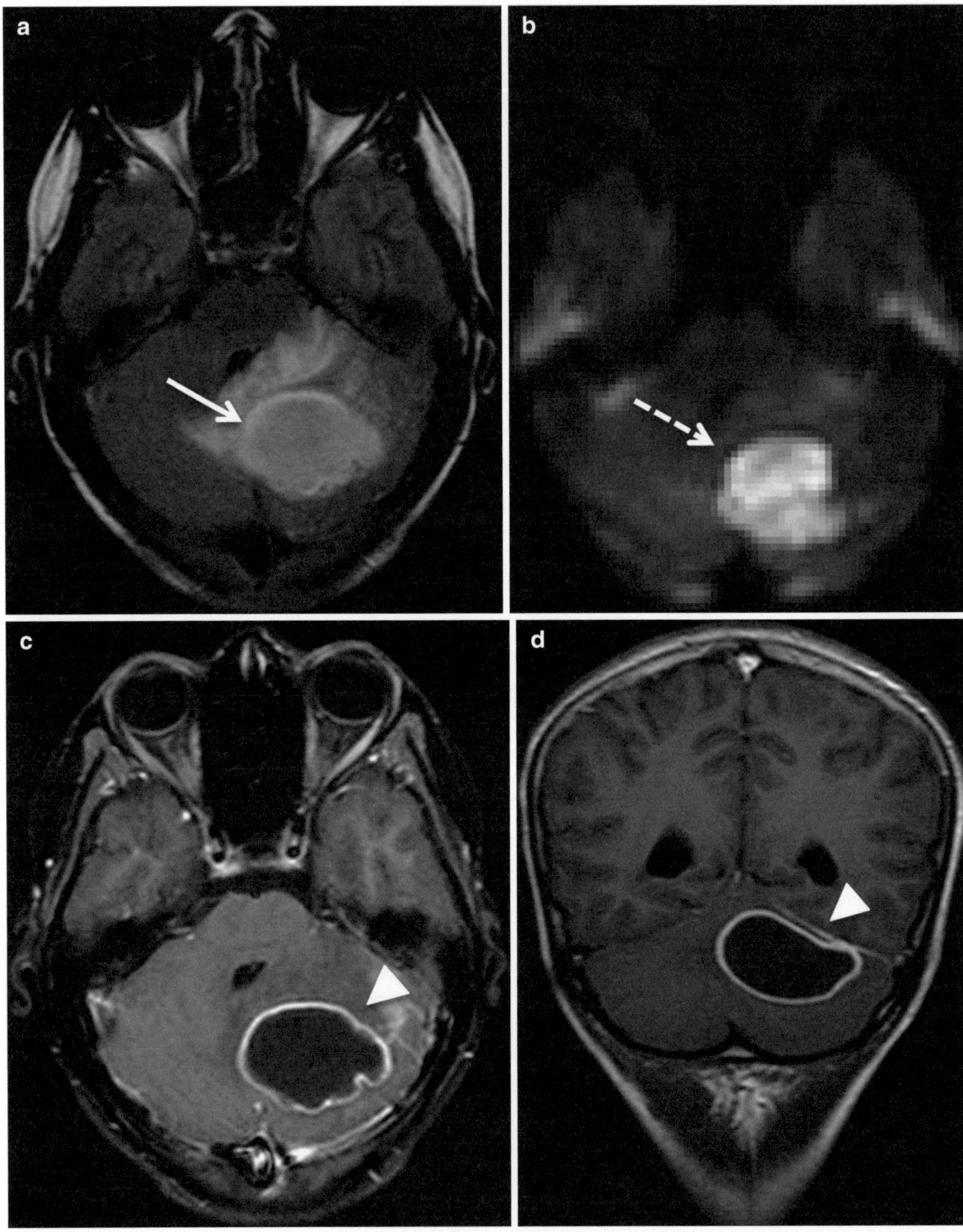

Fig. 16.3 Cerebellar pyogenic abscess. (**a**) Axial FLAIR image depicts the central hyperintense signal (*arrow*) corresponding to the pus cavity and surrounding vasogenic edema. (**b**) Axial DWI shows restricted diffusion on DWI within the abscess cavity (*dashed arrow*). (**c**, **d**) Axial and coronal postcontrast T1WI sequences demonstrate the typical thin and smooth ring of enhancement (*arrowheads*)

Table 16.2 Imaging findings according to development stage

Development stage	Phase	Imaging findings
Early cerebritis	1–3 days	CT demonstrates low attenuation, ill-defined area with subtle mass effect. MR images show hyperintense T2 and FLAIR lesion indistinguishable of edema. Generally no contrast enhancement is present
Late cerebritis	4–9 days	The central area becomes more hypodense due to necrosis. The same findings as above are observed on T1WI, but the periphery may demonstrate an isointense or slight hyperintense rim. On T2WI, the rim is isointense or hypointense and the central area is hyperintense; peripherally to the rim is a hyperintense vasogenic area of edema (target lesion). The central area of necrosis has restricted water diffusion on DWI. After contrast administration, the enhancement can be nodular or ringlikes
Early capsule	10–14 days	The capsule formation is complete. CT demonstrates a demarcated isodense capsule or slight hyperdense margin, interposed between the hypodense central area of necrosis and hypodense surrounding edema. MR demonstrates better defined margins that are markedly hypointense on T2WI, probably due to collagen or paramagnetic free radicals within macrophages and less probably due to hemorrhage that will show hyperintensity on T1WI and hypointensity on T2* images due to susceptibility effects. SWI may show the dual rim sign. The abscess capsule is thinner on its ventricular side than on its cortical side
Late capsule	Beyond the 14th day	The central necrotic cavity decreases in size and the capsule loses the hypointensity on T2WI. Contrast enhancement may persist and progressively decreases

characteristic and suggests underlying infectious disease. On the other hand, neoplastic spread and fungal agents typically produce thicker, lumpy, or nodular enhancement [3]. As cranial sonography is an important tool for assessing ventriculitis in newborns, it is reasonable to recognize that an irregular and echogenic ependyma and presence of intraventricular debris often associated with ventricular dilatation are suggestive of ventriculitis in the right clinical setting [1].

Subdural empyema has two major differential diagnoses. As is subdural empyema, sterile effusions are also commonly associated with bacterial meningitis. Nonetheless, MRI can help to differentiate between them. Effusion is a simply fluid collection that shows CSF-like signal on all conventional MIR pulse sequences and no often peripheral contrast enhancement. Sometimes a sterile effusion may show FLAIR hyperintensity but DWI helps to differentiate it from infected subdural collections as previously mentioned. Subdural hematoma may resemble subdural empyema in view of its morphology and relation to dural reflections. However, T2* or susceptibility-weighted imaging (SWI) depicts blood products within it. The use of DWI for this purpose may be tricky as blood products may cause high signal intensity due to susceptibility magnetic artifacts which may simulate the restricted diffusion of pus. "Shaken baby" syndrome and Menkes disease should be contemplated in the differential diagnosis in children with subdural collection without fever or infectious symptoms [24].

Differential diagnosis of cerebritis is vast and includes encephalitis that also presents with restricted diffusion on DWI affecting a nonvascular territory. Viral infections are the major cause of encephalitis, HSV-1, mumps virus, varicella, and arbovirus being the most common ones [1]. Generally, herpes encephalitis in patients older than 6 month is secondary to HSV-1. Neuroimaging shows the characteristically tropism for the limbic system. Varicella-zoster virus (VZV) infection is common during childhood and CNS complications occur in less than 0.1 % of children. These patients may present with focal neurologic deficit 1–4 months after initial skin rash caused by infarction of basal ganglia due angitis induced by VZV [1]. Involvement of the middle cerebral artery with basal ganglia infarcts is typical.

Differential diagnosis for brain abscess in pediatric population may also be assessed by the *MAGICAL DR* mnemonic, where "M" standing for metastasis, "A" for abscess, "G" for gliomas, "I" for infarction (subacute), "C" for contusion (resolving hematoma), "A" for AIDS (opportunistic infections such as toxoplasmosis and cryptococcosis), "L" for lymphoma (particularly in immunocompromised patients), "D" for demyelination, and "R" for radiation necrosis. Children rarely develop opportunistic CNS complications when compared to adults [1]. In children with cerebellar abscesses, consider an infected dermoid/epidermoid.

Clinical history and advanced MRI techniques help in the diagnostic workflow. A ring-enhancing lesion presenting with a smooth and linear peripheral enhancement and restricted diffusion on DWI within its content is highly suggestive of a pyogenic abscess. Absence of increased perfusion, dual rim sign on SWI, and the presence of lactate (1.3) and amino acids (acetate and succinate predominantly at 0.9 ppm) on MRS may aid to confirm the diagnosis [13, 16].

Tips

- Frequently, anesthesia is needed to perform a MRI in children. Supplemental oxygen administration is a common cause of subarachnoid FLAIR hyperintensity. Sagittal T1WI can easily depict the oropharyngeal aperture, helping identify cannulas used to deliver supplemental oxygen. Besides, in this situation, CSF in the ventricles is usually of normal signal as the ependymal is impervious to oxygen while the pia is not.
- Do not forget to include postcontrast FLAIR sequence in the MRI protocol. It is the most sensitive sequence to depict leptomeningeal enhancement.
- Meningeal enhancement is nonspecific and can be seen in meningitis of any cause, including noninfectious processes.
- Leptomeningeal thickening and enhancement that is centered within the basal cisterns is suggestive of tuberculous meningitis in endemic areas.
- Restricted diffusion on DWI within a centrally T2 hyperintense ring-enhancing mass is nearly always characteristic of a pyogenic brain abscess.
- *MAGICAL DR* mnemonic helps to remember the potential causes of a cerebral ring-enhancing lesion. Clinical history and advanced imaging techniques may help narrow the differential diagnosis.

References

1. Parmar H, Ibrahim M. Pediatric intracranial infections. Neuroimaging Clin N Am. 2012;22(4):707–25.
2. Curtis S, Stobart K, Vandermeer B, Simel DL, Klassen T. Clinical features suggestive of meningitis in children: a systematic review of prospective data. Pediatrics. 2010;126(5):952–60.
3. Mohan S, Jain KK, Arabi M, Shah GV. Imaging of meningitis and ventriculitis. Neuroimaging Clin N Am. 2012;22(4):557–83.
4. Frush DP. Justification and optimization of CT in children: how are we performing? Pediatr Radiol. 2011;41(Suppl 2(S2)):467–71.
5. Heth JA. Neurosurgical aspects of central nervous system infections. Neuroimaging Clin N Am. 2012;22(4):791–9.
6. Riddle J, Shuman EK. Epidemiology of central nervous system infection. Neuroimaging Clin N Am. Elsevier Inc; 2020;22(4):543–56.
7. Chatterjee S. Brain tuberculomas, tubercular meningitis, and post-tubercular hydrocephalus in children. J Pediatr Neurosci. 2011;6(3):96.
8. Steele RW, McConnell JR, Jacobs RF, Mawk JR. Recurrent bacterial meningitis: coronal thin-section cranial computed tomography to delineate anatomic defects. Pediatrics. 1985;76(6):950–3.
9. Willmann O, Ahmad-Nejad P, Neumaier M, Hennerici MG, Fatar M. Toll-like receptor 3 immune deficiency

may be causative for HSV-2-associated mollaret meningitis. Eur Neurol. 2010;63(4):249–51.
10. Barkovich AJ. Pediatric neuroimaging. Philadelphia: Lippincott Williams & Wilkins; 2005. 1 p.
11. Chang KH, Han MH, Roh JK, Kim IO, Han MC, Kim CW. Gd-DTPA-enhanced MR imaging of the brain in patients with meningitis: comparison with CT. Am J Roentgenol. 1990;154(4):809–16.
12. Strauss KJ, Kaste SC. The ALARA (as low as reasonably achievable) concept in pediatric interventional and fluoroscopic imaging: striving to keep radiation doses as low as possible during fluoroscopy of pediatric patients – a white paper executive summary. Radiology. 2006;240(3):621–2.
13. Kim YJ, Chang KH, Song IC, Kim HD, Seong SO, Kim YH, et al. Brain abscess and necrotic or cystic brain tumor: discrimination with signal intensity on diffusion-weighted MR imaging. Am J Roentgenol. 1998;171(6):1487–90.
14. Luthra G, Parihar A, Nath K, Jaiswal S, Prasad KN, Husain N, et al. Comparative evaluation of fungal, tubercular, and pyogenic brain abscesses with conventional and diffusion MR imaging and proton MR spectroscopy. Am J Neuroradiol. 2007;28(7):1332–8.
15. Pal D, Bhattacharyya A, Husain M, Prasad KN, Pandey CM, Gupta RK. In vivo proton MR spectroscopy evaluation of pyogenic brain abscesses: a report of 194 cases. AJNR Am J Neuroradiol. 2010;31(2): 360–6.
16. Toh CH, Wei KC, Ng SH, Wan YL, Lin CP, Castillo M. Differentiation of brain abscesses from necrotic glioblastomas and cystic metastatic brain tumors with diffusion tensor imaging. Am J Neuroradiol. 2011;32(9):1646–51.
17. Gasparetto EL, Cabral RF, da Cruz LCH, Domingues RC. Diffusion imaging in brain infections. Neuroimaging Clin N Am. 2011;21(1):89–113. -viii.
18. Fukuoka H, Hirai T, Okuda T, Shigematsu Y, Sasao A, Kimura E, et al. Comparison of the added value of contrast-enhanced 3D fluid-attenuated inversion recovery and magnetization-prepared rapid acquisition of gradient echo sequences in relation to conventional postcontrast T1-weighted images for the evaluation of leptomeningeal diseases at 3T. AJNR Am J Neuroradiol. 2010;31(5):868–73.
19. Maia AC, Guedes BV, Lucas A Jr, da Rocha AJ. Diffusion MR imaging for monitoring treatment response. Neuroimaging Clin N Am. Elsevier Ltd; 2011;21(1):153–78.
20. Rath TJ, Hughes M, Arabi M, Shah GV. Imaging of cerebritis, encephalitis, and brain abscess. Neuroimaging Clin N Am. 2012;22(4):585–607.
21. Cartes-Zumelzu FW, Stavrou I, Castillo M, Eisenhuber E, Knosp E, Thurnher MM. Diffusion-weighted imaging in the assessment of brain abscesses therapy. Am J Neuroradiol. 2004;25(8):1310–7.
22. Burtscher IM, Holtås S. In vivo proton MR spectroscopy of untreated and treated brain abscesses. Am J Neuroradiol. 1999;20(6):1049–53.
23. Stuckey SL, Goh TD, Heffernan T, Rowan D. Hyperintensity in the subarachnoid space on FLAIR MRI. Am J Roentgenol. 2007;189(4):913–21.
24. da Rocha AJ, Vedolin L, Mendonça RA. Encéfalo. Rio de Janeiro: Elsevier; 2012. 1 p.

Acute Disseminated Encephalomyelitis (ADEM)

17

Ana Lorena Abello and Renato Hoffmann Nunes

Abstract

Acute disseminated encephalomyelitis (ADEM) is an immune-mediated inflammatory disorder of the central nervous system characterized by widespread demyelination that predominantly involves white matter in the brain and spinal cord. It is characteristically a monophasic illness that is commonly associated with a trigger event (e.g., febrile illness or vaccination). In cases of recurrent or multiphasic ADEM, the possibility of developing multiple sclerosis is of concern.

Background

Acute disseminated encephalomyelitis (ADEM) is an immunologically mediated inflammatory disease resulting in multifocal demyelinating lesions affecting the gray and white matter of the brain and spinal cord [1].

ADEM can occur at any age, but it is more common in pediatric patients than in adults. The mean age at presentation ranges from 5 to 8 years. A seasonal distribution with increased prevalence of cases in the winter and spring months has been found [2]. The incidence is variable in different countries. In the United States, this is estimated to be 0.4 per 100,000 in individuals younger than 20 years [3].

ADEM is classically described as a monophasic disorder, which typically begins within 2 days to 4 weeks after an antigenic exposure. Approximately 70–77 % of patients report a clinically evident prior infection or vaccination a few weeks before the onset of ADEM. Typical symptoms and signs of ADEM include a rapid-onset encephalopathy associated with a combination of multifocal neurologic deficits. The clinical course is rapidly progressive and usually develops over hours to maximum deficits within days (mean, 4.5 days). Frequent neurologic symptoms and signs include unilateral or bilateral pyramidal signs, acute hemiplegia, ataxia, cranial nerve palsies, visual loss due to optic neuritis, seizures, spinal cord involvement, impairment of speech, and hemipares-

A.L. Abello, MD (✉)
Department of Radiology,
University of North Carolina, Chapel Hill, NC, USA
e-mail: anaabellop@hotmail.com

R. Hoffmann Nunes, MD
Division of Neuroradiology,
Santa Casa de São Paulo, São Paulo, Brazil
e-mail: renatohn@hotmail.com

R. Hoffmann Nunes et al. (eds.), *Critical Findings in Neuroradiology*,
DOI 10.1007/978-3-319-27987-9_17

thesias, with invariable involvement of mental status, ranging from lethargy to coma. Occasionally, ADEM can present as a subtle disease, with nonspecific irritability, headache, and somnolence [1, 2, 4].

Cerebrospinal fluid (CSF) is normal in up to 61.5 % of patients. If patients are found to have abnormal CSF parameters, these are usually minor and nonspecific. A lymphocyte pleocytosis (usually between 50 and 180 cells/mm^2), elevated protein (commonly 0.5–1.0 g/dL), and/or oligoclonal bands can be seen but less commonly than in multiple sclerosis (MS) [1, 4, 5].

In 2007, The International MS Study Group defined the diagnostic criteria for monophasic ADEM. One of the most significant changes proposed by this classification was the mandatory inclusion of encephalopathy as a symptom in patients presenting with ADEM. These criteria are summarized in Table 17.1 [5].

Based on the presumed autoimmune etiology of ADEM, the common treatment consists of intravenous and oral corticosteroids. In cases of insufficient response or contraindications to corticosteroids, intravenous immunoglobulin is an option. For severe or life-threatening cases, plasmapheresis should be considered. Decompressive craniectomy has been reported to be a life-saving measure for ADEM patients with severe intracranial hypertension [6].

Complete resolution of the disease has been noted in up to 70 % of patients within a few months of presentation; however, residual deficits may persist in up to one-third of patients 2 years after the onset of ADEM [1].

Table 17.1 International MS study group monophasic ADEM criteria

No history of prior demyelinating event
First clinical event with presumed inflammatory or demyelinating cause
Acute or subacute onset
Affects multifocal areas of central nervous system
Must be polysymptomatic
Must include encephalopathy (e.g., behavioral change or altered level of consciousness)
Neuroimaging shows focal/multifocal lesion(s) predominantly affecting white matter
No neuroimaging evidence of previous destructive white matter changes
Event should be followed by clinical/radiologic improvements (although may be residual deficits)
No other etiology can explain the event
New or fluctuating symptoms, signs, or MRI findings occurring within 3 months are considered part of the acute event

Key Points

Etiology

ADEM is characterized histologically by perivenular infiltrates of T cells and macrophages, associated with perivenular demyelination [2, 7].

The precise mechanisms implicated in the development ADEM are not well known. The seasonal distribution of ADEM supports an etiological link with infectious diseases. Viruses that have been implicated in promoting the immune response responsible for ADEM include herpes simplex virus, human immunodeficiency virus, HHV-6, mumps, measles, rubella, varicella, influenza, enterovirus, hepatitis A, coxsackie, EBV, and cytomegalovirus. Other infectious agents that have been linked to ADEM include group A B-hemolytic streptococcal infection, *Bordetella pertussis*, *Mycoplasma pneumoniae*, *Borrelia burgdorferi*, Legionella, Rickettsiae, *Plasmodium falciparum*, *Plasmodium vivax*, and malaria. However, the majority of patients have a preceding infection of the upper respiratory tract, where the actual organism is not identified. Vaccines for influenza, rabies, Japanese B encephalitis, and smallpox have been reported to precipitate ADEM [1, 8].

There are two basic mechanisms proposed to cause ADEM, both of which rely on the exposure of the immune system to an antigenic challenge as follows:

1. *Molecular mimicry theory*: This theory relies on the idea that myelin antigens (e.g., myelin basic protein) share a structural similarity with antigenic determinants on the infecting pathogen. The infected host mounts an immune response producing antiviral antibodies that are thought to cross-react with myelin antigens that share a similar structure, inadvertently producing an autoimmune response.
2. *Inflammatory cascade theory*: Nervous system tissue is thought to be damaged secondary to viral infection, resulting in the leakage of myelin-based antigens into the systemic circulation through an impaired blood–brain barrier. These antigens promote a T-cell response which in turn causes secondary damage to the nervous system tissue through an inflammatory response [1].

Best Imaging Modality

Magnetic resonance imaging (MRI): MRI of the brain is the most important imaging modality available in the diagnosis of ADEM, it also helps to distinguish it from other inflammatory and non-inflammatory neurologic diseases [1, 9, 10]. Fluid-attenuated inversion recovery (FLAIR) and T2-weighted images (T2WI) demonstrate the abnormalities more readily than T1-weighted images (T1WI) [8].

Diffusion-weighted imaging (DWI) and MR spectroscopy are sensitive depending on the stage of the disease. MR perfusion may help to differentiate it from high-grade tumors [1].

Computed tomography (CT): CT is insensitive in detecting small demyelinating lesions compared with MRI and, therefore, may yield false-negative results in the presence of ADEM [1, 9]. Dale et al. reported abnormalities in 59 % of the CT scans in patients with ADEM, whereas all MRI brain scans demonstrated lesions [8].

Major Findings

The typical MRI findings described in ADEM are widespread, bilateral, asymmetric patchy areas of homogeneous or slightly inhomogeneous increased signal intensity on T2WI and FLAIR within the white matter, deep gray nuclei, and spinal cord. Within the white matter, juxtacortical and deep white matter is involved more frequently than is the periventricular white matter. Lesions confined to the corpus callosum are less common. Large demyelinating lesions may extend into the corpus callosum and cross into the contralateral hemisphere [1]. Bilateral middle cerebellar peduncle involvement has been demonstrated [11]. With respect to lesion size and morphology, variation is common ranging from small, round lesions to large, amorphous, and irregular lesions [1].

Four patterns of cerebral involvement have been proposed to describe the MRI findings in ADEM: [2, 4, 8, 12]

1. ADEM with small lesions (<5 mm).
2. ADEM with large (>1 cm), confluent, or tumefactive lesions with frequent extensive perilesional edema and mass effect (Fig. 17.1).
3. ADEM with additional symmetric bithalamic involvement (Fig. 17.2).
4. Acute hemorrhagic encephalomyelitis (AHEM) (Weston–Hurst disease) when hemorrhage can be identified in large demyelinating lesions. The clinical course of AHEM is more fulminant than that of the usual ADEM (Fig. 17.3).

The incidence of gadolinium-enhancing lesions on T1WI is variable in ADEM and depends on the stage of inflammation. Gadolinium-enhancing lesions have been described in 30 % of patients. Different patterns of enhancement have been described: complete or incomplete ring-shaped, nodular, gyral, or diffuse patchy (Fig. 17.1) [1, 2]. Meningeal enhancement is unusual [2].

ADEM rarely presents as a solitary brain stem lesion without evidence of disseminated lesions (monofocal presentation). Patients presenting

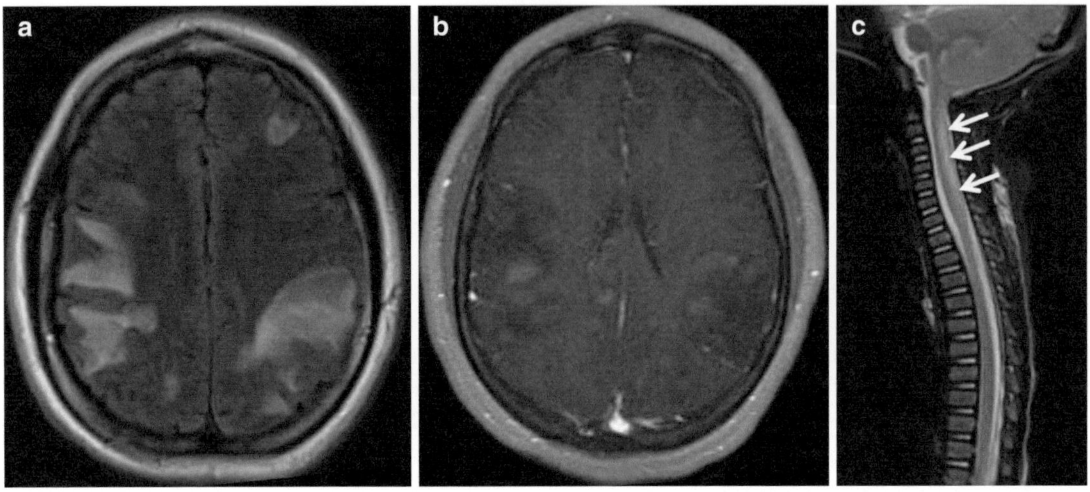

Fig. 17.1 Acute disseminated encephalomyelitis. Large bilateral and asymmetric hyperintense lesions in the white matter of the center semiovale. (**a**) Axial FLAIR image shows hyperintense lesions in both cerebral hemispheres with mass effect. (**b**) Postcontrast axial T1WI at the same level depicts slightly nodular enhancement. (**c**) Sagittal STIR shows an extensive compromise of the posterior cervical spinal cord (*arrows*)

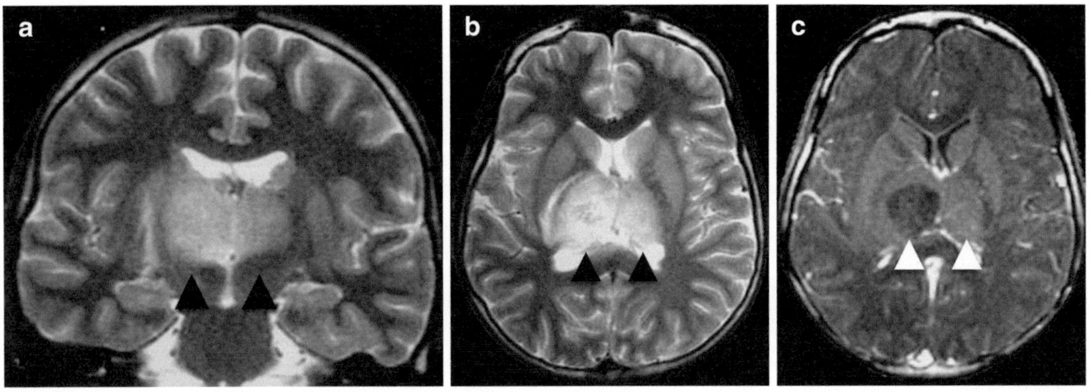

Fig. 17.2 Bithalamic involvement in ADEM. An 8-year-old patient presenting with left hemiparesis and reduced level of consciousness. (**a**, **b**) Coronal and axial T2WI, respectively, show symmetric hyperintense bilateral thalamic lesions (*arrowheads*). (**c**) Postcontrast axial T1-magnetic transfer contrast (MTC) depicts a hypointense lesion in the right thalamus and absence of abnormal enhancement (*arrowheads*)

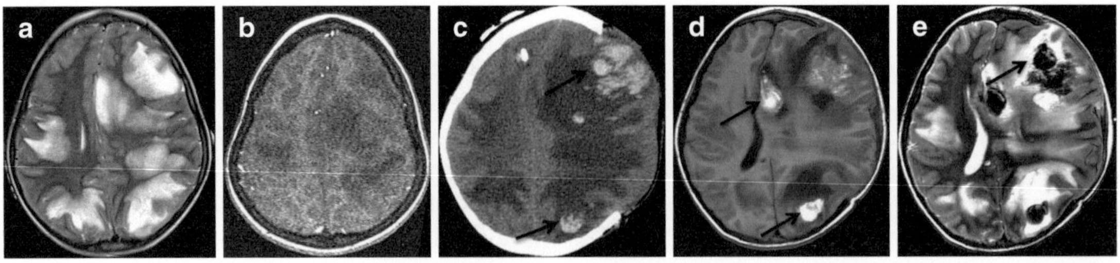

Fig. 17.3 Acute hemorrhagic encephalomyelitis. (**a**) Axial T2WI shows extensive compromise of the hemispheric white matter with mass effect and right-sided subfalcine herniation. (**b**) On postcontrast T1WI, the lesions do not show enhancement. (**c**) Axial CT, D. axial T1WI, and E. axial T2WI 8 days after decompressive hemicraniectomy. The patient developed hemorrhagic lesions and worsening of mass effect. Hemorrhagic foci correspond to hyperdense lesions on CT (**c**), as well as hyperintense and hypointense lesions on T1WI and T2WI, respectively (**d**, **e**) (*arrows*) (Images courtesy of Ramon Figueroa, MD. Augusta, GA (USA))

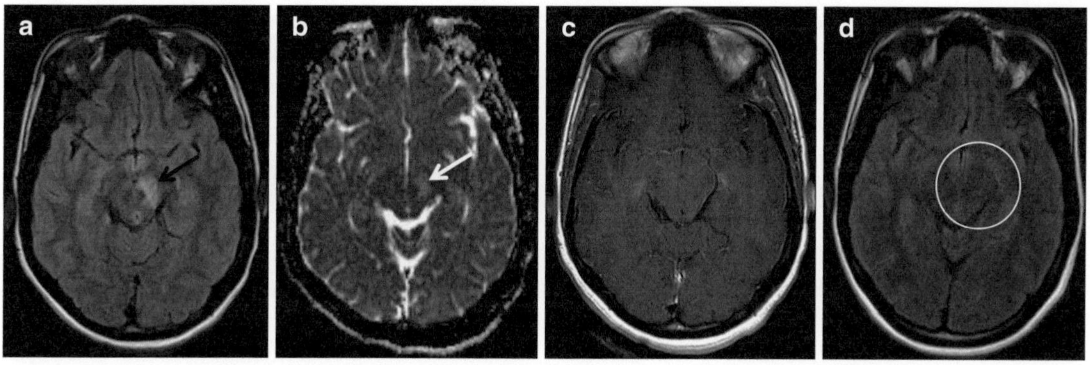

Fig. 17.4 Presumed ADEM compromising the brain stem. (**a**) Axial FLAIR shows a hyperintense lesion in the left middle cerebral peduncle (*black arrow*). The patient presented right hemiparesis and a mildly reduced level of consciousness. (**b**) ADC map depicts high diffusion compatible with vasogenic edema (*white arrow*). (**c**) There is no enhancement on postcontrast T1WI. (**d**) Follow-up imaging 1 month later after complete clinical recovery demonstrates resolution of the lesion (*circle*) on this FLAIR image

with only a brain stem lesion are more challenging to diagnose because the imaging findings that are characteristic of ADEM are not present. Clinically, these patients may or may not have an encephalopathy (Fig. 17.4) [10].

Complete resolution of the lesions occurs in up to 70 % of patients within months of presentation (Fig. 17.4). Residual deficits may persist in up to one-third of patients 2 years after the onset of ADEM [1]. Resolution of MRI abnormalities is related to resorption of abnormally increased interstitial water and remyelination. Some lesions remain visible on MRI as areas of T2 prolongation and probably represent astrocytic hyperplasia and gliosis known to occur in late stages of ADEM [4].

If DWI is obtained within 7 days of the clinical onset, a pattern of restricted diffusion may be seen which subsequently changes to increased diffusion consistent with vasogenic edema (Fig. 17.4) [1, 10, 13].

Within the acute phase, MR spectroscopy shows that N-acetylaspartate (NAA) and choline values are normal. As the disease progresses, there is reduction of NAA and increase in choline (with corresponding reductions in NAA/creatine and NAA/choline ratios) in regions corresponding to areas of high signal intensity on T2WI. These abnormalities resolved after normalization of clinical and MRI findings [1, 2, 14].

Table 17.2 ADEM MRI appearance

White matter > gray matter, but usually both affected
Bilateral asymmetric white matter involvement
Bilateral symmetric gray matter involvement
Deep/juxtacortical white matter > periventricular white matter
Both supratentorial and infratentorial lesions, but more supratentorial
Small>medium>large, but often all sizes are present in same patient
Variable contrast enhancement

The summary of the more frequent imaging findings is found in Table 17.2 [1].

Spinal cord involvement in ADEM has been described in 11–28 % of patients. Typical spinal cord lesions are large and swollen, show variable enhancement, and predominantly affect the thoracic region. Skip lesions with intervening segments of cord that appear normal are typical (Fig. 17.1) [2].

Imaging Follow-Up

Sequential MRI scanning during the follow-up period plays an important role in establishing the diagnosis of ADEM. Monophasic ADEM is not associated with development of new lesions. Complete resolution of MRI abnormalities after treatment has been described in 37–75 % of patients and partial resolution in 25–53 % of them. There are no clear criteria documenting how long to continue to image patients after a single ADEM episode. Some authors suggest reassessing patients with at least two additional MRI studies after the first normal MRI over a period of 5 years from the initial episode as the best way to confirm the absence of ongoing lesions [2].

The 2007 consensus (see above) also defined recurrent and multiphasic ADEM in children who experience subsequent events after an initial ADEM illness not associated with a lifelong disorder characterized by an ongoing demyelinating process. The distinction between multiphasic and recurrent rests on whether the second ADEM illness involves new brain regions (multiphasic) or whether the second event is a recapitulation of the prior illness (recurrent). In both instances, the new event must meet clinical criteria for ADEM, including the presence of encephalopathy [5].

Main Differential Diagnosis

The first priority in a patient presenting with neurologic signs and symptoms and encephalopathy, particularly in presence of a preceding febrile illness, is to rule out a *bacterial or viral infection* of the central nervous system (CNS). A diagnosis of meningoencephalitis can be suggested by leptomeningeal enhancement on postcontrast MRI or CT (which is an unusual feature of ADEM) or the typical involvement of limbic structures in herpes encephalitis [1, 2].

When the MRI shows large *focal tumorlike lesions*, one should consider brain tumors, brain abscesses, or tumefactive demyelinating disease [2, 10].

The presence of *complete ring-enhanced lesions* in the cerebral white matter is unusual in ADEM, and brain neoplasias, abscess, tuberculomas, neurocysticercosis, toxoplasmosis, and histoplasmosis should be excluded [1, 2].

An MRI pattern with *symmetric bithalamic involvement* may be seen in children with deep cerebral venous thrombosis, hypernatremia, and extrapontine myelinolysis, as well as in children with viral encephalitis [2]. Symmetric, hemorrhagic, brain necrosis in the thalami and brain stem may also be seen in acute necrotizing encephalopathy which is a more severe, life-threatening form of influenza-associated encephalopathy with variable genetic components. It is characterized by high fever, seizures, and rapid clinical deterioration within 2 or 3 days after symptom onset. The disease is often fatal and most cases occur in children or young adults. *Basal ganglia involvement* may also be consistent with organic aciduria, or infantile bilateral striatal necrosis [2].

In patients presenting with only a *brain stem lesion,* one should rule out glioma, CNS involvement by connective tissue disorders, brain stem ischemic lesions, and central pontine myelinolysis. Low ADC values in the acute stage are an important feature of central pontine myelinolysis [10].

The *leukodystrophies* should be considered when symmetrical white matter abnormalities are seen [8, 10].

Multiple sclerosis: MS in children can initially present with symptoms and signs that are indistinguishable from ADEM. Subsequent neurologic events or changes on MRI typical of MS lead to the correct diagnosis (Table 17.3) (Fig. 17.5) [2, 5, 15]. Serial MRI in patients with multiphasic ADEM, obtained following resolution of the second demyelinating event, should show a complete or partial resolution of the lesions compared to patients with MS who typically demonstrate ongoing accrual of asymptomatic lesions. Furthermore, high titers of myelin oligodendrocyte glycoprotein (MOG) antibodies are related to other inflammatory demyelinating diseases different from MS [16, 17].

Table 17.3 Differences between typical features of ADEM and MS

Criteria	ADEM	MS
Age	<10 years	>10 years
Gender	Male = female	Female > male
Prior influenza	Very frequent	Variable
Encephalopathy	Required	Rare
Attacks	A single event can fluctuate over the course of 12 weeks	Discrete events separated by at least 4 weeks
Large lesions > 2 cm	Frequent	Rare
Lesion margins	Poorly defined	Well defined
Periventricular white matter compromise	Variable	Frequent
Deep gray matter	Frequently involved	Rarely involved
Spinal cord lesions	Extensive	Small
Longitudinal MRI	Resolution	New lesions
CFS white blood cell count > $50/mm^3$	Frequent	Very rare
CSF oligoclonal bands	Variable	Frequently
MOG atb	Frequent	Rare

Tips

- Bilateral and asymmetric lesions of increased signal intensity on T2WI and FLAIR in white matter and/or symmetric increased signal in both thalami are suggestive of ADEM.
- Monophasic ADEM is typically characterized by lesions at the same stage.
- Incidence and pattern of contrast enhancement are variable. Prominent contrast enhancement is not common.
- A pattern of increased diffusion consistent with vasogenic edema is a common presentation; some ADEM lesions show restricted diffusion in the first week of onset.
- Complete resolution of ADEM is documented in more than 70 % of patients.
- Presence of encephalopathy is necessary to diagnose ADEM.
- Several episodes of ADEM should make or suspect the diagnosis of MS.

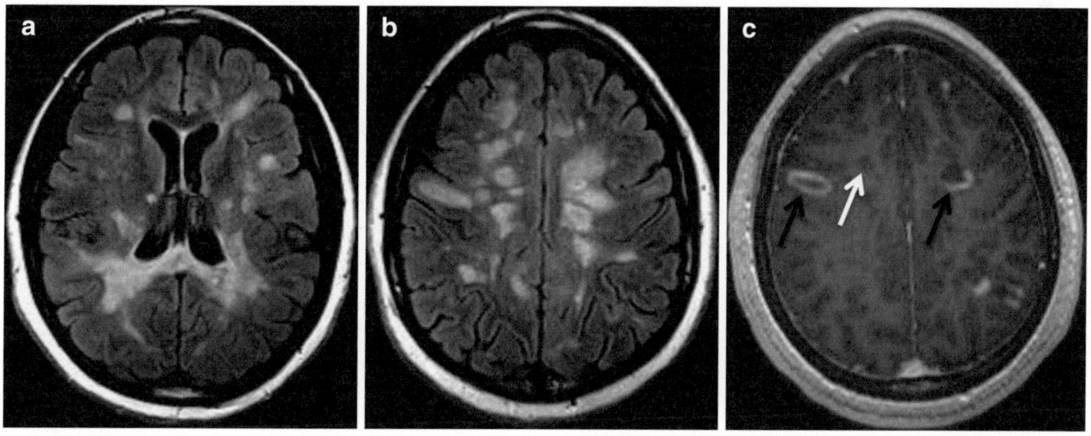

Fig. 17.5 Multiple sclerosis in a pediatric patient. (**a**, **b**) Axial FLAIR at the level of the lateral ventricles and semiovale centers show extensive compromise of the periventricular white matter and juxtacortical ellipsoid lesions characteristic of MS. (**c**) Axial postcontrast T1WI depicts some lesions with complete and incomplete ring enhancement (*black arrows*) as well as non-enhancing hypointense lesions (black holes) (*white arrow*) all related to acute and chronic involvement

References

1. Marin SE, Callen DJ. The magnetic resonance imaging appearance of monophasic acute disseminated encephalomyelitis: an update post application of the 2007 consensus criteria. Neuroimaging Clin N Am. 2013;23(2):245–66.
2. Tenembaum S, Chitnis T, Ness J, Hahn JS, International Pediatric MSSG. Acute disseminated encephalomyelitis. Neurology. 2007;68(16 Suppl 2):S23–36.
3. Leake JA, Albani S, Kao AS, Senac MO, Billman GF, Nespeca MP, et al. Acute disseminated encephalomyelitis in childhood: epidemiologic, clinical and laboratory features. Pediatr Infect Dis J. 2004;23(8):756–64.
4. Baum PA, Barkovich AJ, Koch TK, Berg BO. Deep gray matter involvement in children with acute disseminated encephalomyelitis. AJNR Am J Neuroradiol. 1994;15(7):1275–83.
5. Krupp LB, Banwell B, Tenembaum S, International Pediatric MSSG. Consensus definitions proposed for pediatric multiple sclerosis and related disorders. Neurology. 2007;68(16 Suppl 2):S7–12.
6. Pohl D, Tenembaum S. Treatment of acute disseminated encephalomyelitis. Curr Treat Options Neurol. 2012;14(3):264–75.
7. Mader I, Stock KW, Ettlin T, Probst A. Acute disseminated encephalomyelitis: MR and CT features. AJNR Am J Neuroradiol. 1996;17(1):104–9.
8. Dale RC, de Sousa C, Chong WK, Cox TC, Harding B, Neville BG. Acute disseminated encephalomyelitis, multiphasic disseminated encephalomyelitis and multiple sclerosis in children. Brain: J Neurol. 2000;123(Pt 12):2407–22.
9. Honkaniemi J, Dastidar P, Kahara V, Haapasalo H. Delayed MR imaging changes in acute disseminated encephalomyelitis. AJNR Am J Neuroradiol. 2001;22(6):1117–24.
10. Alper G, Sreedher G, Zuccoli G. Isolated brain stem lesion in children: is it acute disseminated encephalomyelitis or not? AJNR Am J Neuroradiol. 2013;34(1):217–20.
11. Okamoto K, Tokiguchi S, Furusawa T, Ishikawa K, Quardery AF, Shinbo S, et al. MR features of diseases involving bilateral middle cerebellar peduncles. AJNR Am J Neuroradiol. 2003;24(10):1946–54.
12. Lee HY, Chang KH, Kim JH, Na DG, Kwon BJ, Lee KW, et al. Serial MR imaging findings of acute hemorrhagic leukoencephalitis: a case report. AJNR Am J Neuroradiol. 2005;26(8):1996–9.
13. Zuccoli G, Panigrahy A, Sreedher G, Bailey A, Laney EJ, La Colla L, et al. Vasogenic edema characterizes pediatric acute disseminated encephalomyelitis. Neuroradiology. 2014;56(8):679–84.
14. Bizzi A, Ulug AM, Crawford TO, Passe T, Bugiani M, Bryan RN, et al. Quantitative proton MR spectroscopic imaging in acute disseminated encephalomyelitis. AJNR Am J Neuroradiol. 2001;22(6):1125–30.
15. Naidich TP. Imaging of the brain. Philadelphia: Saunders/Elsevier; 2013. Available from: http://getitatduke.library.duke.edu/?sid=sersol&SS_jc=TC0000823014&title=Imaging of the brain.
16. Hacohen Y, Absoud M, Deiva K, Hemingway C, Nytrova P, Woodhall M, et al. Myelin oligodendrocyte glycoprotein antibodies are associated with a non-MS course in children. Neurol Neuroimmunol Neuroinflamm. 2015;2(2):e81.
17. Reindl M, Di Pauli F, Rostasy K, Berger T. The spectrum of MOG autoantibody-associated demyelinating diseases. Nat Rev Neurol. 2013;9(8):455–61.

Metabolic Brain Disorders in Children

18

Antonio Carlos Martins Maia Jr.,
Antônio José da Rocha, and Renato Hoffmann Nunes

Abstract

Although rare, metabolic brain disorders account for a substantial portion of childhood and adult encephalopathy cases and may cause significant morbidity and mortality. Most of these disorders are inborn errors of metabolism, and brain injury results from the accumulation of endogenous toxic substances or a lack of production of necessary biochemicals. Inborn errors of metabolism can occur at nearly any age, and their clinical signs and symptoms are almost invariably nonspecific. Some of them, especially at neonatal period, manifest with acute encephalopathy and a life-threatening episode of metabolic decompensation, whereas later-onset disorders have a more manageable clinical course with variable outcomes.

A.C.M. Maia Jr., MD, PhD (✉)
A.J. da Rocha, MD, PhD
Division of Neuroradiology, Hospital Santa Casa de Misericóridia de São Paulo, Rua Dr. Cesário Motta Junior 112, Vila Buarque, Sao Paulo, SP 01221-020, Brazil

Division of Neuroradiology, Grupo Fleury, Rua Cincinato Braga, 282 Paraíso, Sao Paulo, SP, Brazil
e-mail: antonio.maia@fleury.com.br; antonio.rocha@grupofleury.com.br

R. Hoffmann Nunes, MD
Division of Neuroradiology, Santa Casa de São Paulo, São Paulo, Brazil
e-mail: renatohn@hotmail.com

Background

Although rare, metabolic brain disorders account for a substantial portion of encephalopathy cases and may cause significant morbidity and mortality. Most of all are inborn errors of metabolism (IEMs), and brain injury results from the accumulation of endogenous toxic substances or a lack of production of necessary biochemicals [1]. In these disorders, an enzyme deficiency blocks a metabolic pathway and results in either a deficiency of the product or in an accumulation of a substrate with damage induced by either storage or toxicity.

IEMs can present at nearly any age, and their clinical signs and symptoms are almost invariably nonspecific. Some of the IEMs, especially in the neonatal period, manifest with acute encephalopathy

R. Hoffmann Nunes et al. (eds.), *Critical Findings in Neuroradiology*,
DOI 10.1007/978-3-319-27987-9_18

and a life-threatening episode of metabolic decompensation, whereas later-onset disorders have variable clinical courses and outcomes [1].

Key Points

Etiology

An exhaustive discussion of IEMs is beyond the scope of this book. Herein we discuss the most common and some rare but devastating diseases where prompt diagnosis is crucial to prevent neurological sequelae or death [1].

Different classification schemes of IEMs exist and include disorders of the biosynthesis and breakdown of complex molecules, energy production disorders, intoxication disorders, and neurotransmitter defects (Table 18.1) [1].

Intoxication Disorders

Urea cycle defects include both enzyme and transporter deficiencies that result in impaired elimination of nitrogen and resultant hyperammonemia. High plasma ammonia leads to high glutamine levels in the central nervous system (CNS) [1, 2].

Maple syrup urine disease (MSUD) is caused by deficiency of a branched-chain keto-acid dehydrogenase enzyme and usually presents at the end of the first week of life with poor feeding, vomiting, and stupor followed by dystonia (rhythmic boxing and cycling movements of the limbs), fluctuating ophthalmoplegia, seizures, and a characteristic urine odor of maple syrup [3]. Early detection is critical, as initiation of therapy within the first 5 days is associated with near normal cognitive outcome [4].

Propionic acidemia is an autosomal recessive inherited IEM that results from absence of mitochondrial enzyme propionyl–CoA carboxylase and leads to multiple metabolic and neurologic abnormalities and the subsequent accumulation of organic amino acids. During metabolic decompensations, patients present with ketoacidosis, hyperglycinemia, and hyperammonemia. Severe acidosis may lead to coma and death. Early-onset disease occurs in the first 3 months of age with vomiting, hypotonia, lethargy, metabolic acidosis, seizures, and coma [1].

Methylmalonic acidemia is related to accumulation of methylmalonic acid that is generated during metabolism of certain amino acids (isoleucine, methionine, threonine, and valine) and odd-chain fatty acids. Defects in methylmalonyl-CoA mutase or its coenzyme, cobalamin (vitamin B12), lead to methylmalonic acidemia (MMA), also called methylmalonic aciduria. It usually presents clinically with nonspecific symptoms such as seizures, psychomotor retardation, poor feeding, respiratory distress, loss of consciousness, and muscle tone abnormalities [5].

Glutaric aciduria type I (GA-1) is an organic aciduria of autosomal recessive origin with deficiency of mitochondrial enzyme glutaryl-CoA dehydrogenase which is involved in the metabolism of tryptophan, lysine, and hydroxylysine. These children may be born macrocephalic but are otherwise normal. At some time, usually during a viral syndrome, they develop an acute "encephalitic-like crisis" characterized by acute necrosis of the caudate and putamen, sometimes also with frontotemporal atrophy, and are left with severe dystonia, choreoathetosis, dyskinesia, seizures, and spasticity [1, 2, 6].

Energy Production Disorders

Primary lactic acidosis is usually related in neonates to pyruvate carboxylase, pyruvate dehydrogenase, and mitochondrial complex IV (cytochrome c oxidase) deficiencies [2, 7, 8]. Lactic acidosis disorders cause defective oxidative metabolism which leads to impaired energy production. Neonatal presentation typically consists of severe muscular hypotonia, lethargy, weak sucking, microcephaly, facial dysmorphic signs, and tachypnea. Seizures occur in about one-third of patients. Marked lactic acidosis with increased level of lactate in blood and CSF or only in CSF is mandatory to make the diagnosis. Bouts of dystonia or ataxia and late-onset generalized epilepsy may result from transient failure of brain energy supply and benefit greatly from the ketogenic diet and sometimes from thiamine [3, 9, 10].

Mitochondrial encephalopathies are several distinct syndromes that are recognized on the

Table 18.1 Classification of devastating metabolic diseases in newborns and young infants

Classification	Type of disorder	Clinical manifestations	Diseases
Intoxication disorders	Organic acid disorders	Most common metabolic disorders causing acute encephalopathy. Variable symptom-free interval after birth because toxic metabolites were metabolized by the mother in utero. Acute symptoms of encephalopathy as a result of accumulated toxic metabolites in brain tissues. Clinical manifestations include vomiting, poor feeding, stupor, and lethargy and eventually lead to coma and death if left untreated. Abnormal muscle tone and epilepsy may also be present. Moreover, apnea or hyperventilation may result from metabolic acidosis or hyperammonemia	Propionic acidemia, MMA, isovaleric acidemia, Canavan disease, multiple carboxylase deficiency, pyroglutamic aciduria
	Amino acid metabolism disorders		Urea cycle defect (citrullinemia, ornithine transcarbamylase deficiency, cabamoyl phosphate synthetase deficiency, argininosuccinic aciduria), MSD, nonketotic hyperglycinemia
Energy production disorders	Primary lactic acidosis	The symptoms tend to be multisystemic and in particular involve tissues with a high metabolic rate such as the brain, heart, and skeletal muscles. Reye-like episodes, hepato-splenomegaly, and cardiomyopathy may lead to sudden death	Pyruvate dehydrogenase deficiency, pyruvate carboxylase deficiency, cytochrome oxidase deficiency, complex succinate dehydrogenase (type II) deficiency
	Fatty acid oxidation disorders		Carnitine cycle defects (carnitine palmitoyletransferase deficiency, carnitine translocase deficiency), mitochondrial β-oxidation disorders, glutaric aciduria type II
	Mitochondrial Encephalopathy		MELAS, MERRF, Kearns–Sayre syndrome, Leber's hereditary optic neuropathy, Alpers' disease, and Leigh's disease
Disorders of the biosynthesis and breakdown of complex molecules	Other metabolic disorders	The symptoms are slowly progressive, permanent, and independent of food intake	Zellweger syndrome, neonatal adrenoleukodystrophy, Krabbe disease, Menkes disease, D-bifunctional protein deficiency, sulfite oxidase deficiency, galactosemia
Neurotransmitter defects		Severe metabolic encephalopathy usually starting in the neonatal period. Drug-resistant seizures are typically seen on presentation	Pyridoxine-dependent epilepsy, nonketotic hyperglycinemia or glycine encephalopathy, creatine deficiency syndromes

MMA methylmalonic acidemia, *MSD* maple syrup urine disease, *MELAS* mitochondrial myopathy, encephalopathy, lactic acidosis, and stroke-like episodes, *MERRF* myoclonus, epilepsy, and ragged red fibers basis of their phenotype, histological, biochemical, or genetic manifestations, sharing unique characteristics of mitochondrial inheritance and deterioration of mitochondrial function with aging. Some well-defined disorders include MELAS (mitochondrial myopathy, encephalopathy, lactic acidosis, and stroke-like episodes), MERRF (myoclonus, epilepsy, and ragged red fibers), Kearns–Sayre syndrome (chronic external ophthalmoplegia plus, with retinal pigment abnormalities), Leber's hereditary optic neuropathy, Alpers' disease (progressive infantile poliodystrophy), and Leigh's disease (subacute necrotizing encephalomyelitis). Usually, each of these is associated with a different point mutation of the mtDNA, causing a defect in the mitochondrial protein synthesis [4, 11].

Disorders of Biosynthesis and Breakdown of Complex Molecules

Krabbe disease is a classic lysosomal storage disease (LSD), also named globoid cell leukodystrophy (GLD), and is a lipidosis that affects the CNS and peripheral nervous system. It is an autosomal recessive neurodegenerative disorder due to mutations in the β-galactocerebrosidase gene. Presence of numerous multinucleated globoid cells in the white matter is a typical finding. The infantile phenotype (95 % of cases) usually has its onset within first 6 months of life and leads to death by age 2 years. Affected neonates typically present with flaccidity, irritability, fever, and hyperactive reflex and usually death within the first few years of life [9, 12].

Zellweger syndrome or cerebrohepatorenal syndrome is a disorder of peroxisomal function that presents in the neonatal period with involvement of multiple organs. Elevated very long-chain fatty acids in plasma and fibroblasts are characteristic [13, 14]. Clinical features of this syndrome are striking and easily recognizable at birth with typical dysmorphic facial features and abnormal vision. Cortical dysplasia, hypomyelination, intrahepatic biliary dysgenesis, and polycystic renal disease are also associated. Affected infants usually present soon after birth with severe muscular hypotonia, poor swallowing and sucking, irritability to environmental stimuli, epileptic seizures, prolonged jaundice, and die within the first year of life [14].

Menkes disease (MD) is an X-linked neurodegenerative disease of impaired copper transport caused by mutation of the P-type ATPase 7 gene and resulting in inactivation of cytochrome c oxidase and leading to apoptotic death [14, 15]. Variable MD phenotypes are related to abnormal collagen and elastin formation which results in skin and hair alterations associated with tortuous and elongated intracranial vessels, in addition to bladder diverticula and bone abnormalities [16, 17]. Patients present with hypotonia, hypothermia, and seizures. Laxity of the skin and joints, coarse and sparse hair with broken ends, and hypopigmentation is observed [18, 19].

Neurotransmitter Defects

Creatine deficiency syndromes are related to lack of creatine in the CNS, causing a severe but treatable neurologic disease. There are three recognized syndromes in humans that include three inherited defects in the biosynthesis and transport of creatine, guanidinoacetate methyltransferase deficiency (GAMT gene) and L-arginine-glycine amidinotransferase deficiency (GATM gene), and creatine transporter deficiencies, an X-linked disorder with SLC6A8 gene mutations. GAMT deficiency may present in the first month of life with seizures. Later there are mental, speech, and language delays, epilepsy, and autistic-like behavior. They can be diagnosed by analysis of the creatine, guanidinoacetate, and creatinine in body fluids [14, 20].

Nonketotic hyperglycinemia (NKH) or glycine encephalopathy is caused by an error in the breakdown of glycine resulting in its accumulation in urine, blood, and cerebrospinal fluid (CSF) [21]. The neurotoxicity of glycine is related to excitatory and inhibitory neuronal effects on glycine and N-methyl-D-aspartate receptors in the telencephalon and brainstem/spinal cord, respectively, and to a disturbance in myelin proteins. The neonatal form is most common and manifests a few days after birth with severe encephalopathy, hypotonia, lethargy, respiratory failure, myoclonic seizures, and hiccups. Neonatal neuroimaging findings include structural and white matter abnormalities [22].

Best Imaging Modality

MRI is the method of choice due to its sensitivity to demonstrate changes in myelin, differentiate diseases with predominant involvement of the cortex or white matter, and detect specific patterns of involvement. In the acute phase of some diseases, brain volume increases and signal abnormalities may arise. Global atrophy is usually observed in the chronic phases of all disorders.

The protocol MRI requires, in addition to conventional structural sequences (T1, T2, and T2*), diffusion-weighted imaging (DWI) and magnetic resonance spectroscopy (MRS). FLAIR sequence is not optimal to evaluate brain abnormalities in neonates due to high water contents, but it is useful when CSF signal must be suppressed to detect extra-axial collections or hemorrhage. DWI is capable of differentiating cytotoxic/myelin edema (both restrict the diffusion of water) from vasogenic/interstitial edema. MRS may detect changes that support a specific diagnosis. MRS may also be helpful for assessing response to treatment and to recognize acute lesions in phases of exacerbations. Table 18.2 summarizes the main findings of MRS in different IMEs.

Major Findings

Intoxication Disorders

Urea cycle defects: Characteristic findings on MRI can be divided into four patterns [23]:

- Type 1 – diffuse severe cerebral edema followed by diffuse atrophy (Fig. 18.1)
- Type 2 – extensive infarct-like abnormalities often presenting as acute hemiplegia
- Type 3 – presumably ischemic lesions in cerebral boundary zones
- Type 4 – reversible symmetric cortical involvement of the cingulate gyri, temporal lobes, and insular cortex with sparing of the perirolandic cortex

Nonmyelinated white matter is more severely affected than myelinated areas. Additionally,

Table 18.2 MRS Findings in IEMs

Disease	MRS findings	Comments
Urea cycle defects	Reduced MI, elevated glutamate/glutamine, and lipids/lactate	Can help assessing treatment response showing and may help to monitor metabolic decompensation
Maple syrup urine disease	Broad peak at chemical shift of 0.9 ppm	Changes in peaks are more exuberant in regions with restricted DWI and may help to monitor the metabolic decompensation
Pyruvate dehydrogenase deficiency	Elevated lactate and pyruvate 3.37 ppm	Specific finding of a pyruvate peak has not been reported for respiratory chain defects or other defects in mitochondrial energy metabolism
Mitochondriopathies	Increased lactate during crisis. May have elevated Cho/Cr ratio and reduced NAA	Can identify metabolic abnormalities even when brain parenchyma appears normal by conventional MRI and can be helpful for both diagnosis and follow-up. MRS should be acquired during episodes of clinical exacerbation, in acute lesions, and in the ventricular CSF
Methylmalonic acidemia	Lactate peak and decreased NAA corresponding to the hyperintensity area on DWI and T2WI. The signal of N-acetyl-aspartate (NAA) was decreased	During treatment clinical symptoms gradually improved in parallel with the normalization of MRI and MRS findings

Table 18.2 (continued)

Disease	MRS findings	Comments
Glutaric aciduria type I	Elevated Cho/Cr ratio and reduced NAA. May have increased lactate during crisis	May help to monitor the metabolic decompensation
Krabbe disease	Elevated choline, myoinositol; moderate NAA reduction and mild lactate accumulation	May add important information regarding the extent of brain damage and before hematopoietic stem cell transplantation or substrate-reduction therapy
Menkes disease	Elevated lactate and reduced NAA/Cr ratio	Can help assessing treatment response showing better spectral relationships without significant changes in conventional sequences
Creatine deficiency syndromes	Markedly reduced or completely absent creatine peak at 3.0 ppm	MRI is usually normal, thus the inclusion of MRS in all cases of progressive encephalopathy is helpful. During therapy, the creatine peak slowly reappears in disorders of creatine synthesis
Nonketotic hyperglycinemia	Peak at the region of 3.56 ppm with a long echo time	Glycine concentration, glycine/creatine ratio, and NAA/glycine ratio correlate with the severity of the clinical presentation and can be a valuable tool in the diagnosis and monitoring of treatment effects

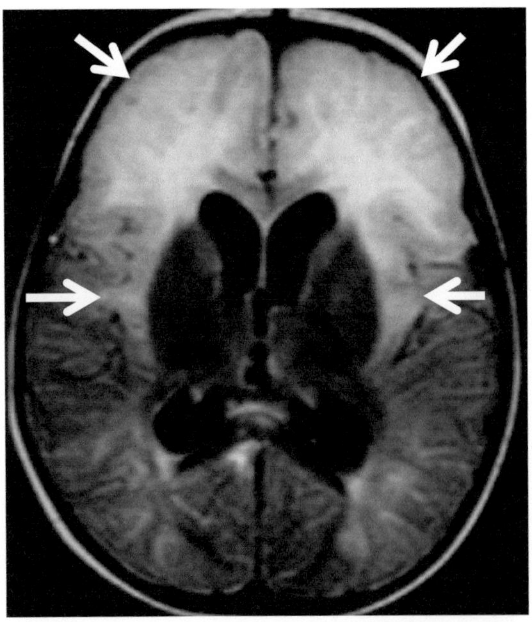

Fig. 18.1 Urea cycle defect. Axial FLAIR displays bilateral extensive hyperintense lesions in the frontal and insular areas (*arrows*). The thalami, perirolandic, and occipital cortices are spared aiding in the differentiation from hypoxic–ischemic injury

when observed, restricted diffusion has been termed metabolic stroke, reflecting tissue injury during a hyperammonemic episode [24].

Maple syrup urine disease: MRI studies show both edema with restricted diffusion characteristically involving the cerebellar white matter, the posterior brainstem, the cerebral peduncles, the posterior limb of the internal capsule, and the posterior centrum semiovale (Fig. 18.2). The diagnosis can be confirmed by the presence of a broad peak from branched chain keto acids at 0.9 ppm on proton MRS with long TE [25, 26].

Propionic acidemia: MRI changes include cortical atrophy, T2 hyperintensities and restricted diffusion in the striatum, white matter T2 hyperintensities, and features suggestive of diffuse cortical edema. In the acute phase, involved areas exhibit restricted and reversible diffusion [27].

Methylmalonic acidemia: The basal ganglia, predominantly globi pallidi, are particularly sensitive to mitochondrial dysfunction and are thus main targets for brain injury in this disease [28]. MRI can demonstrate hyperintensity in globi pallidi both on T2-weighted image (T2WI) and DWI during acute episodes (Fig. 18.3). Low apparent diffusion coefficient (ADC) may reflect intracellular edema but is reversible early on with little cell damage [29].

Glutaric aciduria type I: Common neuroimaging findings included frontotemporal atrophy, subependymal pseudocysts, delayed myelination,

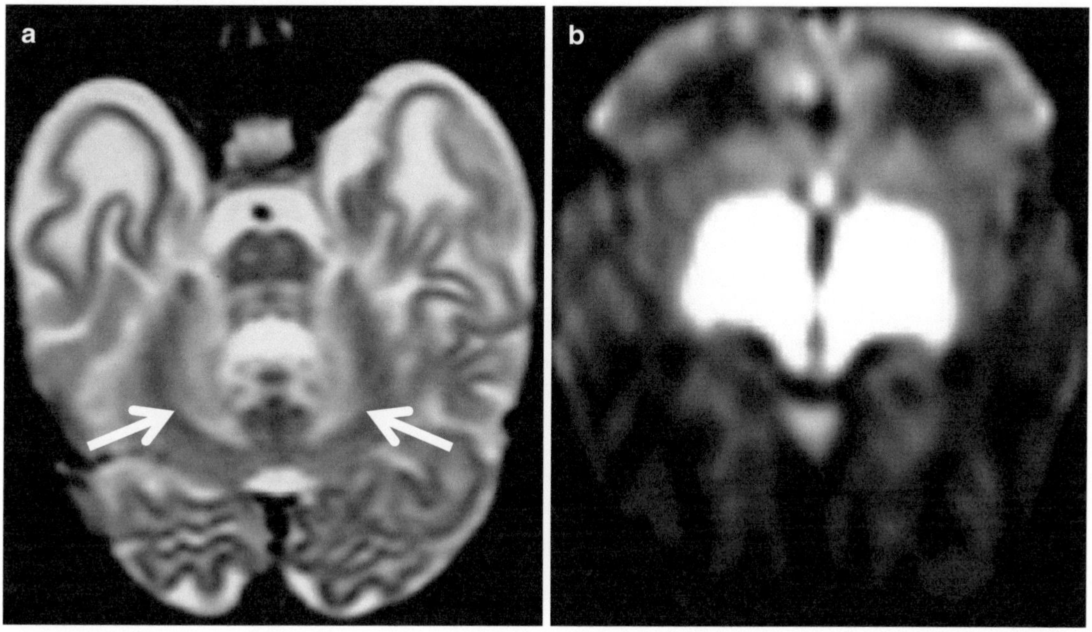

Fig. 18.2 Maple syrup urine disease. (**a**) Axial T2WI shows bilateral and symmetrical hyperintense areas in the cerebellar white matter (*arrows*), dorsal pons, and cerebral peduncles. (**b**) Some of the lesions demonstrate a striking hyperintense signal on axial DWI including the corticospinal tracts and basal ganglia

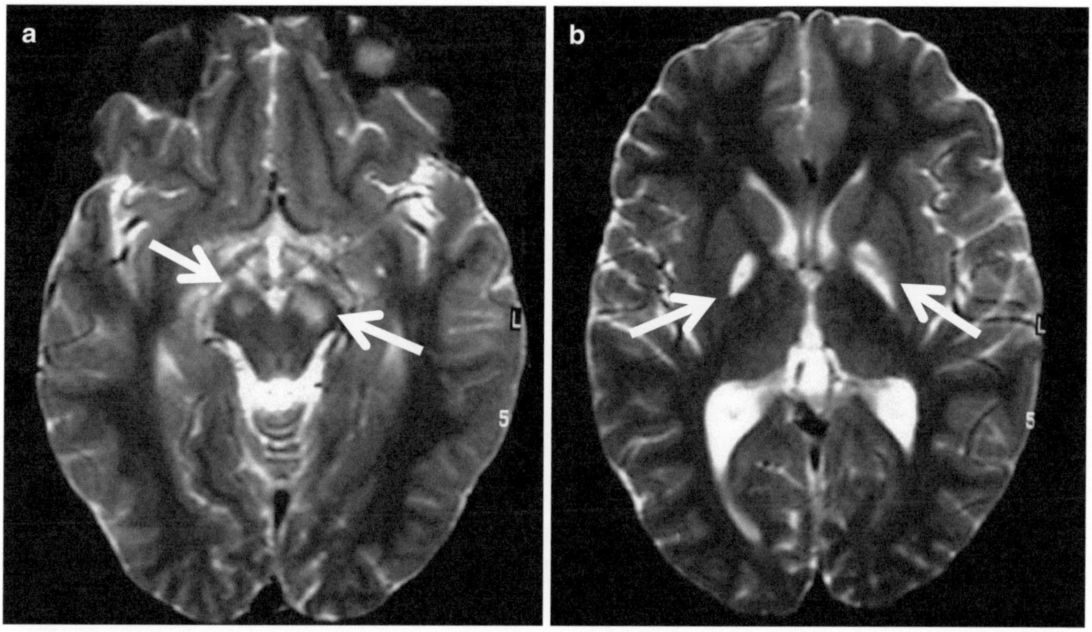

Fig. 18.3 Methylmalonic acidemia. (**a**, **b**) Axial T2WI shows bilateral and symmetrical hyperintensities in the cerebral peduncles and globi pallidi (*arrows*)

basal ganglia T2WI high signal and/or atrophy, chronic subdural effusions, and hematomas (Fig. 18.4). Widening of the Sylvian fissures, mesencephalic cisterns, and expansion of CSF spaces anterior to the temporal lobes are also signs of GA-1. Metabolic treatment does not improve neurologic disease, although it may prevent deterioration [30].

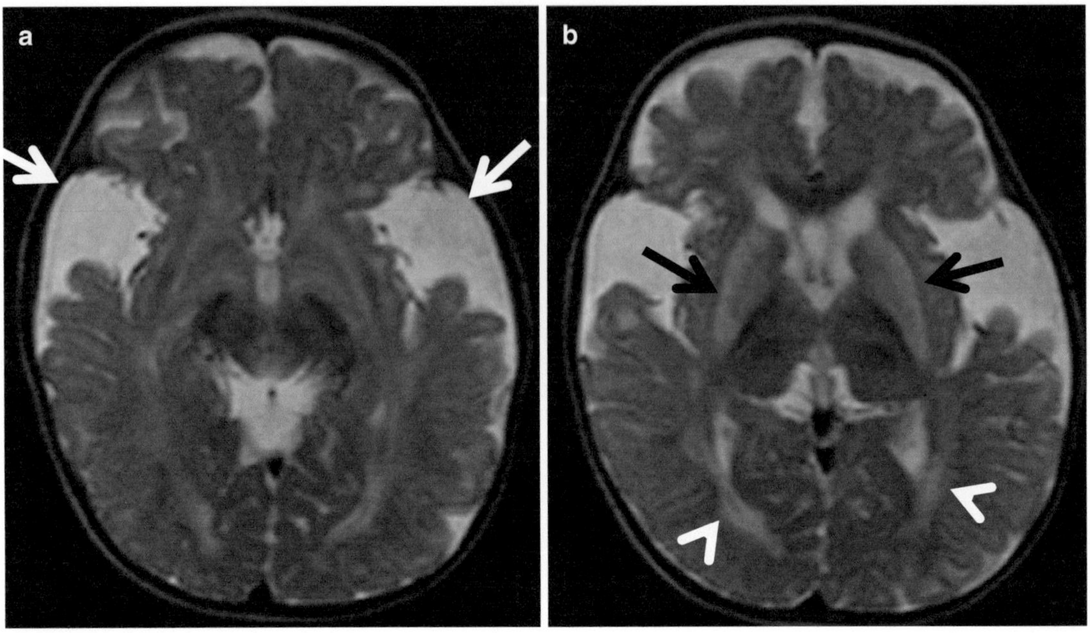

Fig. 18.4 Glutaric aciduria type I. (**a**, **b**) Axial T2WI demonstrates bilateral and symmetrical widening of the Sylvian fissures (*white arrows*). The caudate nucleus and the lentiform nucleus have abnormal increased signal intensity (*black arrows*). Note increased posterior periventricular white matter signal sparing the optic radiations bilaterally (*arrowheads*)

Energy Production Disorders

Primary lactic acidosis: Prenatal energy failure may account for malformations and neonatal encephalopathy, and neuroimaging may show dysgenesis of the corpus callosum, mega cisterna magna, subcortical heterotopias, pachygyria, germinolytic cysts, cortical atrophy, and T2-hyperintense lesions in the basal ganglia (particularly in the putamen) and white matter (cerebellum, posterior limb of the internal capsule, associated with increased ADC values) (Fig. 18.5) [10]. MRI findings may be similar to those of hypoxic ischemic encephalopathy. At MRS, a prominent inverted lactate doublet (TE = 134 msec) is characteristic of lactic acidosis even in normal-appearing parenchyma. However, lactate is not specific for primary lactic acidosis and may be present in other IEMs [2].

Mitochondrial encephalopathies: MRI findings in Kearns–Sayre syndrome are considered specific and include signal changes in the globi pallidus, subcortical white matter, and pontine tegmentum (Fig. 18.6). Other affected sites are the caudate and dentate nuclei, thalami, and red nuclei. Typical findings of Leigh's disease are bilateral and symmetrical. Involvement of the white matter is often observed, which may be edematous during the acute phase and show cystic degeneration in the chronic phase (Fig. 18.7). There may also be involvement of the globi pallidus, substantia nigra, periaqueductal gray matter, and spinal cord. Ventricular dilatation and cerebellar hypoplasia have been described and caused by deficiency of the pyruvate dehydrogenase complex. The most frequently reported findings in MELAS are ischemic lesions without specific vascular distributions, nonspecific white matter lesions, and chronic calcifications in basal ganglia (Fig. 18.8) [1, 11]. MRS is an important complementary tool for the detection of mitochondrial disorders mostly by virtue of showing lactate elevation. This technique is most helpful during episodes of exacerbation [11].

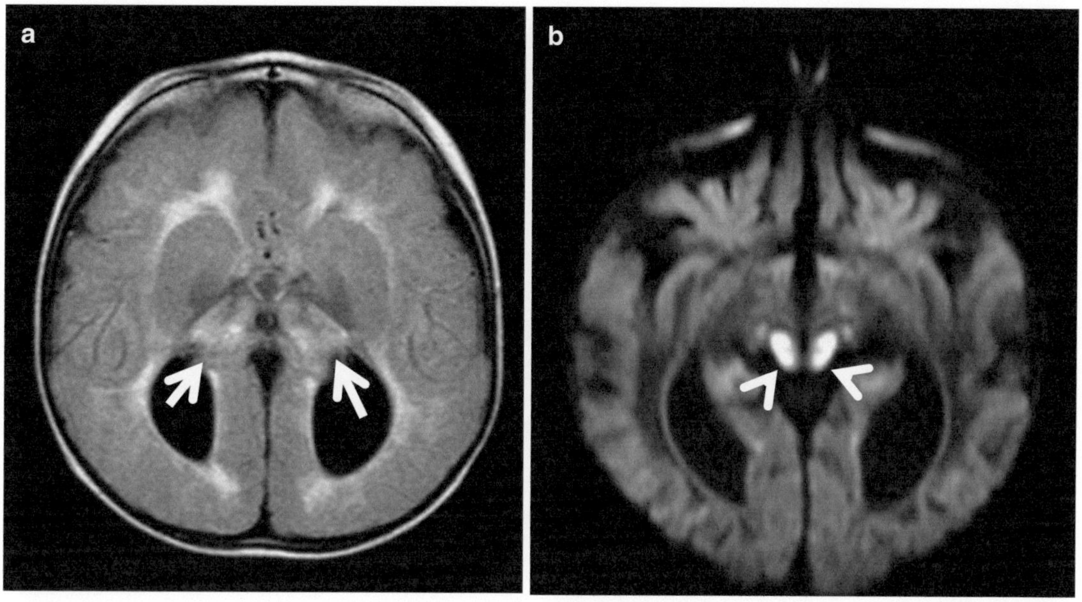

Fig. 18.5 Pyruvate dehydrogenase deficiency. (**a**) Bilateral and symmetrical thalamic (*arrows*), anterior and posterior limbs of the internal capsule, and periventricular white matter involvement are seen on FLAIR. (**b**) DWI ($b = 1000$ s/mm^2) displays striking hypersignal in the peri-aqueductal area (*arrowheads*) (Courtesy of Dr. Lazaro do Amaral, MD – São Paulo, Brazil)

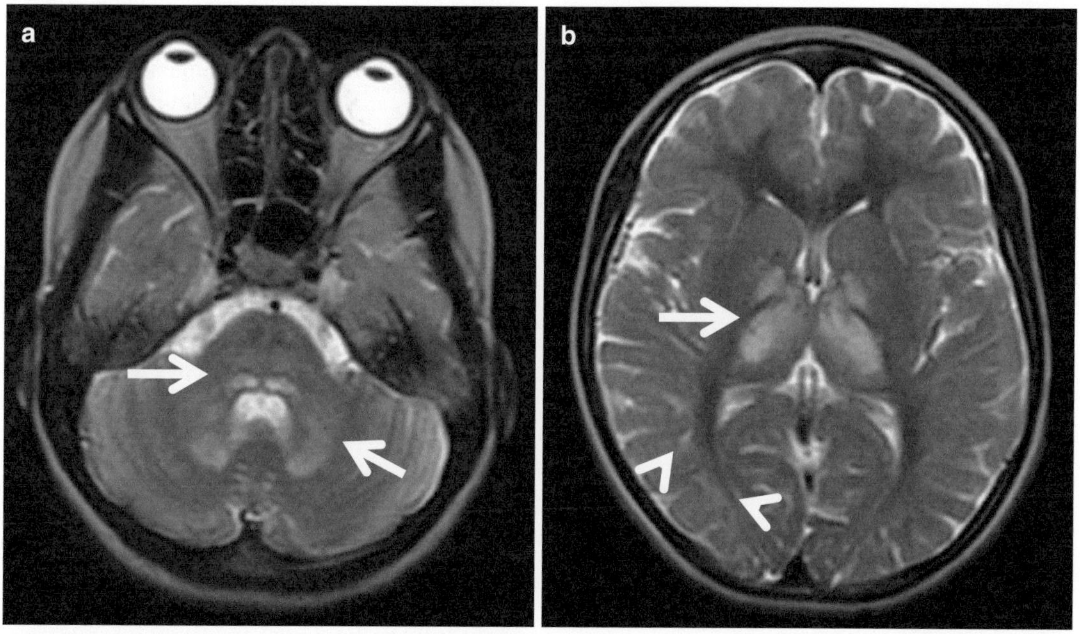

Fig. 18.6 Kearns–Sayre syndrome. (**a**, **b**) Axial T2WI demonstrates bilateral abnormal increased signal intensity in the dentate nuclei and dorsal pons (*arrows*). Foci of abnormal signal intensity are seen bilaterally within the thalamus, globi pallidi, and the corticospinal tracts on (**b**) (*arrows*). Note the subtle loss of myelin arborization into the subcortical U fibers (*arrow heads*)

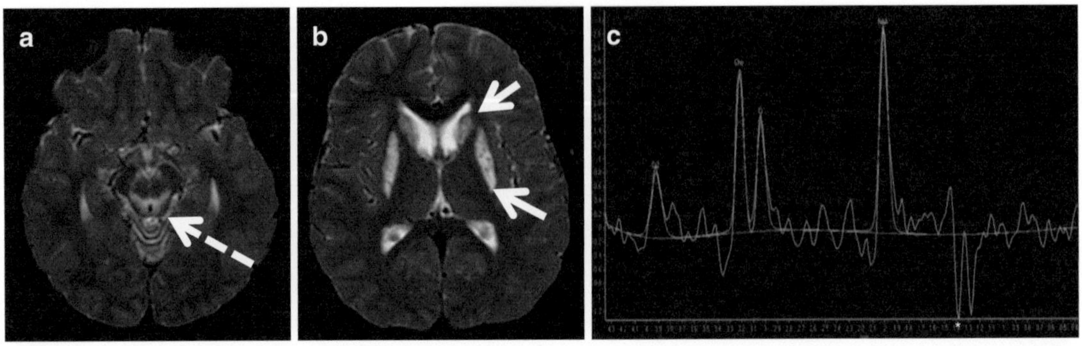

Fig. 18.7 Leigh syndrome. (**a**, **b**) Axial T2WI in an infant with hypotonia and encephalopathy shows bilateral and symmetrical involvement of the caudate heads (*short arrow*) and putaminal (*long arrows*). Note also the abnormal hyperintensity in the midbrain tegmentum, including the periaqueductal gray matter (*white dashed arrow*). (**c**) Single-voxel MRS (PRESS/TE = 144 ms) shows a typical lactate peak at 1.33 ppm (*star*)

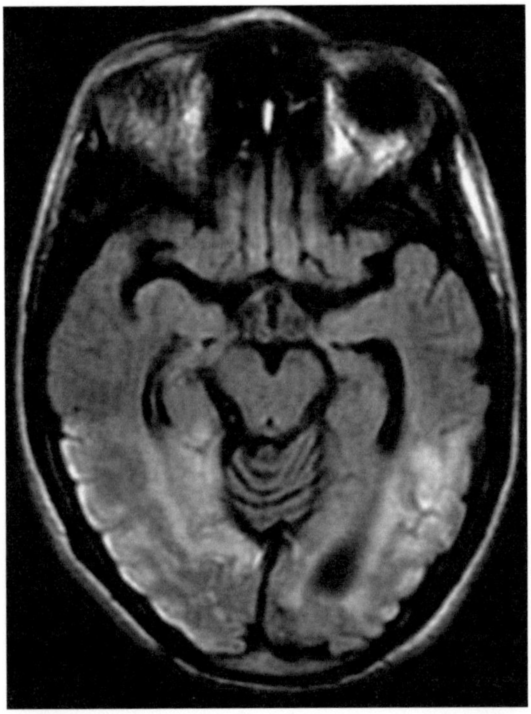

Fig. 18.8 MELAS. Axial FLAIR demonstrates bilateral hyperintense lesions in the cortex and white matter of the parieto-occipital regions without a typical vascular distribution

Disorders of the Biosynthesis and Breakdown of Complex Molecules

Krabbe disease: In the early-onset form of Krabbe disease, imaging findings are signal abnormalities in cerebellar white matter, deep gray nuclei, parieto-occipital white matter, corpus callosum, and the pyramidal tracts. CT can demonstrate high-attenuation in the thalami, posterior limb of the internal capsules, caudate nuclei, brainstem, cerebellar dentate nuclei, and centrum semiovale. MRI reveals demyelination that is prominent in the periventricular areas and centrum semiovale with sparing of the subcortical U fibers. T2WI shows hyperintensity in periventricular white matter, thalami, basal ganglia, and dentate nuclei (Fig. 18.9) [31]. In late-onset disease, MRI shows signal abnormalities in the pyramidal tracts, posterior corpus callosum, and parieto-occipital white matter [12]. Marked enlargement of the intracranial optic nerves can also be seen [13].

Zellweger syndrome: MRI findings include cortical abnormalities and hypomyelination. Cortical malformations consist of polymicrogyria particularly in the perisylvian regions, but it may also be more generalized, affecting the parieto-temporal-occipital lobes. Pachygyria is most often frontoparietal [16]. Periventricular heterotopias and subependymal germinolytic cysts have also been reported [14, 18].

Menkes disease: MRI performed during the early postnatal period may be unremarkable except for presence of tortuous cerebral blood vessels and progressive white matter lesions predominantly in the frontal and temporal areas, and progressive brain atrophy with subdural hemorrhages that may mimic injuries related to abuse can be seen in older patients (Fig. 18.10) [2]. A transient temporal vasogenic edema is as an early finding possibly due to energy metabolism failure induced by seizures [32].

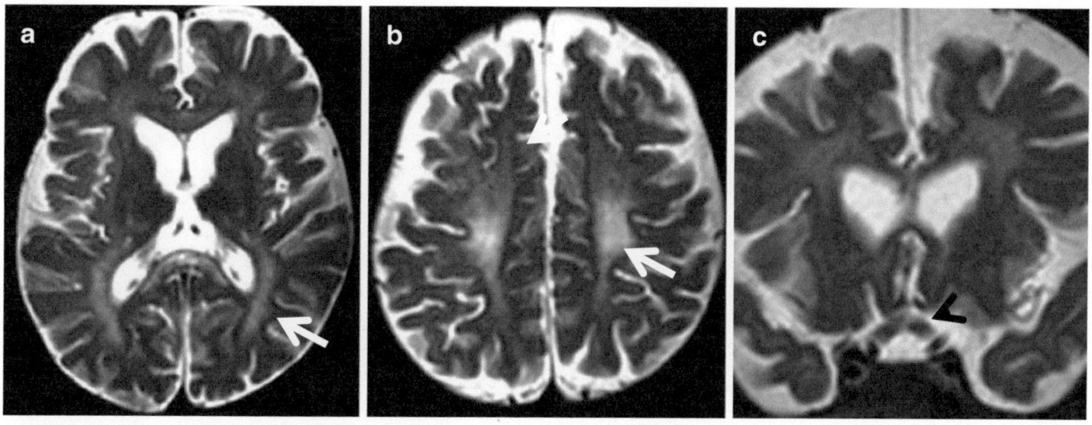

Fig. 18.9 Krabbe disease. (**a–c**) Axial and coronal T2WI of a patient with Krabbe disease reveal abnormal bilateral T2 hyperintensities in the deep and periventricular white matter sparing the subcortical white matter (*arrows*). The white matter involvement typically starts along the corticospinal tracts (*arrow* on **b**). Note the enlargement of the intracranial optic nerves (*arrowhead* on **c**)

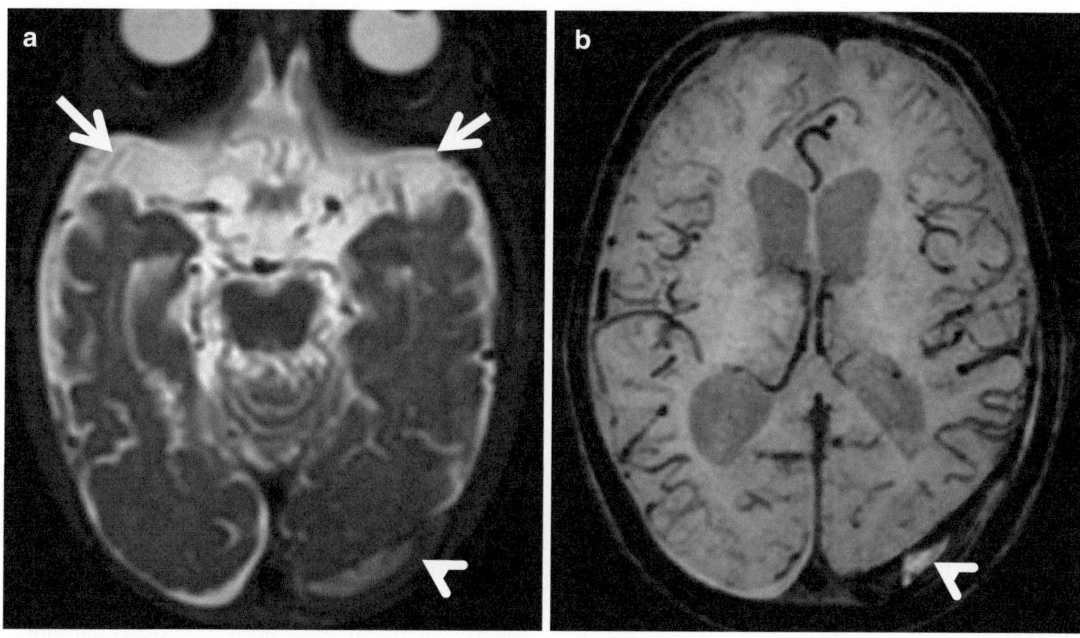

Fig. 18.10 Menkes disease. (**a**, **b**) Axial T2WI (**a**) and susceptibility-weighted imaging (**b**) show the typical vessel tortuosity and symmetrical white matter signal changes. Marked cerebral atrophy and cyst-like lesions are seen at the temporal poles (*arrows*). Also note a subdural hematoma in the left occipital region (*arrowheads*)

Neurotransmitter Defects

Creatine deficiency syndromes: MRI is usually normal, while MRS shows a markedly reduced or absent creatine peak [20]. Disorders of creatine synthesis may be treated by creatine supplementation. After initiation of therapy, the creatine peak slowly reappears in disorders of creatine synthesis, but not when its transport is impaired [33].

Nonketotic hyperglycinemia: Typical findings in NKH include reduction of telencephalic gray matter and white matter, thinning of corpus callosum, and cerebellar hypoplasia. Restricted diffusion in myelinated white matter tracts is evidenced by low ADC values due to myelin vacuoles secondary to the splitting of myelin sheets (Fig. 18.11) [21]. MRS typically displays

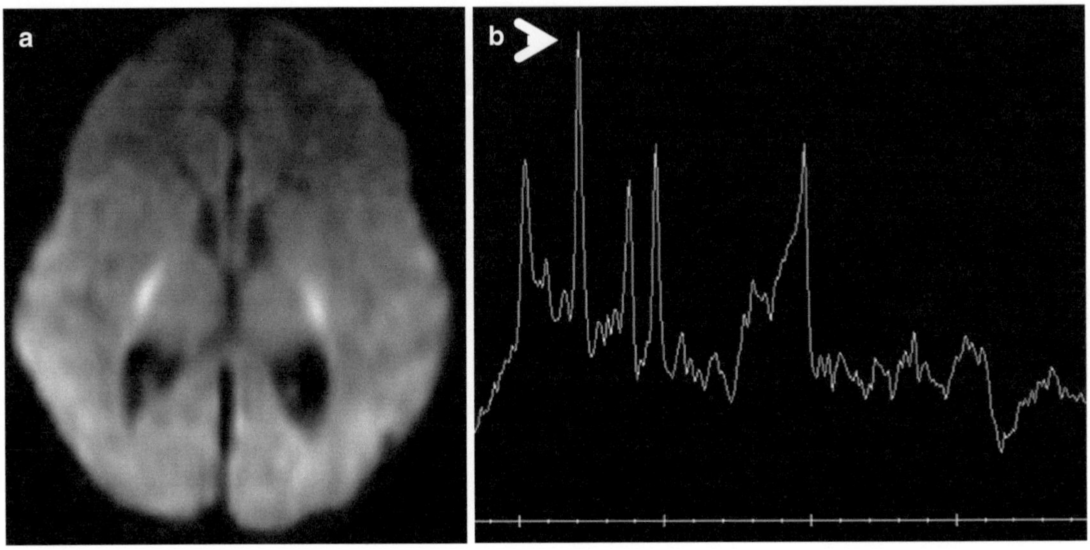

Fig. 18.11 Nonketotic hyperglycinemia. (**a**) DWI image reveals bilateral high-signal lesions along the corticospinal tracts confined to the posterior limbs of the internal capsules. (**b**) MRS displays an abnormal peak of glycine at 3.56 ppm (*arrowhead*) (Courtesy of Dr. Leonardo Vedolin, MD, PhD – Porto Alegre, Brazil)

a peak at the region of 3.56 ppm (TE = 135–166 milliseconds) corresponding to glycine [34].

Imaging Follow-Up

The follow-up of these diseases is mainly clinical. MRI findings tend to progress to marked atrophy and lesion confluence. MRS is an important tool in the follow-up of some of the IEMs, as the detection of abnormal peaks during the treatment course may precede structural imaging findings and clinical manifestations indicating treatment failure (Table 18.2) [1, 2].

Main Differential Diagnosis

Hypoxic ischemic encephalopathy: May present with selective injury of white and deep gray matter and have similar imaging findings to nonketotic hyperglycinemia, primary lactic acidosis, urea cycle disorders, Krabbe disease, and maple syrup urine disease. Lack of perinatal asphyxia and late onset of symptoms (several days or weeks after birth) should raise suspicion for the possibility of a metabolic disorder. At neuroimaging, excessive vasogenic edema that predominantly involves nonmyelinated white matter is characteristic of urea cycle disorders, hyperattenuating thalami on CT may be seen with Krabbe disease, and a hypoplastic corpus callosum is typical of nonketotic hyperglycinemia. MRS may help to narrow the differential diagnosis (Table 18.2) [2].

Child abuse: Menkes disease or any metabolic disease with brain atrophy and subdural hemorrhages may mimic intracranial injuries related to child abuse. Findings that may be associated with abusive head trauma include multistage subdural hemorrhages over the convexities, interhemispheric hemorrhages, posterior fossa subdural hemorrhages, hypoxic–ischemic injury, and cerebral edema. The presence of tortuous blood vessels at MRI and MR angiography may suggest Menkes disease [2].

Bilirubin encephalopathy: Several organic acid disorders have similar MRI findings to bilirubin encephalopathy. However, unconjugated bilirubin deposited in the brain typically involves the globi pallidi, subthalamic nuclei, and hippocampi [2].

Tips

Patients usually present with acute encephalopathy and diverse abnormal laboratory findings. Although nonspecific, brain edema, lack of myelination, and atrophy are common imaging findings in IEMs and several specific patterns of brain involvement may be identified. DWI and MRS provide physiologic information and improve the imaging diagnosis.

- DWI depicts early parenchymal lesions and may help differentiate different types of edema using ADC.
- Metabolites that are specific in certain disorders are glycine in nonketotic hyperglycinemia and branched chain amino acids (e.g., L-leucine, L-isoleucine, and valine) in maple syrup urine disease.
- Nonketotic hyperglycinemia, primary lactic acidosis, urea cycle disorders, Krabbe disease, and maple syrup urine disease may have similar MRI findings to those of hypoxic ischemic encephalopathy with selective injury of white and deep gray matter.
- Menkes disease and metabolic diseases with brain atrophy and subdural hemorrhage may mimic intracranial injuries related to child abuse.

References

1. Cakir B, Teksam M, Kosehan D, et al. Inborn errors of metabolism presenting in childhood. J Neuroimaging. 2011;212:e117–33.
2. Yoon HJ, Kim JH, Jeon TY, et al. Devastating metabolic brain disorders of newborns and young infants. Radiographics. 2014;345:1257–72.
3. Morton DH, Strauss KA, Robinson DL, et al. Diagnosis and treatment of maple syrup disease: a study of 36 patients. Pediatrics. 2002;1096: 999–1008.
4. Simon E, Fingerhut R, Baumkötter J, et al. Maple syrup urine disease: favourable effect of early diagnosis by newborn screening on the neonatal course of the disease. J Inherit Metab Dis. 2006;294: 532–7.
5. Matsui SM, Mahoney MJ, Rosenberg LE. The natural history of the inherited methylmalonic acidemias. N Engl J Med. 1983;30815:857–61.
6. Filiano JJ. Neurometabolic diseases in the newborn. Clin Perinatol. 2006;332:411–79.
7. Gropman A. Brain imaging in urea cycle disorders. Mol Genet Metab. 2010;100S:S20–30.
8. Mumtaz HA, Gupta V, Singh P, et al. MR imaging findings of glutaric aciduria type II. Singap Med J. 2010;514:e69–71.
9. Graziano ACE, Cardile V. History, genetic, and recent advances on Krabbe disease. Gene. 2015;5551:2–13.
10. Barnerias C, Saudubray J-M, Touati G, et al. Pyruvate dehydrogenase complex deficiency: four neurological phenotypes with differing pathogenesis. Dev Med Child Neurol. 2010;522:e1–9.
11. José da Rocha A, Túlio Braga F, Carlos Martins Maia Jr A, et al. Lactate detection by MRS in mitochondrial encephalopathy: optimization of technical parameters. J Neuroimaging. 2008;181:1–8.
12. Kamate M, Hattiholi V. Predominant corticospinal tract involvement in early-onset Krabbe disease. Pediatr Neurol. 2011;442:155–6.
13. Jones BV, Barron TF, Towfighi J. Optic nerve enlargement in Krabbe's disease. AJNR Am J Neuroradiol. 1999;207:1228–31.
14. Barkovich AJ, Peck WW. MR of Zellweger syndrome. AJNR Am J Neuroradiol. 1997;186:1163–70.
15. Cosimo QC, Daniela L, Elsa B, et al. Kinky hair, kinky vessels, and bladder diverticula in Menkes disease. J Neuroimaging. 2011;212:e114–6.
16. Weller S, Rosewich H, Gärtner J. Cerebral MRI as a valuable diagnostic tool in Zellweger spectrum patients. J Inherit Metab Dis. 2008;312:270–80.
17. Rego JIMD, Rocha AJD, Segatelli V, et al. Imaging features that allow for the recognition of Menkes disease. Arq Neuropsiquiatr. 2014;725:396.
18. van der Knaap MS, Valk J. The MR spectrum of peroxisomal disorders. Neuroradiology. 1991;331:30–7.
19. Jain P, Kannan L, Chakrabarty B, et al. Menkes disease – an important cause of early onset refractory seizures. J Pediatr Neurosci. 2014;91:11–6.
20. Clark JF, Cecil KM. Diagnostic methods and recommendations for the cerebral creatine deficiency syndromes. Pediatr Res. 2015;77(3):398–405.
21. Sener RN. Nonketotic hyperglycinemia: diffusion magnetic resonance imaging findings. J Comput Assist Tomogr. 2003;274:538–40.
22. Ichinohe A, Kure S, Mikawa S, et al. Glycine cleavage system in neurogenic regions. Eur J Neurosci. 2004;199:2365–70.
23. Takanashi J-I, Barkovich AJ, Cheng SF, et al. Brain MR imaging in neonatal hyperammonemic encephalopathy resulting from proximal urea cycle disorders. AJNR Am J Neuroradiol. 2003;246:1184–7.

24. Bireley WR, Hove JLK, Gallagher RC, et al. Urea cycle disorders: brain MRI and neurological outcome. Pediatr Radiol. 2011;424:455–62.
25. Cavalleri F, Berardi A, Burlina AB, et al. Diffusion-weighted MRI of maple syrup urine disease encephalopathy. Neuroradiology. 2002;446:499–502.
26. Barkovich AJ. An approach to MRI of metabolic disorders in children. J Neuroradiol. 2007;342:75–88.
27. Kandel A, Amatya SK, Yeh EA. Reversible diffusion weighted imaging changes in propionic acidemia. J Child Neurol. 2013;281:128–31.
28. Yeşildağ A, Ayata A, Baykal B, et al. Magnetic resonance imaging and diffusion weighted imaging in methylmalonic acidemia. Acta Radiol. 2005;461:101–3.
29. Takeuchi M, Harada M, Matsuzaki K, et al. Magnetic resonance imaging and spectroscopy in a patient with treated methylmalonic acidemia. J Comput Assist Tomogr. 2003;274:547–51.
30. Hoffmann GF, Athanassopoulos S, Burlina AB, et al. Clinical course, early diagnosis, treatment, and prevention of disease in glutaryl-CoA dehydrogenase deficiency. Neuropediatrics. 1996;273:115–23.
31. Choi S, Enzmann DR. Infantile Krabbe disease: complementary CT and MR findings. AJNR Am J Neuroradiol. 1993;145:1164–6.
32. Ekici B, Calışkan M, Tatlı B. Reversible temporal lobe edema: an early MRI finding in Menkes disease. J Pediatr Neurosci. 2012;72:160–1.
33. Arias A, Ormazabal A, Moreno J, et al. Methods for the diagnosis of creatine deficiency syndromes: a comparative study. J Neurosci Methods. 2006; 156(1–2):305–9.
34. Gabis L, Parton P, Roche P, et al. In vivo 1H magnetic resonance spectroscopic measurement of brain glycine levels in nonketotic hyperglycinemia. J Neuroimaging. 2001;112:209–11.

19 Basal Ganglia and Thalamic Lesions

Bruno de Vasconcelos Sobreira Guedes,
Antônio José da Rocha,
and Renato Hoffmann Nunes

Abstract

A wide variety of diseases may involve the basal ganglia and thalami, and neuroimaging plays a major role in their diagnosis. The causes of abnormalities in deep gray structures in adults may be broadly classified as toxic, acquired metabolic disorders, inflammatory and infectious diseases, vascular and neoplasms, and many of them represent emergencies and must be promptly reported.

Background

The thalami and basal ganglia (comprised primarily by the caudate nuclei, putamina, and globus pallidi) are part of the most important and better demonstrated deep gray matter structures on neuroimaging, especially on magnetic resonance imaging (MRI).

The basal ganglia are part of the extrapyramidal motor system, participating in the production of movement, but they are also involved in memory, emotion, and other cognitive functions. Clinical signs and symptoms related to lesions in these structures may vary from movement disorders (dystonia, bradykinesia, chorea, tremors) to coma [1].

The thalami are crucial in regulating consciousness, sleep, and alertness, also being responsible for relaying sensory and motor signals to and from the cerebral cortex. Lesions affecting the thalami often result in disorders of consciousness and sensory disturbances [2].

B.de.V.S. Guedes, MD (✉)
Department of Radiology, Multiscan Imagem e Diagnóstico, Rua José Teixeira, 316, Vitoria, ES 29055-310, Brazil
e-mail: b_guedes@hotmail.com

A.J. da Rocha, MD, PhD
Division of Neuroradiology, Hospital Santa Casa de Misericórdia de São Paulo, Rua Dr. Cesário Motta Junior 112, Vila Buarque, Sao Paulo, SP 01221-020, Brazil

Division of Neuroradiology, Grupo Fleury, Rua Dr. Cesário Motta Junior 112, Vila Buarque, Sao Paulo, SP 01221-020, Brazil
e-mail: antonio.rocha@grupofleury.com.br

R. Hoffmann Nunes, MD
Division of Neuroradiology, Santa Casa de São Paulo, São Paulo, Brazil
e-mail: renatohn@hotmail.com

R. Hoffmann Nunes et al. (eds.), *Critical Findings in Neuroradiology*,
DOI 10.1007/978-3-319-27987-9_19

A wide variety of diseases may involve the basal ganglia and thalami, and neuroimaging plays a major role in their diagnosis. The causes of abnormalities in deep gray structures in adults may be classified as toxic, acquired metabolic disorders, inflammatory and infectious diseases, vascular and neoplasms [3].

Key Points

Etiology

Toxic Encephalopathies

Carbon monoxide (CO) poisoning: Brain damage after CO exposure results from complex and partially unknown mechanisms, but is mostly related to hypoxia. Typically it affects the globus pallidi and the caudate nucleus; injuries to the thalami and putamina are unlikely [4].

Methanol intoxication: It is a rare accidental or suicidal condition, which has also been described as a result of fraudulent adulteration of alcoholic drinks. Symptoms as headache, dizziness, weakness, and visual disturbances (due to optic nerve necrosis and/or demyelination) are prominent in acute intoxication. Toxicity may result from metabolism of methanol to formic acid [5].

Acquired Metabolic Disorders

Wernicke encephalopathy: It is a life-threatening condition that results from vitamin B1 (thiamine) deficiency and is characterized by the classic clinical triad of changes in consciousness, ocular dysfunction, and ataxia. Wernicke encephalopathy is often associated with chronic alcohol abuse, but many other conditions can also cause it (so-called nonalcoholic Wernicke) such as celiac and Crohn's disease, hyperemesis gravidarum, and parenteral nutrition [3].

Manganese accumulation: In patients with cirrhosis or portalsystemic shunts, serum manganese is elevated and transferred to the brain. Manganese neurotoxicity ("manganism") is characterized by psychological and neurologic abnormalities, similar to Parkinsonism (hypokinesia, rigidity, and tremor). Manganese has a preferential deposition in the central nervous system at the level of the globus pallidi, subthalamic nuclei, and substantia nigra [6]. Moreover, manganese accumulation has been described in other conditions such as maintenance hemodialysis, total parenteral nutrition, occupation exposure to manganese from welding, non-cirrhotic portal vein thrombosis, and congenital portalsystemic bypass with no intrinsic hepatocellular disease [6, 7].

Hyperammonemia: Acute brain damage may occur when the serum ammonia concentration suddenly increases especially in patients with chronic cirrhosis and manifests as hepatic encephalopathy [6].

Nonketotic hyperglycemia: It is an uncommon cause of chorea-ballismus in diabetic patients. Pathophysiologic mechanisms remain controversial, but include petechial hemorrhages, myelin breakdown products, or hyperviscosity, leading to T1 shortening of the putamen and head of caudate nucleus on MRI [8].

Osmotic myelinolysis: It is associated with rapid overcorrection of hyponatremia and may be seen in chronic alcoholic patients, malnourished patients, or chronically debilitated organ transplant recipients. Symptoms are usually related to a brainstem lesion and include seizures, disturbed consciousness, gait disturbances, and decrease or cessation of respiratory function [9].

Hypoglycemia: Typically occurs in diabetic patients who accidentally overdose while receiving treatment with oral hypoglycemic agents. Involvement of the basal ganglia seems to portend a poor prognosis [10].

Inflammatory and Infectious Diseases

Behçet disease: It is a recurrent multisystem vasculitis of unknown origin, and its classical triad includes oral and genital ulcerations with uveitis. The CNS is affected in 4–49 % of patients, and the most commonly reported findings are a preference for brainstem–diencephalic involvement with a tendency to resolve over time [11].

Viral encephalitis: The family of flaviviruses typically affects the subcortical gray matter, including thalami, basal ganglia, substantia nigra, and also the cerebellum. The geographic distributions are characteristic, with Japanese encephalitis being common in Asia, West Nile fever in Middle East, and Murray Valley fever in Australia [12].

Creutzfeldt–Jakob disease (CJD): It is a spongiform encephalopathy caused by an infectious protein (prion) characterized by progressive dementia, myoclonus, and periodic discharges on the electroencephalogram. Usually CJD leads to death within 1 year of disease onset [13, 14].

Vascular Disorders

Bithalamic stroke: The artery of Percheron is an uncommon anatomic variant, in which a single dominant thalamoperforating artery supplies both medial thalami with variable contributions to the rostral midbrain. Occlusion results in bilateral paramedian thalamic infarcts with or without midbrain involvement. Typical clinical onset is the triad of altered mental status, vertical gaze palsy, and memory impairment [9].

Spectacular shrinking deficit: Refers to a sudden major hemispheric stroke syndrome followed by rapid improvement within a few hours period, leaving mild or no deficits. In it there is selective neuronal death and it has been called "incomplete infarction" [15].

Deep venous occlusion: Thrombosis of the internal cerebral veins, basal veins, vein of Galen, or straight sinus is less common than that affecting the superficial sinuses with most patients presenting symptoms of elevated intracranial pressure that may rapidly progress to coma [9].

Hypoxic-ischemic injury: Severe hypoxic-ischemic injury in adults primarily affects the gray matter structures, including the basal ganglia, thalami, cerebral cortex (perirolandic and visual cortex), cerebellum, and hippocampi [16].

Neoplasms

Bilateral thalamic glioma: This rare glioma, usually an astrocytoma, is characterized by bilateral thalamic involvement and may affect children and young adults presenting with behavioral impairment. Despite its low-grade classification (World Health Organization grade II), the prognosis is poor [9].

Best Imaging Modality

MRI is the modality of choice for evaluating these pathologic conditions affecting the deep gray matter structures. Computed tomography (CT) may be used as the first diagnostic tool especially in an emergency setting [3].

T2-weighted imaging (T2WI) is the best MRI sequence to study abnormalities in the deep gray matter since most diseases demonstrate increased signal intensity. In specific cases, T1-weighted imaging (T1WI) may be informative, showing high signal areas in basal ganglia or thalamus and helping to narrow the differential diagnosis. The role of diffusion-weighted images (DWI) in the detection of acute cytotoxic brain damage in acute infarction, hypoxia, hypoglycemia, CJD, and Wernicke encephalopathy is critical and has been well described [3].

Calcifications present in metabolic conditions, such as Fahr disease and parathyroid disorders and hemorrhage can be found in poisoning, venous infarctions, and encephalitis, are easily detected using non-contrasted CT or MRI susceptibility-weighted imaging (SWI) phase sequences [3].

The MRI protocol must include fluid-attenuated inversion recovery (FLAIR), T2WI and T1WI, gradient echo (GRE), or SWI and DWI, and intravenous gadolinium administration is required when lesions are identified. In some situations, advanced MRI sequences, such as perfusion-weighted imaging (PWI) and MR spectroscopy (MRS), may help to distinguish a neoplastic from a nonneoplastic condition [3].

With regard to vascular disorders such as Percheron artery infarct, basilar artery occlusion, or deep venous thrombosis, MR angiography/venography and CT angiography/venography are alternatives to detect the sites of occlusions and collaterals. Conventional catheter angiography is reserved for doubtful cases [3, 9].

Major Findings

Most of the disorders that affect the basal ganglia and thalami show hyperintensity on T2WI. However, a constellation of imaging findings may help narrow the differential diagnosis as follows.

Toxic Encephalopathies

CO poisoning: The typical findings on MRI are bilateral hyperintensities in the globus pallidi and cerebral white matter on T2WI resulting from necrosis and demyelination (Fig. 19.1). Damage to the caudate nucleus, thalamus, or putamen is unlikely in this condition. The globus pallidi often show findings related to hemorrhagic infarction. DWI frequently demonstrates areas of restricted diffusion in the acute stage. Delayed leukoencephalopathy and T1 shortening in the globus pallidi may be found in chronic stages [4].

Methanol intoxication: The classic MRI findings are bilateral putaminal necrosis with varying degrees of hemorrhage. White matter edema, especially in the frontal lobes, and edema and contrast enhancement of optic nerves are additional imaging features [5].

Acquired Metabolic Disorders

Wernicke encephalopathy: MRI demonstrates symmetric lesions in the medial thalami and the periventricular area of the third ventricle [3]. Symmetric alterations in the mammillary bodies have been observed in 57 % of patients (Fig. 19.2). There is a powerful correlation between contrast enhancement in the mammillary bodies and chronic alcohol consumption [17].

CNS manganese accumulation: Characteristically the globus pallidi, subthalamic nuclei, and substantia nigra exhibit bilateral symmetric high signal intensity on T1WI (Fig. 19.2) [6]. The signal abnormality usually disappears after liver transplantation [6, 7]. Similar findings can

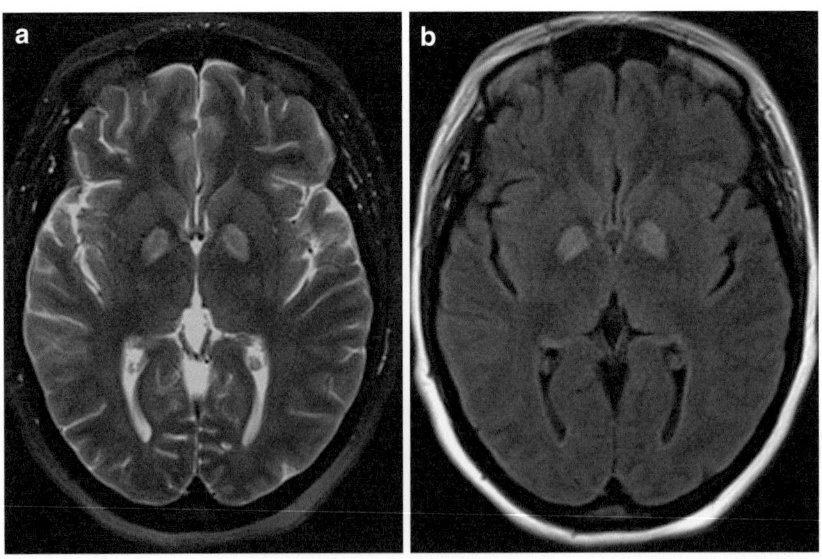

Fig. 19.1 Carbon monoxide (CO) poisoning. Axial T2WI (**a**) and FLAIR (**b**) demonstrate abnormal bilateral hyperintensities in the globus pallidi

be seen in patients with hereditary hemorrhagic telangiectasias, liver vascular shunts, and anemia and may be symptomatic.

Hyperammonemia: It presents as bilateral brain swelling and hyperintensity on FLAIR and T2WI as well as restricted diffusion in the basal ganglia, insular cortex, and cingulate gyrus. MRS characteristically demonstrates decreased levels of myoinositiol (3.5 ppm) and choline (3.2 ppm) and increased levels of glutamine (glutamate/glutamine peak at 2.2–2.4 ppm) (Fig. 19.3) [6].

Nonketotic hyperglycemia: It is characterized by hyperdense changes in the putamen on CT that correspond to increased signal intensity on

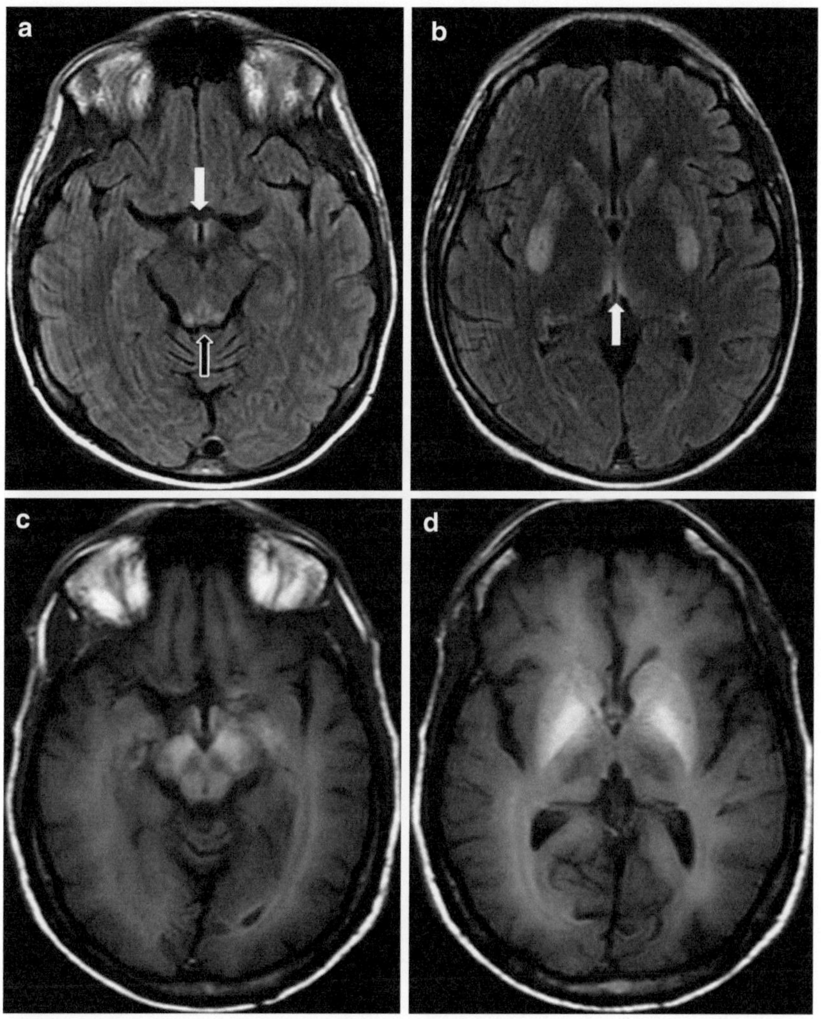

Fig. 19.2 Different patterns of two common metabolic disorders. Wernicke's encephalopathy in a patient with chronic alcohol abuse. (**a**, **b**) Axial FLAIR images show involvement of the mammillary bodies (*white arrow* on **a**) and of the periaqueductal gray matter (*black arrow* on **a**). There is also bilateral putaminal involvement and symmetric lesions involving the medial aspect of the thalami and the periventricular area around the third ventricle (*white arrow* on **b**). (**c**, **d**) A 46-year-old cirrhotic man presents with Parkinsonism due to CNS manganese accumulation. Axial T1WI demonstrate symmetric increased signal in the globus pallidi and substantia nigra

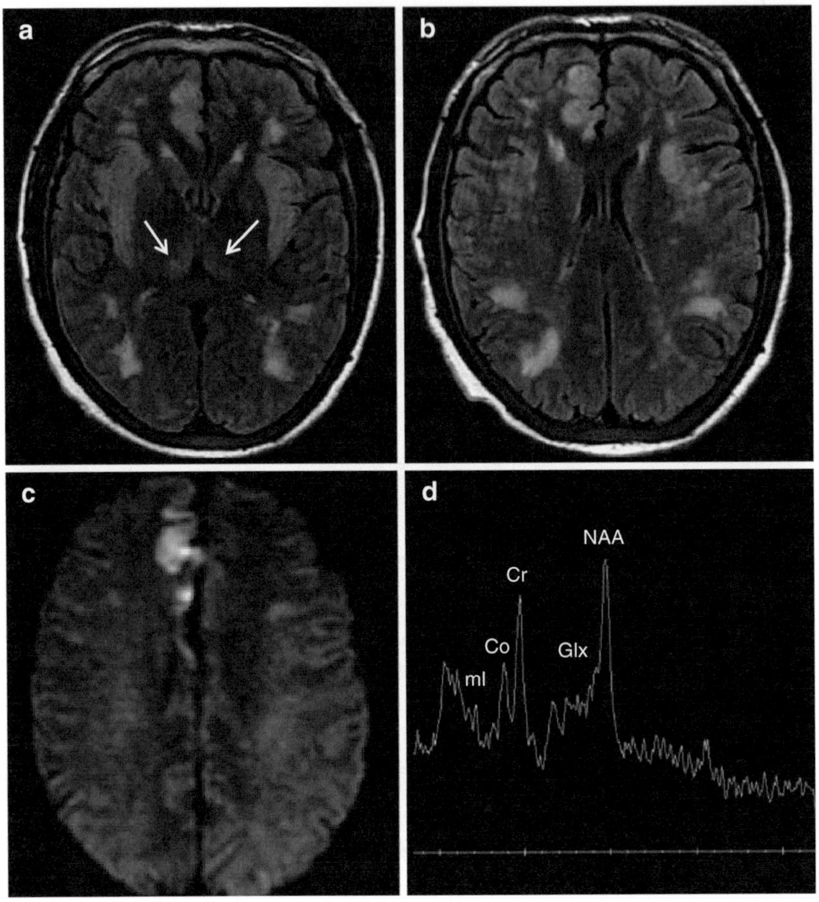

Fig. 19.3 A 50-year-old man with chronic liver disease and hyperammonemic encephalopathy. (**a–c**) FLAIR images (**a**, **b**) depict swelling and areas of increased signal in the insular cortex and cingulate gyrus. There are bilateral thalamic lesions (*arrows* on **a**). (**c**) Areas of cortical restricted diffusion are demonstrated on DWI (**c**). (**d**) MRS demonstrates decreased levels of myoinositiol (mI) (3.5 ppm) and choline (Co) (3.2 ppm) and increased levels of glutamine (Glx) (glutamate/glutamine peak at 2.2–2.4 ppm). NAA= n-acetyl aspartate which is also low

T1WI (Fig. 19.4). The process is either unilateral or bilateral, and, if unilateral, the imaging findings are typically contralateral to the affected hemibody. It has been reported that they usually resolve within a few months after glucose level normalization [8].

Osmotic myelinolysis: The classic described symmetric trident-shaped or bat-shaped area of increased T2 signal in the pons may be associated with extra-pontine lesions involving symmetrically and bilaterally the deep gray matter (basal ganglia and thalami) as well as the white matter (Fig. 19.4). The affected areas may show restricted diffusion in the early stages [9].

Hypoglycemia: The MRI presentation is broad and includes bilateral and symmetric T2 prolongation and restricted diffusion in the cerebral cortex, basal ganglia, subcortical white matter, posterior limb of internal capsule, and splenium of the corpus callosum (Fig. 19.4) [10].

Inflammatory and Infectious Diseases

Behçet disease: Bilateral basal ganglia and midbrain involvement occurs in one-third of patients, and these lesions are hyperintense on T2WI, hypointense in T1WI, enhance after contrast administration, and are typically associated with vasogenic edema (Fig. 19.5) [12].

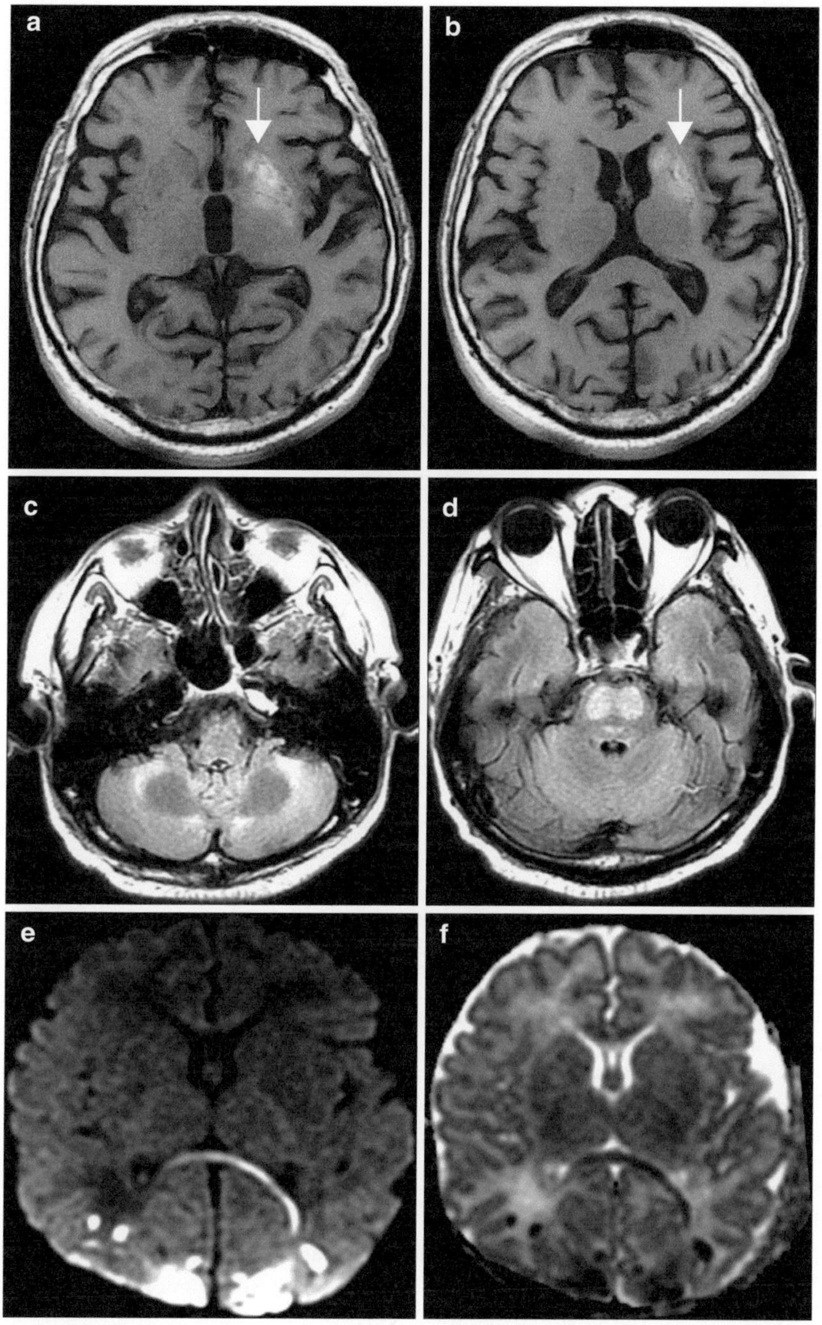

Fig. 19.4 Acquired metabolic disorders. (**a, b**) A diabetic patient presenting with nonketotic hyperglycemia. There is abnormal hyperintensity on T1WI involving the left putamen and caudate nucleus (*arrows*). (**c, d**) Osmotic myelinolysis after a rapid overcorrection of hyponatremia. FLAIR images show abnormal hyperintensities areas in the cerebellar white matter (**c**) and central pons, typically sparing the peripheral fibers (**d**). (**e, f**) Hypoglycemia in a newborn. Axial DWI demonstrating multifocal lesions (restricted diffusion) in the parieto-occipital cortex and white matter. Notice the restricted diffusion in the splenium of corpus callosum as a consequence of excitatory mechanisms

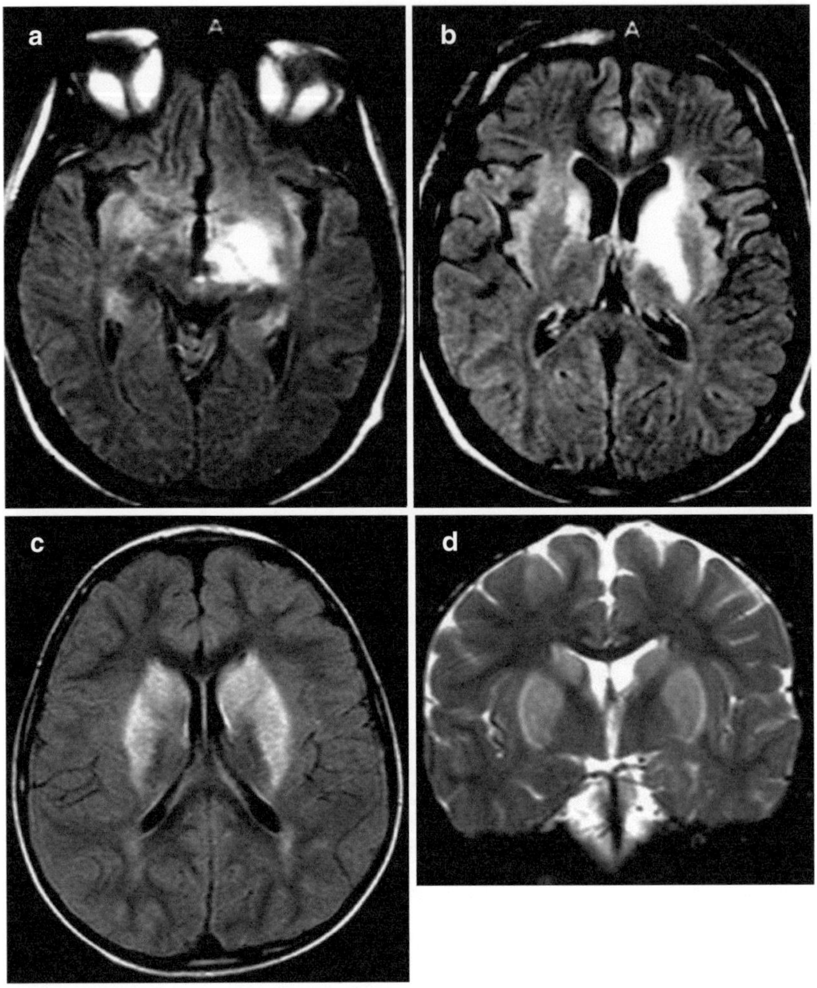

Fig. 19.5 Neuro-Beçhet and flavivirus encephalitis. (**a**, **b**) Relapsing-remitting neuro-Behçet disease. Axial FLAIR images depict a left diencephalic–midbrain junction lesion and affecting the basal ganglia and the internal capsules. (**c**, **d**) Epstein-Barr virus encephalitis in 5-year old boy with selective bilateral abnormal hyperintensity in the basal ganglia on axial FLAIR (**c**) and coronal T2WI (**d**)

Viral encephalitis: Flaviviruses typically affect the subcortical gray matter, including thalami, basal ganglia, substantia nigra, and cerebellum manifesting as T2WI hyperintensities in involved areas (Fig. 19.5). Intralesional hemorrhages and restricted diffusion have also been reported. Common patterns may raise suspicions for specific etiologies as follows: Epstein–Barr virus typically presents as bilateral striatal encephalitis. Western Nile virus and Japanese encephalitis usually manifest as bithalamic hyperintensities on T2WI/FLAIR also affecting the substantia nigra [12].

CJD: Initially MRI demonstrates restricted diffusion usually limited to cerebral cortex and sometimes caudate nuclei, and over time this abnormality may spread to the anterior portion of putamina or involve them entirely (Fig. 19.6). In late stages, restricted diffusion may disappear and there may be abnormal T2 hyperintense areas in the cerebral cortex and basal ganglia and rapidly progressive brain atrophy. The classic described "hockey stick sign" (restricted diffusion in the bilateral pulvinar and medial aspects of the thalami) was described in the variant form of the disease, but can also be seen in the sporadic form [13, 14].

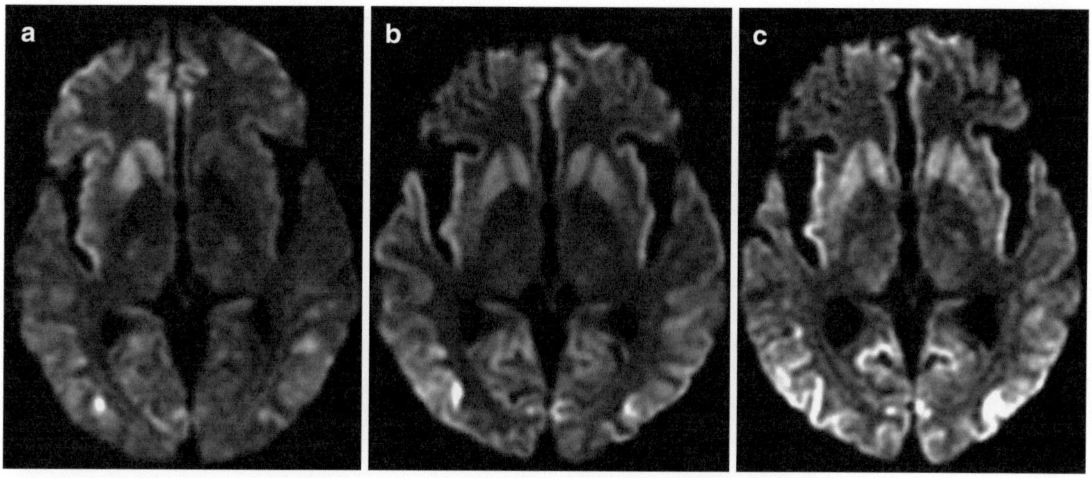

Fig. 19.6 Spongiform encephalopathy. A 62-year-old man presenting with a rapidly progressive dementia and myoclonus diagnosed with Creutzfeldt–Jakob disease. (**a–c**) Axial DWI acquired respectively after 2 (**a**), 4 (**b**), and 6 (**c**) months from the symptoms onset show progressive hyperintensities in the cortex and basal ganglia

Vascular Disorders

Bithalamic stroke: Percheron artery occlusion results in bilateral paramedian thalamic infarcts with or without midbrain involvement [9]. This condition shows restricted diffusion in the affected areas and a distinct pattern of V-shaped hyperintensity on axial FLAIR and/or DWI might be seen along the anterior pial surface of the midbrain adjacent to the interpeduncular fossa (Fig. 19.7) [18].

Spectacular shrinking deficit: This condition is characterized on MRI by persistent hyperintense signal in the basal ganglia on T1WI and relative hypointensity on T2WI 7–10 days from the ictus (Fig. 19.8). The hyperintensity on T1WI gradually subsides with time, and the affected structures show atrophy over time [15].

Deep venous occlusion: Thalamic edema, characterized by increased signal on T2WI and FLAIR, is the imaging hallmark of this condition, and abnormalities may extend to the caudate nuclei and deep white matter. MR venography demonstrates absent flow in the deep venous structures (Fig. 19.9). Hemorrhage and areas of restricted diffusion are seen in some cases [9].

Hypoxic-ischemic injury: DWI demonstrates bilateral and symmetric restricted diffusion in gray matter structures including basal ganglia, thalami, perirolandic and visual cortex, as well as cerebellum and hippocampi usually within the first few hours after a hypoxic-ischemic event (Fig. 19.10). At the same time, T1WI and T2WI are often normal or demonstrate only subtle abnormalities. T2WI become positive in the early subacute stage (24 h to 2 weeks), showing hyperintensity and swelling. DWI abnormalities usually pseudonormalize by the end of the first week [16].

Neoplasms

Bilateral thalamic glioma: MRI and CT demonstrate a mass that enlarges and infiltrates bilaterally the thalami, usually with no contrast enhancement (Fig. 19.11) [9].

Imaging Follow-Up

There is no consensus for a standardized imaging follow-up for all deep gray matter lesions, and it should be clinically determined based on the initial diagnosis and evolution of the patients' symptoms [3].

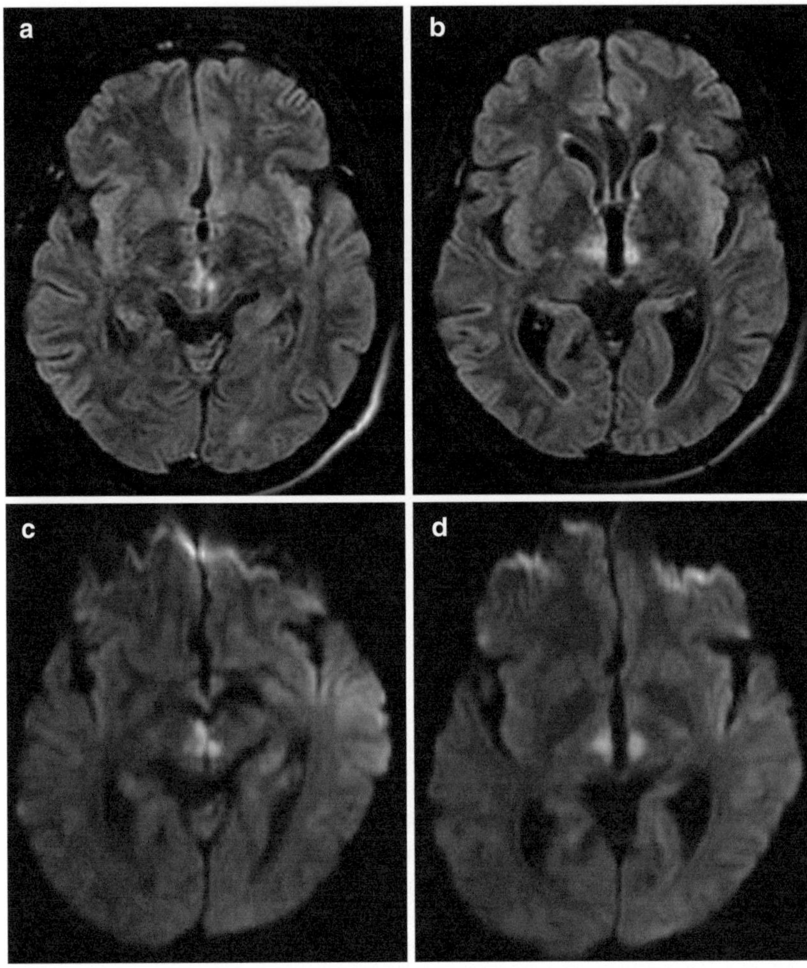

Fig. 19.7 Acute infarct in Percheron artery territory. (**a**, **b**) Axial FLAIR and (**c**, **d**) DWI demonstrate bilateral paramedian thalamic infarcts with involvement of the rostral midbrain

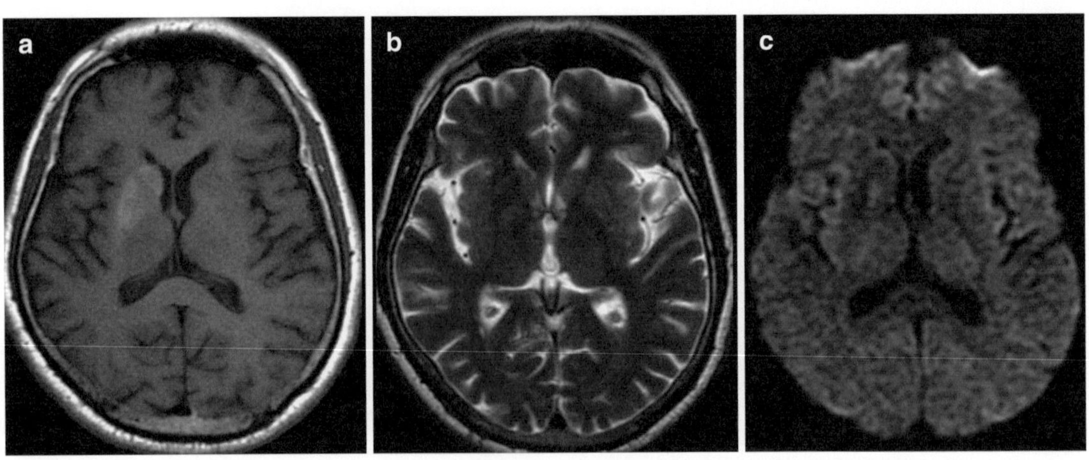

Fig. 19.8 Spectacular shrinking deficit. A 62-year-old man suddenly developed *left* hemiplegia and paresthesias that improved within 20 min suggestive of a transient ischemic attack. (**a**–**c**) The *right* putamen and caudate nucleus are mildly hyperintense on T1WI (**a**) and hypointense on T2WI (**b**). There are no significant changes on DWI (**c**)

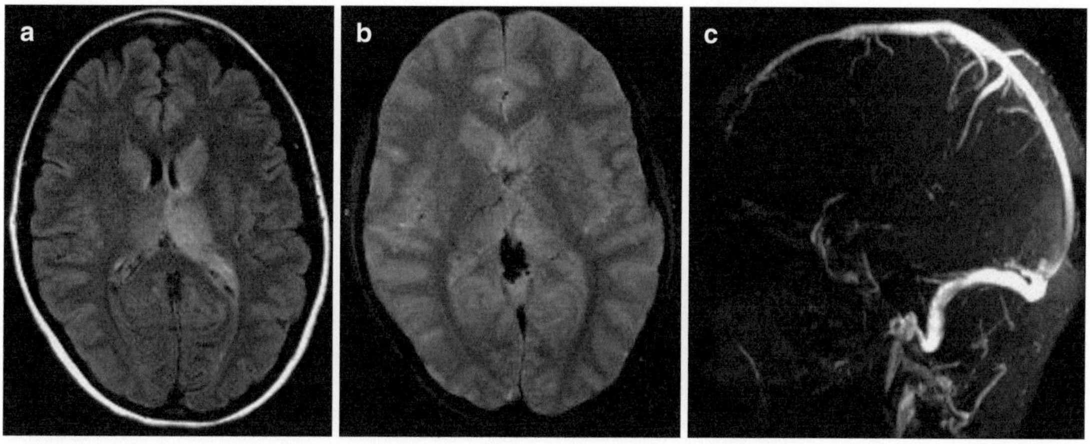

Fig. 19.9 Deep venous occlusion. A 32-year-old woman using oral contraceptives presents with decreased level of consciousness. (**a–c**) Edema is depicted on FLAIR (**a**) especially in the left caudate nucleus and thalamus associated with hypointensity in the internal cerebral veins and straight sinuses on a T2*-weighted image (**b**). (**c**) MR venography shows absent flow in the deep venous system confirming the diagnosis of deep venous thrombosis

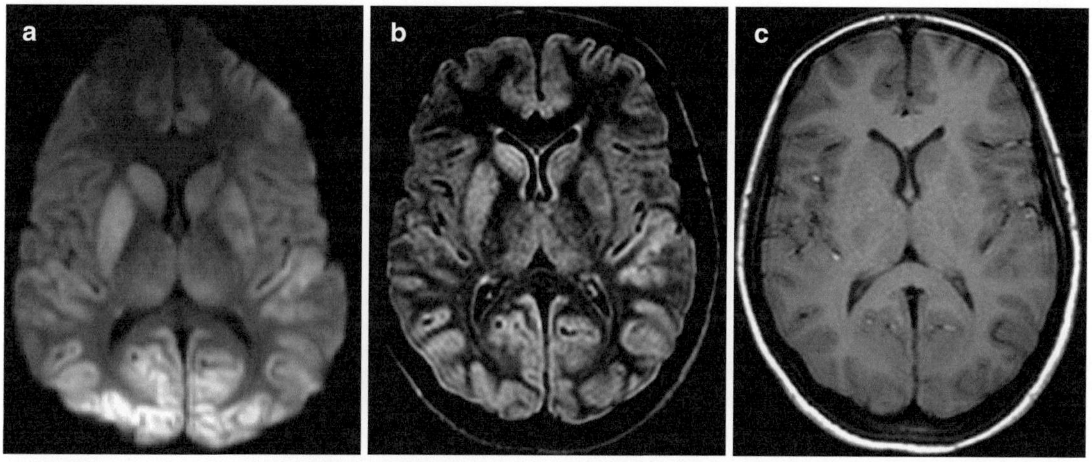

Fig. 19.10 Hypoxic-ischemic injury. 35-year-old man 2 days after a cardiac arrest (**a**, **b**). Basal ganglia and posterior cortical involvement are seen on axial DWI (**a**) and FLAIR images (**b**). (**c**) Axial T1-weighted image only depicted a faint bilateral hypointensity in the basal ganglia

Main Differential Diagnosis

Although inherited metabolic disorders are not the focus of this chapter, they should be remembered as an important differential diagnosis for basal ganglia lesions in young adults, due to its classical presentation and good response to early treatment [19]. *Wilson's disease* is a rare genetic condition in which copper accumulates in tissues, particularly in the liver and brain. Levels of copper might be at levels sufficient to destroy nerve cells. Kayser–Fleischer rings are a pathognomonic sign and are seen as deposits of copper in a ringlike fashion around the cornea. The most common brain finding among patients with neurologic symptoms is bilateral high T2 signal intensity in the striatum. In addition, the occurrence of high T1 signal intensity in the globus pallidus, putamen, and mesencephalon is associated with hepatic dysfunction [19].

Enlarged perivascular spaces (Virchow–Robin spaces) are very common along lenticulostriate arteries through the basal ganglia and become more prominent with age. On

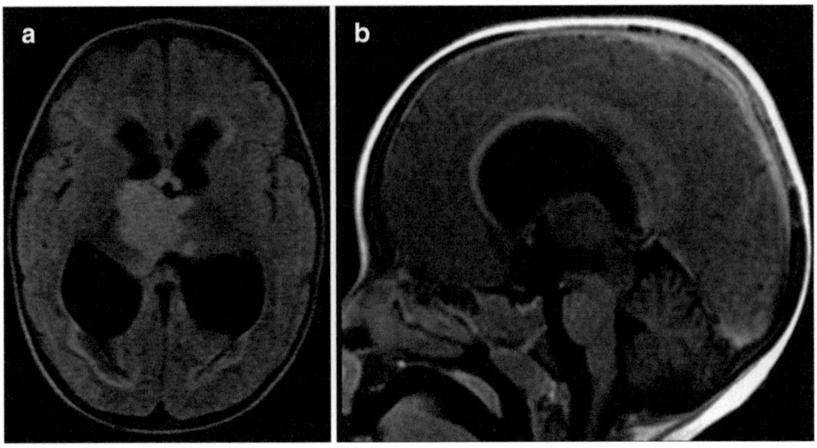

Fig. 19.11 Bilateral thalamic glioma in a 6-year-old boy. (**a**, **b**) Axial FLAIR (**a**) and sagittal T1WI (**b**) show a large bilateral asymmetric thalamic tumor with hydrocephalus

imaging, they characteristically display similar signal to cerebral spinal fluid (CSF) in all sequences and no surrounding gliosis unless giant (>10 mm) [20].

Globus pallidi *calcifications* are more frequently seen in older patients and are considered a normal incidental and idiopathic finding. It is important to remember that basal ganglia calcification may demonstrate high signal on T1WI mimicking manganese deposition due to calcium, reducing the relaxation of adjacent water molecules. SWI or GRE sequences can easily differentiate between them as calcium typically displays blooming effect not seen with manganese [21].

Progressive *iron deposition* in the brain also accompanies normal aging. In healthy adults, the maximum iron concentration is found in the globus pallidus, red nucleus, and pars reticulate of the substantia nigra. However, it is important to recognize that excessive brain iron deposits may be related to many neurodegenerative diseases [22].

Tips

- Correlation of imaging findings with clinical and laboratory data is critical to make the correct diagnosis.
- Putaminal necrosis typically occurs in methanol intoxication.
- Bithalamic symmetric lesions hyperintense on T2WI are commonly seen in Wernicke's encephalopathy. However, they may also be seen in gangliosidosis and ADEM.
- Bilateral and symmetrical globus pallidi lesions in adults may be related to CO poisoning (hyperintense on T2WI) and manganism (hyperintense on T1WI).
- Unilateral striatal T1 hyperintensity may be seen in the spectacular shrinking deficit and nonketotic hyperglycemia. Increased serum glucose level helps to distinguish these conditions.
- Mammillary body involvement is typically seen in Wernicke's encephalopathy and often in association with lesions in the medial thalami and periventricular areas of the third ventricle.
- Symmetric abnormalities involving the thalami and substantia nigra may be seen in viral encephalitis (specially Western Nile virus and Japanese encephalitis).
- Relapsing asymmetric lesions in the midbrain and diencephalon has been described in Behçet disease.
- Bilateral basal ganglia and/or thalamic lesions may be associated with cortical lesions and restricted diffusion in hypoxic-ischemic encephalopathy, hypoglycemia, and CJD, which can be differentiated by their clinical presentations.

References

1. Milton WJ, Atlas SW, Lexa FJ, Mozley PD, Gur RE. Deep gray matter hypointensity patterns with aging in healthy adults: MR imaging at 1.5 T. Radiology. 1991;181(3):715–9. doi:10.1148/radiology.181.3.1947087.
2. Schmahmann JD. Vascular syndromes of the thalamus. Stroke J Cereb Circ. 2003;34(9):2264–78. doi:10.1161/01.STR.0000087786.38997.9E.
3. Hegde AN, Mohan S, Lath N, Lim CC. Differential diagnosis for bilateral abnormalities of the basal ganglia and thalamus. Radiograph: Rev Publ Radiol Soc N Am Inc. 2011;31(1):5–30. doi:10.1148/rg.311105041.
4. Beppu T. The role of MR imaging in assessment of brain damage from carbon monoxide poisoning: a review of the literature. AJNR Am J Neuroradiol. 2014;35(4):625–31. doi:10.3174/ajnr.A3489.
5. Blanco M, Casado R, Vazquez F, Pumar JM. CT and MR imaging findings in methanol intoxication. AJNR Am J Neuroradiol. 2006;27(2):452–4.
6. Rovira A, Alonso J, Cordoba J. MR imaging findings in hepatic encephalopathy. AJNR Am J Neuroradiol. 2008;29(9):1612–21. doi:10.3174/ajnr.A1139.
7. da Silva CJ, da Rocha AJ, Jeronymo S, Mendes MF, Milani FT, Maia Jr AC, Braga FT, Sens YA, Miorin LA. A preliminary study revealing a new association in patients undergoing maintenance hemodialysis: manganism symptoms and T1 hyperintense changes in the basal ganglia. AJNR Am J Neuroradiol. 2007;28(8):1474–9. doi:10.3174/ajnr.A0600.
8. Wintermark M, Fischbein NJ, Mukherjee P, Yuh EL, Dillon WP. Unilateral putaminal CT, MR, and diffusion abnormalities secondary to nonketotic hyperglycemia in the setting of acute neurologic symptoms mimicking stroke. AJNR Am J Neuroradiol. 2004;25(6):975–6.
9. Smith AB, Smirniotopoulos JG, Rushing EJ, Goldstein SJ. Bilateral thalamic lesions. AJR Am J Roentgenol. 2009;192(2):W53–62. doi:10.2214/AJR.08.1585.
10. Johkura K, Nakae Y, Kudo Y, Yoshida TN, Kuroiwa Y. Early diffusion MR imaging findings and short-term outcome in comatose patients with hypoglycemia. AJNR Am J Neuroradiol. 2012;33(5):904–9. doi:10.3174/ajnr.A2903.
11. Kocer N, Islak C, Siva A, Saip S, Akman C, Kantarci O, Hamuryudan V. CNS involvement in neuro-Behcet syndrome: an MR study. AJNR Am J Neuroradiol. 1999;20(6):1015–24.
12. Gupta RK, Jain KK, Kumar S. Imaging of nonspecific (nonherpetic) acute viral infections. Neuroimaging Clin N Am. 2008;18(1):41–52; vii. doi:10.1016/j.nic.2007.12.004.
13. Ukisu R, Kushihashi T, Tanaka E, Baba M, Usui N, Fujisawa H, Takenaka H. Diffusion-weighted MR imaging of early-stage Creutzfeldt-Jakob disease: typical and atypical manifestations. Radiograph: Rev Publ Radiol Soc N Am Inc. 2006;26 Suppl 1:S191–204. doi:10.1148/rg.26si065503.
14. Ukisu R, Kushihashi T, Kitanosono T, Fujisawa H, Takenaka H, Ohgiya Y, Gokan T, Munechika H. Serial diffusion-weighted MRI of Creutzfeldt-Jakob disease. AJR Am J Roentgenol. 2005;184(2):560–6. doi:10.2214/ajr.184.2.01840560.
15. Fujioka M, Taoka T, Hiramatsu KI, Sakaguchi S, Sakaki T. Delayed ischemic hyperintensity on T1-weighted MRI in the caudoputamen and cerebral cortex of humans after spectacular shrinking deficit. Stroke J Cereb Circ. 1999;30(5):1038–42.
16. Huang BY, Castillo M. Hypoxic-ischemic brain injury: imaging findings from birth to adulthood. Radiograph: Rev Publ Radiol Soc N Am Inc. 2008;28(2):417–39. doi:10.1148/rg.282075066; quiz 617.
17. Zuccoli G, Gallucci M, Capellades J, Regnicolo L, Tumiati B, Giadas TC, Bottari W, Mandrioli J, Bertolini M. Wernicke encephalopathy: MR findings at clinical presentation in twenty-six alcoholic and nonalcoholic patients. AJNR Am J Neuroradiol. 2007;28(7):1328–31. doi:10.3174/ajnr.A0544.
18. Lazzaro NA, Wright B, Castillo M, Fischbein NJ, Glastonbury CM, Hildenbrand PG, Wiggins RH, Quigley EP, Osborn AG. Artery of percheron infarction: imaging patterns and clinical spectrum. AJNR Am J Neuroradiol. 2010;31(7):1283–9. doi:10.3174/ajnr.A2044.
19. Kim TJ, Kim IO, Kim WS, Cheon JE, Moon SG, Kwon JW, Seo JK, Yeon KM. MR imaging of the brain in Wilson disease of childhood: findings before and after treatment with clinical correlation. AJNR Am J Neuroradiol. 2006;27(6):1373–8.
20. Kwee RM, Kwee TC. Virchow-Robin spaces at MR imaging. Radiograph: Rev Publ Radiol Soc N Am Inc. 2007;27(4):1071–86. doi:10.1148/rg.274065722.
21. Adams AE. Basal ganglia calcification. Characteristics of CT scans and clinical findings. Neurosurg Rev. 1980;3(3):201–3.
22. Aquino D, Bizzi A, Grisoli M, Garavaglia B, Bruzzone MG, Nardocci N, Savoiardo M, Chiapparini L. Age-related iron deposition in the basal ganglia: quantitative analysis in healthy subjects. Radiology. 2009;252(1):165–72. doi:10.1148/radiol.2522081399.

Acute Temporal Lobe Lesions

20

Bruna Garbugio Dutra, Antônio José da Rocha, and Renato Hoffmann Nunes

Abstract

Several diseases may involve the temporal lobe, including benign and malignant ones. Each disorder may result in a distinct imaging pattern, helping to narrow the differential diagnoses. Clinical manifestations depend on the specific site involved. Magnetic resonance imaging allows a detailed structural evaluation usually demonstrating T2 hyperintense lesions, and advanced sequences aid in reaching a definite diagnosis.

Background

A variety of diseases may involve the temporal lobes (TL), including benign and malignant ones. Each disorder may produce a distinct imaging pattern narrowing the differential diagnosis [1].

B.G. Dutra, MD (✉) • A.J. da Rocha, MD, PhD
Division of Neuroradiology, Hospital Santa Casa de Misericórdia de São Paulo, Rua Dr. Cesário Motta Junior 112, Vila Buarque, Sao Paulo, SP 01221-020, Brazil

Division of Neuroradiology, Grupo Fleury, Sao Paulo, SP, Brazil
e-mail: bruna.gdutra@gmail.com; antonio.rocha@grupofleury.com.br

R. Hoffmann Nunes, MD
Division of Neuroradiology, Santa Casa de São Paulo, São Paulo, Brazil
e-mail: renatohn@hotmail.com

Clinical manifestations depend on the site of involvement. Generalized involvement of both TL leads to emotional and behavior changes, as well as auditory hallucinations. Mesial/hippocampal involvement often leads to seizures, amnesia, behavioral, and psychiatric manifestations. Left-sided TL lesions may cause speech disturbances, while right-sided TL lesions cause perception of music or quality of speech disorders [2].

Key Points

Etiology

Infection: Many infections involve the TL, uni- or bilaterally, but the most common one is viral encephalitis. Herpes virus family accounts for the most frequent etiology, especially *Herpes simplex* virus type 1 (HSV-1) [1, 3, 4]. Herpes simplex encephalitis (HSE) as a primary infection or

R. Hoffmann Nunes et al. (eds.), *Critical Findings in Neuroradiology*,
DOI 10.1007/978-3-319-27987-9_20

as a reactivation of a latent HSV-1 causes significant morbidity and mortality which justify early intervention with antiretroviral treatments even before actual disease confirmation [3, 4]. Others viruses causing TL involvement include HSV-6 and Japanese encephalitis virus, the former mostly associated to post-allogeneic hematopoietic stem-cell transplants [3]. Bacterial and fungal infections may also affect the TL with the most common being *Treponema pallidum* which is mostly seen in the elderly or in HIV/AIDS patients [4–6].

Limbic encephalitis (*LE*): LE is the most common autoimmune-mediated encephalitis characterized by presence of antibodies against neuronal and cell membrane antigens. Based on a potential association with underlying tumors, LE is classified as paraneoplastic (PLE) or non-paraneoplastic (NPLE). Diagnosis depends on clinical presentation, presence of antibodies or underlying tumor diagnosed within 5 years of clinical onset, and morphological evidence of limbic system involvement as demonstrated on imaging studies [7–10].

Neoplasia: Primary and secondary tumors may involve the TL, the more common ones are glial tumors, gangliogliomas (GG), dysembryoplastic neuroepithelial tumors (DNT), and pleomorphic xanthoastrocytoma (PXA) [11].

Ischemic stroke: The majority of the arterial supply to the TL is from branches of the middle cerebral artery (MCA) and the anterior choroidal artery. The inferior portion of the TL is supplied by the posterior cerebral artery (PCA). Rapid-onset neurological deficits determined by the involved vascular territories are the typical clinical presentation. DWI is useful to demonstrate cytotoxic edema thus confirming acute ischemia although similar findings may be seen in acute seizures [2].

Seizure-related limbic disorders: Postictal states can be seen with recurrent or prolonged focal or febrile seizures. MRI features may distinguish reversible abnormalities related to seizures from structural lesions causing epilepsy [2].

Transient global amnesia (*TGA*): It is clinically defined as sudden onset of amnesia with preserved alertness, attention, and personal identity which lasts no more than 24 h and has no long-term sequelae. Pathogenesis is uncertain and includes ischemia, migraine, seizures, venous congestion, and psychological disturbances [4].

Best Imaging Modality

CT is the modality of choice for screening and it is considered useful in an emergency setting. CT identifies hemorrhages, gross structural malformations, large tumors, and calcified lesions. In nonemergency situations, MRI is more sensitive and is the imaging method of choice [2].

MRI provides detailed anatomic information as well as physiological evaluation of the brain. Patients with TL abnormalities frequently present with seizures, and subtle lesions may be missed if a specific MRI protocol is not employed. This protocol includes T1-weighted image (T1WI) sequences with thin-slice thickness (1.5-mm) and no intervening gap acquired as a three-dimensional volume, allowing reformatting of images in multiple planes. The protocol should also include multiplanar thin slices or 3D sequences using FLAIR and T2WI. When the coronal plane is acquired, it must be in an oblique plane perpendicular to the long axis of the hippocampus allowing for better visualization of its internal structures. Susceptibility-weighted imaging (SWI) or gradient-echo (GRE) sequences are recommended in order to identify calcifications and blood products. Intravenous gadolinium administration is required when a structural lesion is identified. In this situation, advanced MRI sequences, such as diffusion-weighted imaging (DWI), perfusion-weighted imaging (PWI), and MR spectroscopy (MRS), may help to distinguish a neoplastic from a nonneoplastic condition [2].

Major Findings

Infections and Inflammatory Lesions

HSV-1 typically affects the TL, initially restricted to its medial–inferior portions with later involvement of the inferior frontal lobes and insulae. Generally, it is unilateral; however, in some patients, it may affect the contralateral side, leading to a bilateral asymmetrical involvement typically sparing the basal ganglia [4]. MRI findings are characterized by hyperintensities on FLAIR/T2WI involving the cortex and white matter, causing mass effect and sometimes containing hemorrhage. Areas of restricted diffusion are seen in the early phases and are sometimes greater than the area of abnormal FLAIR/T2WI. Leptomeningeal and cortical enhancement may also occur (Fig. 20.1) [2, 4].

Neurosyphilis has a broad spectrum of imaging presentations. The most common MRI findings occur in the TL and include cortical and subcortical hyperintensities on T2WI/FLAIR affecting the mesial TL leading to subsequent atrophy in 37 % of patients [6]. Gadolinium enhancement is rare and may appear as a focal meningeal or meningovascular process (Fig. 20.2) [5].

Limbic encephalitis is characterized by bilateral or unilateral mesial TL hyperintensities on FLAIR/T2WI, usually asymmetric. Contrast enhancement is rare and restricted diffusion often occurs in the acute phase [8, 9]. Imaging follow-up shows atrophy of the previously affected areas [7].

Neoplasia

Glial tumors are the most common primary diffuse neoplasia that involve the TL and can be divided into low-grade gliomas (LGGs) and high-grade gliomas (HGGs). All are infiltrative lesions involving cortex and adjacent white matter with hypo-/isointensity on T1WI and hyperintensity on FLAIR/T2WI. HGGs are more heterogeneous than LGG due to presence of necrosis, cysts, hemorrhage, and neovascularization. Contrast enhancement is rare in LGG (Fig. 20.3) and is common in HGG manifesting as thick and irregular zones. On PWI, relative cerebral blood volume (rCBV) values greater than 1.75 are suggestive of HGG. In glial tumors, MRS shows choline (Cho) elevation and *N*-acetylaspartate/creatine (NAA) reduction. In HGG, these changes are prominent and lipid/lactate peaks are present and related to necrosis/ischemia. In LGG, myoinositol to creatine ratio (Myo/Cr) may be high [2, 11, 12]. A peculiar and rare type of glial tumor that might also affect the TL is gliomatosis cerebri (GC) and is characterized by an extensive diffuse brain infiltration involving at least two lobes with relative preservation of the underlying architecture [2, 13].

Ischemic stroke: TL ischemic stroke usually is characterized by cortical and subcortical hyperin-

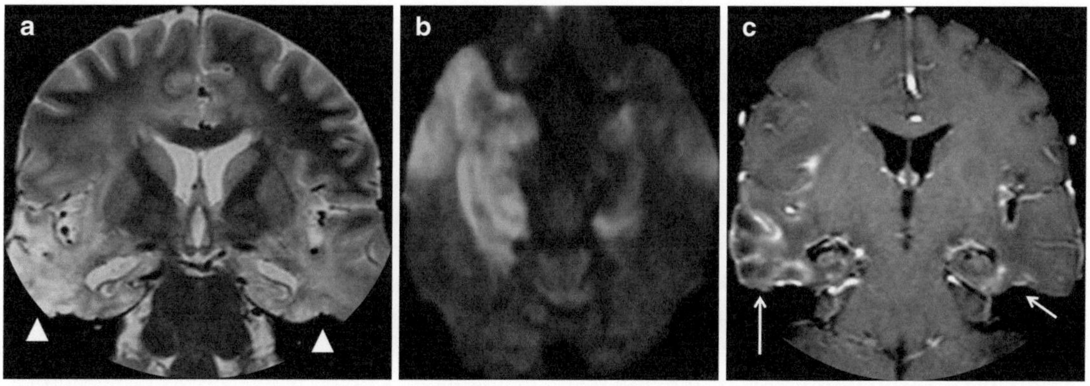

Fig. 20.1 Herpes simplex encephalitis. (**a**–**c**) Coronal T2WI, axial DWI, and postcontrast T1WI. (**a**) Extensive area of hyperintensity on T2WI (**a**) and DWI (**b**) involves the cortex and the white matter of both temporal lobes (*arrowheads*) and insulas, typically sparing the basal ganglia. Cortical and leptomeningeal enhancement are also seen in the temporal lobes (*arrows*) and insulas, especially in the right (**c**)

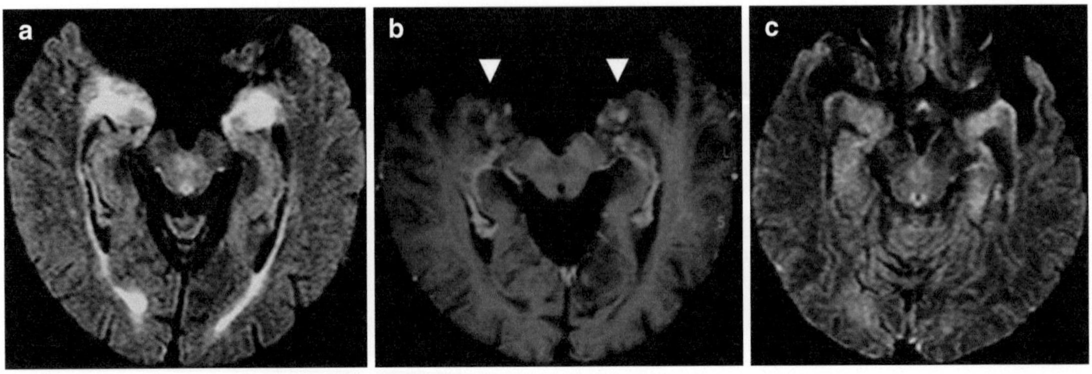

Fig. 20.2 Patient diagnosed with neurosyphilis. (**a**, **b**) Acute/inflammatory phase. (**a**) Axial FLAIR image shows hyperintense areas affecting the mesial aspect of the temporal lobes. (**b**) Axial postcontrast T1WI displays faint enhancement in the affected regions (*arrowheads*). (**c**) Chronic phase. Axial FLAIR image depicts bilateral temporal lobe atrophy and high signal intensity particularly on the left side

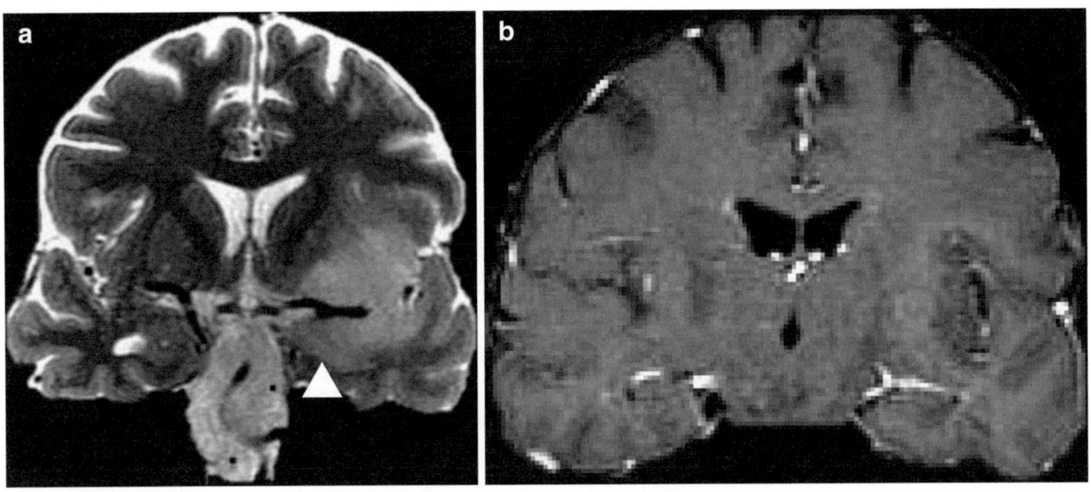

Fig. 20.3 Low-grade glioma. (**a**) Coronal T2WI demonstrates hyperintense lesion infiltrating and expanding the cortex and the white matter of the left mesial temporal lobe (*arrowhead*) as well as the ipsilateral insula and basal ganglia. (**b**) Coronal postcontrast T1WI reveals no enhancement

tense areas on T2WI/FLAIR with restricted diffusion in the early phases and decreased blood flow on PWI. These abnormal areas generally correspond to an arterial vascular territory (either MCA or PCA). Ipsilateral basal ganglia involvement is a finding not expected in HSE and frequently occurs with obstruction of the proximal branches of the MCA [2]. Isolated hippocampus stroke is rare and shows focal restricted diffusion and is due to a PCA and anterior choroidal artery territory infarcts [2, 4].

Seizure-related limbic disorders: Postictal signal changes can manifest as focal or multifocal reversible signal abnormalities on T2WI/FLAIR with restricted DWI associated with morphologic abnormalities in the hippocampus or neocortical structures usually (Fig. 20.4). Mild mass effect is present and contrast enhancement is rare. In the

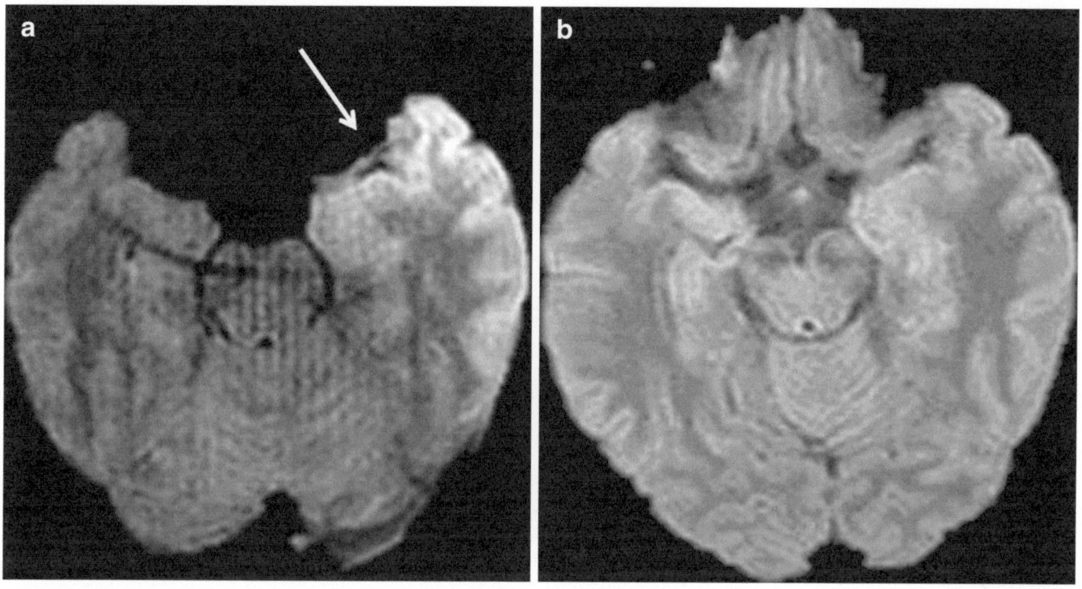

Fig. 20.4 Seizure-related limbic disorders. (**a**) Patient with a frontal lobe metastasis (not shown) presenting with seizures. Axial FLAIR image shows increased signal cortical hyperintensity affecting the cortical and subcortical white matter in the left temporal lobe (*arrow*). (**b**) Resolution of the FLAIR abnormalities from the same patient after 10 days

acute phase, PWI may demonstrate increased cerebral blood flow which may help in differentiating it from an infarct [2, 14].

Transient global amnesia: It usually manifests as subacute small and punctate (1–3 mm) hyperintensities on DWI involving the lateral portion of the hippocampi better depicted 24–72 h after the clinical presentation (Fig. 20.5) [15].

Imaging Follow-Up

There is no consensus for a standardized imaging follow-up for all TL lesions. It should be based on the initial diagnosis and it is usually clinically determined.

Main Differential Diagnosis

The main diseases that affect the TL were described above. Some additional disorders should be remembered when considering the major differential diagnoses including the following.

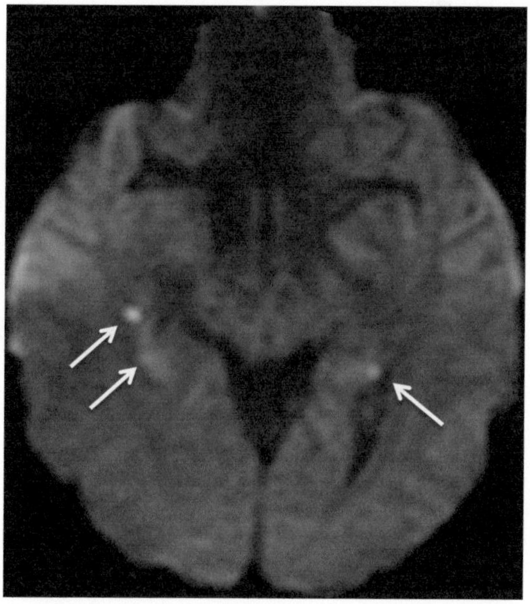

Fig. 20.5 Transient global amnesia. Axial DWI demonstrates punctate hyperintense lesions on the lateral aspect of both hippocampi (*arrows*)

CSF collections: Perivascular spaces (PVS) and choroidal fissure cysts (CFCs) are cystic findings that are isointense to cerebrospinal fluid (CSF) on all imaging sequences. PVS or Virchow–Robin (VR) dilated spaces are seen in subcortical white matter of the anterior TL, which could exhibit linear or punctate enhancement within the cyst, representing a blood vessel. CFC are located lateral to the hippocampus, between the *cornu ammonis* and the dentate gyrus. While PVS tend to be bilateral, CFC tends to be unilateral [2].

Mesial temporal sclerosis: Also known as hippocampal sclerosis, it is the most common cause of refractory TL epilepsy. Histologically, it is characterized by neuronal loss in the hippocampus. It results from insults to the developing brain [16]. On MRI, it shows atrophy and hyperintensity on T2WI/FLAIR predominantly in the hippocampus. Secondary findings include loss of normal internal hippocampal architecture, TL volume loss, subcortical temporal pole hyperintensity on T2WI/FLAIR, dilatation of the temporal horn, and narrowed collateral gyrus white matter, as well as a smaller fornix and an atrophic mammillary body, all of them on the same side of the atrophic hippocampus [4, 16].

Gangliogliomas: Are solid–cystic or solid tumors that frequently present calcifications (Fig. 20.6) [11]. The typical tumor is isointense to gray matter on T1WI without prominent mass effect and located in the medial TL in young patients with TL epilepsy [17].

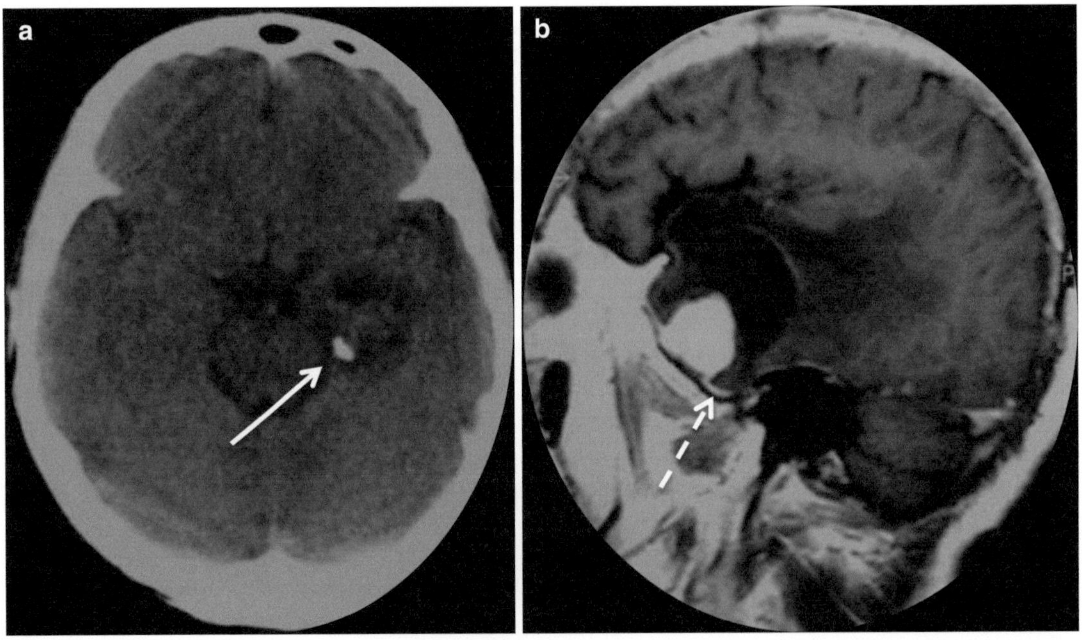

Fig. 20.6 Focal temporal lobe mass. (**a**) Ganglioglioma. Axial non-enhanced CT image shows hypoattenuated lesion in the left hippocampus with a focal course calcification (*arrow*). (**b**) Pleomorphic xanthoastrocytoma. Sagittal postcontrast T1WI demonstrates a temporal lobe solid–cystic mass with leptomeningeal enhancement (*arrow*)

Pleomorphic xanthoastrocytomas: Classically appear as circumscribed cystic tumors with a mural nodule attached to the cortex and adjacent to the leptomeninges [11]. After contrast administration, enhancement of the mural nodule and the adjacent leptomeninges is usually seen (Fig. 20.6). Calcifications are rare [11, 18].

Dysembryoplastic neuroepithelial tumors: Are well-demarcated, wedge-shaped masses characterized by hyperintense signal on T2WI and a "bubbly" intracortical appearance due to multiple cysts. Contrast enhancement is seen in about 30 % of cases [11].

Metastases: Imaging features are similar to those of primary tumors with large amounts of vasogenic edema. Commonly, there are other lesions [2].

Neurodegenerative disorders: Some diseases that may involve TL include Alzheimer disease (AD) and frontotemporal dementia (FTD). Hippocampal atrophy is the most common imaging biomarker of AD, while an asymmetrical frontal and/or temporal lobe atrophy associated to white matter hyperintensity on T2WI/FLAIR is the most common finding in FTD [4].

Cerebral autosomal dominant arteriopathy with subcortical infarcts and leukoencephalopathy (*CADASIL*): It results in recurrent subcortical strokes often complicated by dementia. Neuroimaging shows both focal lacunar infarcts and diffuse white matter ischemic changes, particularly involving the bilateral subcortical white matter regions of the anterior TLs and external capsules [4].

Myotonic dystrophy type 1: It is a disorder with autosomal dominant inheritance presenting with facial and distal muscle weakness, hearing impairment, cataracts, and testicular atrophy. On MRI, the findings are bilateral hyperintensity on T2WI/FLAIR in the subcortical anterior TLs and periventricular white matter as well as VR dilated spaces [4].

Hippocampal malrotation: In this setting, hippocampus is abnormally rounded in shape, with blurred inner structures, and has a more vertical collateral sulcus angle and downwardly displaced fornix [19].

Neurocutaneous melanosis: The typical TL finding is focal, rounded, T1WI shortening in the amygdalae due to melanin deposits. Patient typically has cutaneous stigma (giant nevus or multiple small nevi) [20].

Tips

- Postictal signal changes can manifest as focal or multifocal reversible signal abnormalities on T2WI/FLAIR.
- MRS, PWI, CSF analysis, autoantibodies panel, EEG, and clinical presentation may help arrive at the correct diagnosis.
- Basal ganglia involvement ipsilateral to other TL abnormalities is a suggestive finding of MCA stroke especially if DWI is abnormal.
- In the clinical setting of encephalitis, it is recommended to initiate antiviral treatment even before imaging is performed in order to prevent neurological sequelae.
- Carefully evaluate additional imaging findings in order to recognize the suggestive imaging patterns (Flowcharts 20.1 and 20.2).

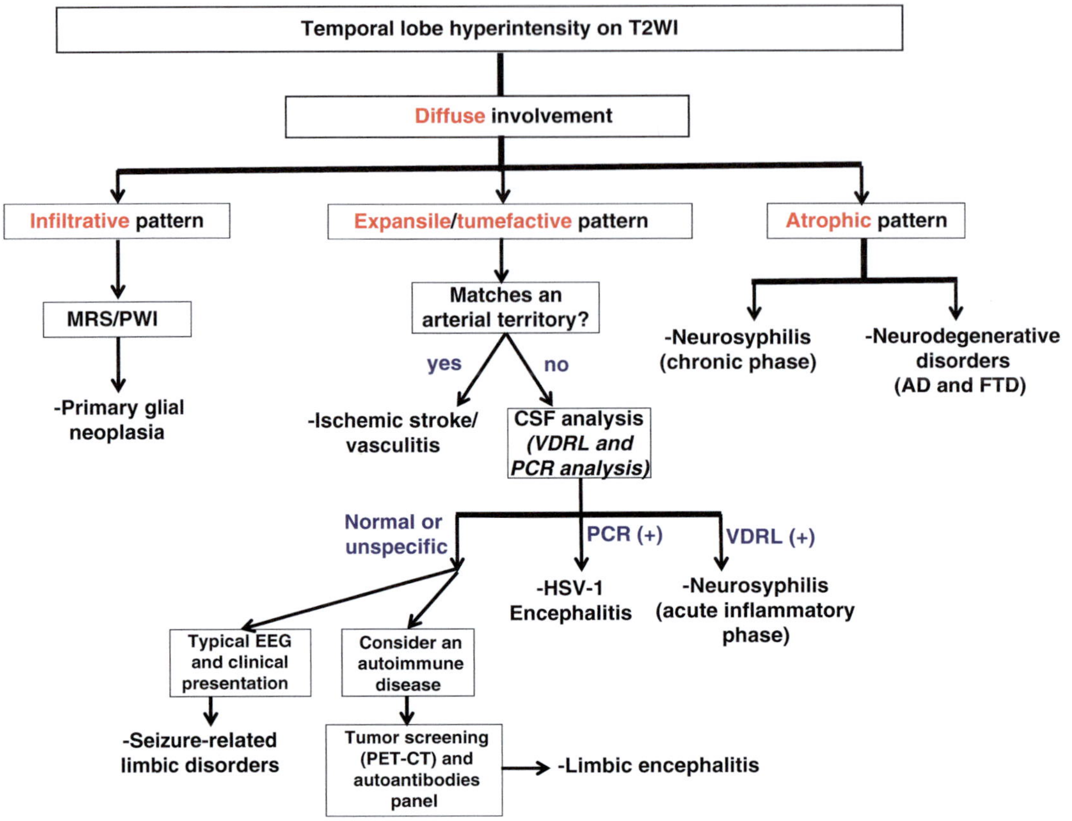

Flowchart 20.1 Recommended approach to diffuse temporal lobe lesions. *WI* weighted image, *MRS* MRI-spectroscopy, *PWI* perfusion WI, *HSV1* herpes simplex type 1, *CSF* cerebrospinal fluid, *EEG* electroencephalogram, *AD* Alzheimer disease, *FTD* frontotemporal dementia, (+) positive

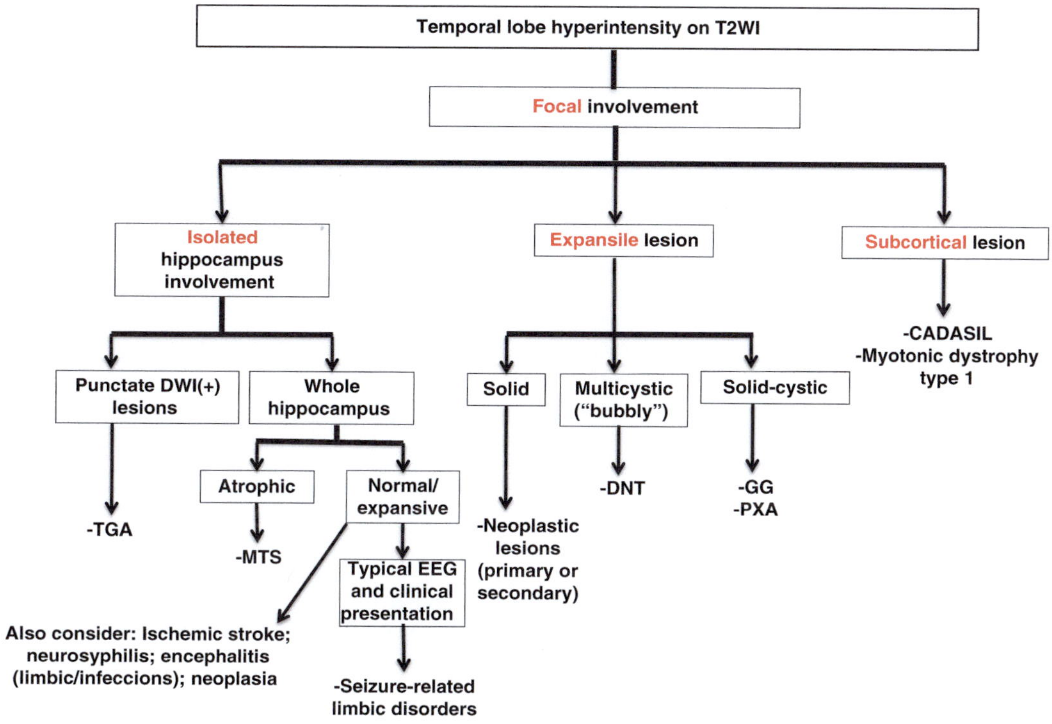

Flowchart 20.2 Recommended approach to focal temporal lobe lesions. *WI* weighted image, *EEG* electroencephalogram, *AD* Alzheimer disease, *MTS* mesial temporal sclerosis, *TGA* transient global amnesia, *GG* ganglioglioma, *PXA* pleomorfic xanthoastrocytoma, *DNT* dysembrioblastic neuroepithelial tumor, *CADASIL* cerebral autosomal-dominant arteriopathy with subcortical infarcts and leukoencephalopathy

References

1. Chow FC, Glaser CA, Sheriff H, Xia D, Messenger S, Whitley R, et al. Use of clinical and neuroimaging characteristics to distinguish temporal lobe herpes simplex encephalitis from its mimics. Clin Infect Dis. 2015;60(9):1377–83. doi:10.1093/cid/civ051.
2. Naidich TP, Castillo M, Cha S, Raybaud C, Smirniotopoulos JG, Kollias S, et al. Imaging of the spine. Elsevier Health Sciences; 2010. 1 p. 629–726.
3. Tunkel AR, Glaser CA, Bloch KC, Sejvar JJ, Marra CM, Roos KL, et al. The management of encephalitis: clinical practice guidelines by the infectious diseases society of America. Clin Infect Dis. 2008;47(3): 303–27.
4. Sureka J, Jakkani RK. Clinico-radiological spectrum of bilateral temporal lobe hyperintensity: a retrospective review. BJR. 2012;85(1017):e782–92.
5. Fadil H, Gonzalez-Toledo E, Kelley BJ, Kelley RE. Neuroimaging findings in neurosyphilis. J Neuroimaging. 2006;16(3):286–9.
6. Brightbill TC, Ihmeidan IH, Post MJ, Berger JR, Katz DA. Neurosyphilis in HIV-positive and HIV-negative patients: neuroimaging findings. AJNR Am J Neuroradiol. 1995;16(4):703–11.
7. Demaerel P, Van Dessel W, Van Paesschen W, Vandenberghe R, Van Laere K, Linn J. Autoimmune-mediated encephalitis. Neuroradiology. 2011;53(11): 837–51.
8. Gultekin SH, Rosenfeld MR, Voltz R, Eichen J, Posner JB, Dalmau J. Paraneoplastic limbic encephalitis: neurological symptoms, immunological findings and tumour association in 50 patients. Brain. 2000; 123(7):1481–94.
9. Tüzün E, Dalmau J. Limbic encephalitis and variants: classification. Diagn Treat Neurologist. 2007;13(5): 261–71.
10. Dalmau J, Rosenfeld MR. Autoimmune encephalitis update. Neuro-Oncology. 2014;16(6):771–8.
11. Giulioni M. Epilepsy associated tumors: review article. WJCC. 2014;2(11):623–20.
12. Law M, Yang S, Wang H, Babb JS, Johnson G, Cha S, Knopp EA, Zagzag D. Glioma grading: sensitivity, specificity, and predictive values of perfusion MR imaging and proton MR spectroscopic imaging compared with conventional MR imaging. AJNR Am J Neuroradiol. 2003;24(10):1989–98.
13. Sun P, Piao H, Guo X, Wang Z, Sui R, Zhang Y, et al. Gliomatosis cerebri mimicking acute viral encephalitis and with malignant transformation of partial lesions: a case report. Exp Ther Med. 2014;8(3): 925–28.
14. Kim JA, Chung JI, Yoon PH, Kim DI, Chung TS, Kim EJ, Jeong EK. Transient MR signal changes in patients with generalized tonicoclonic seizure or status epilepticus: perictal diffusion-weighted imaging. AJNR Am J Neuroradiol. 2001;22(6):1149–60.
15. Weon YC, Kim JH, Lee JS, Kim SY. Optimal diffusion-weighted imaging protocol for lesion detection in transient global amnesia. Am J Neuroradiol. 2008;29(7):1324–8.
16. Bronen R. Commentary: MR of mesial temporal sclerosis: how much is enough? AJNR Am J Neuroradiol. 1998;19(1):15–8.
17. Adachi Y, Yagishita A. Gangliogliomas: characteristic imaging findings and role in the temporal lobe epilepsy. Neuroradiology. 2008;50(10):829–34.
18. Crespo-Rodríguez AM, Smirniotopoulos JG, Rushing EJ. MR and CT imaging of 24 pleomorphic xanthoastrocytomas (PXA) and a review of the literature. Neuroradiology. 2007;49(4):307–15.
19. Gamss RP, Slasky SE, Bello JA, Miller TS, Shinnar S. Prevalence of hippocampal malrotation in a population without seizures. Am J Neuroradiol. 2009; 30(8):1571–3.
20. Bekiesińska-Figatowska M. Giant congenital melanocytic nevi: selected aspects of diagnostics and treatment. Med Sci Monit. 2015;21:123–32.

Traumatic Brain Injuries

21

Andrés Felipe Rodríguez

Abstract

Traumatic brain injury is the most common cause of death and disability in young individuals. Contusions and diffuse axonal injuries are the primary brain lesions that are most common in the setting of head trauma. CT and MRI are the most commonly used imaging techniques in patients who suffered brain trauma. CT is the initial modality due to its availability and high sensitivity in detecting injuries which require immediate and life-saving surgical treatment. MRI is the most sensitive modality for detecting imaging diffuse axonal injury and small foci of hemorrhage that may not be seen on CT. Advanced imaging techniques as diffusion-weighted imaging, spectroscopy, and diffusion tensor imaging can provide useful information in the acute setting and prognosis of these patients but with the exception of diffusion-weighted imaging the others are not routinely used or needed.

Background

Traumatic brain injuries are the most common cause of death and disability among young people [1, 2]. Each year they account for an important number of deaths and permanent disabilities. They are most often secondary to a blow or jolt to the head or to penetrating trauma [3].

According the Center for Disease Control (CDC), approximately 1.4 million people suffer from traumatic brain injury every year in the United States. Almost half of the cases are secondary to falls and motor vehicle accidents, and the former are more common in the children and adults aged 65 and older, while the latter is seen among all age groups [1, 3, 4]. The rate among men is almost twice as women, mostly attributed to risk-taking behavior and high-risk jobs [3, 5].

An early indicator of prognosis is the Glasgow Coma Scale (GCS). Depending on its score, traumatic brain injury is classified clinically as mild (GCS 13–15), moderate (GCS 9–12), and severe (GCS 3–8). Additional prognostic factors for poor outcome is age (>60 years), hypotension at admission, as well as pupils that are fixed and

A.F. Rodríguez, MD
Departamento de Radiología, Escuela de Medicina, Pontificia Universidad Javeriana, Calle 140 #6-30, Bogotá, Colombia
e-mail: afr100@gmail.com

R. Hoffmann Nunes et al. (eds.), *Critical Findings in Neuroradiology*,
DOI 10.1007/978-3-319-27987-9_21

dilated [2, 6]. Despite most of the traumatic brain injuries being classified as mild, a considerable number of these patients will have permanent neurologic deficits [1].

Key Points

Etiology

Intra-axial injuries can be classified as contusions and diffuse axonal injuries (DAI) [7]. When an individual suffers a traumatic brain injury, forces exerted on the brain (acceleration, linear translation, rotational and angular acceleration) within the cranial vault result in deformation and distortion of the parenchyma according to the force of the impact, its direction, and tissue resistance [8, 9]. When these forces stress the brain past its structural tolerance, injury results. The primary parenchymal injury involves axons, glial cells, and vascular cells that lead to irreversible damage. These epicenters are secondary to the force applied to a specific area resulting in different grades of damage. Not all brain cells and structures are equally vulnerable. The most vulnerable are the axons and the more resistant are the blood vessels [1, 8, 9]. Surrounding the epicenter of the lesion is the penumbra, an area that contains cells that have sustained reversible damage and where most of the deleterious secondary biochemical changes will occur. Reversible lesions can turn in to irreversible ones, and this is the reason why some of them become apparent only after the initial scan [1, 8]. Necrotic cells release intracellular substances that provoke a secondary injury response. The primary lesion also affects microvessels leading to extravasation of blood and loss of function of those vessels resulting in ischemia [10].

Contusions. Cortical contusions are bruises and/or lacerations of the brain parenchyma secondary to the different acceleration rates between the calvarium and the brain. Contusions occur in coup or contrecoup sites. Coup injuries are located at the same site where the external force was applied and may be associated with dural tears. Contrecoup lesions occur at the opposite site of where the force was applied and usually these lesions are more severe than coup ones [1, 4, 5, 7]. In contrecoup lesions, the relatively denser cerebrospinal fluid (CSF) shifts toward the impact zone, while the brain parenchyma is displaced to the opposite side striking the inner surface of the calvarium [4, 9].

Diffuse axonal injury. DAI typically occurs when the head is subjected to shearing forces due to impact or non-impact trauma. The occurrence, localization, and severity of the lesions are mainly determined by two factors: the direction and magnitude of rotational acceleration and deceleration forces and the differences in density and rigidity between two adjacent tissues. Most lesions occur at the interfaces where the brain has different densities such the gray–white matter junctions [1, 11, 12]. Shearing forces produce axonal stretching and rupture with microvascular damage that leads to multiple hemorrhagic and nonhemorrhagic lesions. There is a cascade of biochemical events that leads to secondary injury in the hours that follow the trauma. Experimental studies have shown delayed cerebral changes characterized by progression of cerebral atrophy [1, 13]. As the severity of the DAI increases, a compromise of deeper structures occurs. Patients with severe DAI usually manifest with coma which are associated with injuries in the brainstem [1, 14].

Best Imaging Modality

Computed Tomography (CT). Not all head trauma requires neuroimaging, and less than 10 % of patients considered to have minor head injuries have positive findings on CT [15, 16]. CT findings can lag behind and the amount and severity of injuries may be underestimated; less than 20 % of all DAIs are macroscopically hemorrhagic and thus obvious on CT [12, 16].

Magnetic Resonance Imaging (MRI). It is seldom performed in the acute phase of traumatic brain injury due to its longer scan time, clinical stability of patients, and inability of many patients to hold still. MRI has a better sensitivity in identifying certain type of acute lesions such as nonhemorrhagic contusions, brainstem injuries, and DAI lesions that are nonhemorrhagic [1].

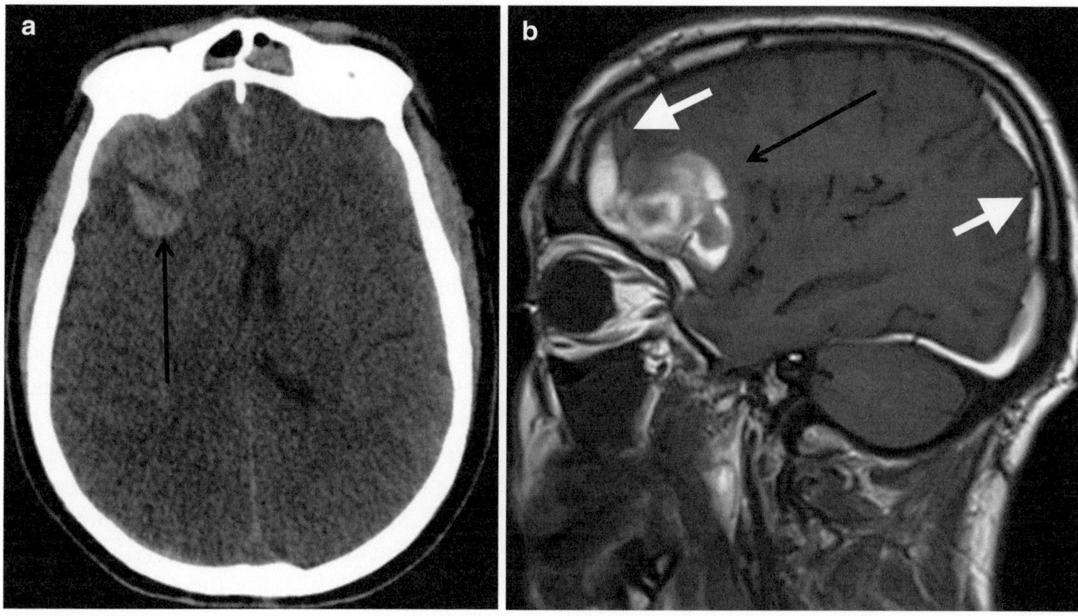

Fig. 21.1 Contusions in a patient with traumatic brain injury. Axial CT (**a**) and sagittal T1WI MRI (**b**) show right frontal hemorrhagic contusion (*black arrows*) with surrounding edema and mild mass effect on the frontal horn of the lateral ventricle. There are frontal and parieto-occipital subdural hematomas (*white arrows* in **b**). The hyperintensity of the lesions in T1WI indicates subacute stage of the blood (methemoglobin)

Gradient-recalled echo (GRE) or susceptibility-weighted image (SWI) sequences should be included since they are very sensitive in the detection of hemosiderin and blood-degrading products.

Diffusion-weighted imaging (DWI) and diffusion tensor imaging (DTI) are widely gaining acceptance for the evaluation of head trauma. DWI in DAI and contusions show restriction of diffusion in areas of acute cell death, and many DAI lesions are easily identified using this technique. Since degree of anisotropy in a white matter region can be viewed as a reflection of the degree of the structural integrity of white matter, DTI may allow detection of damaged white matter which appears normal on conventional anatomic imaging and may help predict prognosis [17]. DTI is, however, not employed in the acute period.

Major Findings

Contusions. Contusions can be focal or multifocal and located in the cortical and subcortical regions depending on the severity of the trauma. They are usually seen in the temporal lobes followed by the frontal lobes especially their basal surfaces. Almost one-half of contusions are hemorrhagic on MRI, but nearly all have associated microscopic hemorrhage. Hemorrhagic contusions can be seen on CT; however, nonhemorrhagic lesions are usually underestimated. MRI has a greater specificity than CT for this type of lesions [1, 4, 5].

Initial CT study may be normal or show small foci of hemorrhage with surrounding edema. These small areas can coalesce to form larger hematomas (Fig. 21.1) [18]. Contusions tend to increase in size in the 72 h that follow the trauma and may develop hemorrhage [1, 4].

MRI findings depend on the age of the lesions as follows: in the acute phase of nonhemorrhagic contusions, T1WI shows the lesions to be isointense, inhomogeneous, and to have mass effect. On FLAIR images and T2WI, the lesions are hyperintense because of vasogenic edema. GRE and SWI improve the detection of small hemorrhagic. Acute nonhemorrhagic contusions may show restriction of diffusion on DWI resulting from cell necrosis.

Hemorrhagic subacute lesions are hyperintense on T1WI and hypointense on T2WI, and as methemoglobin becomes extracellular, they show high signal intensity on T2WI. In the chronic stage due to deposition of hemosiderin, T1WI and T2WI show all previously hemorrhagic lesions to be hypointense (Fig. 21.1) [1, 4, 18].

DAI. These lesions are characterized by punctate hemorrhagic or nonhemorrhagic foci commonly found in the white matter tracts. These lesions tend to be small (1–15 mm), ovoid with their long axis parallel to the white matter tracts. The most common locations for this type of lesions are gray–white matter junctions of the cerebral cortex, the corpus callosum, and the dorsal brainstem. The gray–white matter junction is the most affected especially frontal and temporal lobes; however, it may affect the cerebellum and other parts of the brain. Corpus callosum lesions are more frequent in the splenium which is presumably secondary to its mobility. DAI is graded depending on its location (Table 21.1) [1, 4].

CT is relatively insensitive for the detection of DAI, and punctate hemorrhages resolve quickly becoming indistinguishable from the brain parenchyma, and less than 20 % of them are initially hemorrhagic. Nonhemorrhagic lesions can be seen as small hypodense foci while hemorrhagic lesions as hyperdense foci [5, 12].

MRI is more sensitive than CT because it detects nonhemorrhagic as well as hemorrhagic lesions [5]. In the acute and subacute phases, T1WI and T2WI can be used to readily detect hemorrhagic lesions. FLAIR and T2WI are more sensitive than T1WI for detecting nonhemorrhagic DAI lesions. Edema and axoplasmic leakage in areas of neuronal disruption are conspicuous on FLAIR and T2WI and seen as zones of high signal intensity [7, 12]. GRE and SWI are sensitive in detecting microhemorrhages (Fig. 21.2). DWI is a sensitive sequence in the acute setting, and lesions show hyperintensity associated with decreased ADC values resulting from axonal damage that affects the cell membranes resulting in leakage of glutamate into the extracellular space. Excessive extracellular glutamate leads to axonal swelling and cytotoxic edema of glial cells (Fig. 21.3) [19]. Large DAI lesions have a nearly "fingerlike" configuration. Studies had found that DWI can predict clinical outcome in DAI patients [11].

Diffusion tensor imaging (DTI) may be more sensitive than conventional MRI sequences and provides additional prognostic information. Decreased fractional anisotropy (FA) values had shown to correlate with the injury severity index, patient disability, and posttraumatic amnesia [4, 11].

Contusions can coexist with DAI and sometimes it may be difficult to distinguish between them. Contusions tend to be more superficial, located along gyral crests. DAI is most commonly found in the white matter tracts such as the internal capsule and corpus callosum [18].

Table 21.1 Classification of diffuse axonal injury [1, 4]

Grade	Anatomic location
Grade I	Gray–white matter junction
Grade II	Corpus callosum in addition to grade I locations
Grade III	Brainstem in addition to grade I and II locations

Imaging Follow-Up

Atrophy after traumatic brain injury is common, and its progression is more significant during the first year after the trauma, and the process continues for up to 3 years but at a slower rate. Another delayed consequence of trauma is encephalomalacia which develops at the sites of previous brain contusions. The location of these areas determines the patient's symptoms. Damage to the cerebral cortex may also result in seizures [4, 13]. Ventricular dilation is the most frequent finding after traumatic brain injury and is due to white matter volume loss and is related to cognitive poor outcome. High signal intensity on T2WI is seen in sites of injury secondary to increased water concentration due to axonal loss and gliosis. DTI images show decreased FA values reflecting axonal damage. MR spectroscopy shows decrease NAA/Cr ratios [13].

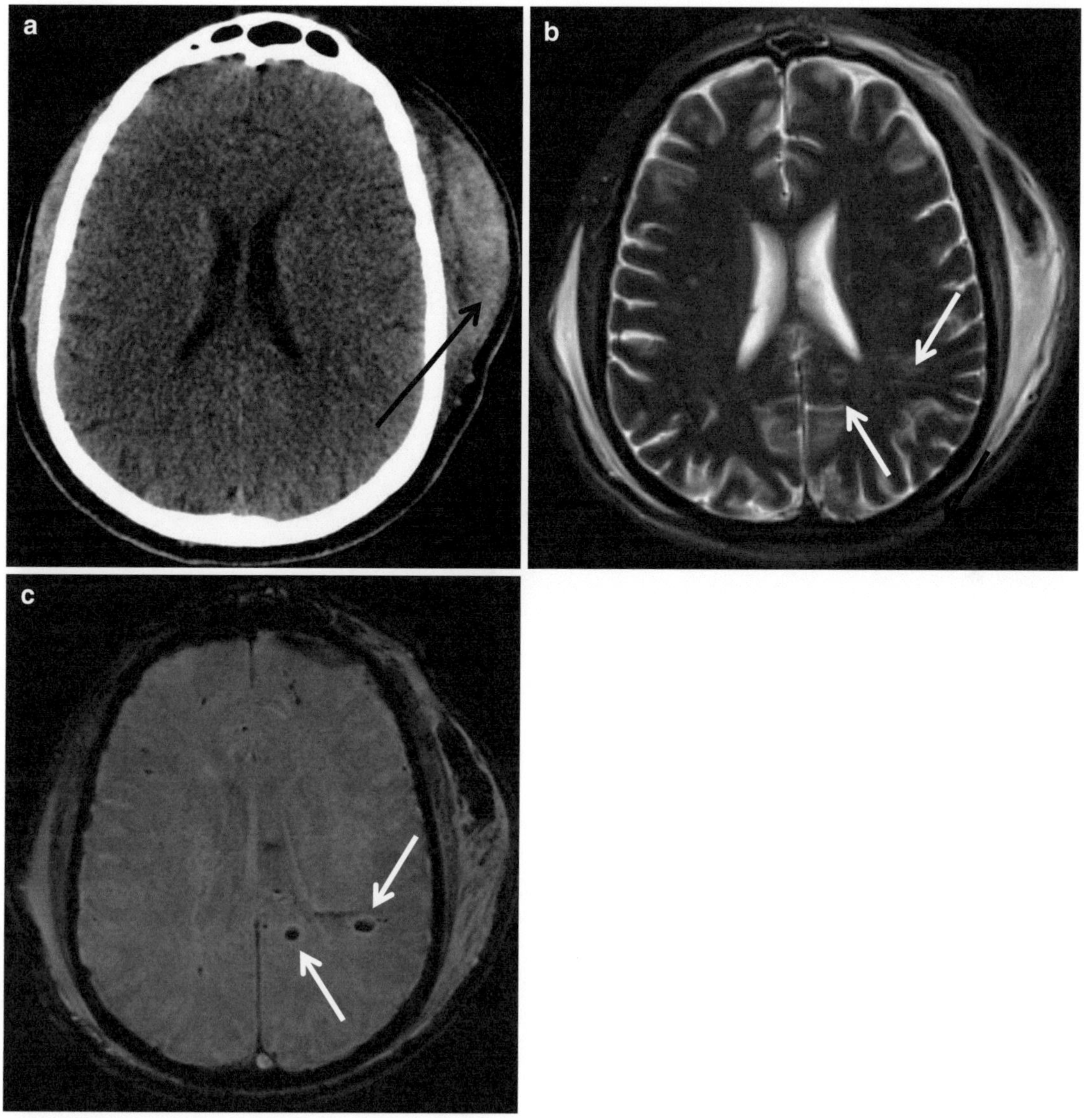

Fig. 21.2 A 47-year-old male involved in motor vehicle accident. (**a**) Axial CT shows a frontotemporal scalp hematoma (*arrow*). There are no intra-axial lesions seen. Axial T2WI (**b**) and SWI (**c**) depict small oval foci of hypointensity with "blooming" effect in SWI on the parietal and frontal lobes and in the splenium of the corpus callosum compatible with DAI (*arrows*)

Main Differential Diagnosis

Multifocal microhemorrhages with blooming on GRE and SWI can be seen in many nontraumatic lesions such as *cerebral amyloid angiopathy* (*CAA*) or *chronic hypertensive encephalopathy* (*CHE*) and should not be mistaken with DAI (Table 21.2) [18, 20].

> **Tips**
> - In head trauma, CT is the initial imaging procedure; however, MRI is more sensitive for the characterization of intraparenchymal lesions.

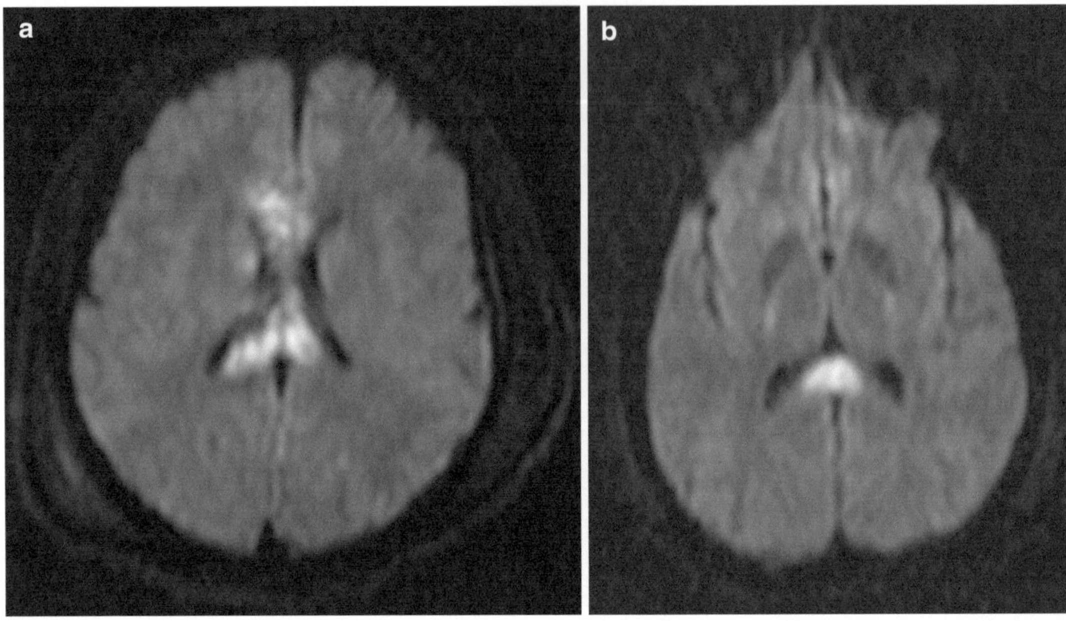

Fig. 21.3 DAI involving the corpus callosum. DWI shows extensive areas of high signal intensity (restricted diffusion on ADC, not shown) in the corpus callosum secondary to DAI

Table 21.2 Different patterns of microhemorrhages in the brain

	DAI	CAA	CHE
Clinical	Transient loss of consciousness Immediate coma	Dementia in elderly patient No history of hypertension	Sudden sensorimotor deficit
Pathophysiology	Rotational acceleration of the head Shearing injury	Deposition of beta amyloid protein in small to medium vessels	Chronic arterial hypertension
Age	15–24 years	>60 years	>50 years
Location of lesions	Gray–white matter interface Corpus callosum Brainstem	Posterior and subcortical (gray–white junction) Lobar hemorrhages	Striatocapsular Thalamus Pons/cerebellum

- Remember that contusions tend to occur in frontal lobe poles, orbital surfaces of the frontal lobes, anterior temporal lobes, and the temporal lobes above the petrous bones. For DAI, look for lesions in gray–white matter interfaces, corpus callosum, and brainstem.
- Check the brain opposite to scalp hematomas and/or skull fractures for contrecoup injuries.
- GRE and SWI images are very useful to detect microhemorrhages that cannot be easily detected in CT.

- In elderly patients with history of trauma and microhemorrhages, remember that cerebral amyloid angiopathy and chronic hypertensive encephalopathy can appear similar to those produced by trauma.

References

1. Bodanapally UK, Sours C, Jiachen Zhuo KS. Imaging of traumatic brain injury. Radiol Clin N Am [Internet]. 2015;53(4):695–71. Elsevier Inc.
2. Ghajar J. Traumatic brain injury. Lancet. 2000; 356(9233):923–9.

3. Faul M, Xu L, Wald MMCV. Traumatic brain injury in the United States: emergency department visits, hospitalizations, and deaths. Atlanta: Centers for Disease Control and Prevention, National Center for Injury Prevention and Control; 2010.
4. Hijaz T a, Cento E a, Walker MT. Imaging of head trauma. Radiol Clin N Am. 2011;49(1):81–103. Elsevier Ltd.
5. Kubal WS. Updated imaging of traumatic brain injury. Radiol Clin N Am. 2012;50(1):15–41. Elsevier Inc.
6. Chesnut RM, Marshall LF, Klauber MR, Blunt BA, Baldwin N, Eisenberg HM, et al. The role of secondary brain injury in determining outcome from severe head injury. J Trauma. 1993;34(2): 216–22.
7. Provenzale J. CT and MR imaging of acute cranial trauma. Emerg Radiol. 2007;14(1):1–12.
8. Besenski N. Traumatic injuries: imaging of head injuries. Eur Radiol. 2002;12(6):1237–52.
9. Drew LB, Drew WE. New perspectives in brain injury the contrecoup–coup phenomenon: a new understanding of the mechanism of closed head injury. Neurocrit Care. 2004;1:385–90.
10. Kurland D, Hong C, Aarabi B, Gerzanich V, Simard JM. Hemorrhagic progression of a contusion after traumatic brain injury: a review. J Neurotrauma. 2012;29(1):19–31.
11. Li X-Y, Feng D-F. Diffuse axonal injury: novel insights into detection and treatment. J Clin Neurosci. 2009;16(5):614–9. Elsevier Ltd.
12. Parizel PM, Özsarlak Ö, Van Goethem JW, Van Den Hauwe L, Dillen C, Verlooy J, et al. Imaging findings in diffuse axonal injury after closed head trauma. Eur Radiol. 1998;965:960–5.
13. Mamere a E, Saraiva L a L, Matos a LM, Carneiro a a O, Santos a C, Evaluation of delayed neuronal and axonal damage secondary to moderate and severe traumatic brain injury using quantitative MR imaging techniques. AJNR Am J Neuroradiol. 2009;30(5):947–52.
14. Smith DH, Meaney DF, Shull WH. Diffuse axonal injury in head trauma. J Head Trauma Rehabil. 2003;18(4):307–16.
15. Saboori M, Ahmadi J, Farajzadegan Z. Indications for brain CT scan in patients with minor head injury. Clin Neurol Neurosurg. 2007;109(5):399–405.
16. Lee B, Newberg A. Neuroimaging in traumatic brain imaging. NeuroRx. 2005;2(2):372–83.
17. Provenzale JM. Imaging of traumatic brain injury: a review of the recent medical literature. Am J Roentgenol. 2010;194(1):16–9.
18. Osborn AG. Osborn's brain: imaging, pathology, and anatomy. 1st ed. Salt Lake City: Amirsys; 2013. 1272 p.
19. Moritani T, Smoker WRK, Sato Y, Numaguchi Y, Westesson P-L. Diffusion-weighted imaging of acute excitotoxic brain injury. AJNR Am J Neuroradiol. 2005;26(2):216–28.
20. Lang EW, Ren Ya Z, Preul C, Hugo HH, Hempelmann RG, Buhl R, et al. Stroke pattern interpretation: the variability of hypertensive versus amyloid angiopathy hemorrhage. Cerebrovasc Dis. 2001;12(2):121–30.

Epidural Hematoma

22

Mauricio Enrique Moreno and Florencia Álamos

Abstract

Epidural hematoma represents bleeding between the dura and the skull. It accounts for 1–4 % of traumatic head injuries. Typically, epidural hematomas have high-attenuation, are biconvex, and are extra-axial blood collections on CT. The margins of the hematoma are anchored at the sutures and they can cross the midline at the vertex. Careful examination of a CT study with bone windows allows identification of a skull fractures in 90 % or more of adults with an epidural hematomas.

22.1 Background

An epidural hematoma (EDH) is due to bleeding between the dura and the skull [1]. Its exact incidence is unknown, but it is found in 1–4 % of traumatic head injuries and in 5–15 % of autopsies [2, 3]. The mean age of patients with EDH is between 20 and 30 years [3].

About one-third of patients present with immediate loss of consciousness caused by concussion and then a lucid interval followed by a relapse into coma with hemiplegia as the EDH expands. The ipsilateral pupil loses reactivity to light because the third cranial nerve is stretched as the midbrain is displaced contralaterally. The pupil then becomes fixed and dilated as the third nerve is compressed by the hippocampal gyrus as it herniates over the free edge of the tentorium [2].

The mortality rate approaches 100 % in untreated patients and ranges from 5 % to 30 % in treated patients. As the interval between injury and the surgical intervention decreases, survival improves. If there is little coexisting brain damage, functional recovery may be excellent [2].

Posterior fossa EDH has an incidence of 4–7 % [4]. It usually is the result of a dural venous sinus injury [5]. Posterior fossa EDHs are generally clinically silent, and when symptoms occur, they are generally nonspecific and thus they are difficult to diagnose. Unless adequate management is prompt, sudden clinical deterioration can be expected in

M.E. Moreno, MD (✉)
Departamento de Radiología, Fundación Santa Fe de Bogotá – Hospital Universitario, Calle 119 No. 7 – 75, Bogotá, Colombia
e-mail: mmorenomejia@hotmail.com

F. Álamos, MD, PhD
Department of Neuroscience, School of Medicine, Universidad Católica de Chile,
Luz Larrain, 3946 Lo Barnechea, Santiago, Chile
e-mail: flopi1987@yahoo.com

R. Hoffmann Nunes et al. (eds.), *Critical Findings in Neuroradiology*,
DOI 10.1007/978-3-319-27987-9_22

most patients [6]. Risk factors in patients with posterior fossa EDHs include pediatric age group, supratentorial extension of the hematoma, major venous sinus tear, low admission Glasgow Coma Score and additional intracranial pathology [6].

22.2 Key Points

22.2.1 Etiology

EDH can be divided in two main groups according to their etiology:

Traumatic: Traffic-related accidents, falls, and assaults account for 53 % of EDH in adults. Most (70–90 %) traumatic EDHs are associated with skull fractures and bleeding from lacerated arteries [1]. The most common location of EDH is temporal. Because the squamosal portion of the temporal bone is thinner than the rest of the skull, it fractures easily often resulting in laceration of the middle meningeal artery [2, 3].

Other causes of EDH include rupture of the middle meningeal vein, diploic veins, or venous sinuses [1].

Posterior fossa EDHs generally are of venous origin (85 %) and are the result of injuries to the transverse or sigmoid sinuses secondary to occipital bone fractures [4, 7, 8].

Nontraumatic: EDHs from a nontraumatic origin are rare. Possible causes include infections (e.g., epidural abscesses), coagulopathy, congenital anomalies, vascular malformations of the dura, hemorrhagic tumors, and complications of neurosurgical procedures. Pregnancy, sickle cell disease, systemic lupus erythematosus, and patients receiving hemodialysis are predisposing conditions [9–14].

22.2.2 Best Imaging Modality

Computed tomography (*CT*): CT is the most widely used imaging method owing to its widespread availability, rapidity of scanning, and compatibility with other medical and life support devices [15]. It has high sensitivity to depict EDH. Early and sometimes repeated CT scanning may be required in cases of clinical neurological deterioration especially in the first 72 h to detect delayed/expanding hematoma and/or associated traumatic brain lesions [15].

Head CT is not conclusive in 8 % of cases possibly due to severe anemia, early scanning (before blood has had time to accumulate), and severe hypotension [16].

Some authors recommend urgent CT scanning in all patients with a suspected fracture of the occipital bone with or without occipital soft tissue swelling to exclude a posterior fossa EDHs [6]. In this situation, imaging findings always occur earlier than clinical changes.

Magnetic resonance imaging (*MRI*): MRI has high sensitivity for the detection of intracranial hemorrhage and is especially useful in the diagnosis of EDH at the vertex [17, 18]. MRI is indicated in situations in which there is a strong clinical suspicion but no evidence of EDH on head CT [16]. Fluid-attenuated inversion recovery (FLAIR) sequence is helpful for imaging small or subacute extra-axial hemorrhages [15]. Gradient-recalled echo (GRE) and susceptibility-weighted image (SWI) sequences are useful in demonstrating small amount of blood even though they are less sensitive in small extra-axial hemorrhages. MRI is less sensitive than CT for the identification of associated skull fractures [19]. Despite this, MRI is not the first line of imaging in patients suspected of harboring EDH; many patients are not stable enough to support the time needed for this examination.

Catheter angiography: It is rarely necessary but may be used to evaluate an underlying vascular lesion such as a dural arteriovenous fistula from the middle meningeal artery which rarely may result in an EDH [20].

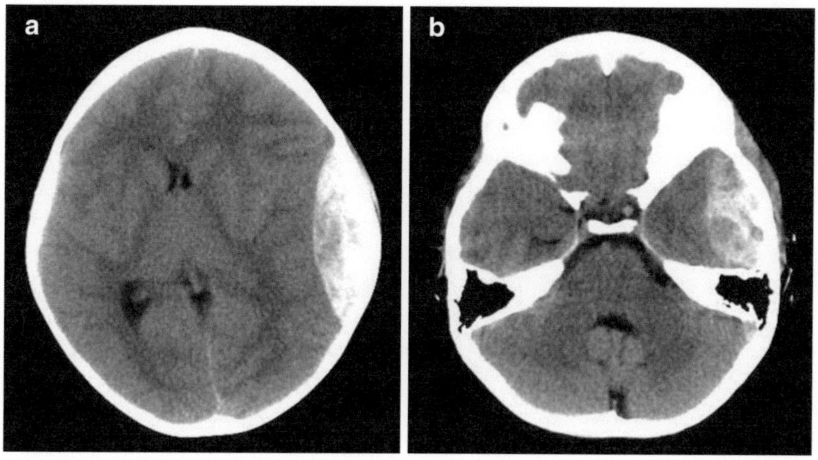

Fig. 22.1 Acute EDH in a 10-year-old boy with history of trauma. Non-contrast head CT at different levels (**a**, **b**) shows a typical high-density, biconvex extra-axial collection in the left temporal region. This hematoma produces mass effect in the adjacent brain parenchyma and shift of the middle line to the right side. This collection is limited anteriorly by the coronal suture

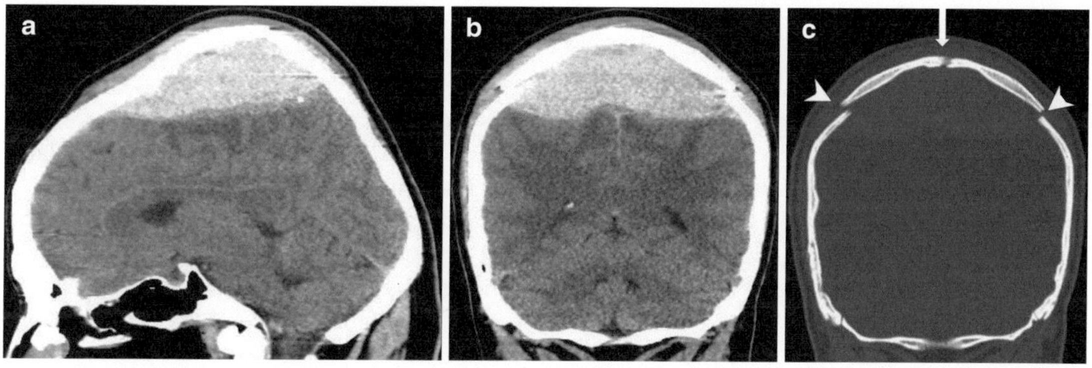

Fig. 22.2 Vertex epidural hematoma. Sagittal (**a**) and coronal (**b**) non-contrast head CT in soft tissue and bone window (**c**) settings. Images show a large EDH at the vertex resulting in significant mass effect on the parietal and frontal lobes. There are bilateral parietal fractures (*arrowheads*) and probable diastasis of the sagittal suture (*arrow*) in (**c**)

22.2.3 Major Findings

- High-attenuation, biconvex, and extra-axial collection in CT (Fig. 22.1). The margins of the hematoma are limited by the bony sutures, and they can cross the midline at the vertex (so-called vertex hematomas which may be difficult to see with axial CT and may necessitate coronal reformations to identify them) (Fig. 22.2).
- EDH may have a heterogeneous appearance, which is a sign of active bleeding. [19]. The low attenuation within the collection represents hyperacute, unclotted blood and is known as the "swirl sign" (Fig. 22.3).
- EDH may cause mass effect and brain herniation (Figs. 22.1 and 22.2).
- Careful examination of the CT at bone windows allows identification of a skull fracture in 90 % or more of adults with an EDH (Fig. 22.4) [21].

- MRI appearance of EDH evolves over time. In hyperacute phase, the clot presents with high signal in T2-weighted images (T2WI) (oxyhemoglobin) followed by low T2 signal (deoxyhemoglobin). Over subsequent weeks, it shows high signal in both T1-weighted images (T1WI) and T2WI secondary to methemoglobin content [22].
- Patients with posterior fossa EDHs can deteriorate rapidly and also develop early obstructive hydrocephalus visible on the CT in 30 % of such patients (Figs. 22.3 and 22.5).

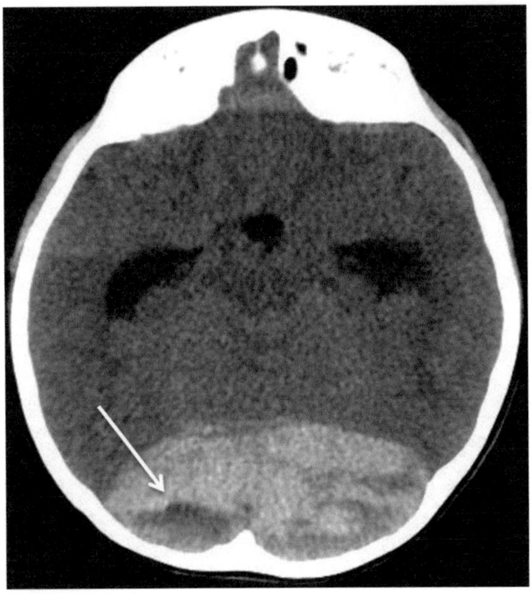

Fig. 22.3 "Swirl sign" in a posterior fossa EDH. A 7-year-old boy with history of trauma. Non-contrast CT shows a heterogeneous high-density extra-axial collection. The area of decreased density (*arrow*) within the collection likely represents unclotted blood from active bleeding ("swirl sign"). There is considerable mass effect in the cerebellar hemispheres with secondary dilatation of the ventricular system

22.2.4 Imaging Follow-Up

Repeat CT scanning may be required in cases of clinical or neurologic deterioration. MRI is indicated in acute head injured patients with suspicions of intra axial lesions.

22.2.5 Main Differential Diagnosis

Subdural hematoma (*SDH*): It is caused by rupture of the bridging veins located within the subdural space. SDH appear as a crescent-shaped extra-axial lesion [19]. Unlike EDHs, SDHs can cross sutural margins, but they do not cross the midline. They can also form along dural reflections such as the falx and the tentorium.

Subarachnoid hemorrhage (*SAH*): Traumatic SAH is usually the result of injury to the small cortical veins passing through the subarachnoid space. Large amounts of SAH may be secondary to extension of intraparenchymal hematoma that dissects into the subarachnoid space [19]. Post-traumatic SAH has a peripheral distribution,

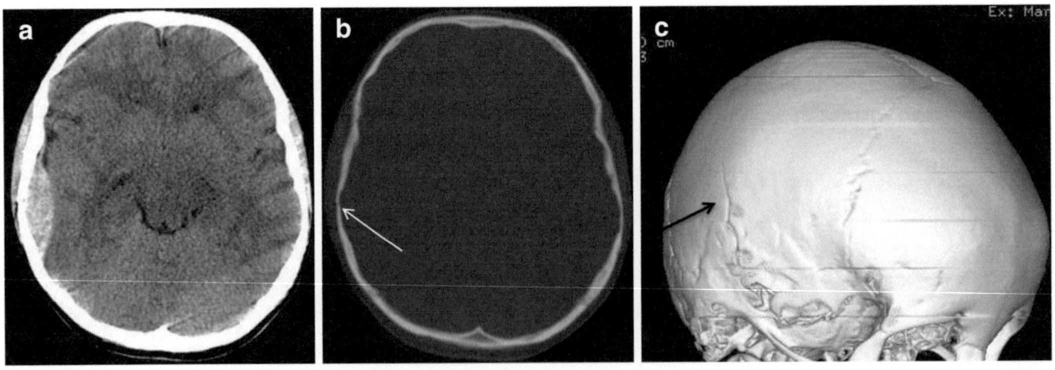

Fig. 22.4 EDH with skull fracture. Axial non-contrast CT in soft tissue (**a**) and bone (**b**) windows show a right middle fossa EDH with compression of the right temporal lobe and a non-displaced linear fracture in the squamosal portion of the bone (*white arrow*). 3D CT reformation of the skull (**c**) shows the right temporal bone fracture (*arrow*)

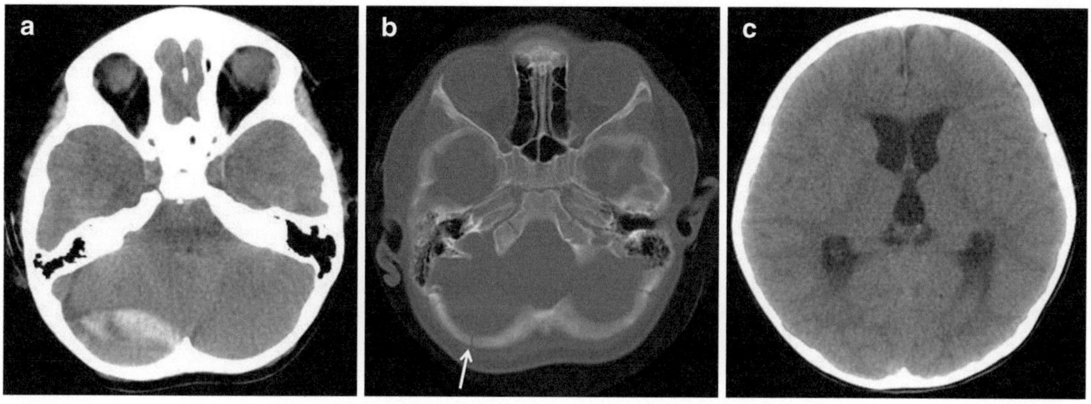

Fig. 22.5 Posterior fossa EDH. Axial non-contrast head CT in soft tissue (**a**) and bone (**b**) windows depict a right posterior fossa EDH with heterogeneous density ("swirl sign"). A fracture in the *right* side (*arrow*) is seen. Axial head CT (**c**), soft tissue window, at more cephalad level shows prominent third ventricle and laterals ventricles secondary to obstructive hydrocephalus

seen as high attenuation conforming to the sulcal spaces. An important clue to differentiate EDH from SAH is that SAH does not cause the significant mass effect that an EDH does.

Tips

- Look for findings that suggest an EDH emergent evacuation:
  - Clot thickness >15 mm.
  - Active bleeding: heterogeneous foci of lower attenuation appear within EDH ("swirl sign").
  - Midline shift >5 mm.
  - Hydrocephalus especially of the opposite lateral ventricle due to occlusion of the foramen of Monro.
- Describe mass effect on the underlying brain (e.g., effacement of ventricles and sulci) and if it is associated with herniation and the type of herniation.

References

1. Daroff RB, Bradley WG. Bradley's neurology in clinical practice. Philadelphia: Elsevier/Saunders; 2012. p. 942–56.
2. Mayer S, Rowland L. Merritt's neurology. Philadelphia: Lippincott Williams & Wilkins; 2012. p. 479–94.
3. Bullock MR, Chesnut R, Ghajar J, et al. Surgical management of acute epidural hematomas. Neurosurgery. 2006;58:S7.
4. Roka YB, Kumar P, Sharma GR, Adhikari P. Traumatic posterior fossa extradural hematoma. JNMA: J Nepal Med Assoc. 2008;47:174–8.
5. Lui T, Lee S, Chang C. Epidural hematomas in the posterior cranial fossa. J Trauma. 1993;34:211–5.
6. Karasu A, Sabanci PA, Izgi N, Imer M, Sencer A, Cansever T, et al. Traumatic epidural hematomas of the posterior cranial fossa. Surg Neurol. 2008;69(3): 247–51.
7. Kawakami Y, Tamiya T, Tanimoto T, Shimamura Y, Hattori S, Ueda T, et al. Nonsurgical treatment of posterior fossa epidural hematoma. Paediatr Neurol. 1990;6:112–8.
8. Bullock MR, Chesnut R, Ghajar J. Surgical management of traumatic brain injury author group: surgical management of posterior fossa mass lesions. Neurosurgery. 2006;58(3 Suppl):47–55.
9. Moonis G, Granados A, Simon SL. Epidural hematoma as a complication of sphenoid sinusitis and epidural abscess: a case report and literature review. Clin Imaging. 2002;26:382.
10. McIver JI, Scheithauer BW, Rydberg CH, Atkinson JL. Metastatic hepatocellular carcinoma presenting as epidural hematoma: case report. Neurosurgery. 2001;49:447.
11. Ng WH, Yeo TT, Seow WT. Non-traumatic spontaneous acute epidural haematoma – report of two cases and review of the literature. J Clin Neurosci. 2004;11(7):791–4.
12. Naran AD, Fontana L. Sickle cell disease with orbital infarction and epidural hematoma. Pediatr Radiol. 2001;31:257.
13. Martínez-Lage JF, Saez V, Requena L, Martínez-Barba E, Poza M. Cranial epidural hematoma in Paget's disease of the bone. Intensive Care Med. 2000;26:1582.

14. Shahlaie K, Fox A, Butani L, Boggan JE. Spontaneous epidural hemorrhage in chronic renal failure. A case report and review. Pediatr Nephrol. 2004;19:1168.
15. American College of Radiology. ACR appropriateness criteria® Clinical condition: head trauma. Reston: American College of Radiology; 2014. Available from: https://acsearch.acr.org/docs/69481/Narrative/. Accessed 20 Nov 2014.
16. Ferri F. Ferri's clinical advisor 2015: 5 books in 1. Philadelphia: Mosby; 2014. p. 428–9.
17. Gentry LR, Godersky JC, Thompson B, Dunn VD. Prospective comparative study of intermediate-field MR and CT in the evaluation of closed head trauma. AJR Am J Roentgenol. 1988;150:673.
18. Miller DJ, Steinmetz M, McCutcheon IE. Vertex epidural hematoma: surgical versus conservative management: two case reports and review of the literature. Neurosurgery. 1999;45:621.
19. Kubal WS. Updated imaging of traumatic brain injury. Radiol Clin North Am. 2012;50(1):15–41.
20. Matsumoto K, Akagi K, Abekura M, Tasaki O. Vertex epidural hematoma associated with traumatic arteriovenous fistula of the middle meningeal artery: a case report. Surg Neurol. 2001;55:302.
21. Zimmerman RA, Bilaniuk LT. Computed tomographic staging of traumatic epidural bleeding. Radiology. 1982;144:809–12.
22. Victor M, Ropper A. Adams and Victor's principles of neurology. 7th ed. New York: McGraw-Hill; 2001. p. 925.

Subdural Hematoma

23

Mauricio Enrique Moreno and Florencia Álamos

Abstract

Subdural hematoma results from bleeding between the dura and the arachnoid membranes. Most cases of subdural hematoma are secondary to tearing of the bridging veins that drain blood from the surface of the brain to the dural sinuses. Head trauma is the most common cause of subdural hematoma. Brain CT is the most widely used imaging study for acute head trauma owing to its speed, accuracy, and widespread availability. Acute subdural hematoma is visualized on CT as a high-density crescentic collection across the hemispheric convexity. Head CT findings that correlate with poor outcome in subdural hematoma include hematoma thickness, the presence and/or degree of midline brain shift, and reduced patency of the basal cisterns.

Background

A subdural hematoma (SDH) usually arises from a venous source, with blood filling the potential space between the dural and arachnoid membranes. Incidence of SDH is estimated to be 11 % of all patients with traumatic brain injury (TBI) [1]. The most common injuries leading to SDH are motor vehicle collisions in the younger population and falls in those older than 75 years [2]. Elderly or alcoholic patients with cerebral atrophy are prone to subdural bleeding. In these patients, large hematomas may result from trivial impacts or even from acceleration–deceleration injuries, such as whiplash. Coagulopathy, including the use of oral anticoagulants, is another important risk factor and is associated with increased mortality [3].

A SDH can be acute or become chronic. Acute SDH is diagnosed within 14 days of TBI [2]. Patients become symptomatic within 72 h of injury, but most patients have neurological symptoms from the moment of impact [3]. Half of all patients with an acute SDH lose consciousness at

M.E. Moreno, MD (✉)
Departamento de Radiología, Fundación Santa Fe de Bogotá – Hospital Universitario, Calle 119 No. 7 – 75, Bogotá, Colombia
e-mail: mmorenomejia@hotmail.com

F. Álamos, MD, PhD
Department of Neuroscience, School of Medicine, Universidad Católica de Chile, Luz larrain, 3946 Lo Barnechea, Santiago, Chile
e-mail: flopi1987@yahoo.com

R. Hoffmann Nunes et al. (eds.), *Critical Findings in Neuroradiology*,
DOI 10.1007/978-3-319-27987-9_23

the time of injury, and 25 % are in coma when they arrive at the hospital. However, approximately 12–38 % of patients have a transient "lucid interval" after the acute injury that is followed by a progressive neurologic decline to coma [4, 5]. Ipsilateral pupillary dilation and contralateral hemiparesis are the most common focal neurologic signs [3].

Chronic SDH contains blood older than 14 days or blood of different ages [2]. Patients generally become symptomatic after 21 days. They are more likely to occur in patients after age 50 years. In 25–50 % of cases, there is no recognized head injury [3]. Global deficits such as disturbances of consciousness are more common than focal deficits after SDH [6]. Other clinical manifestations are insidious onset of headaches, light-headedness, cognitive impairment, apathy, somnolence, and occasionally seizures [7].

Symptomatic acute and chronic SDHs with significant mass effect should be evacuated. Outcome after surgical evacuation depends primarily on the severity of the initial deficit and the interval from injury to surgery [3]. Mortality among patients who arrive at the hospital in a coma and undergo surgical evacuation is between 57 and 68 % [2].

Key Points

Etiology

In most cases, the bleeding is caused by displacement of the brain from the skull leading to stretching and tearing of "bridging" veins that drain blood from the surface of the brain to the dural sinuses [3]. Arterial rupture can also result in SDH, and this source accounts for approximately 20–30 % of SDH cases [8, 9]. Most SDHs are located over the lateral cerebral convexities, but subdural blood may also collect along the medial surface of the hemisphere, between the tentorium and occipital lobes, between the temporal lobe and the base of the skull, or in the posterior fossa [2].

Best Imaging Modality

Computed tomography (CT): CT is the first choice of examination in the acute phase after head injury and provides essential diagnostic information with therapeutic implications. Its advantages include the availability to estimate hemorrhage location and mass effect and evaluate ventricular size and configuration. Early and sometimes repeated CT scanning may be required in cases of clinical or neurological deterioration, especially in the first 72 h after head injury, to detect delayed SDH [10].

Brain CT is also a helpful tool to evaluate SDHs in different ages. In cases of subacute isodense hematoma, contrast enhancement of its membranes can improve its visualization on CT [11].

Computer-generated reformatted images are useful in the setting of hemorrhage along bone surfaces, which approximate the transverse plane of axial images.

Magnetic resonance imaging (MRI): MRI is more sensitive than CT for detection of small, isodense, tentorial, and interhemispheric SDHs. MRI is used for situations in which there is suspicion for SDH or other intracranial hemorrhage, but no clear evidence of hematoma by CT. MRI can diagnose SDHs of varying age by showing blood in different oxidation states which may be important in cases of child abuse.

MRI of head trauma is hindered by its limited availability in the acute trauma setting, long imaging times, sensitivity to patient motion, and incompatibility with various medical and life support devices.

Catheter angiography: Under some unusual conditions, noninvasive angiography (magnetic resonance angiography or computed tomography angiography) or even catheter cerebral angiography may be indicated for evaluation of SDH, particularly when there is no history of trauma and no obvious cause (e.g., intracranial aneurysmal rupture may occasionally produce SDH) [12].

Major Findings

Acute SDH is readily visualized on head CT as a uniform high-density crescentic collection across the hemispheric convexity (Fig. 23.1). It can cross bony suture but not the midline.

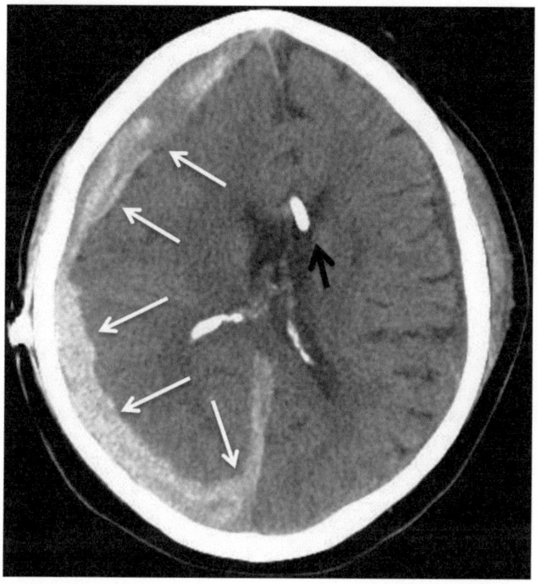

Fig. 23.1 Hemispheric acute SDH. Axial CT image showing an acute right hemispheric SDH caused by blunt head trauma in a 76-year-old patient. Note the typical crescentic configuration (*white arrows*). Also is seen midline shift and the tip of ventriculostomy catheter (*black arrow*)

Subacute and chronic SDHs appear as isodense or hypodense crescent-shaped lesions that deform the surface of the brain (Fig. 23.2). Isodense SDHs may be more difficult to visualize on CT; look for the inward buckling of the gray–white interface and effacement of the cerebral sulci (Fig. 23.2).

Acute blood is hypointense on T2-weighted images (T2WI) due to the presence of deoxyhemoglobin. Over subsequent weeks, deoxyhemoglobin degrades to extracellular methemoglobin, which appears bright on both T1-weighted images (TIWI) and T2WI (Fig. 23.3).

Chronic subdural hematomas can have a complex appearance. Frequently they have septations and fluid levels (Figs. 23.3 and 23.4).

Imaging Follow-Up

The first follow-up head CT scan should be obtained within 6–8 h of the initial scan for patients with acute traumatic SDH who are managed nonoperatively [13]. This is done to access any unexpected growth especially in patients that cannot be adequately clinically examined.

Furthermore, serial follow-up head CT should be obtained during the first 36 h after injury, as there is a high incidence of clot expansion during

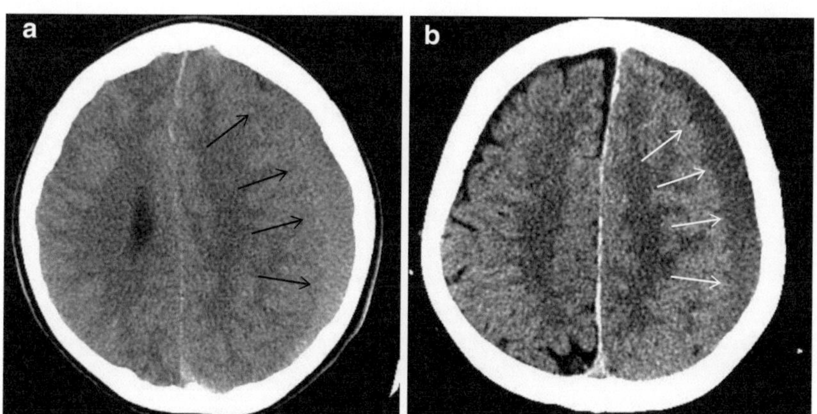

Fig. 23.2 Subacute and chronic subdural hematomas. (**a**) Axial CT showing a left frontoparietal subacute SDH isodense to brain (*arrows*). (**b**) Axial CT in another patient shows a chronic SDH hypodense to brain (*arrows*). These collections deform the surface of the brain and produce sulci effacement more prominent in (**a**)

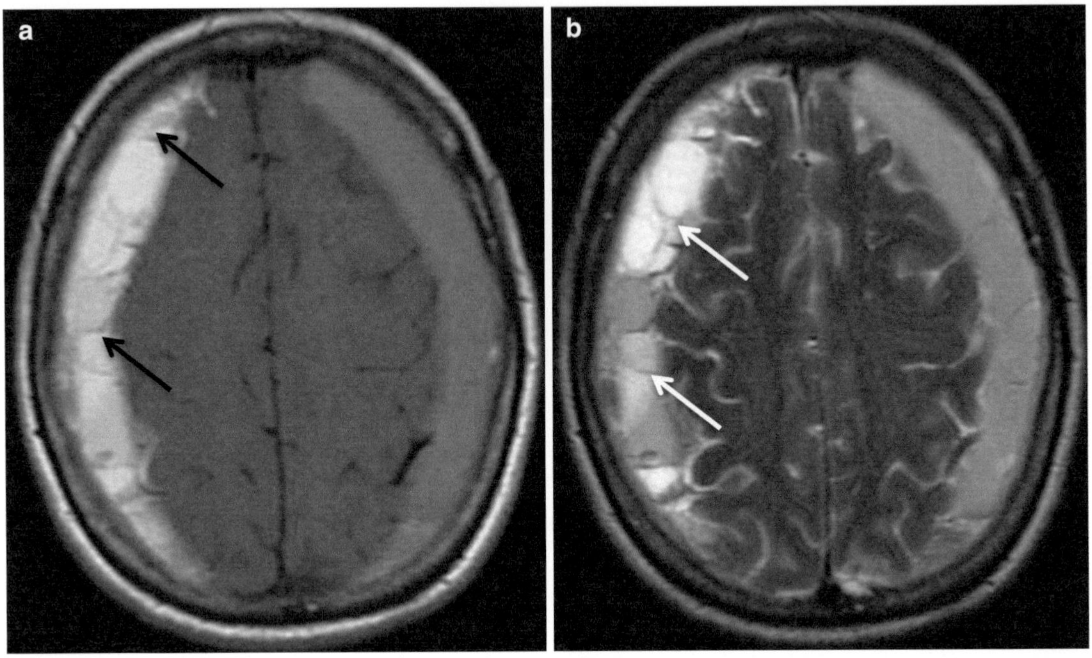

Fig. 23.3 Late subacute SDH. (**a**) Axial T1WI and (**b**) T2WI show bilateral hemispheric SDH with high signal in both images, in the right side brighter than in the left side indicating more antique hematoma in the former. Note septa and complex internal appearance in the right-sided SDH (*arrows* in **a** and **b**)

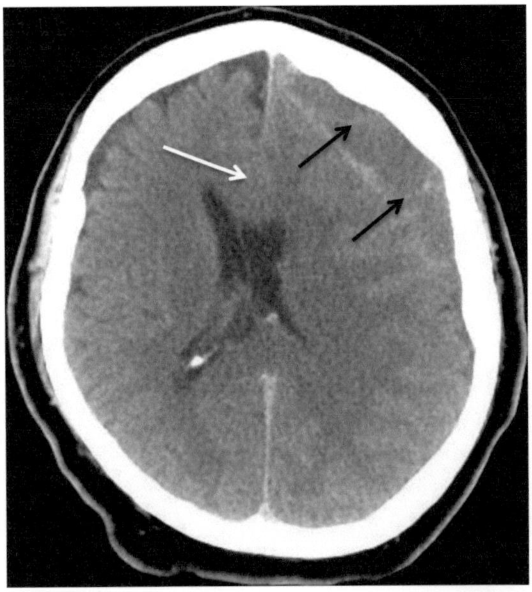

Fig. 23.4 A 68-year-old man with headache. Axial CT image showing subacute on chronic *left* frontal subdural hematoma. Note the septations (*black arrows*) and the varying densities within the collection. There is subfalcine herniation associated (*white arrow*)

this interval [14, 15]. Swelling of underlying brain with progressive midline shift may also occur.

Main Differential Diagnosis

Epidural hematoma (*EDH*): Epidural hematomas arise in the potential space between the dura and the skull. Typically their appearance in CT is a hyperdense extra-axial fluid collection, lens-shaped, that does not cross calvarial sutures but can cross the midline. SDH can cross bony sutures but not the midline. (See previous chapter.)

Subdural hygroma: Similar to a SDH, a hygroma is crescentic shape and results in mass effect. However, it is of low density, similar to that of normal cerebrospinal fluid. It is due to extravasation of non-bloody fluid into the subdural space. Most are post-traumatic in etiology.

Subarachnoid hemorrhage (*SAH*): Trauma is the most common cause of subarachnoid hemorrhage. Traumatic SAH most often occurs in

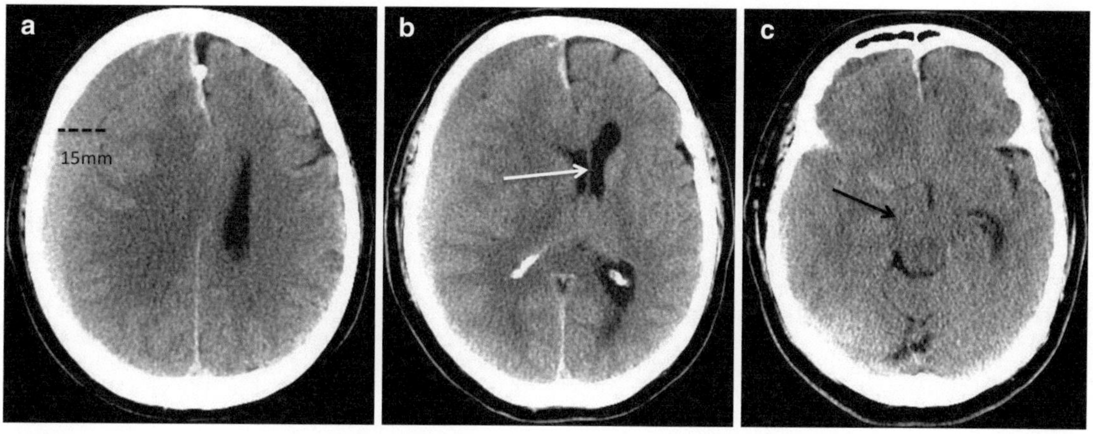

Fig. 23.5 Right subacute SDH. Axial CT at different levels shows right SDH and findings that indicate surgery. (**a**) Clot thickness >15 mm, (**b**) midline shift >5 mm, in this case associated to subfalcine herniation (*arrow*), and (**c**) compression of the ambiens cistern and right uncal herniation (*arrow*)

superficial cerebral sulci near calvarial fractures or cerebral contusions. In the acute and subacute phases, CT shows hyperattenuation in sulci and basal cisterns and occasionally also in portions of the ventricular system. Differentiation of SAH from subdural hematoma (SDH) can be difficult in specific locations, particularly along the tentorium cerebelli. A useful tip to differentiate SAH from SDH is extension of the blood into the cerebral sulci in case of SAH.

Tips

- The majority of SDH requiring surgery are complicated by associated intracranial and/or extracranial injuries. Concurrent brain lesions such as contusions, edema, subarachnoid hemorrhage, and epidural hematoma should be looked for.
- Hematoma expansion may be even more likely when the patient presents with additional intracranial injuries.
- Several studies have identified head CT findings that correlate with poor outcome after SDH, including the following: hematoma thickness > 10 mm, midline brain shift >5 mm, and reduced patency of the basal cisterns (Fig. 23.5) [1, 16].
- Hematoma thickness >10 mm and midline brain shift >5 mm are considered as indications for surgery.

References

1. Servadei F, Nasi MT, Giuliani G, et al. CT prognostic factors in acute subdural haematomas: the value of the "worst" CT scan. Br J Neurosurg. 2000;14:110–6.
2. Daroff RB, Bradley WG. Bradley's neurology in clinical practice. Philadelphia: Elsevier/Saunders; 2012. p. 942–56.
3. Mayer S, Rowland L. Merritt's neurology. Philadelphia: Lippincott Williams & Wilkins; 2012. p. 479–94.
4. Victor M, Ropper A. Craniocerebral trauma. In: Victor M, Ropper A, editors. Adams and Victor's principles of neurology. 7th ed. New York: McGraw-Hill; 2001. p. 925.
5. Bullock MR, Chesnut R, Ghajar J, et al. Surgical management of acute subdural hematomas. Neurosurgery. 2006;58(3 Suppl):S16.
6. Schulz U, Malhotra A, Rothwell P. Oxford case histories in TIA and stroke. New York: Oxford University Press; 2012. p. 256–7.

7. Williamson MA, Snyder LM. Wallach's interpretation of diagnostic tests: pathways to arriving at a clinical diagnosis. Philadelphia: Lippincott Williams & Wilkins; 2014.
8. Gennarelli TA, Thibault LE. Biomechanics of acute subdural hematoma. J Trauma. 1982;22(8):680.
9. Maxeiner H, Wolff M. Pure subdural hematomas: a postmortem analysis of their form and bleeding points. Neurosurgery. 2002;50(3):503.
10. Stein SC, Spettell C, Young G, et al. Delayed and progressive brain injury in closed-head trauma: radiological demonstration. Neurosurgery. 1993;32(1): 25–30; discussion 30–21.
11. Kubal WS. Updated imaging of traumatic brain injury. Radiol Clin N Am. 2012;50(1):15–41.
12. Koerbel A, Ernemann U, Freudenstein D. Acute subdural haematoma without subarachnoid haemorrhage caused by rupture of an internal carotid artery bifurcation aneurysm: case report and review of literature. Br J Radiol. 2005;78:646.
13. Servadei F, Nasi MT, Cremonini AM, et al. Importance of a reliable admission Glasgow Coma Scale score for determining the need for evacuation of posttraumatic subdural hematomas: a prospective study of 65 patients. J Trauma. 1998;44:868.
14. Givner A, Gurney J, O'Connor D, et al. Reimaging in pediatric neurotrauma: factors associated with progression of intracranial injury. J Pediatr Surg. 2002;37:381.
15. Oertel M, Kelly DF, McArthur D, et al. Progressive hemorrhage after head trauma: predictors and consequences of the evolving injury. J Neurosurg. 2002;96:109.
16. Huang YH, Deng YH, Lee TC, et al. Rotterdam computed tomography score as a prognosticator in head-injured patients undergoing decompressive craniectomy. Neurosurgery. 2012;71(1):80–5.

24 Pneumocephalus

Ana Lorena Abello

Abstract

Pneumocephalus is defined as the presence of air inside the cranial vault. It is usually associated with previous neurosurgery, basilar skull fractures, sinus fractures, nasopharyngeal tumors, meningitis, and barotrauma among other causes. Most cases of pneumocephalus resolve spontaneously, and conservative management is all that is needed. CT is the modality of choice for delineation of the location, extent, and etiology of intracranial air, and usually it is easy to identify it as areas with air density distributed in the epidural, subdural, or subarachnoid spaces. "Mount Fuji sign" and "air bubble sign" are indicators of tension pneumocephalus and may be neurosurgical emergencies.

Background

Pneumocephalus is defined as the presence of air inside the cranial vault. Gas collections can occur in several compartments: extradural, subdural, subarachnoid, intraventricular (pneumoventricle), and intraparenchymal (pneumatocele) [1, 2].

It is usually associated with neurosurgical procedures, basilar skull fractures, sinus fractures, nasopharyngeal tumor invasion of the skull base, meningitis, and barotrauma, and in some cases it is idiopathic [2]. Clinical manifestations of pneumocephalus are usually minor but occasionally may be serious. Presenting signs and symptoms include headache, nausea and vomiting, dizziness, depressed neurological status, rhinorrhea or otorrhea, seizures, and "succussion splash" (a sound elicited by shaking the head of a person who has intracranial free fluid and air). Other findings in pneumocephalus may include tympany on percussion of the skull and papilledema on fundoscopic examination. Presence of intracranial hypertension or focal parenchymal gas collections may give rise to confusion, subtle weakness, reflex abnormalities, or frank hemiparesis [1, 3].

Most cases of pneumocephalus resolve spontaneously and conservative management suffices. Nonoperative management involves oxygen therapy, head elevation, antibiotics, and analgesia

A.L. Abello, MD
Department of Radiology,
University of North Carolina, Chapel Hill, NC, USA
e-mail: anaabellop@hotmail.com

R. Hoffmann Nunes et al. (eds.), *Critical Findings in Neuroradiology*,
DOI 10.1007/978-3-319-27987-9_24

[2, 3]. Surgical treatment is indicated when there is recurrent pneumocephalus or signs of increasing intracranial pressure suggesting development of tension pneumocephalus [1, 4, 5].

Key Points

Etiology

Trauma: The majority of cases of pneumocephalus are due to trauma (75–90 %) although only 0.5–1 % of all episodes of head trauma result in pneumocephalus. The presence of intracranial gas in a patient with recent head trauma is suggestive of a basal skull fracture. Regardless of the location of the intracranial air, one should alert the physician in charge of the patient [1]. Air entering the epidural space as a result of basal skull fractures originates in the paranasal sinuses and generally collects in the floor of the anterior or middle cranial fossa or the orbits. If the dura is breached, air will reach the subdural space, which occurs in about 28 % of cases of pneumocephalus, and tearing of the arachnoid allows air to enter the subarachnoid space. The distinction between subdural and subarachnoid air can be difficult to make, and the two may coexist. The pathophysiology of each of these types of pneumocephalus usually involves one of the following two mechanisms: (1). It may involve a ball-valve effect, with air being forced through a craniodural defect by coughing, sneezing, or other sudden changes in nasopharyngeal pressure. (2) It may be also due to excessive leakage of cerebrospinal fluid (CSF) causing a negative intracranial pressure, and as a result, air is drawn into the cranial cavity [1, 6].

Surgery: Pneumocephalus is commonly observed after intracranial surgery. The amount of intracranial air may vary, but it is usually benign in nature and takes approximately 2–3 weeks to completely reabsorb. Presence of pneumocephalus in a patient requiring surgery is of special concern to the anesthesiologist because of the possible development of tension pneumocephalus secondary to the use of nitrous oxide as its administration can lead to expansion of any trapped air thereby increasing intracranial pressure [7].

Infection: In the presence of persistent or progressive pneumocephalus several weeks after intracranial surgery, intracranial infection needs to be excluded [8].

Tumors: Pneumocephalus can be caused by tumors with the most common being frontal and ethmoidal sinus osteomas. Osteomas breach the posterior wall of the frontal sinus creating a one-way valve through which air enters the intracranial cavity. Other tumors that have been associated with the production for pneumocephalus are the skull base metastasis, nasopharyngeal tumors, and pituitary adenomas [6, 9].

Other causes: Spontaneous otogenic pneumocephalus is a rare event. Raised pressure in the middle ear by nose blowing, sneezing, swallowing, coughing, or Valsalva maneuver can create a positive-pressure gradient forcing air into the intracranial space in susceptible individuals (i.e., those with congenital defects of the tegmen tympani or with hyperpneumatization of the mastoid air cells) [10].

Venous air emboli from intravenous catheterization: Thompson et al. demonstrated a 6 % rate of iatrogenic pneumocephalus following venous catheterizations [11]. One explanation is that peripherally injected air ascends passively within the venous system in response to gravitational forces countercurrent to jugular venous flow. Gas bubbles can then be found in the internal jugular vein, subclavian vein, anterior neck veins, dural sinuses, ophthalmic veins, and trabeculated venous spaces of the cavernous sinuses [12, 13].

Cerebral air embolism also can be produced by positive-pressure maneuvers performed during cardiac procedures, resuscitation, lung biopsies and in diving-related decompression illness [14].

Delayed shunt-related pneumocephalus is a rare complication that appears to have two requirements for its development: (1) the presence of a CSF diversion system that causes decreased intracranial pressure and (2) the existence of a craniodural defect with or without obvious CSF leak. Large negative intracranial pressure can develop by a siphoning phenomenon in these patients. The negative pressure and the displaced volume of CSF allow the entry of air that is trapped leading to headache and decreased level of consciousness. A detailed search for the CSF leak must be performed on these patients [15].

Best Imaging Modality

Computed tomography (CT): CT is the modality of choice for delineation of the location, extent, and etiology of intracranial air. CT is extremely sensitive and can identify as little as 0.5 cc of air in the intracranial spaces. Air has an extremely low attenuation coefficient (−1000 HU) and therefore appears as a region of very low density that is surrounded by a white rim which is artifactual [16].

Magnetic resonance imaging (MRI): On MRI, the diagnosis may be trickier as there is no "objective" density measurement. Air will appear completely black on all sequences but, depending on the location and morphology, can be mistaken for blood product or flow voids [17]. MRI should not be used for the initial evaluation of patients suspected of harboring pneumocephalus.

Major Findings

Trauma and surgery are the most common cause of epidural air collections and a frequent cause of air in other intracranial spaces [1]. When pneumocephalus is of important volume, it is easy to identify areas with air density usually distributed in epidural, subdural, or subarachnoid spaces. Evidence of trauma or surgery may also be evident on CT. Presence of tiny bubbles of gas may also be related to a fracture or infection (Fig. 24.1).

Tension pneumocephalus occurs after drainage of subdural hematomas. There are two signs that suggest increased tension of the subdural air: (1). Subdural air separates and compresses the frontal lobes creating a widened interhemispheric space between the tips of the frontal lobes that mimics the silhouette of Mount Fuji in Japan called the "Mount Fuji sign" [1–5, 18]. (2) Presence of multiple small air bubbles scattered through several cisterns called the "air bubble sign" [3]. These air bubbles enter the subarachnoid space through a tear in the arachnoid membrane caused by high-pressure air in the subdural space. Presence of tension pneumocephalus on CT of head trauma and postoperative patients is a critical finding. Identification of this sign can

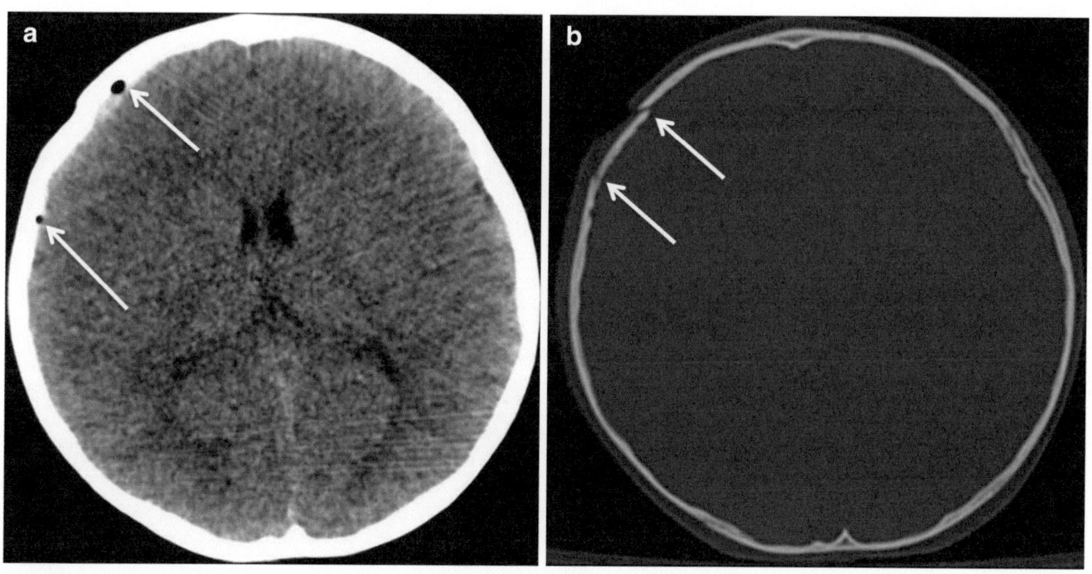

Fig. 24.1 Post-traumatic pneumocephalus. Axial CT soft tissue window (**a**) and bone window (**b**) show tiny gas bubbles in the epidural space associated to thin epidural hematoma (*arrows* in **a**). Fractures are seen in the frontal bone (*arrows* in **b**)

have immediate and important impact on patient care and outcome (Fig. 24.2) [4].

Intracerebral pneumatocele is gas collection within the brain. Pneumatoceles may result from head trauma, infection and surgery, erosion from skull base tumors, and radiotherapy. Air gets trapped in the brain by a ball valve mechanism caused by fragments of bone, dural flap, foreign bodies, sinus mucosa, granulation tissues, or a collapsible fistulous track that behaves as a valve. Air is toxic to neurons causing further damage to the already trauma-compromised parenchyma and leads to cerebral edema. Progression of pneumocephalus is aided by expansion of air at body temperature and ease of dissection of white matter tracts by the air. On imaging, a pneumatocele is usually round or oval in configuration measuring on average 3–4 cm in diameter and surrounded by brain. It is usually found in a location abutting the fronto-ethmoidal sinuses, and a funnel may be visualized connecting the cavity to a paranasal sinus. An important differential diagnosis is an abscess containing gas-producing bacteria in which a mottled gas collection may be seen surrounded by an enhancing rim after contrast administration (Fig. 24.3) [19].

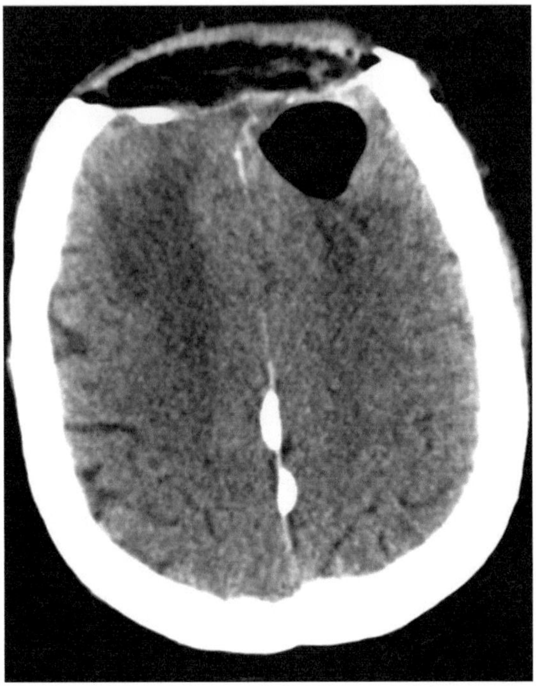

Fig. 24.3 Pneumatocele. Axial CT shows a rounded air bubble in the left frontal lobe. At fat graft is seen filling the frontal defect. Note differences in density between the air and the fat

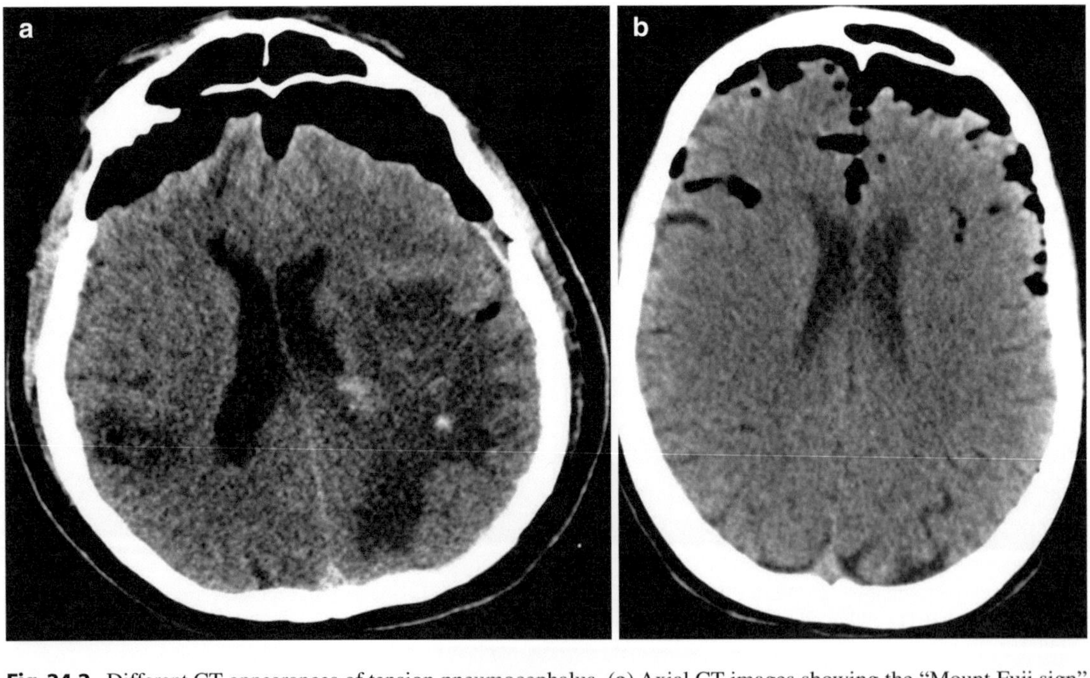

Fig. 24.2 Different CT appearances of tension pneumocephalus. (**a**) Axial CT images showing the "Mount Fuji sign" and (**b**). The "air bubble sign" in two different postoperative patients

Cerebral air embolism can be displayed in venous or arterial structures depending on the mechanism of embolism. In the presence of air in the jugular vein and distant blood vessels in the brain, one should consider the possibility iatrogenic intravenous embolism (Fig. 24.4) [13].

Imaging Follow-Up

After surgery, the most important study is the clinical neurological examination to check for progression of pneumocephalus expected after surgery that evolves into tension pneumocephalus. Serial CT of the brain has been recommended, but there is no evidence supporting its use.

Main Differential Diagnosis

The main differential diagnoses include a *fatty (ossified) falx cerebri*, *intracranial lipoma,* and the *rupture of a dermoid cyst* (Fig. 24.5). All these conditions result in areas of very low density in different intracranial spaces which can be distinguished from pneumocephalus measuring their Hounsfield Units (HU) and recalling that the fat has densities between – 60 and – 120 HU and the air below has density of −1000 HU or less [20].

Fat is frequently encountered in the form of *fat grafts* after skull base surgery and can appear very dark on standard soft tissue CT windows, and thus it may be misdiagnosed as pneumocephalus [3] (Fig. 24.3).

Tips

- Immediately report tension pneumocephalus as evidenced by the "Mount Fuji" sign, "air bubble" sign or subdural pneumocephalus causing mass effect and subfalcine herniation. Tension pneumocephalus may be a neurosurgical emergency [20].
- Rule out skull fractures in the presence of intracranial gas in a trauma patient. If

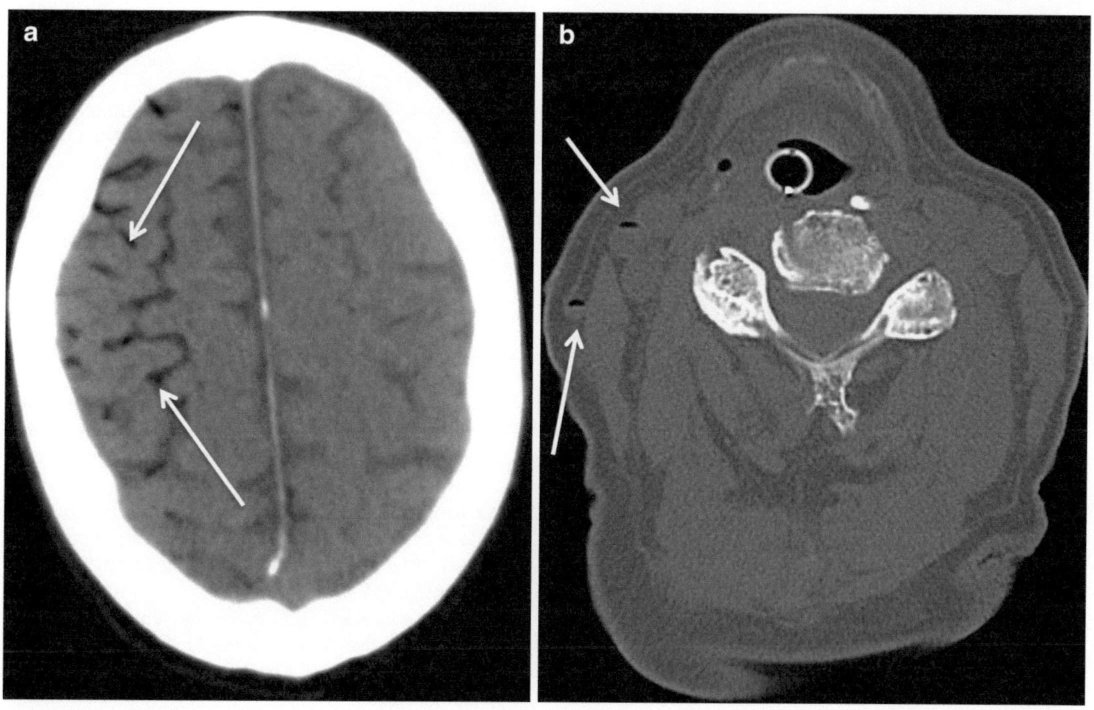

Fig. 24.4 Intravascular gas. Axial CT (**a**) shows gas in the distal veins (*arrows*) and in (**b**) air in the neck veins (*arrows*)

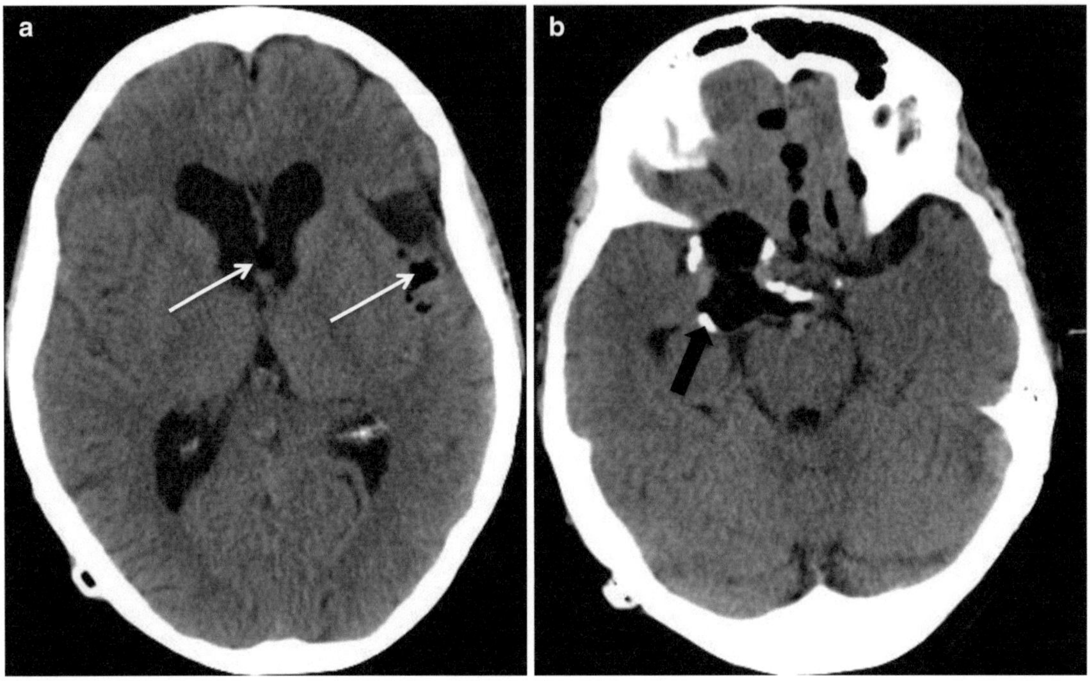

Fig. 24.5 Fat simulating intracranial air. (**a**) Hypodense nearly "drop-like" abnormalities (*arrows*) are present in the left Sylvian fissure and ventricles. These correspond to fat due to a dermoid cyst rupture located at the skull base that has peripheral calcifications (*black arrow*) in (**b**)

not repaired, they may lead to future CSF leaks and meningitis.

- Suspect iatrogenic cerebral air embolism in the presence of intravascular (especially venous) gas.
- Persistent or progressive pneumocephalus several weeks after intracranial surgery should heighten suspicion of intracranial infection and CSF leak.
- Keep in mind that fat particles may be confused with pneumocephalus, so it is necessary to measure their density to avoid misdiagnoses.

References

1. Leong KM, Vijayananthan A, Sia SF, Waran V. Pneumocephalus: an uncommon finding in trauma. Med J Malaysia. 2008;63(3):256–8.
2. Aguilar-Shea AL, Manas-Gallardo N, Romero-Pisonero E. Post-traumatic pneumocephalus. Int J Emerg Med. 2009;2(2):129–30.
3. Schirmer CM, Heilman CB, Bhardwaj A. Pneumocephalus: case illustrations and review. Neurocrit Care. 2010;13(1):152–8.
4. Michel SJ. The Mount Fuji sign. Radiology. 2004;232(2):449–50.
5. Heckmann JG, Ganslandt O. Images in clinical medicine. The Mount Fuji sign. N Engl J Med. 2004; 350(18):1881.
6. Mahabir RC, Szymczak A, Sutherland GR. Intracerebral pneumatocele presenting after air travel. J Neurosurg. 2004;101(2):340–2.
7. Satapathy GC, Dash HH. Tension pneumocephalus after neurosurgery in the supine position. Br J Anaesth. 2000;84(1):115–7.
8. Sarkiss CA, Soleymani T, Caplan JM, Dorsi MJ, Huang J. Intracerebral abscess with dissecting pneumocephalus caused by a gas-producing gram-positive rod following craniotomy for glioblastoma multiforme resection. J Clin Neurosci: Off J Neurosurg Soc Australas. 2013;20(11):1625–7.
9. Lehmer LM, Kissel P, Ragsdale BD. Frontal sinus osteoma with osteoblastoma-like histology and associated intracranial pneumatocele. Head Neck Pathol. 2012;6(3):384–8.
10. Singh A, Alvarez J. Spontaneous otogenic intracerebral pneumocephalus. West J Emerg Med. 2010;11(1):107.
11. Thompson TP, Levy E, Kanal E, Lunsford LD. Iatrogenic pneumocephalus secondary to intravenous catheterization. Case Rep J Neurosurg. 1999;91(5):878–80.

12. Rubinstein D, Symonds D. Gas in the cavernous sinus. AJNR Am J Neuroradiol. 1994;15(3):561–6.
13. Syed ON, Weintraub D, DeLaPaz R, Connolly ES. Venous air emboli from intravenous catheterization: a report of iatrogenic intravascular pneumocephalus. J Clin Neurosci: Off J Neurosurg Soc Australas. 2009;16(10):1361–2.
14. Dutra M, Massumoto C. Images in clinical medicine. Cerebral air embolism. N Engl J Med. 2012;367(9): 850.
15. Ugarriza LF, Cabezudo JM, Lorenzana LM, Porras LF, Garcia-Yague LM. Delayed pneumocephalus in shunted patients. Report of three cases and review of the literature. Br J Neurosurg. 2001;15(2):161–7.
16. Osborn AG, Daines JH, Wing SD, Anderson RE. Intracranial air on computerized tomography. J Neurosurg. 1978;48(3):355–9.
17. Palma JA, Zubieta JL, Dominguez PD, Garcia-Eulate R. Pneumocephalus mimicking cerebral cavernous malformations in MR susceptibility-weighted imaging. AJNR Am J Neuroradiol. 2009;30(6):e83; author reply e4.
18. Ho M-L, Eisenberg RL. Neuroradiology signs. 1st Ed. Mc Graw Hill Education. 2014. 470 p.
19. Venkatesh SK, Bhargava V. Clinics in diagnostic imaging (119). Post-traumatic intracerebral pneumatocele. Singapore Med J. 2007;48(11):1055–9; quiz 60.
20. Sinclair AG, Scoffings DJ. Imaging of the post-operative cranium. Radiographics: A Rev Publ Radiol Soc North Am Inc. 2010;30(2):461–82.

Child Abuse

25

Tito Navarro and Ana Lorena Abello

Abstract

Abusive head trauma includes inflicted skull, cerebral and vascular injuries resulting from blunt force trauma, shaking, or a combination of these forces. Lesions that arise from abusive head trauma include subdural hemorrhage, epidural hemorrhage, subarachnoid hemorrhage, subdural hygromas, cerebral edema, cerebral ischemia, diffuse axonal injury, cerebral contusion, skull fractures, retinal hemorrhages, and scalp swelling. There is no gold standard diagnostic test for child abuse. The diagnosis relies on clinical and imaging features as well as supporting social and child welfare information. Several imaging tools, including CT, MRI, skull radiography, and ultrasonography are often needed to confirm a suspected diagnosis of child abuse.

Background

Abusive head trauma (AHT) includes inflicted cranial and cerebral injuries resulting from blunt force trauma, shaking, or a combination of these forces. It is the most serious form of physical child abuse (CA) with an associated mortality of 30 % and morbidity in 50 % of survivors. While the annual incidence of AHT is estimated at 24–34 per 100,000 children younger than 1 year of age, this is likely underestimated because many cases are not brought to medical attention and others are not recognized as abuse [1–5].

In inflicted head injuries, the history may be vague or may vary with time, and a mechanism of injury that is incompatible with the developmental capacity of the child is commonly described. Common symptoms include lethargy, irritability, seizures, increased or decreased tone, impaired consciousness, vomiting, poor feeding, breathing abnormalities, and apnea. Approximately one-half of all patients with the shaking–impact syndrome have severe neurological impairment, are

T. Navarro, MD
Departamento de Radiología,
Instituto Nacional de Enfermedades Neoplásicas,
Av. Gregorio Escobedo 426, Jesús María, Lima, Peru
e-mail: tinaro12345@hotmail.com

A.L. Abello, MD (✉)
Department of Radiology,
University of North Carolina, Chapel Hill, NC, USA
e-mail: anaabellop@hotmail.com

R. Hoffmann Nunes et al. (eds.), *Critical Findings in Neuroradiology*,
DOI 10.1007/978-3-319-27987-9_25

unresponsive, have opisthotonos, or are moribund at presentation. Seizures are reported in 40–70 % of patients [1, 5].

Many conditions may be associated with AHT including subdural hemorrhage, epidural hemorrhage, subarachnoid hemorrhage, subdural hygromas, cerebral edema, cerebral ischemia, diffuse axonal injury, cerebral contusion, skull fractures, retinal hemorrhages, and scalp swelling [1–5].

Key Points

Etiology

Biomechanics

The term "whiplash shaken-baby syndrome" was coined by Caffey in 1972 to explain infantile subdural and subarachnoid hemorrhages, traction type of metaphyseal fractures, and retinal hemorrhages and was based on evidence of sudden angular (rotational) deceleration forces [6]. The forceful striking of the head against a surface is responsible for most severe inflicted brain injuries, including diffuse axonal injury and subdural hematomas [2, 5].

Secondary mechanisms of hypoxic–ischemic injury probably are due to aspiration or strangulation. Severe abusive head trauma may damage the brainstem or spinal cord, including the respiratory centers (possibly from hyperflexion/hyperextension injury), which initiates widespread secondary hypoxia, leading to global hypoxia [1, 7]. Seizures may be related to the hypoxia and exacerbate further damage to the brain through excitotoxic mechanisms or by inducing further respiratory insufficiency [8].

Best Imaging Modality

There is no gold standard diagnostic test for child abuse. The diagnosis relies on clinical and imaging features as well as supporting social and child welfare information [3]. Several imaging tools, including non-enhanced computed tomography (CT), magnetic resonance imaging (MRI), skull radiography, and ultrasonography are often needed to confirm a suspected diagnosis of child abuse [1].

Controversial information has been reported as to whether CT and MRI can differentiate between accidental and inflicted brain injury. A recent review on the diagnostic value of CT and MRI reported additional information in 25 % of cases when MRI was acquired after an abnormal early CT examination. MRI also helped demonstrate recurrent episodes of injury [9].

According to the American College of Radiology recommendations, neuroimaging indications depend on the child's age and type of presentation (Diagram 25.1) [10].

Non-enhanced computed tomography: CT is widely accepted as the modality of first choice in an acutely ill child with neurological symptoms. Therefore, CT of the head is usually the initial radiologic examination used in suspected AHT [1]. CT provides information regarding intracranial hemorrhage, cerebral edema, early brain herniation, and bone injuries [4, 6]. The finding of a scalp swelling must be carefully examined with bone or intermediate windowing, as it indicates the point of impact. Old fractures (without scalp swelling) may be difficult to differentiate from accessory fissures and sutures [1].

Magnetic resonance imaging: When neurological signs are absent, MRI should be preferred to CT because of its higher sensitivity to detect smaller parenchymal injuries of different ages which may prove critical in diagnosis and legal proceedings [1].

Small accumulations of subdural, subarachnoid, intraventricular and intraparenchymal blood can be identified by using gradient-echo (GRE) MRI or susceptibility weighted imaging (SWI) sequences as well as retinal hemorrhages especially when a high-resolution SWI protocol is performed [11]. Diffusion-weighted imaging (DWI) is sensitive in early detection of hypoxic–ischemic injury. Fluid-attenuated inversion recovery imaging (FLAIR) is particularly helpful in detecting cerebral edema, contusions, shearing injuries (diffuse axonal injury), parenchymal lacerations, and small subdural hematomas [4]. Vascular complications,

Diagram 25.1 Protocol in suspected child abuse according to the American College of Radiology

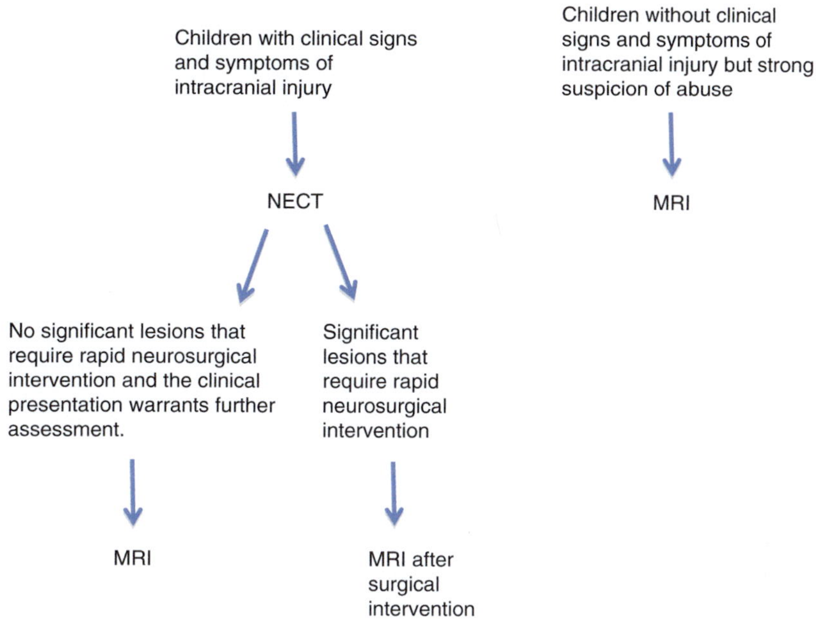

including stroke and vessel dissection, are better seen with magnetic resonance angiography and venography. MR venography performed following intravenous contrast can detect thrombi in superficial and deep venous structures [1].

Skull radiography: AHT may be the only condition in which a skull radiography is indicated in children. It is useful to detect possible fractures that are missed on CT because of their location in the same plane of scanning. Skull radiography, usually part of the skeletal survey, should include anteroposterior and lateral views [12].

Color Doppler ultrasound: It is useful in children under 6 months with increased cranial perimeter to detect subdural collections and should only be used as a screening method [13].

Cervical spine MRI: Another important contribution of MRI is the evaluation of the craniovertebral junction for the detection of atlantoaxial separation, ligamentous injury, vertebral body compression, and epidural and intradural hemorrhages all of which can be seen in child abuse [14]. Kadom et al. found that the prevalence of cervical injury in children with abusive head trauma and diffuse hypoxic–ischemic cerebral injuries was high suggesting a causal relationship [15].

Major Findings

Subdural hemorrhages: It is significantly associated with AHT, and these are commonly localized interhemispherically, in the posterior fossa, or over the hemispheric convexity. The association of AHT with multiple subdural hematomas of differing attenuation has been interpreted as indicative of repetitive inflicted head injury. MRI is more sensitive than CT in the identification of membranes within the subdural collections, and presence of these membranes is a useful indicator for older hemorrhages. As the blood ages, there is a transition from hyperintensity in T1-weighted images (T1WI), T2-weighted images (T2WI), and FLAIR to hypointensity on T1WI and T2WI (Figs. 25.1 and 25.3) [1, 3, 16, 17]. Bridging vein thrombosis may be the origin of subdural hemorrhages since bridging veins have little muscle in their walls and the segments that penetrate the dural border cell layer can have a thickness of only 10 μm, whereas the wall thickness of their subarachnoid portions ranges between 50 and 200 μm. Thus, increased fragility of the dural segment of a bridging vein is presumed to be the site of rupture. This may explain why subdural hemorrhages are more common than

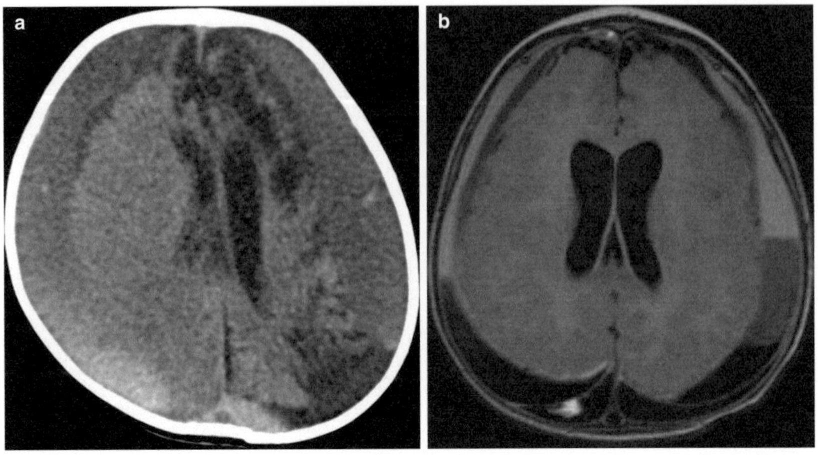

Fig. 25.1 Two different patients with AHT. (**a**) CT shows bilateral subdural hemorrhages with different attenuation indicating blood products in different stages. (**b**) T1WI MRI showing blood with different signal intensities and levels in bilateral subdural spaces

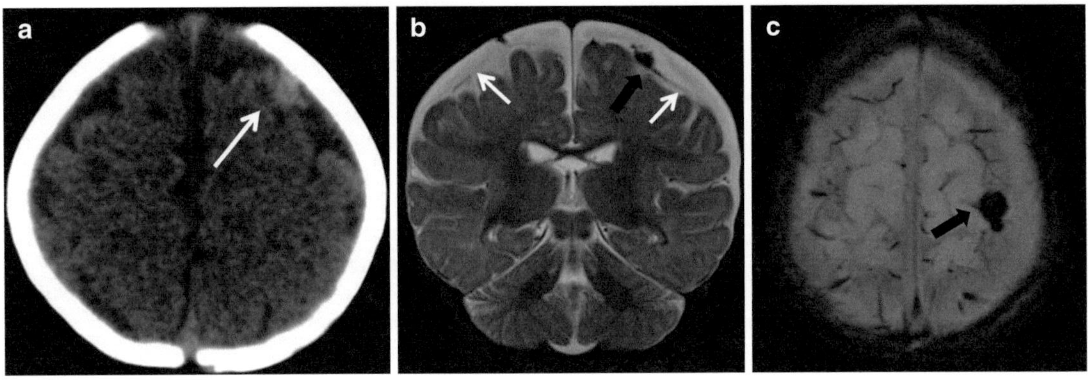

Fig. 25.2 A 5-month-old boy with child abuse history. (**a**) Axial CT shows left focal frontal acute extra-axial hemorrhage, probably due to bringing vein thrombosis, the "tadpole sign" (*arrow*). (**b**) Coronal T2WI MRI and (**c**) axial SWI MRI demonstrate "blooming" area indicating in the area of acute blood (*black arrows*). Subdural hygromas with CSF signal are evident in T2WI (*white arrows* in **b**)

subarachnoid hemorrhages in CA cases. Bridging vein thrombosis may resemble a tadpole, with an oval- to round-shaped "body" representing thrombotic material and a bent "tail" reflecting a torn bridging vein expanded by clotted blood. Accordingly this shape is called the "tadpole sign" (Fig. 25.2) [18].

Epidural hemorrhages: Occur significantly more often with unintentional head trauma than with AHT. They usually result from a fall which produces a hemorrhage without other associated injuries, except for retinal hemorrhages [1, 3, 16].

Subdural hygromas: Traumatic subdural hygromas arise from tears in the arachnoid membrane with subsequent leakage of CSF into the subdural compartment. They typically appear 3 or more days after head trauma. On CT they have attenuation identical to CSF and may be indistinguishable from chronic subdural hematomas. MRI can discriminate between these two entities because hygromas have CSF signal intensity on all sequences. Chronic subdural hemorrhages, in contrast, have loss of signal due to hemosiderin deposition. In most cases, hygromas are asymptomatic (Fig. 25.2) [19]. Color Doppler ultrasound can depict the bridging veins traversing the extra-axial spaces ("positive cortical vein sign") that are typical of benign enlargement of the subarachnoid spaces thus differentiating them from true subdural collections [13].

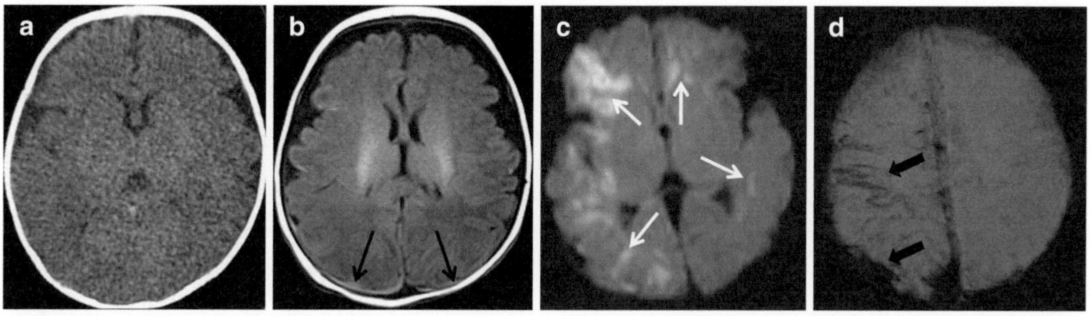

Fig. 25.3 A 6-week-old girl with hypoxic–ischemic injury due to child abuse. (**a**) Axial CT shows loss of gray matter differentiation. (**b**) Axial T1WI depicts hyperintensity in the subdural parietal spaces compatible with subdural hemorrhages (*arrows*). (**c**) Axial DWI shows diffuse cortical and subcortical diffusion abnormalities involving both hemispheres concerning infarctions (*arrows*) and (**d**). Axial SWI demonstrating low signal in the subarachnoid and subdural spaces compatible with subarachnoid and subdural blood (*arrows*)

Subarachnoid hemorrhage: Subarachnoid hemorrhage is observed in less than 50 % child abuse cases and is usually hyperdense in CT in acute stage. "Blooming" with hypointensity surrounded by hyperintense cerebrospinal fluid (CSF) can be identified on GRE and SWI sequences (Fig. 25.3) [20].

Hypoxic–ischemic injury and cerebral edema: These findings have a significant association with CA [3, 16]. On premature babies in whom abuse is common, white matter edema may be difficult to appreciate on MRI; nevertheless, edema appears hyperintense on T2WI. DWI has been used to detect early cytotoxic edema in ATH when findings on MRI performed with other pulse sequences are normal. Areas of restricted water diffusion appear bright on DWI [2]. Lesions with restricted diffusion are more common in the posterior watershed territories, a distribution that is considered typical of abusive trauma. Global ischemia shows diffuse loss of gray-white matter differentiation in CT with decreased attenuation in the cortex and relative sparing of thalami, basal ganglia, cerebellum, and brainstem, which therefore appear hyperdense "reversal sign" or "white cerebellum sign" (Fig. 25.3) [1] (also see Chap. 6).

Diffuse axonal injury: Traumatic axonal injuries result from rotational acceleration of the head. Because different tissues in the brain accelerate at different rates, shear forces develop between them and disrupt the axons, which are particularly vulnerable to stretch injury. CT is relatively insensitive for diffuse axonal injury and is positive in only 19 % of nonhemorrhagic axonal shear injuries. MRI is superior to CT for detecting diffuse axonal injury. The superiority of FLAIR for diffuse axonal injury detection is related to its nulling of CSF signal intensity. GRE and SWI are useful for detecting small hemorrhages that may be visible as areas of decreased signal intensity for years after the injury [19]. A recent literature meta-analysis showed that in the absence of any significant clinical history, the finding previously mentioned was significantly associated with CA [3] (also see Chap. 21).

Cerebral contusion: Refers to a focal hemorrhage in the brain parenchyma (usually the cortex) that results from direct contact forces. Such injuries are rare in infants. Commonly contused areas are the frontal lobes, temporal lobes, and parafalcine cortex (Fig. 25.4) [1].

Retinal hemorrhages: Have individual significant association with CA [3]. SWI is sensitive to signal heterogeneities within the magnetic field induced by paramagnetic or diamagnetic materials such as hemosiderin and calcium among others. The signal intensity from such paramagnetic materials "blooms" on SWI. When compared with GRE sequences, SWI enhances small changes in susceptibility across a voxel as signal intensity losses. This improves the morphological delineation of paramagnetic and diamagnetic

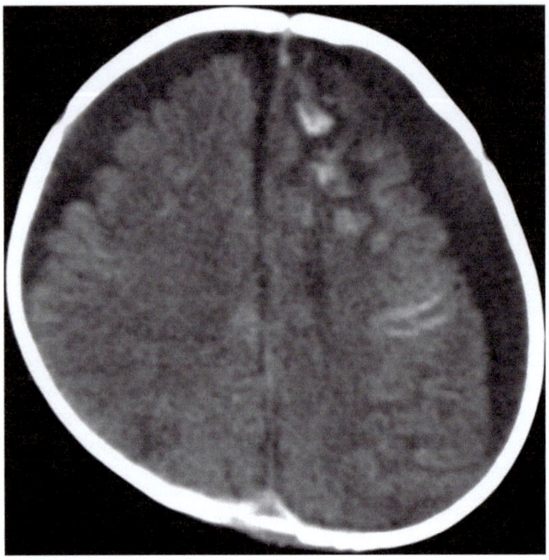

Fig. 25.4 Axial CT shows hyperdensities in the left frontal and parietal cortex compatible with brain contusions. Bilateral chronic extra-axial fluid collections are also seen

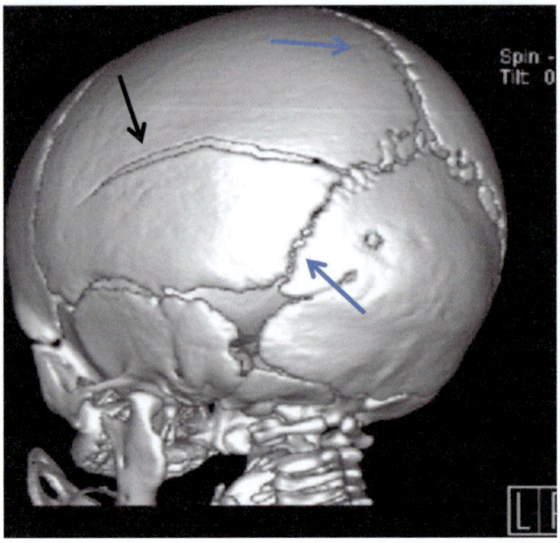

Fig. 25.5 3D CT cranial images in a 3-month-old boy with child abuse show a horizontal temporal fracture (*black arrow*). Sagittal and lambdoid sutures are normal (*blue arrows*)

materials. Nonhemorrhagic paramagnetic or diamagnetic materials such as dystrophic calcifications may be mistakenly identified as retinal hemorrhages on SWI [11].

Skull fractures: The infant's skull is very resistant to trauma, so any fracture that is inconsistent with the clinical history should raise the question of CA.

Skull fracture(s) in conjunction with intracranial injuries are significantly associated with CA [3]. Patterns of skull fractures in AHT are simple, multiple "eggshell" fractures, bilateral fractures, occipital impression fractures, fractures crossing sutures, and diastatic fractures (Fig. 25.5) [21, 22].

A summary of the abovementioned findings can be found in Table 25.1.

Imaging Follow-Up

There is no evidence-based approach for the imaging follow-up of abusive head trauma patients. Repeat CT and MRI are both currently used, but the literature on this approach is inconclusive. Injuries may be evaluated 7–10 days after the acute injury with repeat CT or better MRI to document laminar cortical necrosis, enlargement of subdural collections, and early development of hydrocephalus. In addition, MRI may be repeated 2–4 months after the initial injury to better evaluate the extent of end damage, prognosis, and medicolegal information [1].

Main Differential Diagnosis

Non-abusive head trauma: It is the principal differential diagnosis. In a recent meta-analysis performed in 2012, Piteau et al. found that the epidural hemorrhage, scalp swelling, and isolated skull fracture(s) were each significantly associated with non-abusive head trauma and must not be assumed to be related to child abuse [3].

Meningitis: Frequently produces subdural sterile fluid collections and empyemas that could be mistaken for subdural collections due to child abuse.

Bleeding dyscrasias: They can cause recurrent subdural hematomas, epidural hematomas following minor trauma, and intracerebral bleeds [20].

Inborn errors of metabolism: Rarely, diseases such as glutaric aciduria type 1 and Menke's kinky hair syndrome can cause retinal hemorrhages and bilateral subdural hematomas [20].

Table 25.1 Radiographic characteristics associated with child abuse

Findings	Best imaging modality	Key points
Subdural hemorrhage	CT MRI	Different densities and signal intensities in CT and MRI indicate blood in different ages
Subdural hygromas	MRI US	Signal intensity similar to CSF in MRI "Positive cortical vein sign" in US rule out AHT
Subarachnoid hemorrhage	MRI CT	Signal hyperintensity in SAS on FLAIR or "blooming" in GRE or SWI
Hypoxic–ischemic injury	MRI	Restricted diffusion in watershed territories
Global cerebral edema	CT	Decreased attenuation in cortex and relative sparing of thalami, basal ganglia, cerebellum, and brainstem
Diffuse axonal injury	MRI	Subcortical, callosal, brainstem lesions of high T2 signal
Cerebral contusion	MRI	Focal hematoma in the cortex
Retinal hemorrhages	MRI	"Blooming" in the globes with GRE and SWI
Skull fractures	Skull radiography CT	Radiographs are ideal for fractures oriented parallel to CT scanning angle

Tips

- Due to medical and legal implications, avoid use of vague or imprecise language in reports to facilitate legal court decisions.
- When findings bring up the possibility of child abuse, always search clinical history for red flags.
- Mention presence or absence of subdural hemorrhages, and describe if there are different densities, indicating the presence of blood at different times of evolution. Bleeds occurring at different times are highly suggestive of abusive head trauma.
- Skull radiographs are a tool to detect skull fractures, and suspected child abuse and documentation of foreign bodies are the only indications for them.
- Always search the ocular globes in SWI or GRE sequences to rule out retinal hemorrhages. Occasionally these may be seen on CT.

References

1. Vazquez E, Delgado I, Sanchez-Montanez A, Fabrega A, Cano P, Martin N. Imaging abusive head trauma: why use both computed tomography and magnetic resonance imaging? Pediatr Radiol. 2014;44 Suppl 4:S589–603.
2. Lonergan GJ, Baker AM, Morey MK, Boos SC. From the archives of the AFIP. Child abuse: radiologic-pathologic correlation. Radiographics: A Rev Publ Radiol Soc N Am Inc. 2003;23(4):811–45.
3. Piteau SJ, Ward MG, Barrowman NJ, Plint AC. Clinical and radiographic characteristics associated with abusive and nonabusive head trauma: a systematic review. Pediatrics. 2012;130(2):315–23.
4. Hedlund GL, Frasier LD. Neuroimaging of abusive head trauma. Forensic Sci Med Pathol. 2009;5(4):280–90.
5. Duhaime AC, Christian CW, Rorke LB, Zimmerman RA. Nonaccidental head injury in infants – the "shaken-baby syndrome". N Engl J Med. 1998;338(25):1822–9.
6. Caffey J. On the theory and practice of shaking infants. Its potential residual effects of permanent brain damage and mental retardation. Am J Dis Child. 1972;124(2):161–9.
7. Geddes JF, Vowles GH, Hackshaw AK, Nickols CD, Scott IS, Whitwell HL. Neuropathology of inflicted head injury in children. II. Microscopic brain injury in infants. Brain: A J Neurol. 2001;124(Pt 7):1299–306.
8. Ichord RN, Naim M, Pollock AN, Nance ML, Margulies SS, Christian CW. Hypoxic-ischemic injury complicates inflicted and accidental traumatic brain injury in young children: the role of diffusion-weighted imaging. J Neurotrauma. 2007;24(1):106–18.
9. Kemp AM, Rajaram S, Mann M, Tempest V, Farewell D, Gawne-Cain ML, et al. What neuroimaging should be performed in children in whom inflicted brain injury (iBI) is suspected? A systematic review. Clin Radiol. 2009;64(5):473–83.
10. Meyer JS, Gunderman R, Coley BD. ACR Appropriateness Criteria® on suspected physical abuse-child. J Am Coll Radiol. 2011;8(2):87–94.

11. Zuccoli G, Panigrahy A, Haldipur A, Willaman D, Squires J, Wolford J, et al. Susceptibility weighted imaging depicts retinal hemorrhages in abusive head trauma. Neuroradiology. 2013;55(7):889–93.
12. Sieswerda-Hoogendoorn T, Boos S, Spivack B, Bilo RA, van Rijn RR. Abusive head trauma Part II: radiological aspects. Eur J Pediatr. 2012;171(4):617–23.
13. Chen CY, Chou TY, Zimmerman RA, Lee CC, Chen FH, Faro SH. Pericerebral fluid collection: differentiation of enlarged subarachnoid spaces from subdural collections with color Doppler US. Radiology. 1996;201(2):389–92.
14. Choudhary AK, Bradford RK, Dias MS, Moore GJ, Boal DK. Spinal subdural hemorrhage in abusive head trauma: a retrospective study. Radiology. 2012;262(1):216–23.
15. Kadom N, Khademian Z, Vezina G, Shalaby-Rana E, Rice A, Hinds T. Usefulness of MRI detection of cervical spine and brain injuries in the evaluation of abusive head trauma. Pediatr Radiol. 2014;44(7):839–48.
16. Kemp AM, Jaspan T, Griffiths J, Stoodley N, Mann MK, Tempest V, et al. Neuroimaging: what neuroradiological features distinguish abusive from non-abusive head trauma? A systematic review. Arch Dis Child. 2011;96(12):1103–12.
17. Vezina G. Assessment of the nature and age of subdural collections in nonaccidental head injury with CT and MRI. Pediatr Radiol. 2009;39(6):586–90.
18. Hahnemann ML, Kinner S, Schweiger B, Bajanowski T, Karger B, Pfeiffer H, et al. Imaging of bridging vein thrombosis in infants with abusive head trauma: the "Tadpole Sign". Eur Radiol. 2015;25(2):299–305.
19. Naidich TP. Imaging of the brain. Philadelphia: Saunders/Elsevier; 2013. Available from: http://VB3LK7EB4T.search.serialssolutions.com/?V=1.0&L=VB3LK7EB4T&S=JCs&C=TC0000823014&T=marc.
20. Osborn AG. Osborn's brain : imaging, pathology, and anatomy. 1st ed. Salt Lake City: Amirsys; 2013. xi, 1272 p. p.
21. Meservy CJ, Towbin R, McLaurin RL, Myers PA, Ball W. Radiographic characteristics of skull fractures resulting from child abuse. AJR Am J Roentgenol. 1987;149(1):173–5.
22. Foerster BR, Petrou M, Lin D, Thurnher MM, Carlson MD, Strouse PJ, et al. Neuroimaging evaluation of non-accidental head trauma with correlation to clinical outcomes: a review of 57 cases. J Pediatr. 2009;154(4):573–7.

Pediatric Skull Fractures

26

Mariana Cardoso Diogo
and Carla Ribeiro Conceição

Abstract

Lesions associated to skull fractures are a leading cause of death and disability in children. Skull fractures can be classified into several types not only by the energy of the trauma and the striking object but also to the characteristics of the developing skull. Some fracture types are specific of infants, such as "ping pong" and growing fractures. CT is the most useful imaging technique in the acute setting, although MRI may be occasionally indicated. Radiographs are no longer routinely used, as detection of isolated skull fractures without evaluation of the underlying brain serves no clinical purpose. Skull radiographs may help search for foreign bodies in cases of trauma or document fractures for legal purposes. Knowledge of the normal skull development and expected pathological findings are essential for correct diagnosis and treatment of these patients.

Background

A skull fracture is a bone discontinuity resulting from a direct calvarial impact. Although they might be clinically silent, a fracture is an indicator that a substantial amount of force has been applied to the head, increasing the possibility of associated traumatic brain injury (TBI), a leading cause of death and disability [1, 2].

Skull fractures are classified as open or closed depending on whether the overlying skin is intact and further divided according to their imaging appearance into linear, diastatic, depressed, and basilar. Combinations of all of these fracture types are possible. The fracture type is determined by the energy and shape of the striking object, direction of the impact force, and the area affected.

Isolated linear and diastatic fractures usually do not require treatment. Fractures depressed

M.C. Diogo, MD (✉)
Departamento de Neurorradiologia, Centro Hospitalar de Lisboa Central, Hospital de São José, Rua José António Serrano, Lisbon 1150, Portugal
e-mail: Mariana_cdiogo@hotmail.com

C.R. Conceição, MD
Departamento de Neurorradiologia, Hospital Dona Estefânia, Centro Hospitalar de Lisboa Central, Rua Jacinta Marto, Lisbon 1169-045, Portugal
e-mail: cribeiroconceicao@gmail.com

R. Hoffmann Nunes et al. (eds.), *Critical Findings in Neuroradiology*,
DOI 10.1007/978-3-319-27987-9_26

more than the full thickness of the skull may require surgical correction to avoid injury to the underlying brain and future cosmetic defects [3].

Uncomplicated skull fractures rarely produce neurological deficits, but the associated TBI may have serious neurological sequelae. Prognosis depends on associated intracranial injuries.

Key Points

Etiology

In children the mechanisms of injury vary with age and mainly include birth trauma, falls, recreational activities, and motor vehicle accidents [4]. Skull fractures arising from minor trauma are more common in infants as the calvarium is softer and thinner and the fracture threshold is lower [1, 5].

Linear fractures are the most common type of skull fracture in children of all ages with the parietal bones involved in over half the cases. They generally result from blunt trauma to the head when the impact force is conveyed over a wide calvarial surface area [6]. They rarely require specific treatment, and in the absence of intracranial lesions, they have good outcomes [7].

Diastatic fractures consist of a traumatic separation of the cranial sutures and are common in children particularly under 3 years of age [6]. Suture size and appearance vary with age, and when evaluating pediatric trauma, patient's knowledge of their normal anatomy is important [8, 9].

In the newborn, in the context of traumatic delivery, separation of the lambdoid suture and outward dislocation of the occipital bone is known as *occipital osteodiastasis* and is often associated with posterior fossa hematomas [5, 10].

Depressed fractures: With increasing impact force applied to a small area, the calvarium fails to rebound and is displaced inwardly, resulting in depressed skull fractures [6]. CT shows multiple fracture lines with inward displacement of bone fragments. These fractures are associated with intracranial lesions and may be open, increasing the risk of infection and cerebrospinal fluid (CSF) leaks.

In very young children, due to the thin and pliable nature of the skull, there may be an inward buckling skull depression without true bone disruption, and this is known as *"ping pong" fracture* [5, 10]. Intracranial complications are less frequent, but surgical correction of the deformity is often necessary.

Basilar skull fractures require a higher impact force than calvarial fractures [6]. They are often associated with TBI and secondary complications such as CSF leaks, vascular injuries, and infections from direct communication with paranasal sinuses and the middle ears.

Growing skull fractures are rare complications of skull fractures and occur almost exclusively (>90 %) in children under the age of 3 years [5]. They ensue when a skull fracture is associated with an underlying dural tear and the torn meninges become interposed between the fracture fragments inhibiting bone healing. CSF pulsations cause the fracture to enlarge [5, 6]. Progressive enlargement may be associated with herniation of meninges and brain tissue through the bone defect.

When a skull fracture communicates with an overlying lacerated scalp, involves the skull base, or violates a paranasal sinus and/or the middle ear structures, the terms *open or compound fractures* are used [3]. These fractures require surgical treatment.

Best Imaging Modality

Non-contrast computed tomography (CT): CT is considered the most valuable neuroimaging test in any posttraumatic setting [1, 5]. Multiplanar reconstructions and 3D reconstructed images can be particularly helpful to help distinguish fractures from normal variants and sutures [1].

Dedicated pediatric protocols adapted to patient size should always be used to minimize radiation exposure dose. Protective gear should be used to protect areas not being imaged, paying special attention to the gonads and thyroid gland [1, 5, 11].

Bone and soft tissue algorithms should be obtained. Because mineralization in young children is minimal, a narrow window may be needed [8].

CT angiography (CTA): CTA may be indicated if a fracture crosses a major vascular structure, such as the carotid canal or a dural venous sinus, and evaluation of these vascular structures is needed.

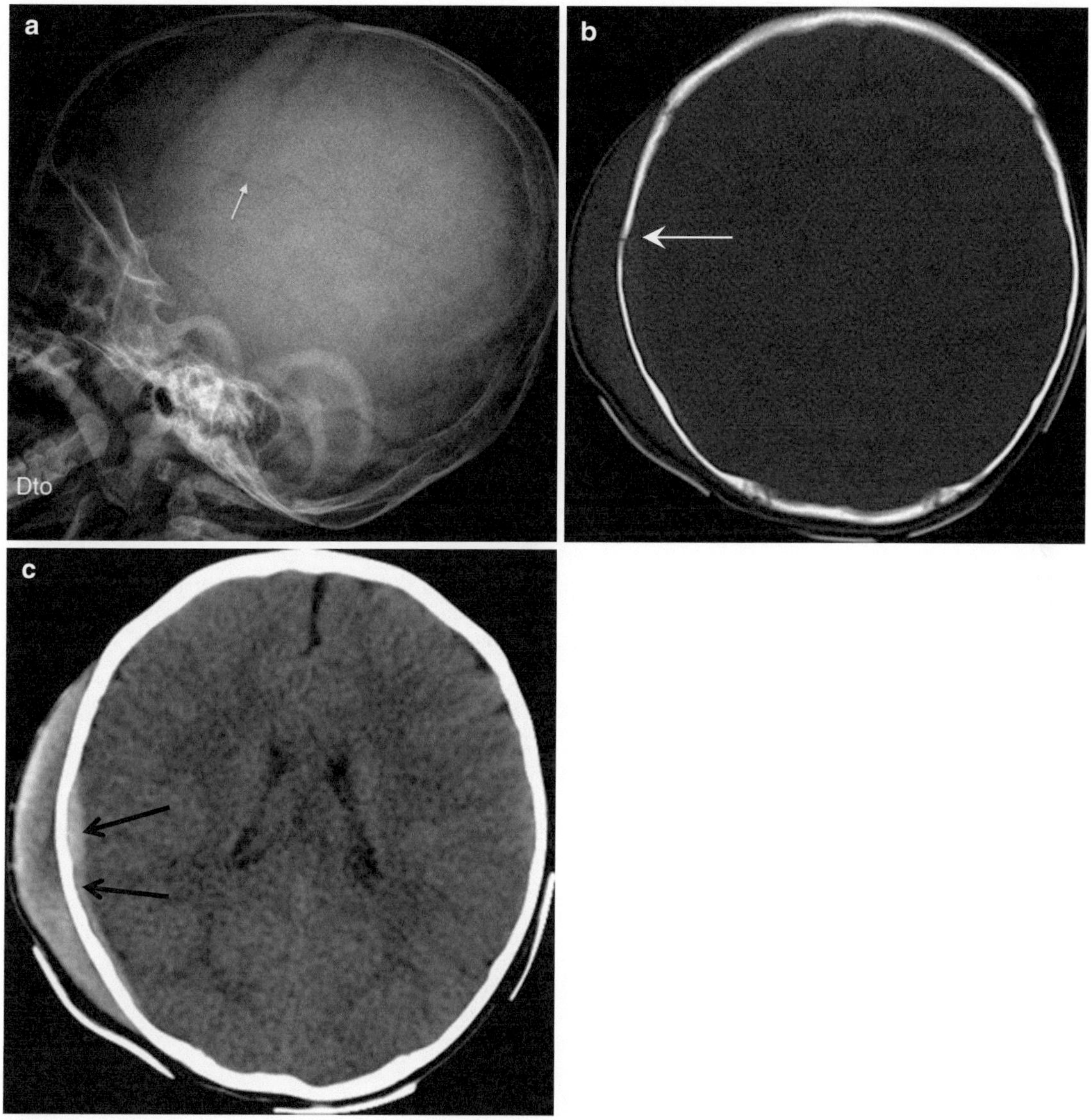

Fig. 26.1 Linear skull fracture. Lateral radiograph (**a**) depicts a linear lucency (*arrow*) also identified in axial CT bone window (**b**). Epicranial hematoma at point of impact is present. Axial CT soft tissue window (**c**) shows a small intracranial subdural hematoma (*arrow*)

Magnetic resonance imaging (*MRI*): MRI has limited indications in the evaluation of acute skull fractures. It is helpful in cases of CFS leaks, growing skull fractures, or when complications such as pseudomeningoceles are suspected. MRI is the imaging modality of choice to evaluate TBI.

Conventional radiographs: The role of skull radiographs in pediatric skull fractures is limited. Conventional radiography is not used except when documenting fractures for medical/legal reasons is necessary or when CT is not available. Radiographs may miss up to 21 % of fractures detectable by CT, and up to 50 % of intracranial injuries in children occur in the absence of fractures [11–13].

Major Findings

Acute fractures present as well-defined, usually *linear*, sharply marginated hypodensities, without sclerotic borders. They are typically unilateral and cross suture lines (Figs. 26.1 and 26.2).

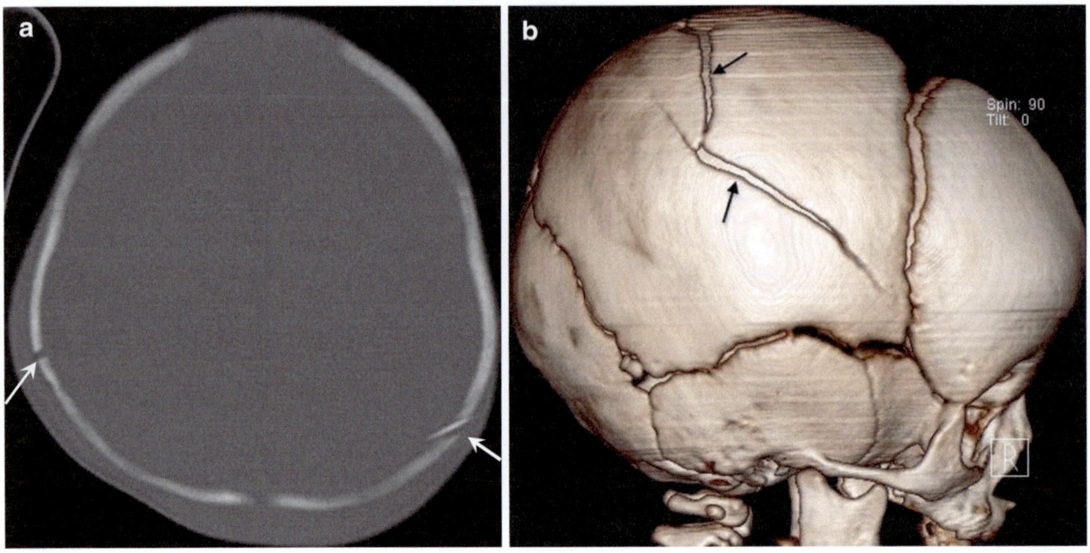

Fig. 26.2 CT of a 5-month-old infant. Axial CT bone window (**a**) shows linear bilateral parietal bone fractures (*arrows*). Right side fracture is aligned, and left side fracture has a small inwardly displaced bone fragment. 3D CT bone reconstruction (**b**) demonstrates typical sharp fracture angulations (*arrows*)

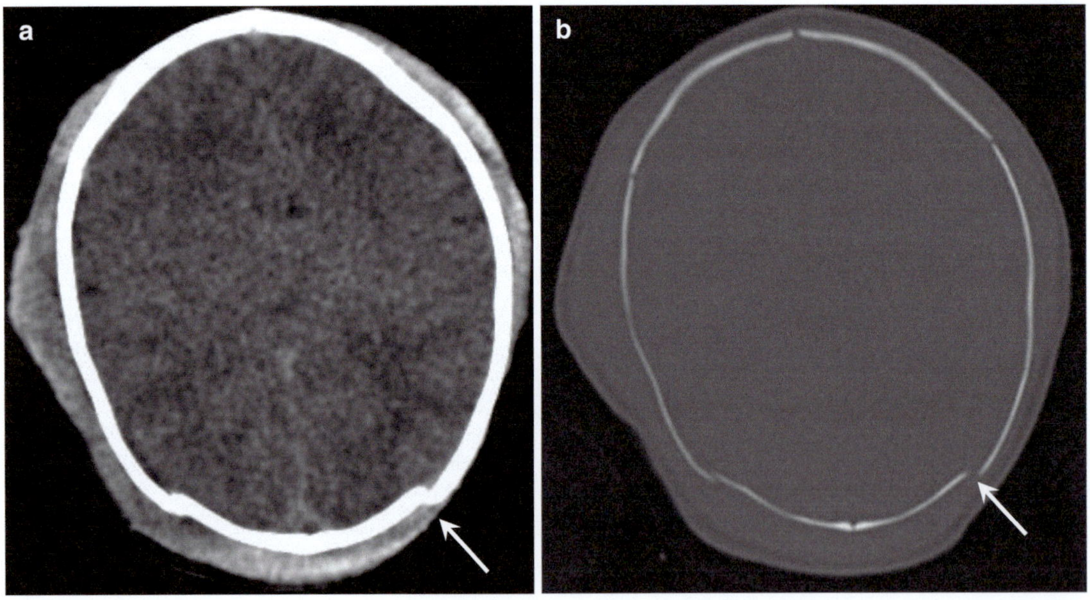

Fig. 26.3 Axial CT in soft tissue (**a**) and bone (**b**) windows of a newborn after traumatic forceps delivery. There is a diffuse thickening and high density of the epicranial soft tissues (a subgaleal hematoma as it crosses sutures) and a slight diastasis of lambdoid sutures (*arrows*) with inward displacement of occipital bone

Diastatic fractures are widened sutures or synchondrosis. In older children and adolescents, a cutoff of 2 mm defines abnormal widening of a suture. In younger children, this threshold is unreliable. As a general rule, the width of all sutures should be harmonious and symmetrical. Anomalies of the underlying or overlying soft tissues can provide clues as the presence of an underlying fracture (Fig. 26.3) [8, 9].

Depressed fractures are typically comminuted, and CT shows inward displacement of bone fragments with the exception of "ping pong" fractures in which inward bone bending occurs without associated true fractures (Figs. 26.4 and 26.5).

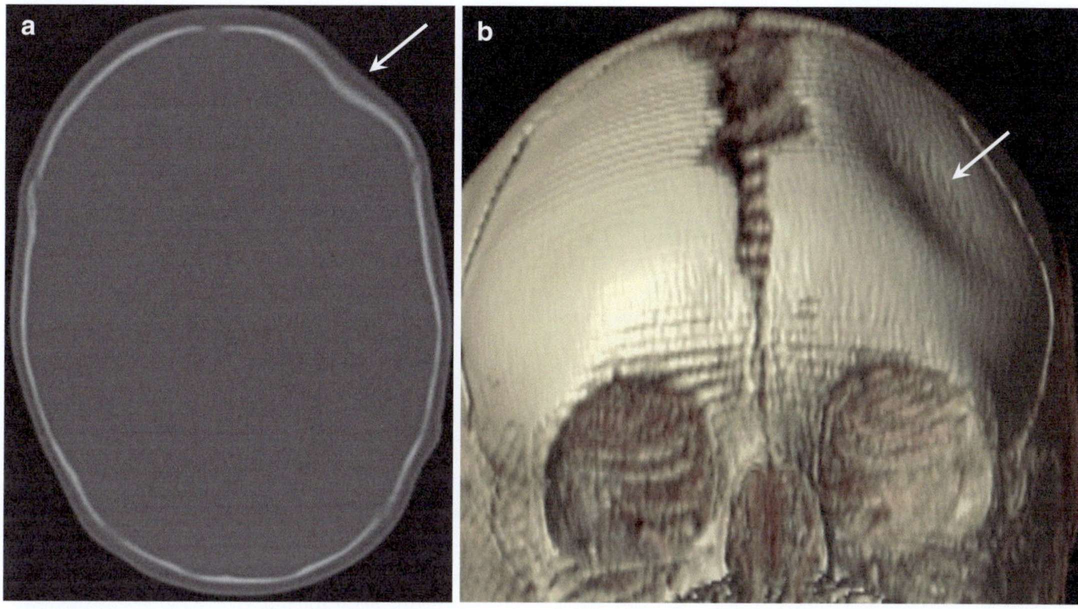

Fig. 26.4 "Ping pong" fracture. Axial CT bone window (**a**) and 3D bone reformation (**b**) depict inward buckling of the left frontal bone without associated true fracture lines (*arrows*)

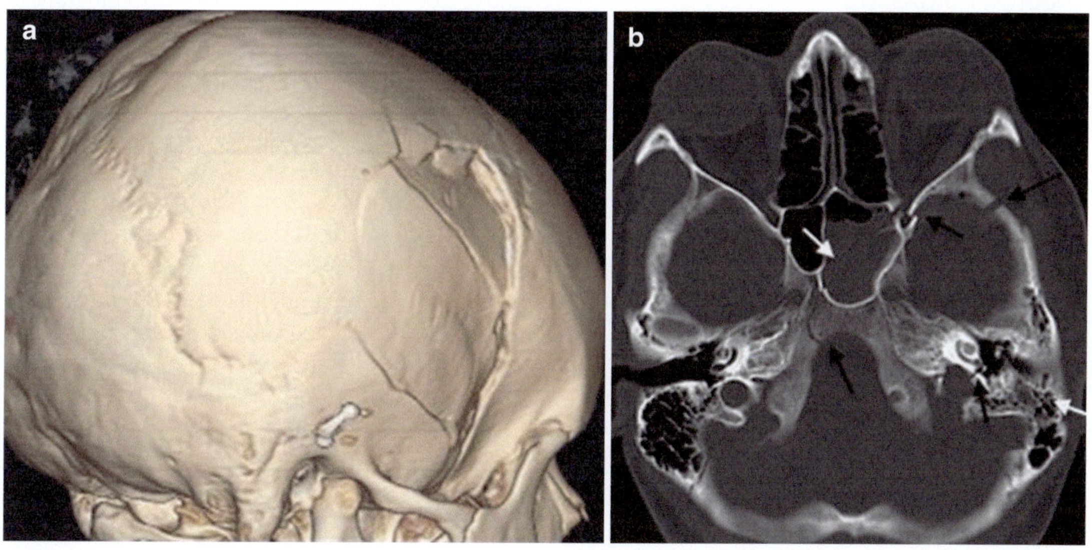

Fig. 26.5 Depressed comminuted skull fracture associated with basilar fracture in an adolescent. CT 3D bone reformation (**a**) shows linear temporal bone fracture with some bone fragments displaced into the skull. Axial CT bone window (**b**) depicts blood filling the left sphenoid sinus and ipsilateral mastoid cells (*white arrows*), secondary to multiple fracture lines at the skull base (*black arrows*)

Growing skull fractures appear as oval areas of bone erosion with smooth, tapered margins. CT detects both the skull defect and the cyst, whose density parallels that of CSF. The cyst may be intracranial, extracranial, or both. In the presence of a growing skull fracture, attempt to classify it according to the type of tissue herniating through the bone defect: type I (leptomeningeal cyst), II (damaged/gliotic brain), or III (porencephalic cyst) (Fig. 26.6) [5].

Opacification of a paranasal sinus and/or the middle ear in a trauma patient can be an indirect sign of *basilar skull fracture* (Fig. 26.5).

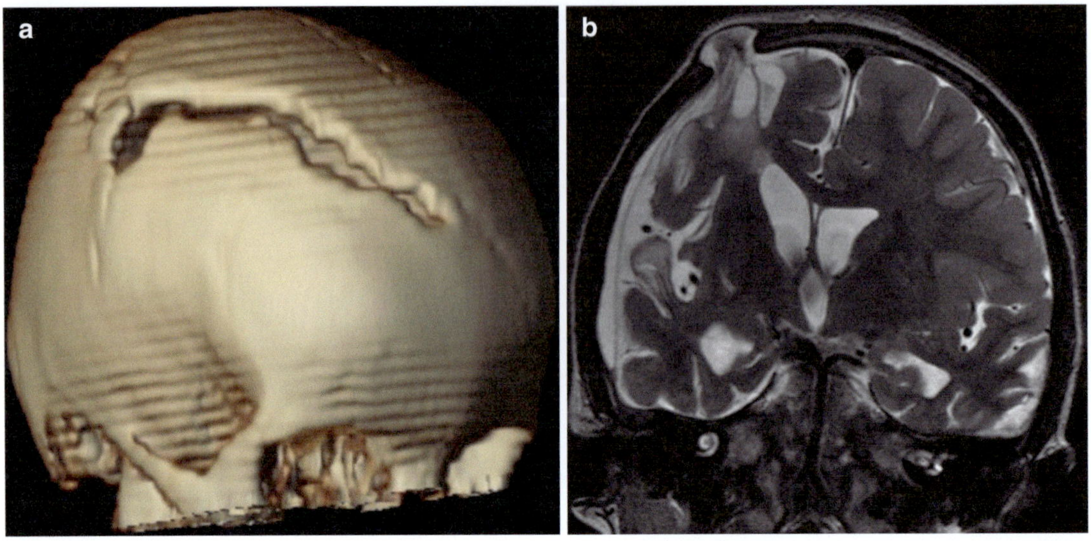

Fig. 26.6 Growing skull fracture in a 5-year-old boy. CT 3D bone reformation (**a**) shows a wide fracture with smooth edges. Coronal T2WI MRI demonstrates damaged brain parenchyma protruding through the bone defect (growing skull fracture type II)

Imaging Follow-Up

Follow-up of skull fractures is usually not needed, unless there are associated intracranial injuries and CSF leaks or a growing fracture is suspected. For the latter, imaging evaluation after 3 and 6 months with radiographs should be considered [5].

Main Differential Diagnosis

Accessory sutures, vascular grooves, and neurovascular channels can be difficult to differentiate from linear fractures.

Sutures evolve with age. In neonates and young children, they have smoothly tapered edges with poor cortical definition. In older children, sutures close and begin to interlock, presenting a "zigzag" pattern, with sclerotic borders. Knowledge of appearance and position of normal sutures and synchondroses is important in distinguishing them from fractures [11]. Their symmetrical distribution is usually helpful in this differentiation.

Vascular grooves are less radiolucent than fractures and tend to be bilateral, have a branching pattern, and are relatively symmetrical. The groove for the posterior branch of the middle meningeal artery should not be confused with a linear skull fracture.

Pathological suture widening associated with increased intracranial pressure (ICP) or secondary tumor infiltration may be confused with diastatic fractures. In raised ICP, suture separation is generalized [8]. Suture infiltration can be secondary to neuroblastoma, leukemia, and lymphoma, and in these cases, the separation is not uniform, and the margins of the affected sutures are indistinct [14].

Lytic calvarial lesions can be mistaken for growing skull fractures. A history of trauma with previous documented skull fracture is the best diagnostic clue.

Tips

- Look at the scalp – overlying soft tissue swelling is a good indicator of the point of impact.
- Scout CT views should be examined if available as some linear skull fractures may be missed on axial CT images. This occurs when fractures are parallel to the

slice angle. Also pay close attention to cervical spine alignment, signs of facial trauma, and foreign bodies.

- Always report the type of fracture and which structures the fracture line crosses, paying special attention to vascular channels (carotid canal in particular) and dural sinuses.
- If a depressed fracture is present, describe the extent of bone displacement and the presence of intracranial complications.
- Look carefully for signs of open fracture, including pneumocephalus and involvement of paranasal sinus or middle ear walls.

References

1. Ryan ME, Palasis S, Saigal G, Singer AD, et al. ACR appropriateness criteria head trauma—child. J Am Coll Radiol. 2014;11:939–47.
2. Schutzman SA, Greenes DS. Pediatric minor head trauma. Ann Emerg Med. 2001;37:65.
3. Gruen A. Surgical management of head trauma. Neuroimaging Clin N Am. 2002;12:339–43.
4. Kraus JF, Fife D, Cox P, et al. Incidence, severity, and external causes of pediatric brain injury. Am J Dis Child. 1986;140:687.
5. Tortori-Donati P, Rossi A. Pediatric neuroradiology. 1st ed. Germany: Springer; 2005.
6. Gean AD. Imaging of head trauma. 1st ed. New York: Raven Press; 1995. p. 27–73.
7. Shane SA, Fuchs SM. Skull fractures in infants and predictors of associated intracranial injury. Pediatr Emerg Care. 1997;13:198.
8. Furuya Y, Edwards MSB, Alpers CE, Tress BM, Ousterhout DK, Norman D. Computerized tomography of cranial sutures part 1: comparison of suture anatomy in children and adults. J Neurosurg. 1984;61:53–8.
9. Mitchell LA, Kitley CA, Armitage TL, et al. Normal sagittal and coronal suture widths by using CT imaging. AJNR Am J Neuroradiol. 2011;32:1801–5.
10. Mohan A, Bowman RM. Birth head trauma. In: Red WH, editor. Youmans neurological surgery. 6th ed. Saunders an imprint of Elsevier Inc. Philadelphia; 2011. p. 2187–91.
11. Kim YI, Cheong JW, Yoon SH. Clinical comparison of the predictive value of the simple skull x-ray and 3 dimensional computed tomography for skull fractures of children. J Korean Neurosurg Soc. 2012;52(6): 528–33.
12. Pinto PS, Poretti A, Meoded A, Tekes A, Huisman TA. The unique features of traumatic brain injury in children. Review of the characteristics of the pediatric skull and brain, mechanisms of trauma, patterns of injury, complications and their imaging findings-part 1. J Neuroimaging. 2012;22(2):e1–17.
13. Nakahara K, Shimizu S, Utsuki S, et al. Linear fractures occult on skull radiographs: a pitfall at radiological screening for mild head injury. J Trauma. 2011;70(1):180–2.
14. Nour-Eldin EA, Abdelmonema O, Tawfika A, Naguiba NN, Klingebield T, Rollee U, Schwabed D, Hartha M, Eltoukhyb MM, Vogla TJ. Pediatric primary and metastatic neuroblastoma: MRI findings pictorial review. Magn Reson Imaging. 2012;30:893–906.

Hydrocephalus in Children

27

Lillian Gonçalves Campos, Rafael Menegatti,
and Leonardo Modesti Vedolin

Abstract

Hydrocephalus can be defined as a process in which the cerebrospinal fluid compartments are actively enlarged at the expense of brain tissue. The clinical presentation depends on the age of the patient. Hydrocephalus is classified as either obstructive, when the drainage pathways is occluded, or communicating, when no clear obstruction can be demonstrated. It can be evaluated using ultrasound, computed tomography, and magnetic resonance imaging. The latter is the best imaging tool to characterize the cause and extension of hydrocephalus and treatment complications. Treatment depends on cause, patient age, and rapidity of onset of the symptoms.

Background

Hydrocephalus (HC) can be defined as a process in which the cerebrospinal fluid (CSF) compartments are actively enlarged at the expense of the brain tissue [1]. In the recent past, HC had a dismal outlook and most often met with mortality [2]. With the advent of an effective shunting device in the 1960s, most children with HC will survive and grow into adulthood, and most adults can be treated [3, 4].

The incidence of hydrocephalus is variable [4, 5]. Older children are more likely to develop HC from tumors, and these remain a possible cause of HC throughout life [6]. The clinical presentation of HC depends on the age of the patient [6]. Before the closing of the sutures (<2 years), the main clinical findings are macrocephaly, conjugate down deviation ("sun setting") of the eyes, developmental delay, and poor feeding [1, 6]. After 2 years of age, neurologic manifestations referable to a primary lesion or intracranial hypertension are common, such as vomiting, headaches, nausea, papilledema, sleepiness, and coma [2, 6].

L.G. Campos, MD, PhD (✉) • R. Menegatti
Postgraduate Program, Clinical Sciences,
Universidade Federal do Rio Grande do Sul,
Rua Ramiro Barcelos, 910 Subsolo 1, Porto Alegre,
RS, Brazil
e-mail: cglillian@yahoo.com.br;
rgmenegatti@yahoo.com.br

L.M. Vedolin, MD, PhD
Hospital de Clinicas e Hospital Moinhos de Vento,
Universidade Federal do Rio Grande do Sul,
Rua Ramiro Barcelos, 910. Subsolo 1, Porto Alegre,
RS, Brazil
e-mail: lvedolin@hcpa.edu.br

R. Hoffmann Nunes et al. (eds.), *Critical Findings in Neuroradiology*,
DOI 10.1007/978-3-319-27987-9_27

HC treatment depends on the cause, patient age, and rapidity of onset of the symptoms [2, 6]. In acute situations, an external ventricular drain is often performed. In subacute or chronic settings, ventriculoperitoneal shunt is the most common form of treatment [2, 6]. An alternative form of treatment in obstructive HC is endoscopic third ventriculostomy. Death from HC still exists, and motor and cognitive sequelae among long-term survivors are frequent and often severe [7, 8].

Key Points

Etiology

Historically, HC has been classified as either obstructive (CSF pathways is occluded) or communicating (no clear obstruction to the CSF flow can be demonstrated) [2, 4]. In obstructive HC, a physical obstruction at or proximal to the fourth ventricular outlet foramina, aqueduct of Sylvius, or foramina of Monro is demonstrated by imaging. It can be congenital or acquired, acute or chronic [2, 9, 10]. The most common acquired cause of HC is tumor, especially posterior fossa neoplasm in children older than 2 years (Fig. 27.1) [2, 4]. Aqueductal stenosis and Chiari II malformation are the most frequent congenital etiologies for HC (Figs. 27.2 and 27.3) [2, 4]. In communicating HC, the free movement of CSF is impaired by arachnoid pathology related to the subarachnoid spaces (Fig. 27.4). Venous hypertension is also a potential cause of HC [2, 4, 11]. Rarely, HC can result from excessive oversecretion of CSF by a choroid plexus papillomas or carcinomas [2]. The most frequent causes are listed in Table 27.1.

Best Imaging Modality

MRI is the best imaging tool to detect and characterize the cause and extension of HC and treat-

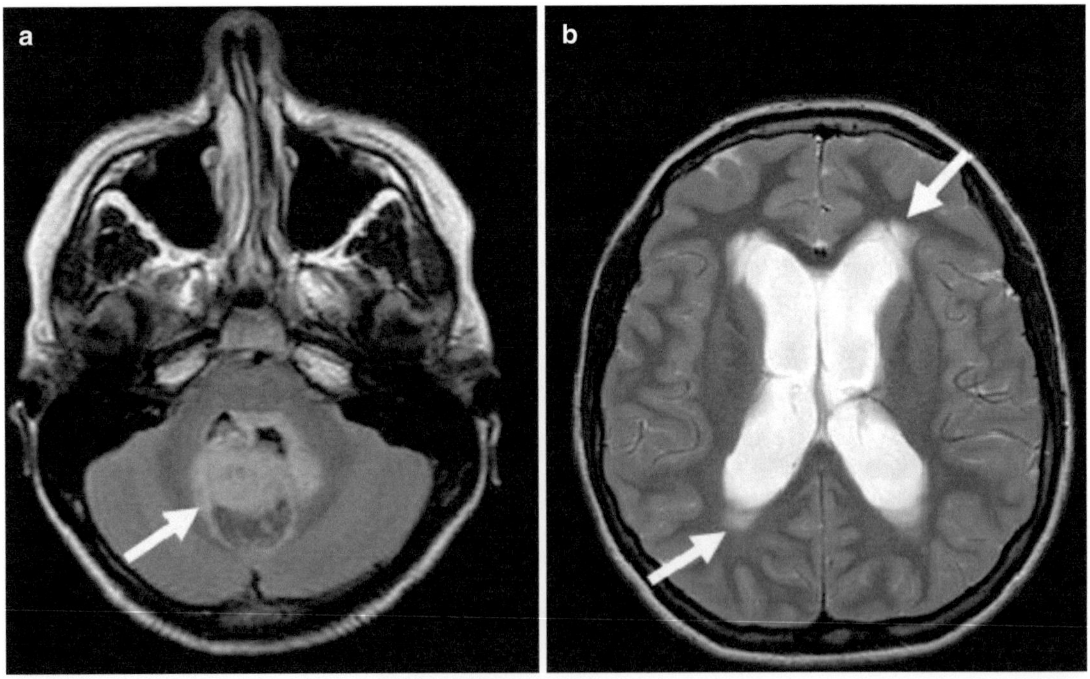

Fig. 27.1 A 7-year-old girl with cerebellar pilocytic astrocytoma and obstructive hydrocephalus. (**a**) Axial FLAIR image shows a hyperintense cerebellar midline lesion that fills the fourth ventricle (*arrow*), surrounded by peritumoral edema. (**b**) Axial T2WI depicts obstructive hydrocephalus with transependymal CSF migration (*arrows*)

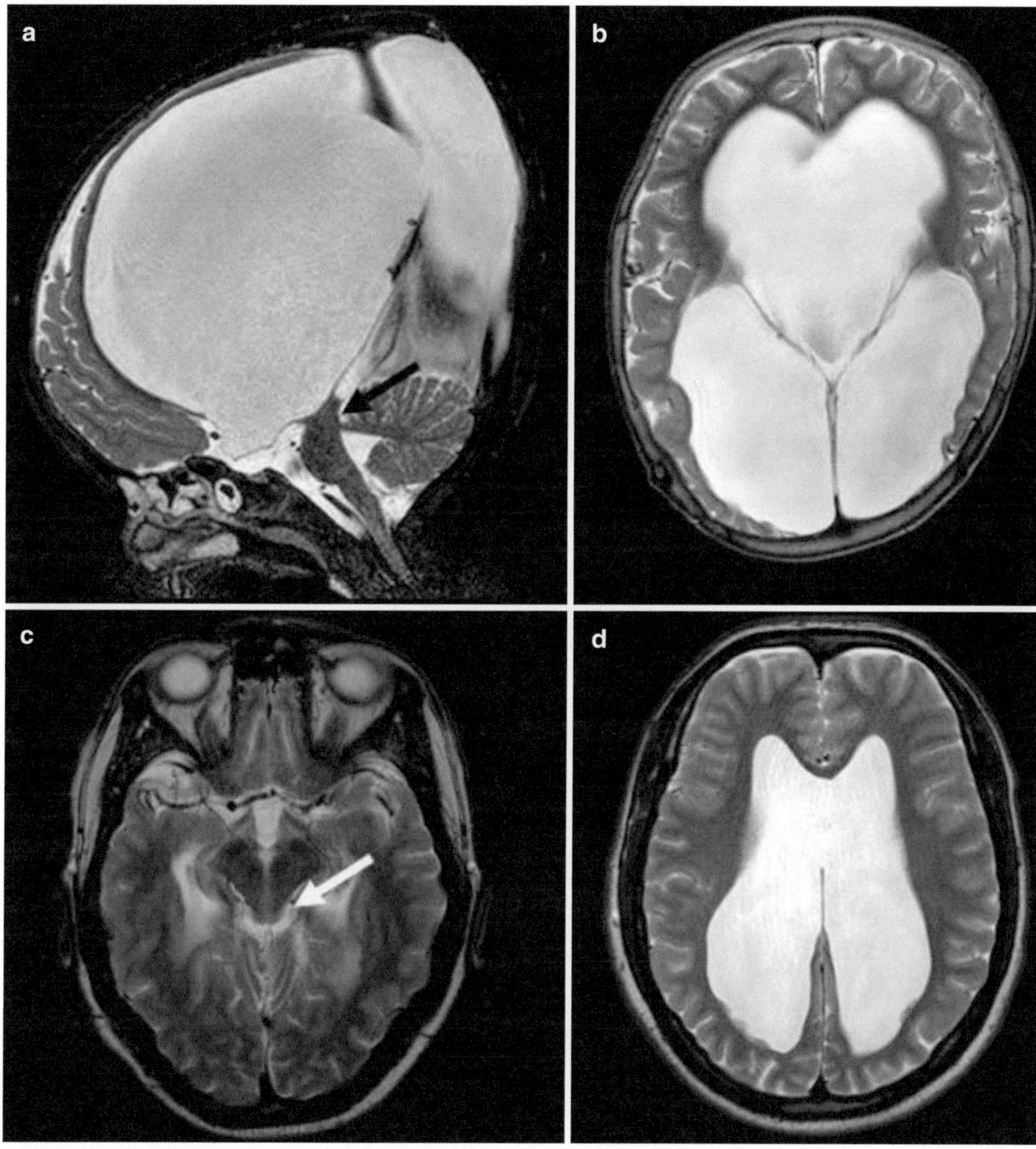

Fig. 27.2 Aqueductal stenosis. (**a**) Sagittal T2WI demonstrates aqueductal stenosis (*arrow*). (**b**) Axial T2WI shows obstructive hydrocephalus with marked enlargement of lateral and third ventricles. Note that the fourth ventricle is not significantly dilated. (**c**, **d**) Axial T2WI reveal a deformed midbrain with no visualization of the aqueduct (*arrow* on **c**) and hydrocephalus (**d**)

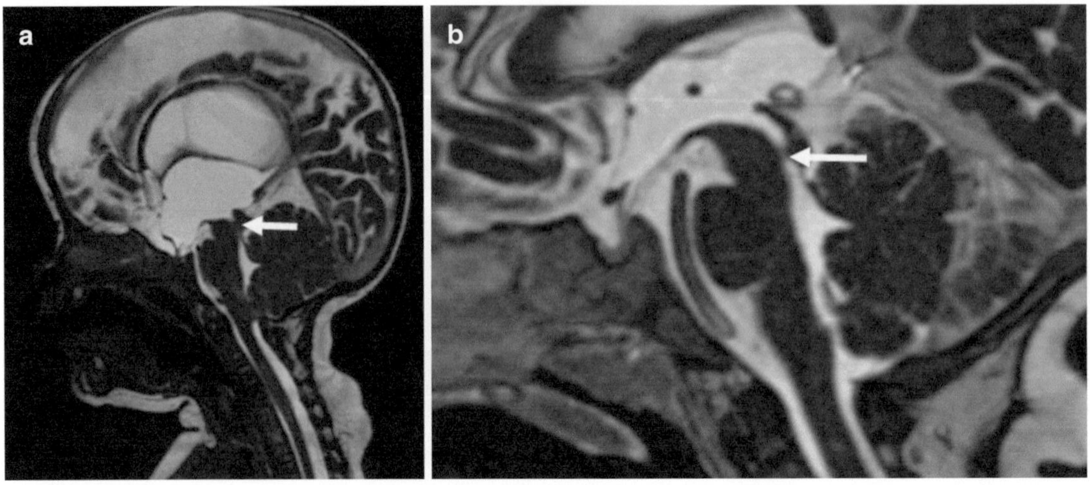

Fig. 27.3 Aqueductal stenosis (**a**, **b**). Sagittal CISS images demonstrates a fibrous band in the aqueduct (*arrows*)

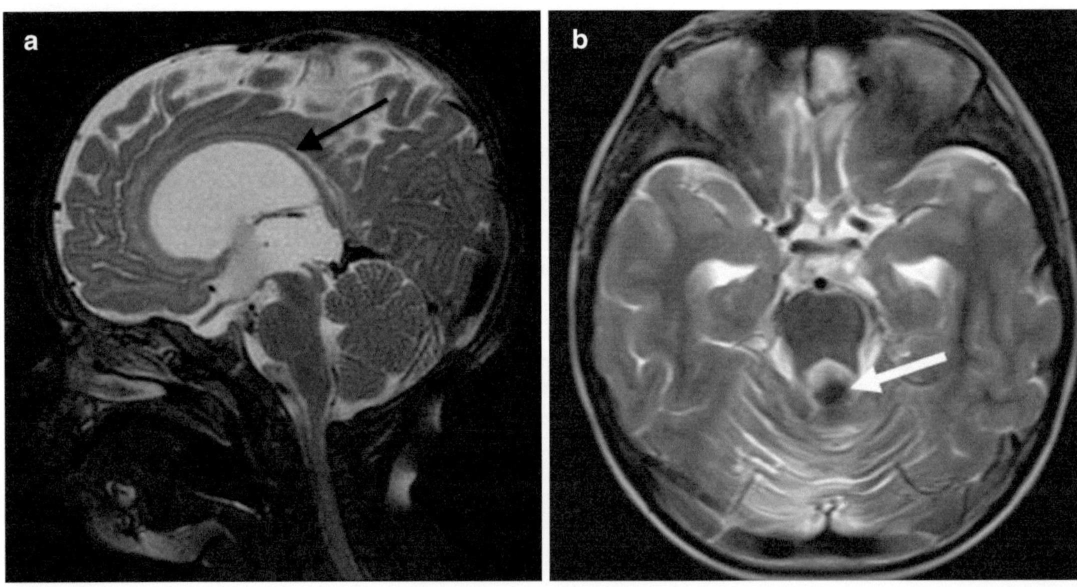

Fig. 27.4 A 2-year-old girl with obstructive hydrocephalus. (**a**) Sagittal T2WI demonstrates dilation of the lateral ventricles. The corpus callosum is stretched, thinned, arched upward (*arrow*). A 10-year-old boy with communicating hydrocephalus. (**b**) Axial T2WI shows the flow-void artifact in the fourth ventricle due to inflow from a patent aqueduct (*arrow*)

ment complications [1, 2, 12]. The recommended initial imaging protocol is as follows [1, 2]:

- T1-weighted image (T1WI) – to assess the anatomy of the ventricular system
- T2-weighted image (T2WI) and fluid-attenuated inversion recovery (FLAIR) image – to diagnose interstitial periventricular edema and flow void within the aqueduct
- Diffusion-weighted image (DWI) – to identify infarcts and infection foci, e.g., ventriculitis
- Gradient echo (GRE) or susceptibility-weighted image (SWI) – to depict hemorrhage, which can be related to previous hemorrhagic events

Table 27.1 Common causes of hydrocephalus

Prematurity (posthemorrhagic hydrocephalus)
Congenital or developmental conditions affecting the brain
Aqueduct stenosis
Dandy–Walker malformation
Arachnoid cysts, interhemispheric cysts
Rhombencephalosynapsis
Chiari II
Brain tumor
Subarachnoid hemorrhage
Congenital or developmental conditions affecting the skull
Crouzon, Pfeiffer syndromes
Achondroplasia
Meningitis

- 3D heavily T2W sequences, such as constructive interference in steady-state imaging (CISS), fast imaging employing steady-state acquisition (FIESTA), and balanced steady-state free precession (BALANCED) – to better delineate the ventricular and extra ventricular anatomy, as well as they are more sensitive to identify obstruction sites [12]
- Postcontrast T1WI – are considered useful in cases of suspected brain tumor and/or infection [1, 2]
- Phase contrast sequence – allow the qualitative and quantitative analysis of CSF flow and may be useful for aqueduct stenosis and normal pressure hydrocephalus [1, 12]

As the fast, simple, and more available imaging modality, CT is the most commonly used technique to evaluate acute HC [13, 14]. In referral centers, low-dose CT scans (reduce ionizing radiation) are performed dedicated to assess the ventricular size in the initial evaluation and for follow-up although recently "fast" MRI using only T2-weighted half-Fourier acquisition single-shot turbo spin-echo (HASTE) (or similar sequences) is being used especially in children who will need multiple assessments throughout their life [15, 16].

Ultrasonography is the primary imaging modality to detect fetal HC. It is noninvasive and can be performed at the bedside [13].

Major Findings

Ventricular System Changes Related to HC

The lateral ventricles (LV) are enlarged and present a round appearance on both axial and coronal images [2, 12]. The ventricular index can be useful to monitor ventricular changes after shunt. The Evans index is the ratio of maximum width of the frontal horns of the lateral ventricles and maximal internal diameter of skull at the same level employed in axial CT and MRI images. The ratio varies with the age and sex; however, when higher than 0.3, it is usually considered increased, consequently, compatible with HC. Periventricular interstitial edema represents a sign of acute HC and manifests as a periventricular band of low density on CT and hyperintensity on T2WI/FLAIR on MRI (Fig. 27.1) [2, 12]. In severe HC, herniation of the ventricular wall (medial atrial diverticula) through the choroidal fissure of the ventricular trigone into the supracerebellar and quadrigeminal cisterns may alter the ventricular anatomy [2, 12].

Ultrasonography is the primary imaging modality to detect fetal HC, showing neonatal ventriculomegaly, which can be quantitatively assessed by the measurement of the atrium of the lateral ventricles (normal – less than 10 mm) [15]. Further assessment may be done with fetal MRI.

Dilatation of the anterior and posterior recesses of the third ventricle (TV) is an important imaging sign of acute HC [2, 12]. On sagittal images, the floor of the TV appears straight, the mamillopontine distance is reduced, and the corpus callosum is stretched (Figs. 27.4 and 27.5) [2, 12]. In severe HC, herniation of the supra-pineal recess of the TV causes compression of the quadrigeminal plate and narrows the aqueduct [2, 12]. Additionally, chronic HC may rupture spontaneously the floor of the TV [2, 12]. The cerebral aqueduct is better demonstrated in the sagittal plane and shows flow void on most T2WI MR sequences [2, 12]. The fourth ventricle usually has a normal or slightly increased diameter in both obstructive and communicating HC (Figs. 27.3 and 27.4) [2, 12].

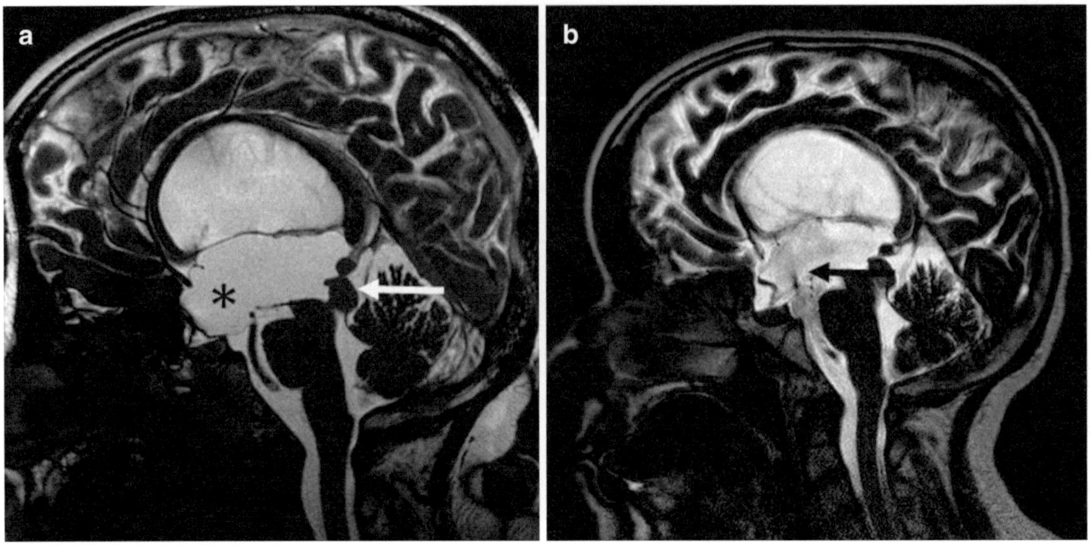

Fig. 27.5 A 7-year-old boy with obstructive hydrocephalus (**a**). Sagittal T2WI demonstrates expansion of the tectal plate resulting in aqueductal stenosis (*arrow*). Observe the downward convexity of the floor (*asterisk*) of the third ventricle (decreased mamillopontine distance) caused by the hydrocephalus. (**b**) The patient was treated with an endoscopic third ventriculostomy. There is a pulsatile jet of CSF passing through the floor of the third ventricle (*arrow*). The downward convexity of the floor of the third ventricle has disappeared

An isolated fourth ventricle (trapped) occurs when the fourth ventricle is hugely dilated in a situation where both its inflow and outflow are blocked [2].

Effacement of the subarachnoid space is a common finding in patients with obstructive HC [2]. When occlusion is cisternal, the cisterns between the occlusion and the ventricular outlets are dilated [1, 2]. 3D heavily T2W sequences can demonstrate linear multiple adhesions/bands of fibrosis within the cisterns as a result of previous hemorrhagic or infectious events [1, 12]. Rarely, a mixed (effaced/dilated) CSF space can appear if specific anatomic/hydrodynamic conditions present, such as in patients with mucopolyssacharidoses [12].

Imaging Signs Related to the Cause of HC

Brain tumors most commonly obstruct the CSF pathways at their narrowest points such as at the foramen of Monro and the cerebral aqueduct (Fig. 27.1) [2]. Aqueductal stenosis by tumor should be distinguished from fibrous tissue caused by acquired or congenital processes (Fig. 27.3). Rarely, tumors of the spine and spinal cord cause HC [12]. In communicating HC, MRI may show signs of extra-axial hemorrhage, meningitis (usually granulomatous) (Fig. 27.6), meningeal carcinomatosis, or venous hypertension [2].

Imaging Signs Related to Treated HC and Resulting Complications

Imaging of shunt malfunction shows increasing ventricular size comparing to previous studies, edema adjacent to the intracerebral segment of the catheter and subgaleal fluid collections [2]. Conventional radiography demonstrates fractures, calcifications, disconnections, or distal catheter migration [2, 12].

Imaging of shunt infection may show irregular leptomeningeal (meningitis) and ventricular (ventriculitis) enhancement and debris on diffusion-weighted imaging [2, 12]. Dural enhancement can persist for months after surgery and should not be confused with a sign of reinfection [2]. Ventricular loculations are pockets of CSF that do not communicate with the shunted ventricular segment and are better demonstrated on 3D heavily T2W sequences [2].

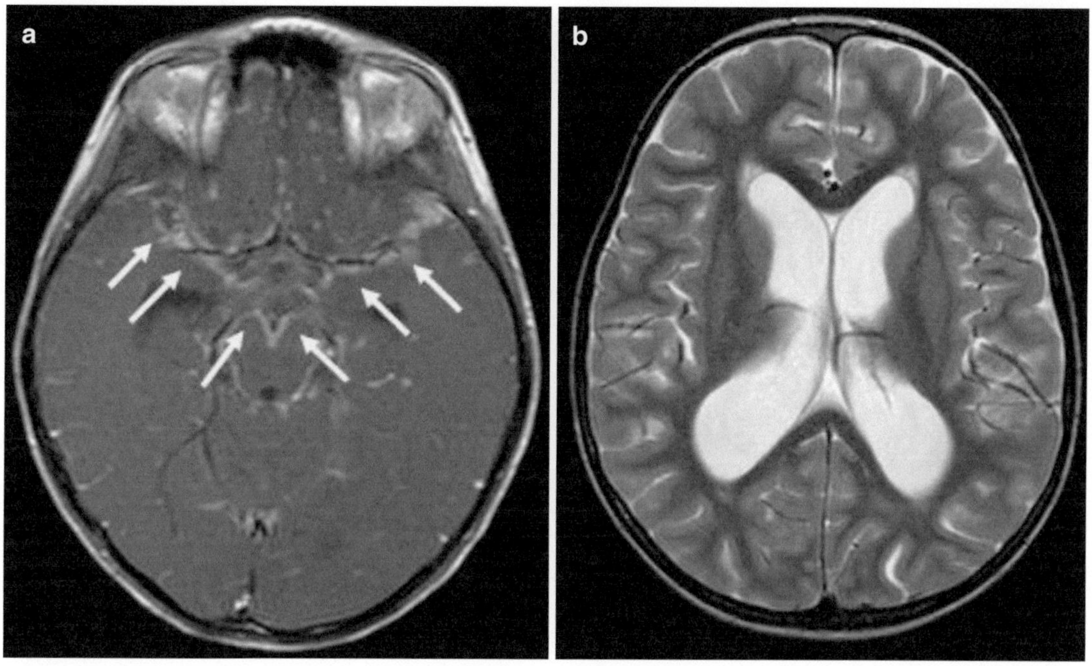

Fig. 27.6 A 6-year-old boy diagnosed with tuberculous meningitis complicated with communicating hydrocephalus. (**a**) Axial postcontrast T1WI shows meningeal enhancement in the basal cisterns (*arrows*), in a typical distribution described in tuberculous meningitis. (**b**) Axial T2WI depicts communicating hydrocephalus

A rapid decrease in the ventricles size after shunting (over-drainage) may lead to subdural hygromas or hematomas [2, 12]. Chronically, a significant number of patients (specially children) present with small slit-like ventricles and a phenomenon called "slit ventricle syndrome" with symptoms of intermittent intracranial hypertension without ventricular dilatation [2, 12].

Small hemorrhages within the ventricular system after shunting are common, but usually self-limited [2]. CSF accumulation within the pleura (ventriculo-pleural shunt), CSF hydrothorax, and ascites can be detected by imaging [2, 12]. Chronic mechanical irritation of the tricuspid valve by an atrial catheter may cause fibrosis, calcification, valvar stenosis, and clot formation [1, 2].

Imaging Follow-Up

Imaging follow-up assesses the integrity of the shunt system, change in ventricular size, and identifies any shunt-related complications [13, 17]. CT is often the preferred technique because of its wide availability, cost, and reduced imaging time [13, 14, 17]. Low-dose CT protocols are recommended and should be an attempt to balance image quality with radiation dose savings [2, 17].

MRI is the best imaging modality for assessment of third ventriculostomy (Fig. 27.5) [2]. A rapid brain MR imaging protocol has been used in pediatric patients with good results, avoiding sedation, and it includes only axial, coronal, and sagittal fast T2-weighted sequences, such as HASTE [2]. MRI is also recommended to access complications of treatment, particularly vascular complications and infection [2].

Conventional radiographs are recommended to detect shunt fracture, calcification, separation at connector locations, or distal catheter migration (Fig. 27.7) [14, 15, 17]. A typical series include frontal and lateral radiography of the head and neck and frontal radiography of the chest and abdomen [14, 15].

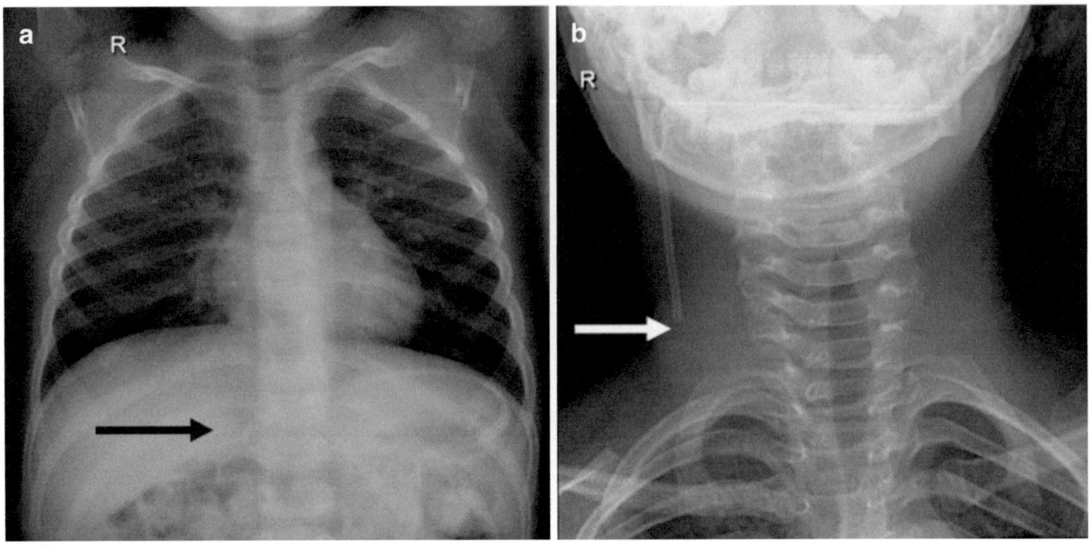

Fig. 27.7 A 10-year-old boy with a ventriculoperitoneal shunt and signs of increased intracranial pressure. (**a**, **b**) Anteroposterior chest (**a**) and cervical spine (**b**) radiographs depict a fracture of the shunt tubing (*arrow* on **b**) and intra-abdominal coiling (*arrow* on **a**) of the distal segment

Main Differential Diagnosis

Brain atrophy: Although rare in children, cerebral atrophy related to degenerative disease can mimic hydrocephalus. In HC the temporal horns are rounded with the choroidal fissures enlarged and the hippocampi compressed and displaced inferomedially [2, 12].

Benign enlargement of the subarachnoid spaces in infants: neurologically normal infants (before 2 years of age) with large CSF spaces, especially around the frontal lobes, frequently presenting with mild macrocephaly [1, 2].

Systemic conditions (ACTH/corticosteroid therapy, dehydration, malnutrition, chemotherapy, and total parental nutrition) can reduce brain volume and increase the CSF spaces, simulating CSF flow disorder [1].

Tips

- Describe imaging findings related to HC (ventriculomegaly, enlargement of the third ventricular recesses and temporal ventricular horns, decreased mamillopontine distance and frontal horn angle, as well as thinning and elevation of the corpus callosum).
- Describe interstitial edema.
- Use imaging findings to distinguish between obstructive from communicant HC (aqueductal flow-void phenomenon and 3D heavily T2W sequences).
- If obstructive, the location and cause of the obstruction should be described.
- Any sign of acute decompensation should be reported.
- Check for complications of HC or shunting.

References

1. Osborne AG. Brain: imaging, pathology and anatomy. 1st ed. Salt Lake City: Amirsys; 2013.
2. Barkovich AJ, Raybaud C. Pediatric neuroimaging. 5th ed. Philadelphia: Lippincott Williams and Wilkins; 2012.
3. Demerdash A, Singh R, Loukas M, Tubbs RS. A historical glimpse into treating childhood hydrocephalus. Childs Nerv Syst. 2015:1–3 [Epub ahead of print]. doi:10.1007/s00381-015-2652-3.

4. Green AL, Pereira EAC, Kelly D, Richards PG, Pike MG. The changing face of paediatric hydrocephalus: a decade's experience. J Clin Neurosci. 2007;14: 1049–54.
5. Garton HJL, Piatt JH. Hydrocephalus. Pediatr Clin N Am. 2004;51:305–25.
6. Corns R, Matin A. Hydrocephalus. Neurosurgery. 2012;30:142–8.
7. Vinchon M, Baroncini M, Delestret I. Adult outcome of pediatric hydrocephalus. Childs Nerv Syst. 2012;28:847–54.
8. Vinchon M, Rekate H, Kulkarni AV. Pediatric hydrocephalus outcomes: a review. Fluids Barriers CNS. 2012;9:18.
9. Rekate HL. The definition and classification of hydrocephalus: a personal recommendation to stimulate debate. Cerebrospinal Fluid Res. 2008;5:1–7.
10. Rekate HL. A contemporary definition and classification of hydrocephalus. Semin Pediatr Neurol. 2009;16:9–15.
11. Kestle JRW. Pediatric hydrocephalus: current management. Neurol Clin N Am. 2003;21:883–95.
12. Tortori-Donati. Pediatric neuroradiology brain. 1st ed. Springer-Verlag Berlin Heidelberg, 2005.
13. Albright AL, Pollack IF. Principles and practice of pediatric neurosurgery. 2nd ed. New York: Thieme Medical Publications; 2008.
14. Randomized trial of cerebrospinal fluid shunt valve design in pediatric hydrocephalus. Neurosurgery 1998:43:294–303.
15. Goeser CD, Mc Leary MS, Young LW. Diagnostic imaging of ventriculoperitoneal shunt malfunctions and complications. RadioGraphics. 1998;18:635–51.
16. Browd SR, Gottfried ON, Ragel BT, Kestle JRW. Failure of cerebrospinal fluid shunts: part II: overdrainage, loculation, and abdominal complications. Pediatr Neurol. 2006;34:171–6.
17. Wallace AN, McConathy J, Menias CO, Bhalla S, Wippold FJ. Imaging evaluation of CSF shunts. Am J Radiol. 2014;202:38–53.

Retained Foreign Bodies

28

Heitor Castelo Branco Rodrigues Alves,
Antônio José da Rocha,
and Renato Hoffmann Nunes

Abstract

Foreign bodies may be ingested, inserted into a body cavity, or deposited into the body by traumatic or iatrogenic injuries. Retained foreign bodies following surgical procedures are a clinically significant problem. The real incidence is unknown since intracranial foreign bodies are seldom reported and the majority consist of materials intentionally left in the cranium. Clinical manifestations may be variable such as acute infections, late-onset seizures, or they remain clinically silent for years. The major role of the radiologist is to recognize these foreign bodies and their potential complications.

Background

Foreign bodies may be ingested, inserted into a body cavity, or deposited into the body by a traumatic or iatrogenic injury [1]. Retained foreign bodies (RFBs) following surgical procedures are a clinically significant problem [2]. The terms *gossypiboma*, *textiloma*, *gauzoma*, and *muslinoma* have been used to describe surgical foreign bodies. However, they should be reserved for those lesions produced by retained cotton surgical sponges accidentally left in the surgical bed. Synthetic reabsorbable and nonreabsorbable materials have now largely replaced cotton and are either inadvertently or deliberately left behind during surgery. Even though the real incidence is unknown, cases of intracranial foreign bodies are seldom reported, and the majority consists in materials intentionally left in the cra-

H.C.B.R. Alves, MD (✉)
Division of Neuroradiology, Hospital Santa Casa de Misericórdia de São Paulo,
Rua Dr. Cesário Motta Junior 112, Vila Buarque, Sao Paulo 01221-020, SP, Brazil
e-mail: heitor.cbra@gmail.com

A.J. da Rocha, MD, PhD
Division of Neuroradiology, Hospital Santa Casa de Misericórdia de São Paulo,
Rua Dr. Cesário Motta Junior 112, Vila Buarque, Sao Paulo 01221-020, SP, Brazil

Division of Neuroradiology, Grupo Fleury,
Rua Dr. Cesário Motta Junior 112, Vila Buarque, Sao Paulo 01221-020, Brazil
e-mail: antonio.rocha@grupofleury.com.br

R. Hoffmann Nunes, MD
Division of Neuroradiology, Santa Casa de São Paulo, São Paulo, Brazil
e-mail: renatohn@hotmail.com

R. Hoffmann Nunes et al. (eds.), *Critical Findings in Neuroradiology*,
DOI 10.1007/978-3-319-27987-9_28

nium, such as wrappings to correct a cerebral aneurysms (*muslinomas*) and/or hemostatic agents [3].

Penetrating head injuries with RFBs are also rare and mainly reported in transorbital penetrating injuries, mostly with wooden (branches, arrows, chopsticks, or pencils), metal (needles or bullets), stones, or fireworks [4, 5].

Contact with a nonphysiological surface leads to local foreign body reaction, which in the central nervous system (CNS) consists mainly of activated glial cells – microglia and astrocytes – characterized by hypertrophy (increase in volume and processes), proliferation (increase in cell number), and chronic inflammatory reactions [6].

Clinical manifestations may be variable such as late-onset seizures [5] or patients remain clinically silent for years [7]. Late-onset seizures can be induced secondary to progressive granulomatous changes or delayed abscess formation and, in cases of penetrating head injuries, secondary to gradual gliosis [8]. Penetrating head injuries commonly have also higher rates of acute infections (almost 70 %) [4] and may be associated with meningitis, cerebritis, and brain abscess.

Key Points

Etiology

Surgery: The hemostatic agents most widely used in contemporary neurosurgical practice include reabsorbable and nonreabsorbable materials. Reabsorbable agents, such as oxidized cellulose, gelatin foam, and microfibrillar collagen, are deliberately left in the CNS to prevent rebleeding after surgical closure and may induce an inflammatory reaction. Nonreabsorbable materials include cotton pledgets and cloth (such as muslin), as well as synthetic rayon hemostats (cottonoids and kites), the latter are removed prior to surgical closure. Muslin which is used to reinforce cerebral aneurysms is left in place [9]. A limited inflammatory reaction secondary to the aneurysm wrapping material is desirable since it is associated with media and adventitia thickening that theoretically results in a reduced likelihood of aneurysm rupture. However, exuberant inflammatory reaction can extend beyond the aneurysm into the adjacent brain parenchyma and produce symptoms [10]. Nonreabsorbable agents have greater occurrence of foreign body reaction following intracranial procedures; however, when compared to those used in general surgery, this type of reaction has been reported less frequently [3, 9].

Endovascular procedures: There are recent isolated reports of foreign body emboli after diagnostic and therapeutic cerebral angiograms [11–14]. Clinically silent emboli are a common known complication of diagnostic cerebral angiograms, but the first foreign body reaction after endovascular therapy (EVT) was published by Fealey et al. [14], and its incidence has increased in recent years likely because magnetic resonance imaging (MRI) and magnetic resonance angiography (MRA) are replacing the use of digital subtraction angiography (DSA) for imaging follow-up [12]. As most of these lesions are restricted to the accessed vascular territory and located in the cortical and subcortical regions and it is reasonable to believe that these lesions represent an embolic phenomenon. Pathology findings of granuloma and microabscess formation suggest a foreign body reaction caused by shedding of hydrophilic catheter coating into the bloodstream [12, 14]. The interval of 3–4 days between coiling and symptom onset as well as the abrupt response to steroid in some patients suggests delayed hypersensitivity to the material at the time of the intervention. There is evidence suggesting that a hypersensitivity reaction related to nickel, possibly in combination with other factors like procedural or genetic ones, may be the underlying causes [11, 15].

Trauma: Patients with RFBs after head trauma are at a higher risk for secondary morbidity and mortality [16]. The most common routes by which foreign bodies penetrate the cranium are through the orbital roof and the superior orbital fissure [17, 18]. Since the bones comprising the orbit are relatively thin, a straight external force easily penetrates them, and foreign bodies may reach the frontal or temporal lobes. RFBs due to transcranial penetrations are rarely reported, most are wood and occur in children after falling down. The risk of late complications increases with organic wooden objects and they frequently lead to infections [4, 5]. Therefore, it is thought that RFBs should be removed at the time of injury if possible or the patient should be monitored for life [5].

Best Imaging Modality

Computerized tomography (CT) is the modality of choice for RFBs detection. Nonreabsorbable surgical sponges have radiopaque filaments readily visible on CT scans [7]. Metal and graphite are often recognized by their characteristic increased attenuation, whereas wood CT appearance is variable but generally appears as air on soft tissue windows and has a striate appearance on bone windows [18]. MRI may be complementary to CT to identify foreign bodies, but it should not be performed if a metallic foreign body is suspected [17]. Susceptibility-weighted imaging (SWI) plays an important role in the differential diagnosis and has higher sensitivity than gradient-echo (GRE) T2-weighted images (T2WI) in detecting most RFBs.

MRA is indicated for muslin-induced foreign bodies after aneurysm treatment and may cause vascular narrowings and infarctions.

Advanced imaging, such as MR perfusion and MR spectroscopy, should be included in the protocol as they might be useful to differentiate tumor from infection/inflammation secondary to RFBs [3].

Major Findings

Surgically placed foreign bodies present with nonspecific neuroimaging findings. Reabsorbable hemostatic agents may be difficult to recognize on CT, especially in the early postoperative phase because of the high density of surrounding blood, whereas most nonreabsorbable surgical sponges have radiopaque filaments readily visible on CT scans and radiographs [7]. MRI displays susceptibility effects on GRE and SWI arising from the RFBs [7, 9]. There are two main types of inflammatory reaction related to RFBs (Table 28.1): one characterized by exudation, resulting in abscess formation typically characterized by a focal area of hyperintense signal on T2WI, restricted diffusion, and rim enhancement (Fig. 28.1) [10]). Alternatively, there can be an aseptic fibrous tissue reaction that does not show restricted diffusion, characterized by a solid-appearing material within the surgical cavity that may present nodular enhancement (Fig. 28.2) [3, 9].

Enhancing lesions following EVT are usually subcortical, multiple, and small with nodular enhancement and perilesional edema in the vascular territory of the previously catheterized artery. Rim enhancement occurs in lesions larger

Table 28.1 Foreign body reaction pathologic and imaging correlation

Foreign body reaction		
	Exudative response	Aseptic fibrous reaction
Pathology	Abscess	Adhesion Encapsulation Granulomatous
Clinical manifestation	Acute	Subacute/chronic
Imaging	Ring enhancement Restricted on DWI	Nodular enhancement DWI – variable

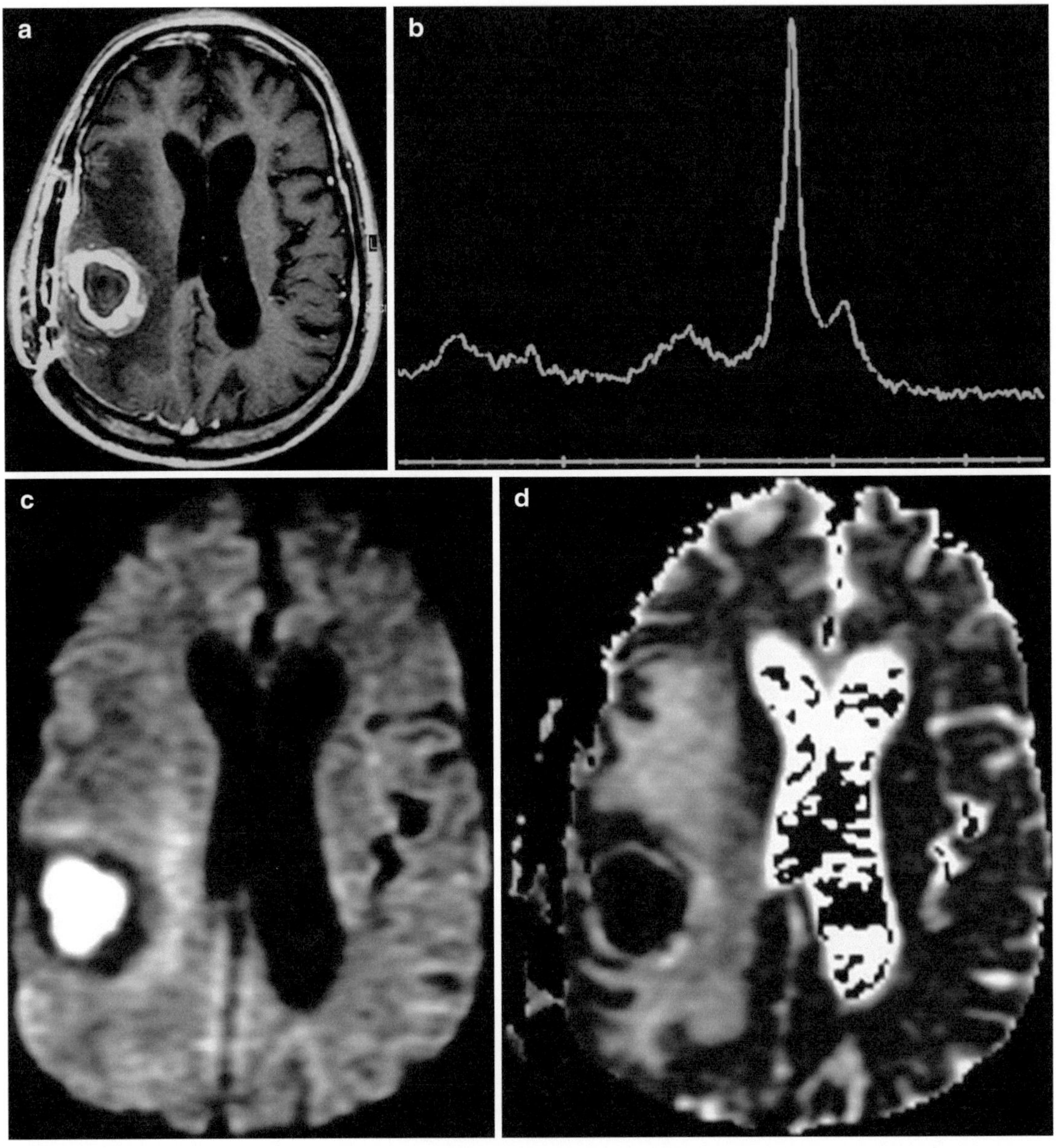

Fig. 28.1 Exudative reaction to a nonreabsorbable RFB. A 42-year-old patient presenting with reduced level of consciousness and seizures after craniotomy. There is a focal rim-enhancement area in the right parietal lobe (**a**). MR spectroscopy revealed only a lipid/lactate peak (**b**) and high signal on DWI (**c**) and restricted ADC (**d**) is observed. Surgery confirmed an abscess secondary to a surgical sponge

than 5 mm, and they may show focal restricted diffusion. Some of the lesions may also show susceptibility effect. The median time from procedure to lesion detection on MRI is approximately 2 months, and the number of lesions usually decreases on follow-up studies (Fig. 28.3) [12, 14].

Penetrating orbital or cranial injuries should be first evaluated with CT when RFBs are suspected. While CT detects metallic and graphite objects, detection of wooden foreign bodies may be challenging. Dry wood, which often displays low attenuation, should not be dismissed as air or artifact, and to accomplish this, bone windows

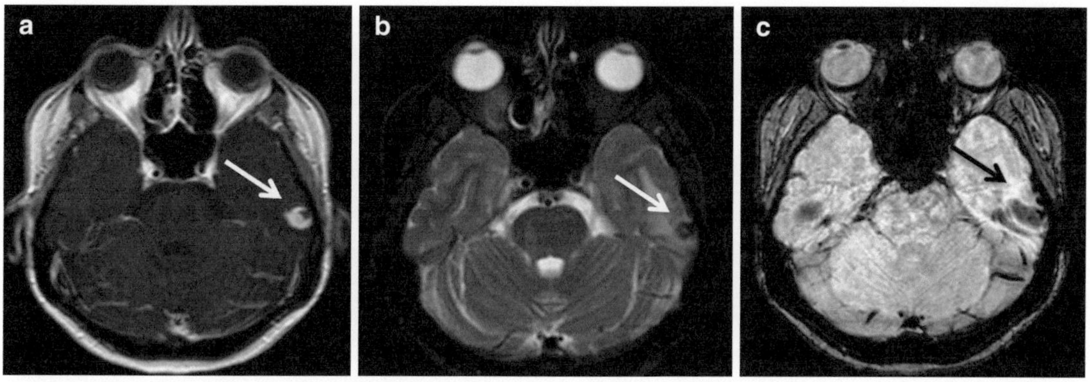

Fig. 28.2 Aseptic fibrous tissue reaction. Patient presented with seizure 3 months after cholesteatoma resection and inadvertent violation of the tegmen tympani. There is a granuloma (*arrows*) characterized by focal area of nodular enhancement (**a**) and hypointensity on T2WI (**b**), which is better seen on SWI (**c**). RFB must be suspected when late-onset seizures develop after surgery

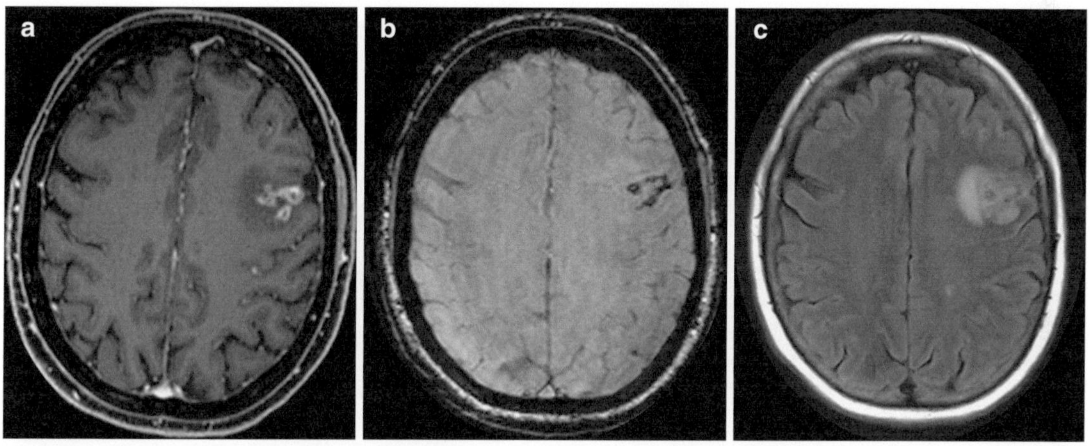

Fig. 28.3 Enhancing lesions after EVT. Patient presenting headaches and incoordination of the right hand 19 days after EVT for an aneurysm of left M2 segment. Multiple small subcortical lesions are noticed after intravenous gadolinium administration (**a**). Most of them show nodular enhancement, but the larger lesions exhibited a ring enhancement. There are susceptibility artifacts on SWI (**b**) and perilesional edema on FLAIR (**c**)

are needed (Fig. 28.4). In subacute and chronic stages, wooden objects absorb water, and their density approaches that of brain tissues. In these cases, MRI can show secondary gliosis, progressive granulomatous changes, and delayed abscess formation [4, 5, 17, 18].

Imaging Follow-Up

Imaging within 24–48 h after most neurosurgical procedures is a routine practice. RFB that are not removed should be monitored for life. Late-onset seizures, focal symptoms, or recurrent infections in a patient with a neurosurgical antecedent or penetrating trauma are suspicious for delayed inflammatory reaction from RFBs [3].

Main Differential Diagnosis

Recurrent tumor or even unrelated primary or metastatic neoplasms can display nodular enhancement after intracranial surgery; however, they usually have high relative cerebral blood volume (rCBV) values on MR perfusion studies

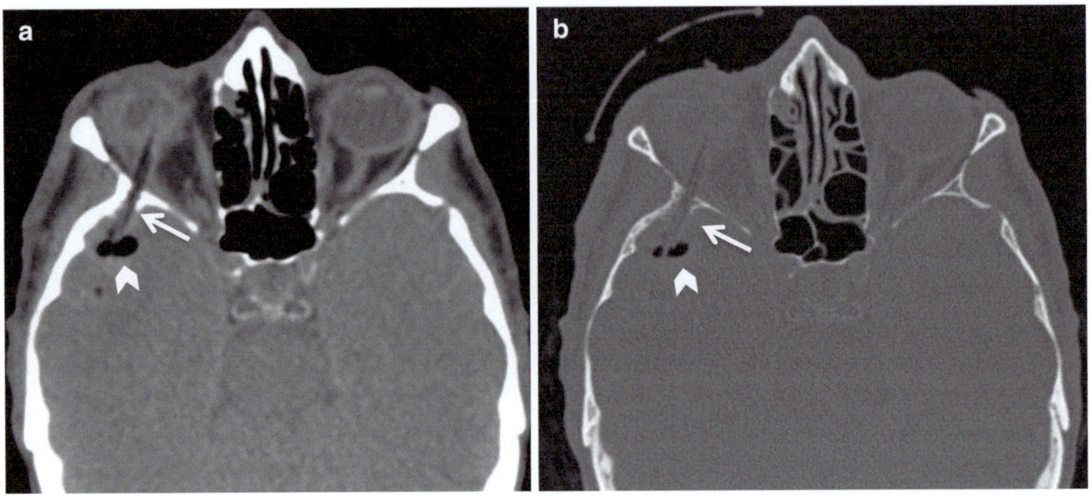

Fig. 28.4 Wooden retained foreign body in the temporal lobe. Wood (*arrow*) in acute stages has low attenuation (**a**) and should not be misdiagnosed as air (*arrow head*). Bone window (**b**) is helpful to differentiate them since air will remain with low attenuation and wood of intermediate density with internal striations

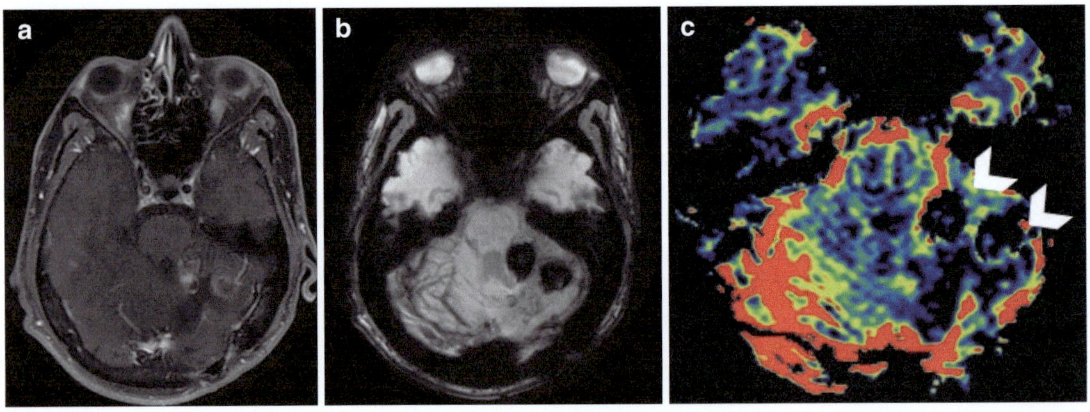

Fig. 28.5 RFB 5 years after pilocytic astrocytoma resection. There are focal areas of nodular and ring enhancement on the left cerebellar hemisphere (**a**). Susceptibility artifacts (**b**) and low rCBV area on perfusion maps are observed (*arrowheads*, **c**), helping to distinguish RFB from recurrent/residual tumor. Surgery confirmed an aseptic fibrous reaction due to nonreabsorbable surgical material

and may show an infiltrative pattern. Susceptibility artifacts within the enhanced area and low rCBV values are suggestive of RFBs in the correct clinical setting (Fig. 28.5) [9, 19].

Radiation necrosis usually shows low rCBV values, similar to RFBs. However, absence of susceptibility effects in the white matter and the presence of a "Swiss cheese" pattern of enhancement favor the diagnosis of radionecrosis [20, 21].

Abscesses not related to RFBs can be indistinguishable from that induced by them. In these cases, the presence of a solid material inside the abscess cavity as well as a serpentine or irregular susceptibility abnormality on GRE or SWI may help one to suspect RFBs [7, 9].

There are rare reports of brain abscesses after aneurysm coiling, and all patients presented with positive biomarkers for CNS infection or pathogens were isolated on cerebral spinal fluid cultures. Focal areas with restricted diffusion may be observed after cerebral angiograms and neuroendovascular procedures, but they disappear in 2 weeks follow-up studies [12].

Tips

- Nonreabsorbable materials often show a characteristic hyperattenuated serpentine configuration on CT and radiographs.
- Clinical manifestations and size progression in RFBs may be subtle. Stable masses or persisting enhancing lesions (over 6 weeks) after trauma or surgical procedures, especially, when displaying susceptibility effect should raise concern for RFB.
- Dry wood displays CT low attenuation on routine brain windows and can mimic air on bone windows, but internal striations suggest the diagnosis [22].
- Persistent enhancing lesions with an embolic distribution after EVT should raise concern for foreign bodies.

References

1. Hunter TB, Taljanovic MS. Foreign bodies1. RadioGraphics. 2003;23(3):731–57.
2. Whang G, Mogel GT, Tsai J, Palmer SL. Left behind: unintentionally retained surgically placed foreign bodies and how to reduce their incidence— pictorial review. Am J Roentgenol. 2009;193(6_supplement):S79–89.
3. Peloquin P, Vannemreddy PSSV, Watkins LM, Byrne RW. Intracranial cotton ball gossypiboma mimicking recurrent meningioma: report of a case with literature review for intentional and unintentional foreign body granulomas. Clin Neurol Neurosurg. 2012;114(7):1039–41.
4. No Authors? A case of delayed brain abscess due to a retained intracranial wooden foreign body: a case report and review of the last 20 years. Acta Neurochir (Wien). 2004;146(8):1–4.
5. Chunhua Q, Qun W. A late-onset seizure due to a retained intracranial foreign body—pencil lead. J Craniofac Surg. 2014;25(2):e109–10.
6. Moshayedi P, Ng G, Kwok JCF, Yeo GSH, Bryant CE, Fawcett JW, et al. The relationship between glial cell mechanosensitivity and foreign body reactions in the central nervous system. Biomaterials. 2014; 35(13):3919–25. Elsevier Ltd.
7. Kim AK, Lee EB, Bagley LJ, Loevner LA. Retained surgical sponges after craniotomies: imaging appearances and complications. Am J Neuroradiol. 2009; 30(6):1270–2.
8. Annegers JF, Hauser WA, Coan SP, Rocca WA. A population-based study of seizures after traumatic brain injuries. N Engl J Med. 1998;338(1):20–4.
9. Ribalta T, McCutcheon IE, Neto AG, Gupta D, Kumar AJ, Biddle DA, et al. Textiloma (gossypiboma) mimicking recurrent intracranial tumor. Arch Pathol Lab Med. 2004;128(7):749–58.
10. Slater L-A, Chandra RV, Holt M, Danks A, Chong W. Long-term MRI findings of muslin-induced foreign body granulomas after aneurysm wrapping. Interv Neuroradiol. 2014;20(1):67.
11. Lobotesis K, Mahady K, Ganesalingam J, Amlani S, Carlton-Jones L, Davies NWS, et al. Coiling-associated delayed cerebral hypersensitivity: is nickel the link? Neurology. 2015;84(1):97–9.
12. Cruz JP, Marotta T, O'Kelly C, Holtmannspotter M, Saliou G, Willinsky R, et al. Enhancing brain lesions after endovascular treatment of aneurysms. AJNR Am J Neuroradiol. 2014;35(10):1954–8.
13. Minks D, Briley D, Schulz U, Küker W. Suspected cerebral foreign body granuloma following endovascular treatment of intracranial aneurysm: imaging features. Neuroradiology. 2014;57(1):71–3.
14. Fealey ME, Edwards WD, Giannini C, Piepgras DG, Cloft H, Rihal CS. Complications of endovascular polymers associated with vascular introducer sheaths and metallic coils in 3 patients, with literature review. Am J Surg Pathol. 2008;32(9):1310–6.
15. Majersik JJ. Comment: nickel-associated delayed cerebral hypersensitivity – recognition is key. Neurology. 2014;84(1):97–7.
16. Fischer BR, Yasin Y, Holling M, Hesselmann V. Good clinical practice in dubious head trauma – the problem of retained intracranial foreign bodies. Int J Gen Med. 2012;5:899–902.
17. Matsumoto S, Hasuo K, Mizushima A, Mihara F, Fukui M, Shirouzu T, et al. Intracranial penetrating

injuries via the optic canal. AJNR Am J Neuroradiol. 1998;19(6):1163–5.

18. Aulino JM, Gyure KA, Morton A, Cole JW. Temporal lobe intraparenchymal retained foreign body from remote orbital trauma. AJNR Am J Neuroradiol. 2005;26(7):1855–7.
19. Barajas RF Jr, Chang JS, Segal MR, Parsa AT. Differentiation of recurrent glioblastoma multiforme from radiation necrosis after external beam radiation therapy with dynamic susceptibility-weighted contrast. Radiology. 2009;253(2):486–96.
20. Miyatake S-I, Nonoguchi N, Furuse M, Yoritsune E, Miyata T, Kawabata S, et al. Pathophysiology, diagnosis, and treatment of radiation necrosis in the brain. Neurol Med Chir (Tokyo). 2015;55(1):50–9.
21. Kumar AJ, Leeds NE, Fuller GN, Van Tassel P, Maor MH, Sawaya RE, et al. Malignant gliomas: MR imaging spectrum of radiation therapy- and chemotherapy-induced necrosis of the brain after treatment. Radiology. 2000;217(2):377–84.
22. Tasneem K, Concannon ES, Abulkhir A, Ryan RS, Barry K. Radiolucent wooden foreign body masquerading as a depressed skull fracture. BMJ Case Rep. 2011; 2011 (dec 20), published online. doi:10.1136/bcr.10.2011.4964.

Part II

Head and Neck

Preseptal Orbital Cellulitis in Children

29

Carlos Jorge da Silva

Abstract

Preseptal cellulitis defines infections limited to the skin and subcutaneous tissues of the eyelid anterior to the orbital septum. Clinically, patients present with erythema and swelling of the eyelid. Although imaging of an isolated preseptal cellulitis is usually not clinically indicated, it can be useful in patients in whom the clinical differentiation of preseptal and postseptal cellulitis is not possible or when the diagnosis is unclear. Contrast-enhanced computed tomography and magnetic resonance imaging demonstrate the anterior location of edema. The prognosis is generally excellent if early diagnosis and correct antibiotic treatment is given.

Background

Preseptal cellulitis is defined as an infection limited to the skin and subcutaneous tissues of the eyelid anterior to the orbital septum [1].

Historically, most cases of preseptal cellulitis are believed to be secondary to paranasal sinus infection (most commonly ethmoidal), typically in children. Other causes include skin trauma, insect bites, as well as the spread of other infections such as from an acute hordeolum and dacryocystitis [1–4].

Clinically, patients present with erythema and swelling of the eyelid. There is no proptosis, chemosis, or ocular motility limitation. At a more advanced stage, chemosis may occur. It is unusual for a preseptal infection to traverse the orbital septum and result in postseptal cellulitis [1–4].

Oral antibiotics are the therapy of choice when the infection remains preseptal in location. Severe infection may require intravenous antibiotics and surgical drainage [3].

Prognosis is generally excellent if early diagnosis is made and correct antibiotic treatment is given. Complications that may result include preseptal abscess, postseptal cellulitis, postseptal abscess, thrombophlebitis of the superior ophthalmic vein and of the cavernous sinus [1–3].

C.J. da Silva, MD, PhD
Division of Head and Neck Radiology, Hospital Santa Casa de Misericórdia de São Paulo, Rua Dr. Cesário Motta Junior 112, Vila Buarque, Sao Paulo, SP 01221-020, Brazil

Division of Neuroradiology, Fleury Medicina e Saúde, Sao Paulo, SP, Brazil
e-mail: carlos.silva@grupofleury.com.br

R. Hoffmann Nunes et al. (eds.), *Critical Findings in Neuroradiology*,
DOI 10.1007/978-3-319-27987-9_29

Key Points

Etiology

Preseptal edema is the first stage of an orbital infection secondary to sinusitis. It is often clinically misdiagnosed as orbital or periorbital cellulitis. The infection in this early stage actually is still confined to the paranasal sinus and the swelling of the eyelids reflects congestion of the venous outflow. Usually the upper medial eyelid is affected, and if untreated, preseptal cellulitis develops. The most common bacteria are *Staphylococcus aureus*, *Streptococcus pyogenes*, *Streptococcus pneumoniae*, and *Haemophilus influenzae* [1–3]. Trauma with foreign bodies also plays a role in its etiology.

Best Imaging Modality

Contrast-enhanced computed tomography (CT) is the preferred imaging modality because of its high resolution, shorter scan times, lower costs, and overall better evaluation of eventual complications as abscesses or postseptal inflammatory extension. It also permits the evaluation of inflammatory sinonasal disease and associated bony structures. Even though magnetic resonance imaging (MRI) is able to better characterize the orbital soft tissues and estimate the extension of the process, the shorter scan time with CT is advantageous in children and may reduce or eliminate the need of sedation [1–3].

Contrast-enhanced CT with slice thickness less than 3 mm through the orbits is recommended and is also helpful in evaluating the presence of paranasal sinus infection (especially ethmoidal) [1–3].

Major Findings

Although CT and MRI of isolated preseptal cellulitis usually are not clinically indicated, these studies can be useful in patients in whom clinical differentiation between preseptal and postseptal cellulitis is impossible or when the diagnosis is unclear [5].

- Contrast-enhanced CT and MRI demonstrate the eyelid edema as a diffuse soft tissue thickening and areas of enhancement anterior to the orbital septum (Fig. 29.1).
- CT and MRI may also demonstrate the causative paranasal sinus infection.

Imaging Follow-Up

- Follow-up for patients with preseptal orbital cellulitis is clinical, and surveillance imaging is generally not indicated unless a patient fails to show an adequate clinical response to therapy or develops progressive symptoms or suspected complications, such as:
  - Postseptal inflammatory extension
  - Preseptal abscess or areas of rim enhancement
  - Bone dehiscence or erosion
  - Subperiosteal abscess or thrombotic complications of the ophthalmic veins and/or cavernous sinus [4, 6]

Main Differential Diagnosis

- *Allergic eyelid edema (angioedema)* is impossible to differentiate from preseptal cellulitis based solely on CT and MRI, particularly if the paranasal sinuses are normal. The clinical history is essential in these patients [1–5].
- *Inflammatory preseptal edema* is sometimes impossible to differentiate from preseptal cellulitis on imaging. Even clinically inflammatory preseptal edema is often misdiagnosed as orbital or periorbital cellulitis. [1–5].
- *Preseptal tumors*, such as lymphoma and squamous cell carcinoma, usually present as an infiltrative lesion with heterogeneous postcontrast enhancement in older patients. They may demonstrate adjacent bone erosions [1–5].

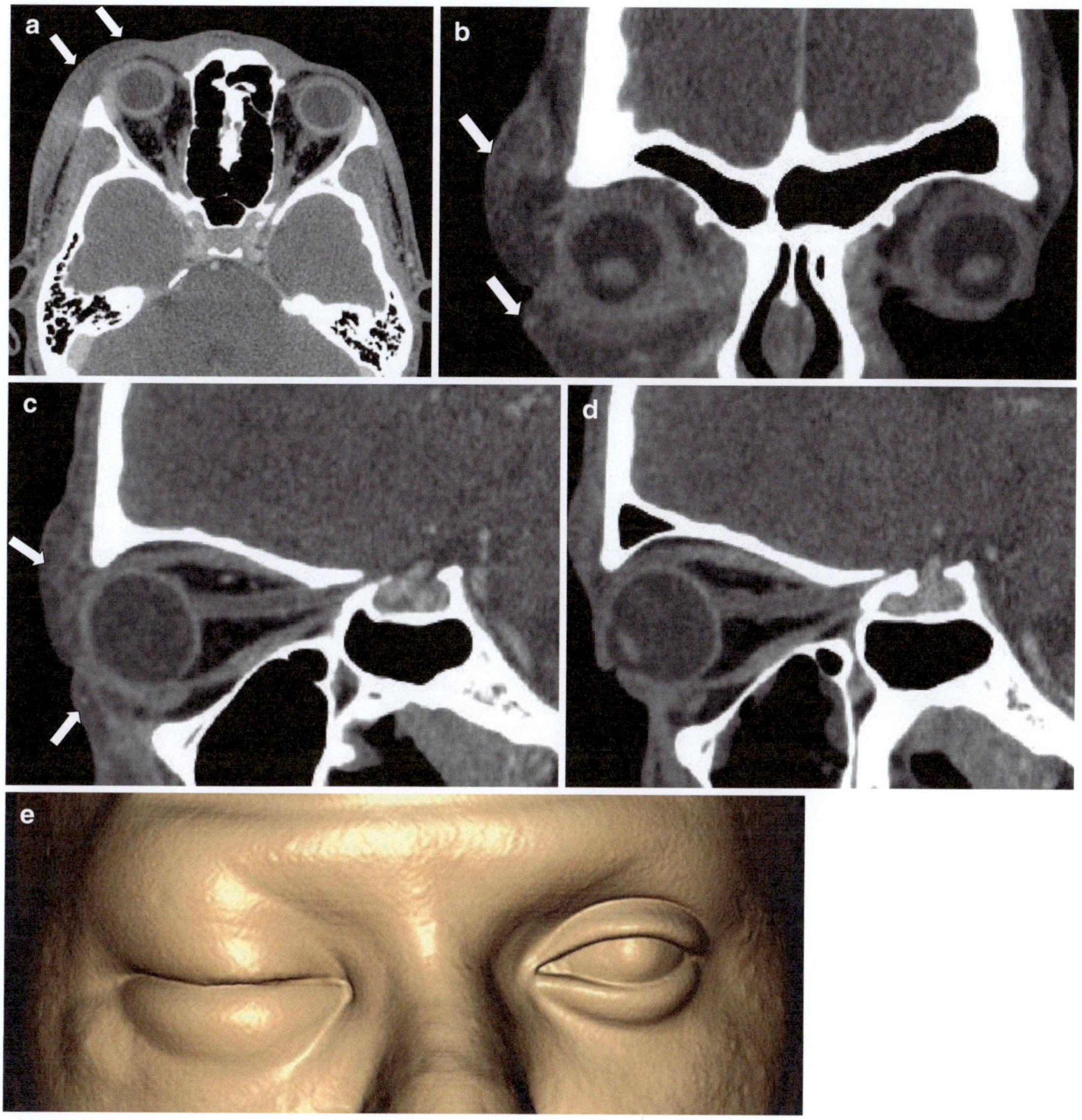

Fig. 29.1 A 14-year-old boy presenting with right orbital erythema and swelling. (**a**–**d**) Axial, coronal, and sagittal oblique postcontrast CT images show signs of preseptal orbital cellulitis without postseptal extension (*arrows*). Note that intra- and extraconal postseptal fat is normal. (**e**) 3D CT-reformatted image demonstrates the swelling of the right eyelids

Tips

- Radiologists should provide a detailed description of the sinonasal inflammatory disease and the eyelid swelling, as well as its relationships with the adjacent structures.
- Look for foreign bodies.
- The report should mention the integrity of the orbital septum and absence of postseptal inflammation in uncomplicated patients. The orbital septum is made up by the reflection of periosteum

and the check ligaments of the eyelids. It completely surrounds the anterior globe and provides a resistant physical barrier. When breached, it is usually the medial aspect that is affected, and infection spreads posteriorly. Many postseptal orbital cellulitis arise from adjacent ethmoid sinus infections. The bones may be intact, and the infection is presumably transmitted via venous channels, resulting in a subperiosteal abscess in the medial orbit. Mostly but not all postseptal infections are accompanied by a preseptal process.

- It is important to look after and describe potential complications as preseptal abscess, postseptal cellulitis and abscess, thrombophlebitis of the superior ophthalmic vein and of the cavernous sinus, and their relationships with the adjacent structures [6].

References

1. Eustis HS, Mafee MF, Walton C, Mondonca J. MR imaging and CT of orbital infections and complications in acute rhinosinusitis. Radiol Clin N Am. 1998;36(6):1165–83, xi.
2. Weber AL, Mikulis DK. Inflammatory disorders of the paraorbital sinuses and their complications. Radiol Clin North Am. 1987;25(3):615–30.
3. Gupta S, Goyal R, Gupta RK. Clinical presentation and outcome of the orbital complications due to acute infective rhino sinusitis. Indian J Otolaryngol Head Neck Surg. 2013;65 Suppl 2:431–4. doi:10.1007/s12070-013-0646-6.
4. Promelle V, Bennai D, Drimbea A, Milazzo S, Bremond-Gignac D. Pediatric orbital cellulitis without sinusitis: report of four cases. J Fr Ophtalmol. 2014;37(2):149–54. doi:10.1016/j.jfo.2013.08.004.
5. Mafee MF, Putterman A, Valvassori GE, Campos M, Capek V. Orbital space-occupying lesions: role of computed tomography and magnetic resonance imaging. An analysis of 145 cases. Radiol Clin North Am. 1987;25(3):529–59.
6. Mathew AV, Craig E, Al-Mahmoud R, Batty R, Raghavan A, Mordekar SR, Chan J, Connolly DJ. Paediatric postseptal and pre-septal cellulitis: 10 years' experience at a tertiary-level children's hospital. Br J Radiol. 2014;87(1033):20130503. doi:10.1259/bjr.20130503.

Postseptal Orbital Cellulitis in Children

30

Carlos Jorge da Silva

Abstract

Postseptal cellulitis is an infectious process that occurs within the orbit and behind the orbital septum. It is considered a possible complication of paranasal sinus infections. Clinically, patients present with eyelid edema, mild proptosis, and chemosis. Imaging studies demonstrate swelling and occasionally a slight enhancement of the postseptal orbital fat. The prognosis is generally excellent if early diagnosis and aggressive treatment are provided.

Background

Postseptal cellulitis is an infectious process that occurs within the orbit, behind the orbital septum, and within the bony walls of the orbit [1]. Historically, postseptal cellulitis is considered to be one of the possible complications of paranasal sinus infection (most commonly ethmoidal). Other causes of postseptal cellulitis include extension of preseptal cellulitis, dacryocystitis, mid-facial or dental infection, hematogenous spread, orbital trauma that penetrates the orbital septum, and postsurgical [1–4].

Postseptal orbital cellulitis is more frequently secondary to inflammatory sinonasal disease (most commonly ethmoidal), and this occurs more frequently in the pediatric population [1–4]. Clinically, the patient has eyelid edema, mild proptosis, and chemosis. In severe cases, there may be generalized limitation of ocular motility. However, visual acuity is generally not impaired. Postseptal cellulitis is probably the most common cause of proptosis in children [1].

Hospital admission with otolaryngological assessment and ophthalmic evaluation is recommended, as well as intravenous antibiotic therapy. Surgical intervention should be considered in the following circumstances: lack of response to antibiotics and subperiosteal or intracranial abscesses [1–5].

Prognosis is generally excellent if early diagnosis and aggressive treatment are provided to the patient. However, complications may result, as follows.

C.J. da Silva, MD, PhD
Division of Head and Neck Radiology, Hospital Santa Casa de Misericórdia de São Paulo, Sao Paulo, Brazil

Division of Neuroradiology, Fleury Medicina e Saúde, Sao Paulo, SP, Brazil
e-mail: carlos.silva@grupofleury.com.br

R. Hoffmann Nunes et al. (eds.), *Critical Findings in Neuroradiology*,
DOI 10.1007/978-3-319-27987-9_30

Ocular complications include exposure keratopathy, raised intraocular pressure, occlusion of the central retinal artery or vein, endophthalmitis, and optic neuropathy. Intracranial complications are rare but serious [5–7].

Key Points

Etiology

Inflammatory edema characterizes the earliest stage of postseptal orbital infection. There is diffuse edema of the orbital contents with inflammatory cells and fluid, but no abscess formation [1]. Swelling of orbital tissues occurs when an increase in sinus venous pressure is transmitted to the orbital vasculature, resulting in transudation and leakage through the vessel walls [1]. The most common causative organisms are *Streptococcus pneumoniae*, *Staphylococcus aureus*, *Streptococcus pyogenes*, and *Haemophilus influenzae* [1–3, 7].

Best Imaging Modality

Postcontrast computed tomography (CT) is the preferred modality because of its high resolution, shorter scan times, lower costs, and overall better evaluation of the possible complications mentioned above. It also permits evaluation of paranasal sinus infection and of the integrity of the orbital walls. Also, the reduced scan time with CT is advantageous in the pediatric population and may reduce or eliminate the need for sedation in infants and young children [1–3, 7].

Contrast-enhanced CT with slice thickness less than 3 mm covering the orbits is the recommended imaging protocol and also serves to evaluate the presence of paranasal sinus infection (mostly ethmoidal) in this setting [1–3, 7].

Magnetic resonance imaging (MRI) is able to better characterize the orbital soft tissues and estimate the extension of the process, especially intracranially [1–3].

Major Findings

Contrast-enhanced CT and MRI studies are usually complementary, for the evaluation of the bone and the soft tissues respectively (Figs. 30.1 and 30.2). Imaging studies may demonstrate [1–4, 7, 8]:

- Swelling and occasionally a slight enhancement of the postseptal fat (Figs. 30.1 and 30.2). In the presence of ethmoid sinusitis, the fat under the medial rectus is involved.
- Mass effect and mild proptosis.
- Poor definition of orbital planes, inflammatory stranding in the intraconal fat, and extraocular muscle edema are typical imaging findings (Figs. 30.1 and 30.2).
- CT and MRI may also demonstrate the causative paranasal sinus infection (Fig. 30.1).
- Complications:
  - Postseptal abscess or areas of rim enhancement (intraorbital abscess) (Fig. 30.3)
  - Bone dehiscence or erosion
  - Subperiosteal abscess
  - Intracranial extension

Imaging Follow-Up

Follow-up for patients with postseptal abscess is clinical and surveillance imaging is generally not indicated unless a patient fails to show an adequate clinical response to therapy or develops progressive symptoms or suspected complications as follows [5–7]:

- Subperiosteal abscess
- Postseptal abscess
- Intracranial complications, such as meningitis, epidural empyema, brain abscess, and cavernous sinus thrombophlebitis

Main Differential Diagnosis

*Postseptal absc*ess is a potential complication and must be differentiated from a non-complicated (phlegmonous) postseptal cellulitis. An abscess

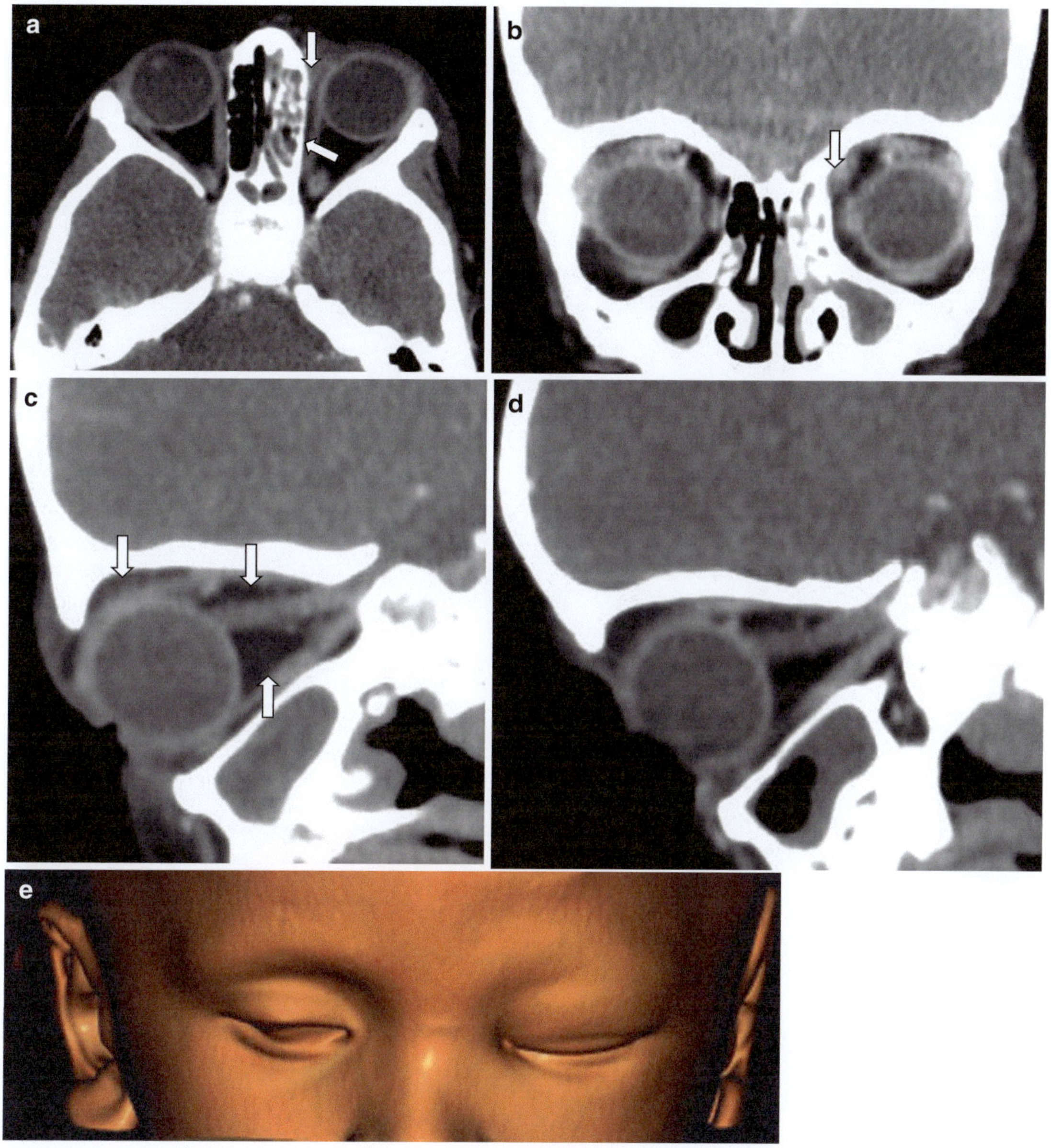

Fig. 30.1 Postseptal cellulitis. A 3-year-old boy with a history of left orbital pain and fever, presenting erythema and swelling in the medial portion of the left eyelids. (**a–c**) Axial and coronal and oblique sagittal reformatted postcontrast CT images show signs of left postseptal cellulitis (*arrows*) without abscess formation. Note left ethmoidal sinusitis. (**d**) Sagittal oblique reformatted postcontrast CT image of the right orbit demonstrates the normal aspect of the postseptal fat for comparison purposes. (**e**) 3D CT reformatted image demonstrates a more pronounced swelling in the medial portion of the left eyelids

usually presents with mass effect and a characteristic rim enhancement on postcontrast CT and MRI, occasionally with air content [1–3, 7].

Subperiosteal abscess is also a potential complication and must be differentiated from a noncomplicated postseptal cellulitis. It is characterized by a lesion displaying rim enhancement in the medial aspect of the extraconal space adjacent to the lamina papyracea. There may or may not be dehiscence of the lamina papyracea

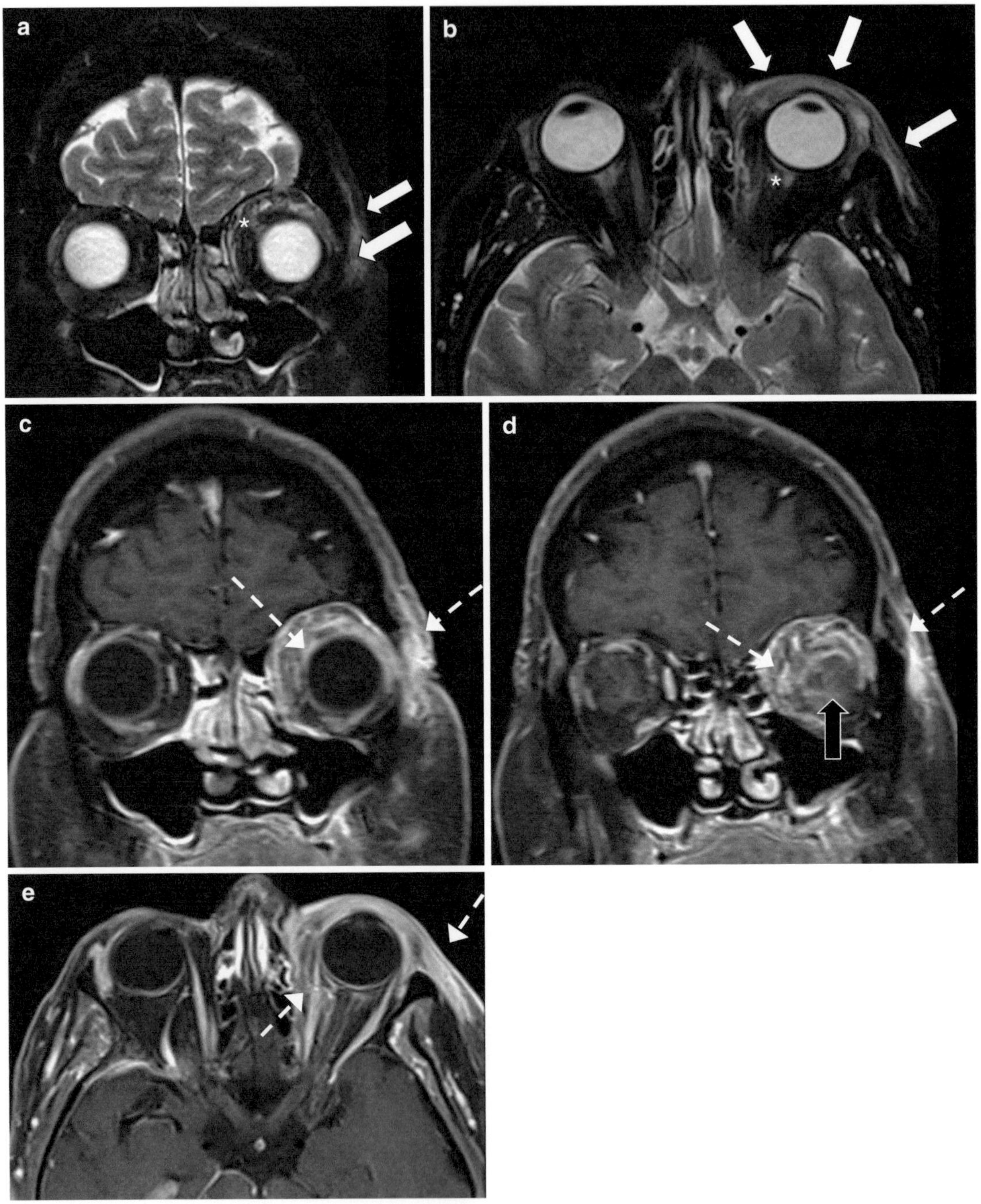

Fig. 30.2 Postseptal cellulitis. A 16-year-old girl with a history of periodontal disease, presenting with left orbital pain and fever. (**a**, **b**) Coronal and axial fat-sat T2WIs show soft tissue swelling and inflammation along the left orbit (*arrows*). The inflammation extends to the left medial and superior rectus muscles and into the intraconal fat side (*stars*), consistent with left postseptal cellulitis without abscess formation. (**c**–**e**) Coronal and axial postcontrast fat-sat T1WIs demonstrate avid abnormal enhancement in these regions (*dashed arrows*), as well as extensive inflammation of the intraconal fat (*black arrow*)

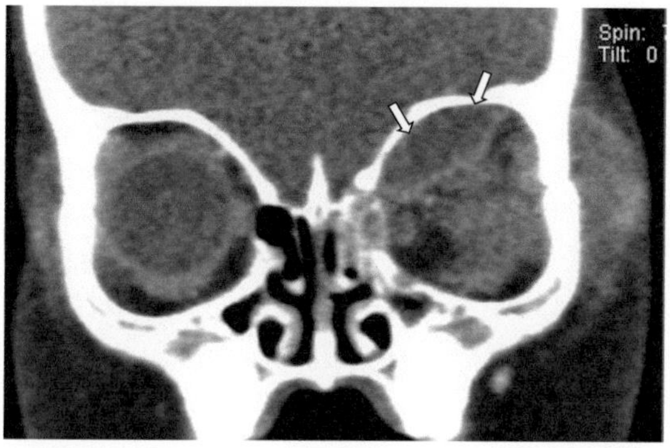

Fig. 30.3 Complicated postseptal cellulitis with abscess formation. A 14-year-old boy with a history of left orbital pain and fever. Postcontrast coronal CT image demonstrates soft tissue swelling and inflammation about the left orbit. The inflammation extends to the left medial and superior rectus muscles and into the intraconal fat on this side. An intraconal abscess (*arrows*) is depicted in the upper medial portion of the left orbit, displacing the intraconal structures

and opacification of the ipsilateral ethmoidal sinus [1–3, 7].

Preseptal cellulitis is another differential diagnosis, although the inflammation is confined anterior to the orbital septum. Postseptal cellulitis may be a complication of preseptal cellulitis; thus, it is not uncommon that both of them may coexist [1–3, 7].

Idiopathic orbital inflammatory disease may mimic postseptal cellulitis. This disease may involve the retrobulbar fat but is frequently associated with a "shaggy" enhancement of the optic nerve sheath and of the posterior uveal–scleral region [1–3, 7]. IgG4-associated disease may display similar findings but is generally accompanied by systemic symptoms.

Tips

Radiologists should provide a detailed description of the sinonasal inflammatory disease and the extension of the postseptal cellulitis.

The radiology report should also include a detailed description of potential complications, as follows:

- Presence of a subperiosteal abscess and any associated bone dehiscences or erosions
- Presence of postseptal abscess
- Meningitis
- Epidural empyema
- Brain abscess
- Superior ophthalmic vein thrombophlebitis or thrombosis
- Cavernous sinus thrombophlebitis or thrombosis

These complications may have relevant implications in the treatment and prognosis of these patients [7].

References

1. Eustis HS, Mafee MF, Walton C, Mondonca J. MR imaging and CT of orbital infections and complications in acute rhinosinusitis. Radiol Clin N Am. 1998;36(6):1165–83. xi.
2. Weber AL, Mikulis DK. Inflammatory disorders of the paraorbital sinuses and their complications. Radiol Clin N Am. 1987;25(3):615–30.
3. Gupta S, Goyal R, Gupta RK. Clinical presentation and outcome of the orbital complications due to acute infective rhino sinusitis. Indian J Otolaryngol Head Neck Surg. 2013;65 Suppl 2:431–4. doi:10.1007/s12070-013-0646-6.
4. Promelle V, Bennai D, Drimbea A, Milazzo S, Bremond-Gignac D. Pediatric orbital cellulitis without sinusitis: report of four cases. J Fr Ophtalmol. 2014;37(2):149–54. doi:10.1016/j.jfo.2013.08.004.
5. Ozkurt FE, Ozkurt ZG, Gul A, Akdag M, Sengul E, Yilmaz B, Yuksel H, Meric F. Management of orbital complications of sinusitis. Arq Bras Oftalmol. 2014; 77(5):293–6.
6. Schmitt NJ, Beatty RL, Kennerdell JS. Superior ophthalmic vein thrombosis in a patient with dacryocystitis-induced orbital cellulitis. Ophthal Plast Reconstr Surg. 2005;21(5):387–9.
7. Mathew AV, Craig E, Al-Mahmoud R, Batty R, Raghavan A, Mordekar SR, Chan J, Connolly DJ. Paediatric post-septal and pre-septal cellulitis: 10 years' experience at a tertiary-level children's hospital. Br J Radiol. 2014;87(1033):20130503. doi:10.1259/bjr.20130503.
8. Mafee MF, Putterman A, Valvassori GE, Campos M, Capek V. Orbital space-occupying lesions: role of computed tomography and magnetic resonance imaging. An analysis of 145 cases. Radiol Clin N Am. 1987;25(3):529–59.

Invasive Fungal Sinusitis

31

Carlos Toyama

Background

Fungal infections of the sinuses are classified as noninvasive and invasive. Most fungal sinusities are noninvasive which can be further subdivided in allergic fungal rhinosinusitis and fungus ball. Invasive fungal sinusitis is subdivided in acute invasive fungal, chronic invasive fungal, and chronic granulomatous invasive fungal sinusitis [1].

Acute invasive fungal sinusitis occurs in immunocompromised and diabetic patients, as well as in neutropenic ones, and it is considered rare in healthy individuals. The infection is rapidly progressive and spreads from the paranasal sinuses to the adjacent orbits and the central nervous system followed by extension into blood vessels resulting in vasculitis, hemorrhage, and tissue infarctions. The nasal cavity is the primary site of infection, and biopsy of the middle turbinate has been proposed as a means of diagnosis. It is the most lethal from of fungal sinusitis and the mortality rate in this setting is reported to be high, ranging from 50 % to 80 %. It is clinically characterized by acute-onset fever; painless, necrotic nasal septal ulceration; sinusitis; and progression to headache and orbital symptoms [2]. Treatment is usually a combination of endonasal surgical debridement and antifungal medications [3].

Chronic invasive fungal sinusitis is a slowly progressive infection that occurs over a period of weeks or months and most commonly affects the ethmoid and sphenoid sinuses. The entity is usually seen in the patients who have history of diabetes mellitus, chronic corticosteroid use, or other immunosuppressive treatment. Patients present with symptoms of chronic sinusitis, such as sinus pain, nasal discharge, low-grade fever, and intermittent epistaxis. Surgery is necessary to confirm the diagnosis and to remove all involved tissue. Systemic antifungal treatment is also warranted. Untreated patients are at risk for complications including visual changes, orbital apex syndrome, and cerebral nervous system involvement [4, 5].

Chronic granulomatous invasive fungal sinusitis is typically of gradual onset and is primary found in Sudan, India, Pakistan, and Saudi Arabia and rarely in the United States. Patients are usually immunocompetent and present with proptosis or an enlarging mass within the orbit, nose, paranasal sinuses, or maxillae. Histopathologically, a noncaseating granuloma with foreign body or Langerhans-type giant cells is found [4, 5].

C. Toyama, MD
Division of Head and Neck Radiology, Hospital Santa Casa de Misericóridia de São Paulo, Sao Paulo, Brazil

Division of Neuroradiology, Fleury Medicina e Saúde, Rua Dr. Cesário Motta Junior 112, Vila Buarque, Sao Paulo, SP, 01221-020, Brazil
e-mail: carlos.toyama@grupofleury.com.br

R. Hoffmann Nunes et al. (eds.), *Critical Findings in Neuroradiology*,
DOI 10.1007/978-3-319-27987-9_31

Key Points

Etiology

The nasal cavity is the primary site of infection of acute invasive fungal sinusitis and the most common causative pathogens are the Zygomycetes and *Aspergillus* species [4, 5].

Chronic invasive fungal sinusitis is usually related to *Aspergillus* species, which is isolated in more than 50 % culture-positive tissue [4, 5].

Chronic granulomatous invasive fungal sinusitis frequently occurs in immunocompetent patients and *Aspergillus flavus* is isolated in almost all cases [4, 5].

Best Imaging Modality

Paranasal sinuses, computed tomography (CT): CT is recommended for evaluation of the paranasal sinuses and bone erosion. Contrast enhancement is recommended for the investigation of extrasinus (adjacent fat, intracranial, intraorbital, periantral) and nasal cavity involvement [6, 7].

Magnetic resonance imaging (MRI) may be considered in the investigation of intraorbital and intracranial extension. However, MRI may be indicated early in patients with clinical suspicion of invasive fungal sinusitis and nonspecific findings obtained with CT. The protocol should cover the paranasal sinuses as well as the orbits and the cavernous sinuses. Postcontrast 3D constructive interference in steady-state (3D-CISS) sequence may better demonstrate cavernous sinus involvement [6, 8].

Computed tomography angiography (CTA) or magnetic resonance angiography (MRA) is recommended for the investigation of vascular involvement (narrowing, dissection, thrombosis, pseudoaneurysm) [6].

Major Findings [7]

- Non-contrast CT demonstrates a hypoattenuated mucosal thickening or an intrasinus and/or intranasal soft tissue attenuation mucosal thickening (nonspecific findings) (Fig. 31.1).
- Intrasinus hyperattenuation suggests fungal infection, dehydrated secretions, and/or high protein content.
- Bone erosion is variable. When severe, it may present as an aggressive osseous destruction usually in the medial aspect of the orbit, followed by intraorbital and/or intracranial extension. In many patients, it is absent.
- Bone erosion and mucosal thickening may sometimes be very subtle and appear insignificant (Fig. 31.1) [2].
- Obliteration of the normal fat density within the periantral regions represents the earliest sign of extrasinus involvement (Fig. 31.1). This may occur even if the bones remain intact.
- Evaluation of the nasal cavity (middle turbinate and septum nasal) may show a non-enhancing turbinate soft tissue, and mucosa is described as the "black turbinate sign" [9] (Figs. 31.1 and 31.2). The lack of enhancement and restricted diffusion occur due to vascular invasion, necrosis, and devitalized tissue [9].
- The loss of contrast enhancement of the wall of the sinus, as well as of the anterior and posterior soft tissue and the inferior rectus muscle, correlates with tissue necrosis [10].
- Cervicofacial tissue infarction is demonstrated as an area of absent contrast enhancement. It may be a relatively common and a characteristic finding of invasive fungal sinusitis. The bone wall of the sinonasal tract and the adjacent fat is frequently intact [11].
- Meningitis, cerebral abscess, cavernous sinus thrombosis, and cerebral infarction are associated with higher mortality (Fig. 31.2) [11].

Imaging Follow-Up

Follow-up for patients with invasive fungal sinusitis is generally clinical. Surveillance imaging is generally indicated if a patient fails to show an adequate clinical response to therapy or develops progressive symptoms or suspected complications. However some imaging findings may guide the follow-up as follows:

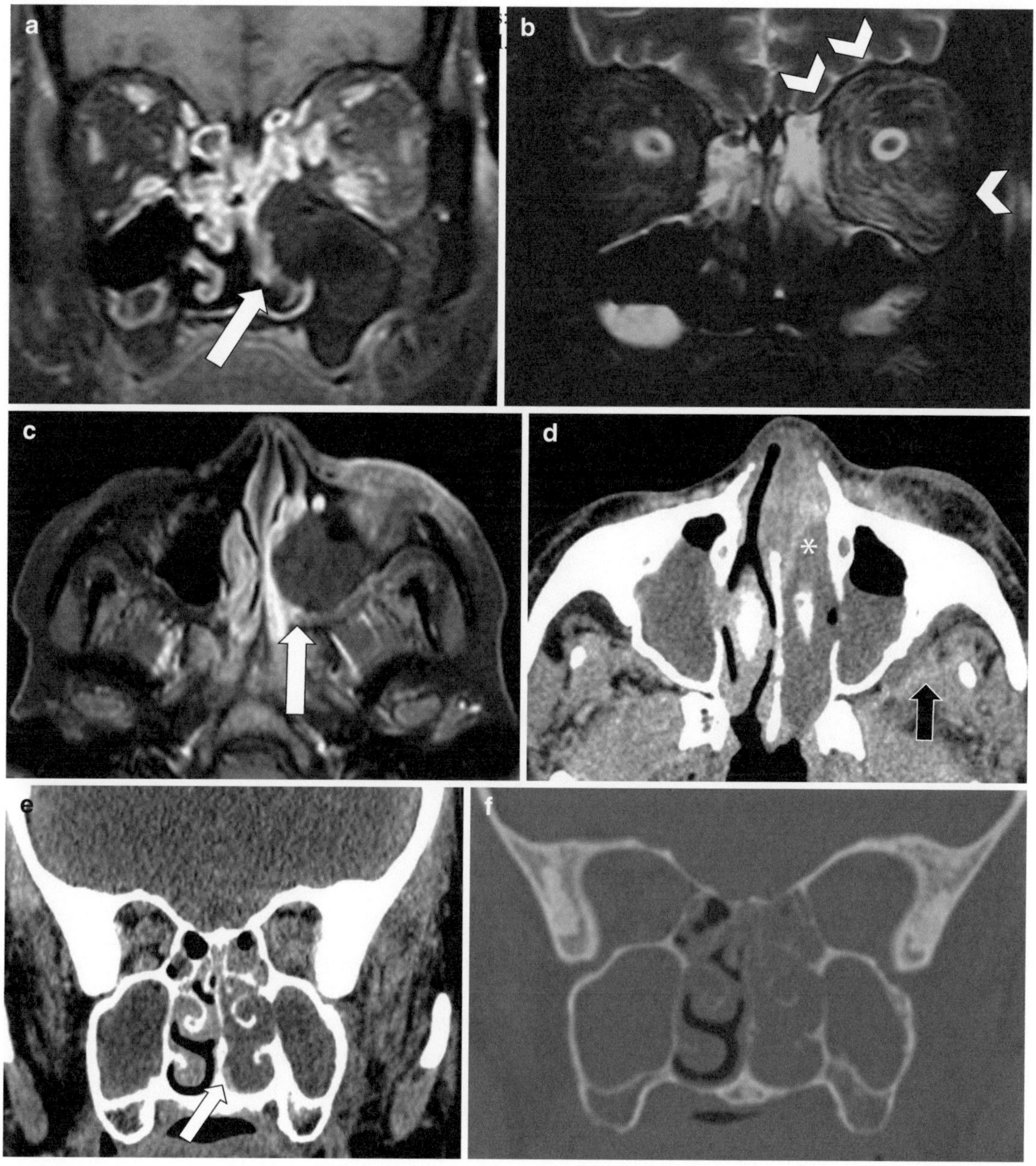

Fig. 31.1 A 45-year-old man with diabetes presents with malaise, left-eye proptosis, and left facial pain. (**a**) Coronal postcontrast T1-weighted image demonstrates a non-enhancing soft tissue within the left maxillary sinus and orbital fat. The mucosa of the left middle and inferior turbinates shows lack of enhancement compatible with the "black turbinate" sign (*arrow*). (**b**) Coronal T2-weighted image shows low signal intensity in the left middle turbinate and the inflamed retrobulbar fat (*arrowheads*). (**c**) Axial postcontrast T1-weighted image confirms the non-enhancing soft tissue within the left maxillary sinus and middle turbinate compatible with the "black turbinate" sign (*arrow*). (**d**) After 6 days, the patient symptoms persist despite treatment for invasive fungal sinusitis, and axial postcontrast CT image depicts opacification of the left maxillary sinus as well as infiltration of the retroantral fat (*arrow*) consistent with fungal spread. There is lack of enhancement of the nasal turbinate mucosa (*star*) and increase enhancement of nasal septum mucosa. (**e**) Coronal contrast-enhanced CT image shows lack of enhancement of the left middle and inferior turbinates compatible with the "black turbinate" sign (*arrow*). (**f**) Coronal CT image on bone window demonstrates almost intact bone walls despite spread to the left orbit. (**g**) After 15 days, axial contrast-enhanced CT demonstrates persistent opacification of the left maxillary sinus and increase of retroantral fat stranding (*arrow*). (**h**) Coronal contrast-enhanced CT image reveals an abscess in the left orbit (*arrowhead*). (**i**) Axial postcontrast-enhanced CT shows left proptosis and thickening of the medial rectus muscles (*white curved arrow*) and optic nerve on that side (*black curved arrow*)

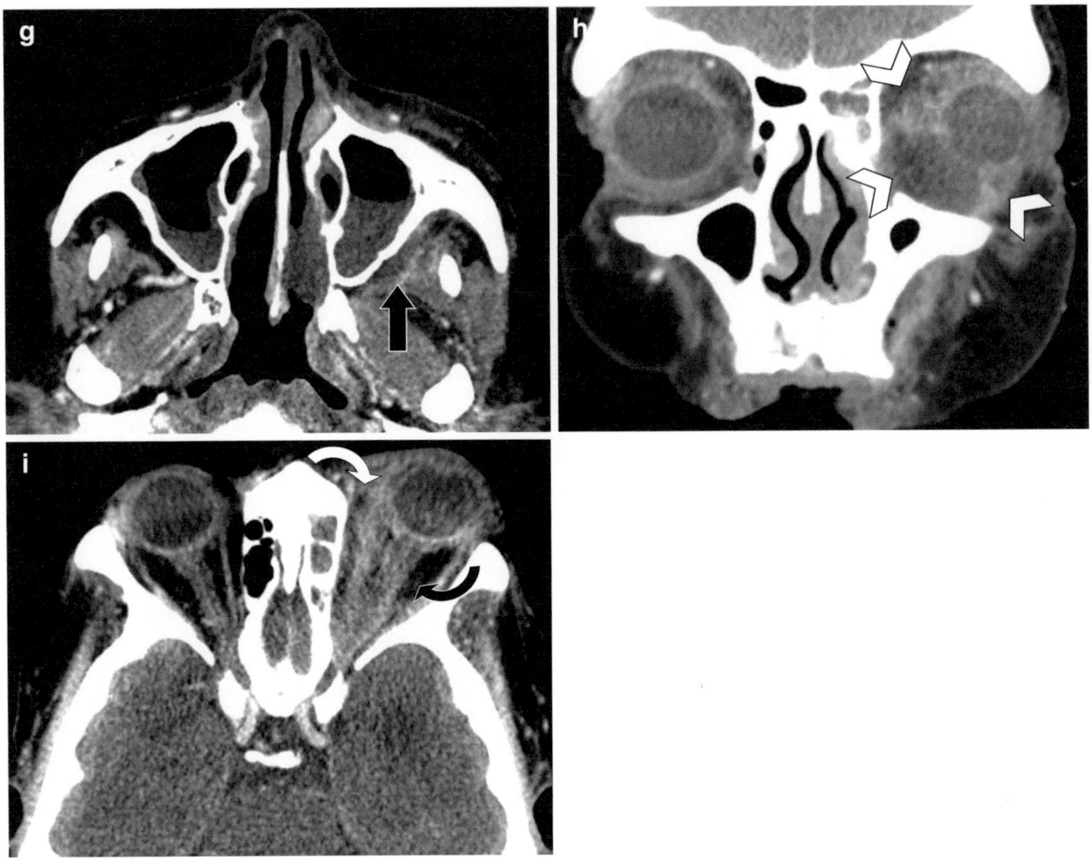

Fig. 31.1 (continued)

- *CT* [6]:
  - Lack of enhancement of the nasal turbinates: MRI may be performed to confirm the finding or biopsy may be considered.
  - Suspected arterial involvement: CTA or MRA should be performed.
  - Suspected orbital and intracranial extension: orbit and brain MRI should be performed.
- *MRI* [6]:
  - Positive "black turbinate sign": biopsy of the turbinate is indicated.

Main Differential Diagnosis

- *Allergic fungal sinusitis* is the most common form of fungal sinusitis and has a strong association with allergic rhinitis and asthma and frequently involves multiple sinuses. Noncontrast CT demonstrates expanded paranasal sinuses with areas of hyperdense opacification and thinning of septae on CT [2].
- *Complications of rhinosinusitis* may be intraorbital and intracranial and may appear similar to invasive fungal sinusitis. Patients may

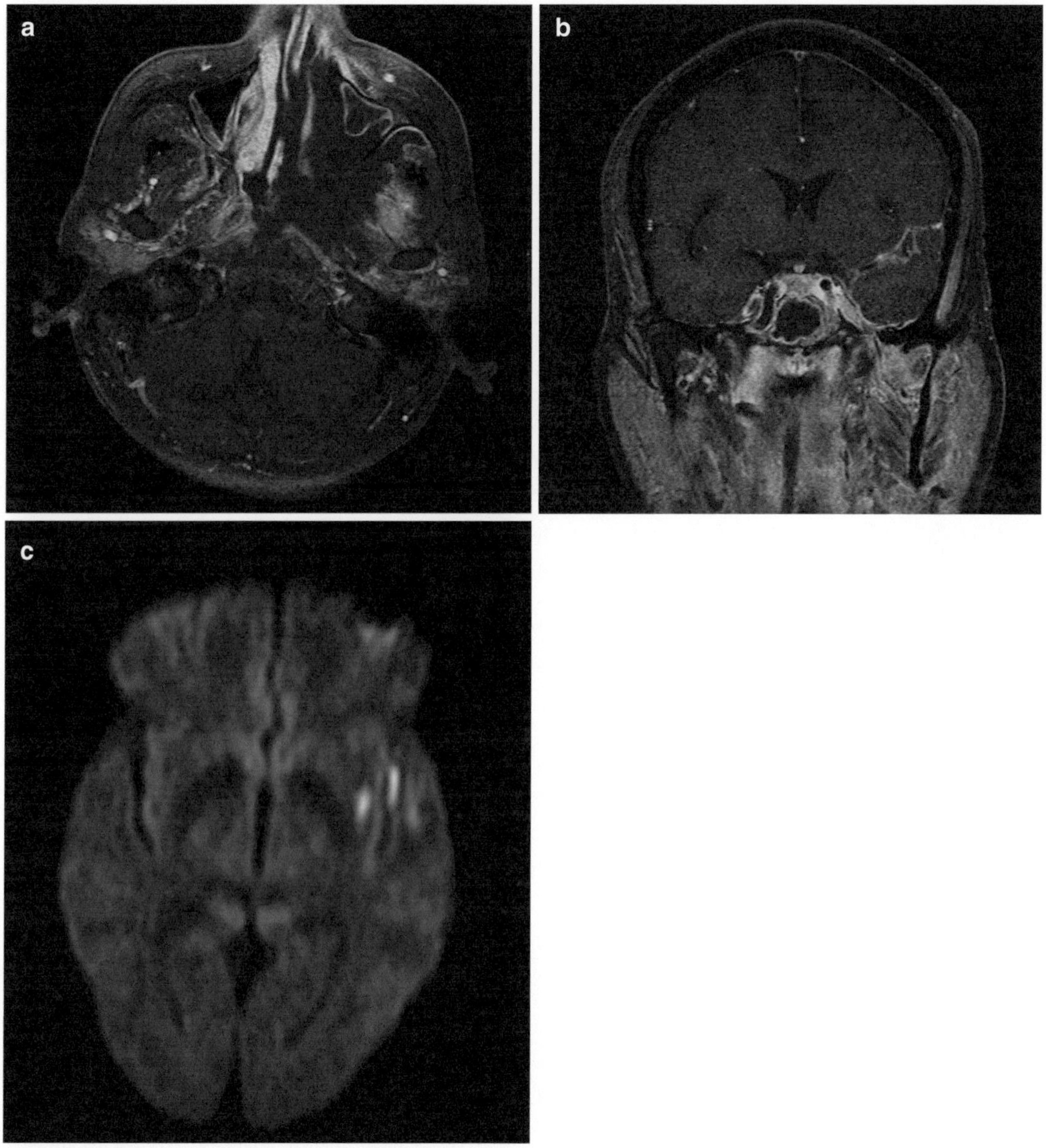

Fig. 31.2 A 64-year-old man with diabetes presents with malaise, left-eye proptosis, diplopia, and facial numbness and weakness. (**a**) Axial postcontrast fat-saturated T1WI demonstrates an extensive non-enhancing lesion within the left maxillary sinus extending to the masticator space, rhinopharynx, as well as the mucosa of the left middle turbinate and nasal septum compatible with the "black turbinate" sign. (**b**) Coronal postcontrast fat-saturated T1WI shows V3 and cavernous sinus involvement on the left. (**c**) Diffusion-weighted imaging depicts multiple hyperintense foci in the left middle cerebral artery territory, compatible with acute embolic infarcts due to carotid artery involvement

not be immunocompromised. Soft tissue involvement and bone erosion are less likely. Involvement is more likely bilateral, and heterogeneity of secretions in non-fungal secretion is less pronounced. Bone wall thickening and sclerosis occur more commonly in chronic bacterial sinusitis [2].

- *Sinonasal squamous cell carcinoma* also occurs in immunocompetent patients and imaging shows a solid mass with osseous erosion. The most frequently localization when it arises in the paranasal sinuses is the maxillary antrum [12].
- *Non-Hodgkin lymphoma* may present as a soft sinonasal mass. T2 hypointensity and marked restricted diffusion also occur in lymphoma due to a high nucleus to cytoplasm ratio and it may mimic fungus. Clinical history and lack of bone erosion may help to distinguish lymphoma from invasive fungal sinusitis [12].
- *Sinonasal Wegener granulomatosis* is an idiopathic necrotizing granulomatous vasculitis. It usually involves the nasal cavity, presenting with turbinate and medial wall destruction, as well as nasal septum perforation. Bone erosion is prominent and orbit and skull base involvement is possible [12].

Tips

- *Always evaluate the extra-sinonasal fat*, because extension beyond the sinuses may occur even with an intact bone wall, as the fungus tends to extend along the blood vessels. This may be the first indication that invasive fungus is present [2].
- *Pay attention to the turbinates* because the lack of enhancement is an early sign which may help increase the likelihood of patient survival.
- *Always evaluate the orbits*. No contrast enhancement of the superior ophthalmic vein may represent thrombosis. Orbital apex involvement increases the risk of intracranial and cavernous sinus spread.
- *Look for intracranial spread* that is considered an isolated predictive factor for high mortality. Dural thickening and enhancement are typical early on; later cerebral infarctions may occur.

References

1. deShazo RD, O'Brien M, Chapin K, Soto-Aguilar M, Gardner L, Swain R. A new classification and diagnostic criteria for invasive fungal sinusitis. Arch Otolaryngol Head Neck Surg. 1997;123(11):1181–8.
2. Aribandi M, McCoy VA, Bazan 3rd C. Imaging features of invasive and noninvasive fungal sinusitis: a review. Radiographics: Rev Publ Radiol Soc N Am Inc. 2007;27(5):1283–96.
3. Kasapoglu F, Coskun H, Ozmen OA, Akalin H, Ener B. Acute invasive fungal rhinosinusitis: evaluation of 26 patients treated with endonasal or open surgical procedures. Otolaryngol Head Neck Surg Off J Am Acad Otolaryngol Head Neck Surg. 2010;143(5):614–20.
4. Gorovoy IR, Kazanjian M, Kersten RC, Kim HJ, Vagefi MR. Fungal rhinosinusitis and imaging modalities. Saudi J Ophthalmol Off J Saudi Ophthalmol Soc. 2012;26(4):419–26.
5. Thompson 3rd GR, Patterson TF. Fungal disease of the nose and paranasal sinuses. J Allergy Clin Immunol. 2012;129(2):321–6.
6. Suslu AE, Ogretmenoglu O, Suslu N, Yucel OT, Onerci TM. Acute invasive fungal rhinosinusitis: our experience with 19 patients. Eur Arch Otorhinolaryngol. 2009;266(1):77–82.
7. Middlebrooks EH, Frost CJ, De Jesus RO, Massini TC, Schmalfuss IM, Mancuso AA. Acute invasive fungal rhinosinusitis: a comprehensive update of CT findings and design of an effective diagnostic imaging model. AJNR Am J Neuroradiol. 2015;36(8):1529–35.
8. Yagi A, Sato N, Takahashi A, Morita H, Amanuma M, Endo K, et al. Added value of contrast-enhanced CISS imaging in relation to conventional MR images for the evaluation of intracavernous cranial nerve lesions. Neuroradiology. 2010;52(12):1101–9.

9. Safder S, Carpenter JS, Roberts TD, Bailey N. The "Black Turbinate" sign: an early MR imaging finding of nasal mucormycosis. AJNR Am J Neuroradiol. 2010;31(4):771–4.
10. Gorovoy IR, Vagefi MR, Russell MS, Gorovoy M, Bloomer MM, Glastonbury CM. Loss of contrast enhancement of the inferior rectus muscle on magnetic resonance imaging in acute fulminant invasive fungal sinusitis. Clin Exp Ophthalmol. 2014;42(9):885–7.
11. Seo J, Kim HJ, Chung SK, Kim E, Lee H, Choi JW, et al. Cervicofacial tissue infarction in patients with acute invasive fungal sinusitis: prevalence and characteristic MR imaging findings. Neuroradiology. 2013; 55(4):467–73.
12. Gomaa MA, Hammad MS, Abdelmoghny A, Elsherif AM, Tawfik HM. Magnetic resonance imaging versus computed tomography and different imaging modalities in evaluation of sinonasal neoplasms diagnosed by histopathology. Clin Med Insights Ear Nose Throat. 2013;6:9–15.

Temporal Bone Infections

32

Kenny Emmanuel Rentas and Benjamin Y. Huang

Abstract

Several inflammatory diseases affect the temporal bones and can potentially lead to permanent neurologic deficits and even death. Mastoiditis is the most common temporal bone infection for which imaging is performed and consists of inflammation of the mastoid air cells. It is the most common suppurative complication of acute otitis media given the contiguity of the middle ear cavity and mastoid air system. If not adequately treated, acute mastoiditis can eventually progress to coalescent mastoiditis, subperiosteal abscess formation, petrous apicitis, labyrinthitis, facial nerve involvement, or subcutaneous abscesses. Intracranial extension can lead to meningitis, intracranial abscess, subdural empyema, dural venous sinus thrombosis, and otitic intracranial hypertension. Patients frequently present with fever and otalgia. Imaging plays a pivotal role in patients who fail to respond to antimicrobial therapy and present with neurological symptoms, subcutaneous findings, or persistent pain, fever, and otorrhea. Treatment ranges from antimicrobial therapy for uncomplicated cases to simple drainage or radical mastoidectomy for advanced disease.

Background

Several inflammatory diseases affect the temporal bones and can potentially lead to permanent neurologic deficits and even death. These diseases are generally classified according to the anatomy: external ear, middle ear and mastoid, inner ear, and petrous apex. As it is the most common temporal bone infection for which imaging is performed, only acute mastoiditis and its complications will be discussed in this chapter.

K.E. Rentas, MD (✉) • B.Y. Huang, MD, MPH
Department of Radiology,
University of North Carolina at Chapel Hill,
101 Manning Dr. Campus, Box 7510,
Chapel Hill, NC 27599-7510, USA
e-mail: Dr.Rentas@gmail.com;
bhuang@med.unc.edu

R. Hoffmann Nunes et al. (eds.), *Critical Findings in Neuroradiology*,
DOI 10.1007/978-3-319-27987-9_32

Mastoiditis refers to inflammation of the mastoid air cells and is a common complication of acute otitis media (AOM). Prior to the introduction of antibiotics, acute mastoiditis (AM) had an incidence of 5–10 % in patients with AOM, whereas currently the incidence ranges from 0.24 to 0.74 % [1, 2]. The close relationship between AOM and AM is not surprising as the middle ear cavity and mastoid air systems communicate freely via the aditus ad antrum, allowing inflammation to easily spread between compartments. If not adequately treated, uncomplicated AM can eventually progress to coalescent mastoiditis, in which mastoid air cells coalesce by a process of demineralization and osteoclastic activity [3]. Subperiosteal abscesses may then develop, facilitated by disease spread through vascular channels or directly through frank bone erosions. Local disease spread in the petrous bone may lead to petrous apicitis, labyrinthitis, and facial nerve involvement.

Intracranial extension of AM is a dreaded complication of AM with an incidence approaching 16 % among hospitalized children and those requiring surgery for mastoiditis [4]. Intracranial spread may manifest as meningitis, intracranial abscess, subdural empyema, or dural venous sinus thrombosis. Once the intracranial venous drainage is impaired, intracranial pressures may become elevated, an entity often referred to as otitic intracranial hypertension [5]. AM can also spread extracranially into the adjacent soft tissues, leading to abscess formation.

Clinically, acute mastoiditis can occur in persons of any age but most commonly affects patients younger than 2 years of age with an average age at presentation of 12 months. Patients frequently present with fever and otalgia; however, this is also a common clinical presentation in patients with uncomplicated AOM. Persistent fever, pain, and otorrhea despite adequate antimicrobial therapy may suggest the presence of acute surgical mastoiditis. Pain tends to be located deep in the ear or over the mastoid process. In infants, signs of infection can include irritability, diarrhea, fever, and poor feeding. A common location for subperiosteal abscess formation is the postauricular region, and abscesses in this region produce the typical clinical appearance of a protruding ear. Inferomedial spread and abscess formation deep to the sternocleidomastoid muscle (Bezold abscess) can be difficult to detect clinically; therefore, imaging plays a crucial role in early detection for adequate treatment. Treatment for uncomplicated acute mastoiditis typically includes antimicrobial agents targeted to common causative pathogens, as is the case for acute otitis media. Mastoidectomy is usually reserved for cases of AOM that have failed to resolve with antibiotics and have progressed to coalescent otomastoiditis.

Key Points

Etiology

Acute mastoiditis most commonly results from untreated AOM, which in turn is usually the sequela of a viral upper respiratory infection that disrupts the mucosal barrier that prevents microorganisms from spreading from the nose and nasopharynx into the middle ear cavity [6]. Due to the direct communication between the middle ear cavity and the mastoid air system, the pathogens involved in AOM and AM tend to be same. In decreasing order of frequency, the most common causative microorganisms are *Streptococcus pneumonia*, *Streptococcus pyogenes*, *Haemophilus influenza*, and *Staphylococcus aureus* [2, 7, 8].

Best Imaging Modality

Computed tomography (*CT*). Acute mastoiditis can usually be diagnosed clinically; however, CT may be performed to confirm the diagnosis. CT is the modality of choice for surgical planning and to evaluate potential complications such as coalescent mastoiditis. Contrast-enhanced CT is more sensitive than unenhanced CT for detection of abscesses. The CT protocol should include high-resolution images through the bilateral temporal bones using a high-spatial-frequency (bone) reconstruction algorithm in axial and coronal planes. Postcontrast images reconstructed with a soft tissue algorithm should also be included in addition to the above mentioned bone algorithm if soft tissue involvement is suspected.

Magnetic resonance imaging (MRI). MRI is superior to CT in visualizing intracranial complications particularly after the administration of intravenous contrast. Magnetic resonance venography (MRV) increases the sensitivity to detect dural venous sinus thrombosis.

Major Findings

Acute mastoiditis: Early stages of mastoiditis with or without periostitis usually manifest on CT or MRI as a mastoid effusion without bone erosion. Most CT studies also show opacification of the middle ear cavity. If periostitis is present, swelling of the postauricular soft tissues may be seen clinically (Fig. 32.1a).

Coalescent mastoiditis: Coalescent mastoiditis is best depicted on CT images as loss of the mastoid trabeculations with opacification of the middle ear and mastoid air cells. If the infection persists for long enough, the mastoid air cells may coalescence into a single mastoid cavity. Careful inspection along the mastoid walls should be performed for evidence of erosions and for the presence of loculated fluid in the adjacent soft tissues. Inflammatory debris may enhance after intravenous contrast administration (Fig. 32.1b).

Subperiosteal abscess: Subperiosteal abscess is commonly found in the postauricular region (suprameatal triangle) as the bone there is particularly thin. These are best demonstrated on contrast-enhanced CT as a crescentic or ovoid rim-enhancing fluid collection typically adjacent to an area of focal osteolysis of the mastoid bone. However cortical erosions along the adjacent mastoid wall are not seen in all cases (Fig. 32.2). The subperiosteal abscess can also extend toward the external auditory canal, posterior to the occipital bone (Citelli abscess), deep to the temporalis muscle (Luc abscess), or into the inferomedial soft tissues (Bezold abscess) [1, 3, 9].

Bezold abscess: Erosion of the mastoid tip with tracking of pus medial to the insertion of the

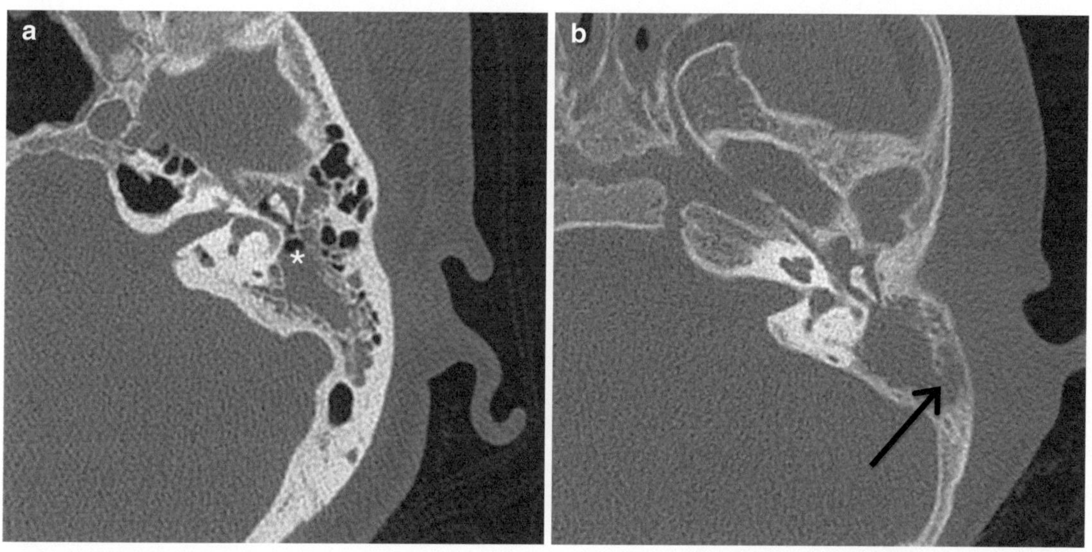

Fig. 32.1 Acute non-coalescent (**a**) and coalescent otomastoiditis (**b**). Axial unenhanced CT images on bone windows (**a**) demonstrate partial opacification of the middle ear cavity and mastoid air cells without erosive changes. Normal mastoid antrum (*). Uncomplicated otomastoiditis was diagnosed clinically. (**b**) CT image shows a diffusely opacified middle ear cavity and mastoid air cells with loss of the trabeculae and subtle cortical erosions (*arrow*) consistent with coalescent otomastoiditis

sternocleidomastoid muscle may form what is known as a Bezold abscess. On postcontrast CT/MRI, the abscess manifests as a rim-enhancing fluid collection inferior to the tip of the mastoid. Because the mastoid tip is usually not well pneumatized in young children, Bezold abscesses are usually found in older children or adults (Fig. 32.3) [7].

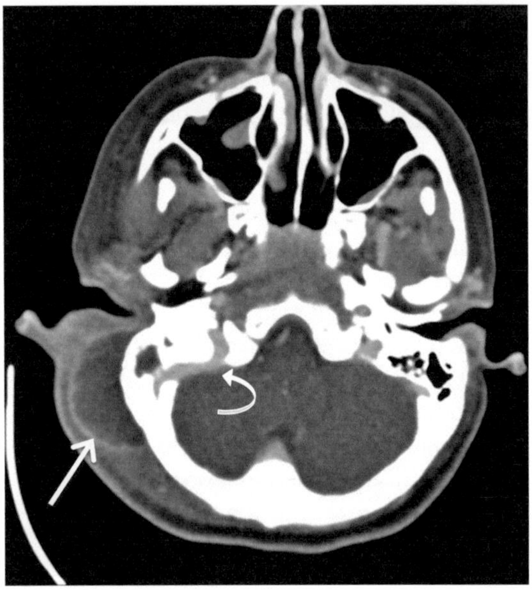

Fig. 32.2 Subperiosteal abscess. Contrast-enhanced axial CT images shows a subperiosteal abscess (*arrow*) in the postauricular region adjacent to a diffusely opacified mastoid bone. Notice the close proximity to the sigmoid dural venous sinus which is patent (*curved arrow*)

Epidural abscess, subdural empyema, and brain abscess: Epidural abscesses in the setting of coalescent mastoiditis are typically due to contagious spread following bone destruction and are most commonly found in the posterior fossa followed by the middle cranial fossa [3]. Epidural abscesses are best evaluated by MRI after intravenous contrast administration, classically have a biconvex shape, and resemble CSF on T2-weighted images (T2WI). However they demonstrate higher signal intensity than CSF on T1-weighted images (T1WI) and FLAIR images. After intravenous contrast administration, epidural abscesses demonstrate a peripheral enhancement on T1WI. On diffusion-weighted imaging (DWI), epidural abscesses may demonstrate reduced diffusion. Breaching of the dura leads to spread of infection into the subdural space, potentially resulting in a subdural empyema, meningitis, and cerebritis. Subdural empyemas may also develop through spread of infection by thrombophlebitis or periphlebitis and tend to show similar imaging features on MRI to epidural abscesses. Subdural empyemas tend to have a crescentic shape and do not extend across dural reflections (Fig. 32.4). Abnormal signal intensity on T2WI or FLAIR sequences

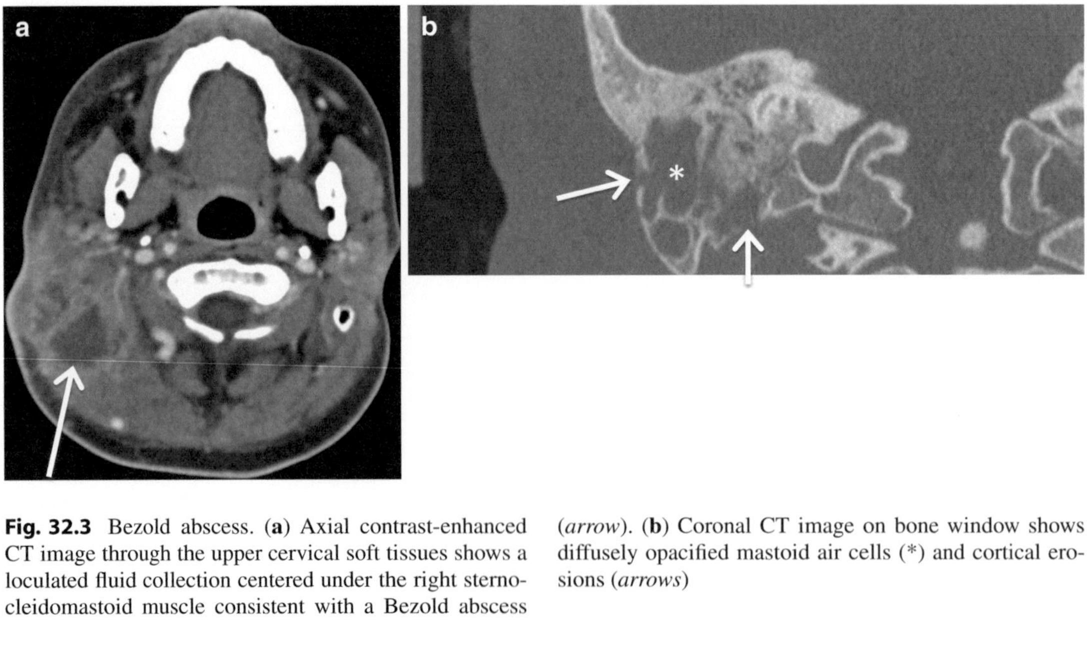

Fig. 32.3 Bezold abscess. (**a**) Axial contrast-enhanced CT image through the upper cervical soft tissues shows a loculated fluid collection centered under the right sternocleidomastoid muscle consistent with a Bezold abscess (*arrow*). (**b**) Coronal CT image on bone window shows diffusely opacified mastoid air cells (*) and cortical erosions (*arrows*)

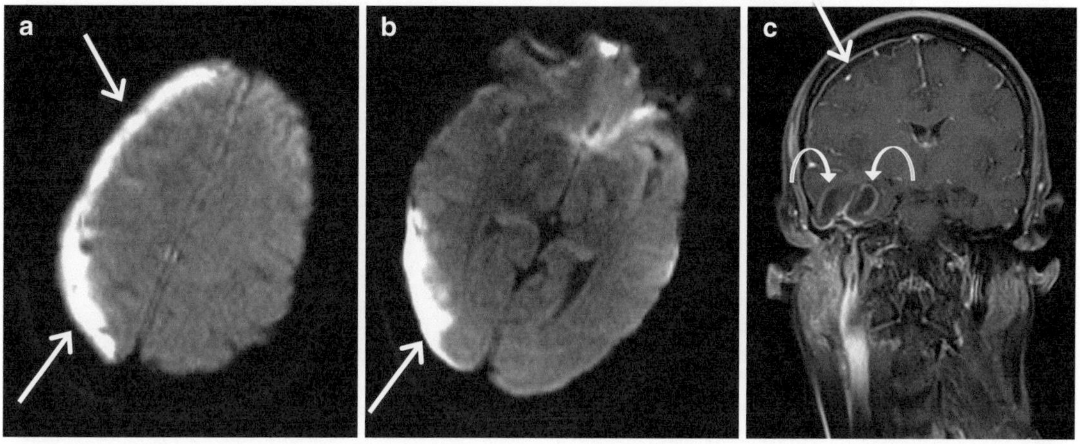

Fig. 32.4 Subdural empyema. (**a**, **b**) DWI demonstrates hyperintense signal along the right frontoparietal and right temporal convexities (*arrows*) consistent with restricted diffusion characteristic of a subdural empyema. (**c**) Coronal postcontrast T1WI shows a peripherally enhancing right cerebral convexity extra-axial fluid collection consistent with a subdural empyema (*arrow*). Two early right temporal lobe abscesses are partially imaged (*curved arrows*)

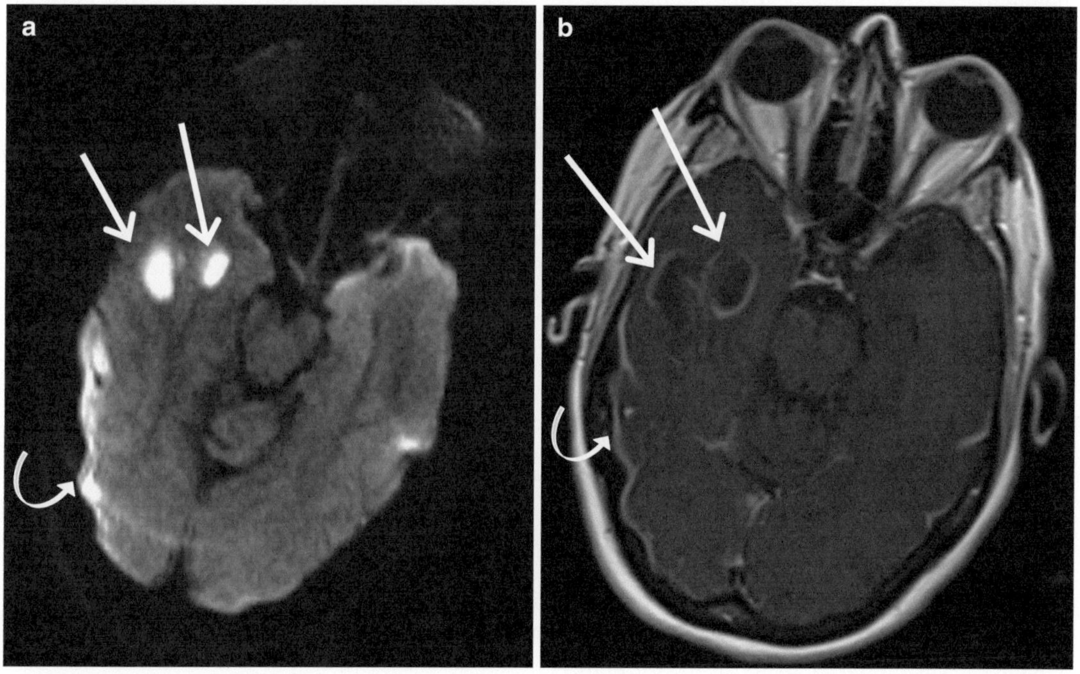

Fig. 32.5 Subdural empyema and brain abscesses. (**a**) Diffusion-weighted image shows two intraparenchymal areas of restricted diffusion in the right temporal lobe (*arrows*) and right temporal convexity (*curved arrow*) consistent with cerebral abscesses and subdural empyema respectively. (**b**) Postcontrast T1WI demonstrates peripheral enhancement of early intraparenchymal abscesses (*arrow*) and right temporal convexity subdural empyema (*curved arrow*)

seen on the adjacent brain parenchyma usually represents cerebritis. Brain abscesses are most commonly found in the temporal lobe and demonstrate similar imaging features as the epidural abscess described above on MRI depending on the pathologic stage (Fig. 32.5).

Meningitis: Imaging studies are usually normal in the setting of clinically diagnosed

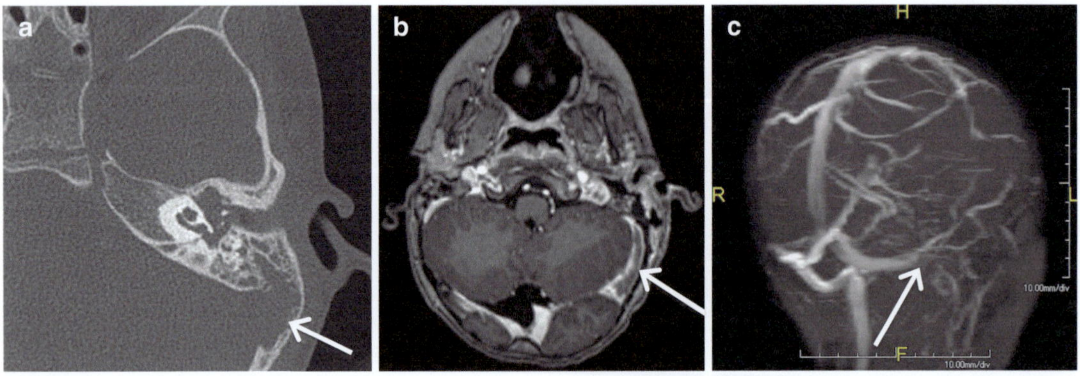

Fig. 32.6 Dural venous sinus thrombosis. (**a**) Axial CT image on bone windows shows a completely opacified mastoid air system and middle ear cavity with associated cortical and trabecular erosions (*arrows*) consistent with coalescent otomastoiditis. (**b**) Axial postcontrast T1WI shows a filling defect in the left sigmoid and transverse sinus (*arrow*). (**c**) Oblique time-of-flight MRV image demonstrates lack of flow-related enhancement in the left sigmoid and internal jugular vein (*arrow*)

meningitis. Non-enhanced CT may show effacement and increased density at the basilar cisterns and sulci, particularly when there is a significant amount of inflammatory debris. On MRI, there may be hyperintense signal in the sulci and basilar cisterns on FLAIR due to the presence of inflammatory debris. Pial enhancement may be seen on magnetic resonance postcontrast T1WI. Hydrocephalus may also develop due to obstruction of CSF absorption.

Dural sinus thrombosis: Dural sinus thrombosis may manifest as high-density material within the occluded sinus on unenhanced CT; however, this finding is only evident in a minority of cases. An intraluminal filling defect is usually evident on CT or MRI after intravenous contrast administration within an occluded sigmoid sinus. On MRI, the presence of sinus thrombosis may be suggested by lack of the normal flow voids typically seen on spin-echo sequences. The signal intensity of the intraluminal thrombus will depend on the clot's age, becoming increasingly hyperintense on T1 and T2WI in the subacute setting. Intraluminal clot will appear markedly hypointense on susceptibility-weighted images (SWI). Time-of-flight MRV will show absence of flow-related enhancement in the involved dural venous sinus; however, a normal appearance may be mistakenly seen within the sinus if the clot has intrinsic hyperintense signal (Fig. 32.6).

Imaging Follow-Up

There are no clear guidelines for imaging follow-up of acute mastoiditis. Patients with evidence of cerebellar, cerebral, or meningeal signs or symptoms should undergo a dedicated head MRI in addition to a high-resolution temporal bone CT to detect potential intracranial complications [10]. Some physicians may opt for medical management and serial imaging follow-up over surgical intervention for small brain abscesses in patients that are neurologically intact.

Main Differential Diagnosis

Acquired cholesteatoma. It can be difficult to distinguish from coalescent mastoiditis, as acquired cholesteatomas may present with ossicular and mastoid trabecular erosions. Both entities can present concomitantly as cholesteatomatous otomastoiditis. Acquired cholesteatomas are usually centered in the epitympanic region and may be accompanied by tympanic membrane retraction

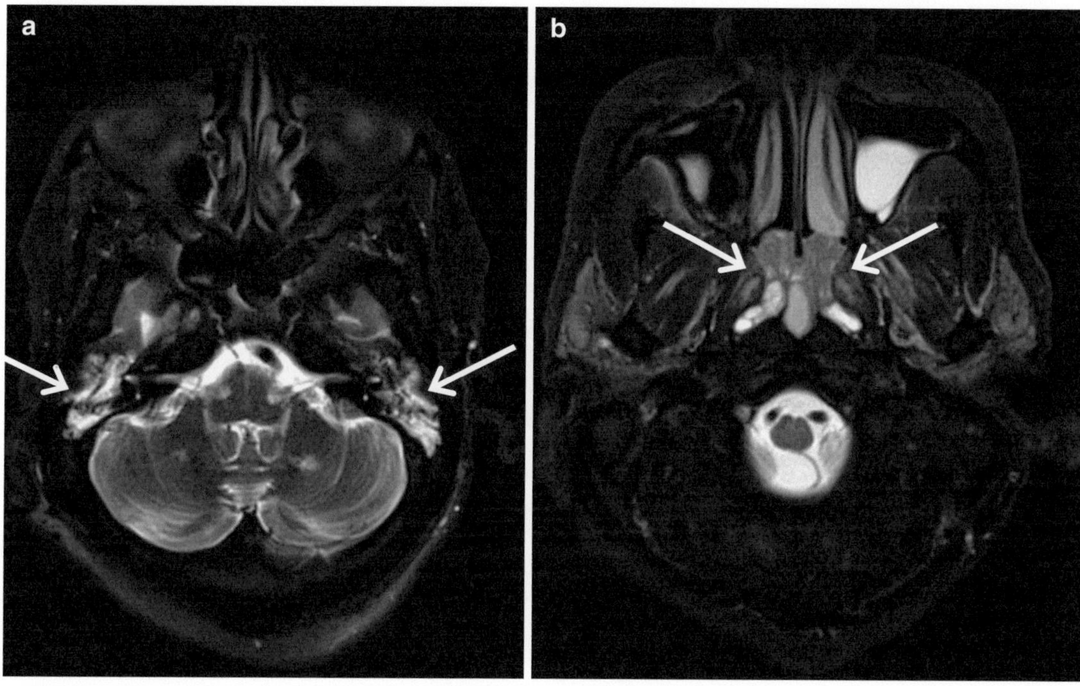

Fig. 32.7 Eustachian tube obstruction. (**a**) Axial T2WI shows bilateral mastoid and middle ear effusions (*arrows*). (**b**) Axial T2WI demonstrates HIV-related adenoidal hypertrophy obstructing the normal drainage of the auditory (Eustachian) tube

or perforation. On MRI, acquired cholesteatomas usually demonstrate lack of enhancement after intravenous contrast administration and hyperintense signal on DWI related to decrease diffusivity.

Tips

- On imaging, it would be erroneous to refer to a middle ear cavity or mastoid effusion as otitis media or mastoiditis without supporting clinical findings.
- Avoid mistaking the normal void of mastoid trabeculation at the mastoid antrum and aditus ad antrum for erosive changes in the setting of diffusely opacified mastoid air cells.
- Some patients may fail to demonstrate the classic signs and symptoms of otitis media and may present late for care with intracranial complications already developed [11].
- Intracranial complications from mastoiditis may occur without macroscopic erosions of the mastoid cortex.
- An intrinsically hyperintense dural venous sinus thrombus may be mistaken for normal flow on time-of-flight MRV images.
- Aberrant arachnoid granulations may simulate filling defects within the sinus on MRV.
- Mastoid fluid can represent retained secretions secondary to an obstructive mass at the nasopharynx obstructing normal drainage of the auditory (Eustachian) tube (Fig. 32.7). Therefore, always scrutinize the nasopharynx in patients with middle ear/mastoid effusions, especially if they occur unilaterally in an adult patient.

References

1. Bluestone C. Clinical course, complications and sequelae of acute otitis media. Pediatr Infect Dis J. 2000;19:S37–46. doi:10.1097/00006454-200005001-00007.
2. Quesnel S, Nguyen M, Pierrot S, et al. Acute mastoiditis in children: a retrospective study of 188 patients. Int J Pediatr Otorhinolaryngol. 2010;74:1388–92. doi:10.1016/j.ijporl.2010.09.013.
3. Vazquez E, Castellote A, Piqueras J, et al. Imaging of complications of acute mastoiditis in children. RadioGraphics. 2003;23:359–72. doi:10.1148/rg.232025076.
4. Zevallos J, Vrabec J, Williamson R, et al. Advanced pediatric mastoiditis with and without intracranial complications. Laryngoscope. 2009;119:1610–5. doi:10.1002/lary.20259.
5. Swartz JD, Hagiwara M. Head and neck imaging. In: Som P, editor. Inflammatory diseases of the temporal bone. 5th ed. St. Louis: Mosby; 2011. p. 1183–97.
6. Phillips G, LoGerfo S, Richardson M, Anzai Y. Interactive web-based learning module on CT of the temporal bone: anatomy and pathology. RadioGraphics. 2012;32:E85–105. doi:10.1148/rg.323115117.
7. Juliano A, Ginat D, Moonis G. Imaging review of the temporal bone: part I. Anat Inflamm Neoplastic Process Radiol. 2013;269:17–33. doi:10.1148/radiol.13120733.
8. Abdel Raouf M, Ashour B, Abdel Gawad A. Updated management strategies for mastoiditis and mastoid abscess. Egypt J Ear Nose Throat Allied Sci. 2012;13:43–8. doi:10.1016/j.ejenta.2012.03.001.
9. Weiss I, Marom T, Goldfarb A, Roth Y. Luc's abscess: the return of an old fellow. Otol Neurotology. 2010;31(5):776–9.
10. Patel K, Almutairi A, Mafee M. Acute otomastoiditis and its complications: role of imaging. Oper Tech Otolaryngol Head Neck Surg. 2014;25:21–8. doi:10.1016/j.otot.2013.11.004.
11. Holt GR, Gates GA. Masked mastoiditis. Laryngoscope. 1983;93(8):1034–7.

Petrous Apicitis

33

Melissa Ann Davis

Abstract

Petrous apicitis can be a serious disease and it is important for the radiologist to recognize the imaging findings and relay this information to the clinician. If this disease is allowed to progress, it will lead to intracranial infection through direct extension.

Background

Common benign lesions include petrous apex effusion, cholesterol granuloma, mucocele, and cholesteatoma. Benign tumors such as meningiomas, schwannomas, paragangliomas, and chondromas are also known to affect the petrous apex. Langerhans cell histiocytosis, nasopharyngeal carcinoma, chondrosarcoma, and chordomas are malignant lesions known to occur in the petrous apex [1]. Apical petrositis is a serious infection of the petrous apex. A well-described, although relatively rare, clinical presentation includes facial pain, cranial nerve six palsy, and ear pain. This is named Gradenigo triad (or syndrome) after Giuseppe Gradenigo, who described this combination of symptoms in 1907 [2]. Although more common in the past, with the advent of antibiotics, petrous apicitis has become increasingly rare.

M.A. Davis, MD
Department of Radiology, University of North Carolina Hospitals, 2006 Old Clinic, CB# 7510, Chapel Hill, NC 27599, USA
e-mail: Melissa.Davis2@unchealth.unc.edu

Major complications include intracranial extension with subsequent meningitis, intracranial abscess, inflammation of the petrous portions of the internal carotid arteries, and dural/cavernous sinus thrombosis. Additional complications include neuropathy and nasopharyngeal extension of inflammation causing abscess [3, 4].

Key Points

Etiology

The petrous apex is pneumatized in approximately 33 % of the population [1, 5]. This pneumatization is usually symmetric but may be asymmetric. There is some debate as to whether pneumatization of the petrous apex is required for the development of petrous apicitis. Debris and inflammation within the petrous apex either seed directly from an infectious otomastoiditis (due to obstruction of the petrous drainage) or via adjacent vasculature in the bone. There is progressive osseous demineralization and resorption

R. Hoffmann Nunes et al. (eds.), *Critical Findings in Neuroradiology*,
DOI 10.1007/978-3-319-27987-9_33

causing a skull base osteomyelitis [3]. Common bacteria causing this disease include *Staphylococcus aureus*, *Streptococcus pneumoniae*, and *Haemophilus influenzae* [4].

Infection of the petrous apex is aggressively treated because progression may lead to disruption of the walls of the petrous apex and intracranial extension of infection posteriorly and nasopharyngeal extension of infection anteriorly. Rarely extension into the facial planes of the neck has also been described. Intracranial extension can lead to significant sequela and is the most complication of petrous apicitis. These patients present with meningitis and abscess formation.

Involvement of the trigeminal ganglion in Meckel's cave can cause facial pain. Involvement of the sixth nerve in Dorello's canal can lead to palsy of the lateral rectus muscle on the affected side [1–5].

Best Imaging Modality

If there is concern, computed tomography (CT) is the initial modality of choice with magnetic resonance imaging (MRI) becoming necessary to assess intracranial extension [5].

Computed tomography. CT of the temporal bone is the best imaging modality for the initial evaluation of the petrous apex. Initial scans are generally performed without contrast. However, if there is concern for soft tissue infiltration, contrast may be administered.

Magnetic resonance imaging. MRI with contrast is crucial to evaluate for intracranial infection and cranial nerve and carotid artery involvement. A protocol focusing on the temporal bone and potentially affected adjacent structures is preferred. T1-weighted images (T1WI) before and after contrast administration should always be obtained. T2-weighted images (T2WI) using a three-dimensional technique centered at the petrous apex – balanced steady-state free-precession sequence (CISS) especially after contrast – are useful in assessing the status of the cavernous sinuses. Diffusion-weighted image (DWI) is extremely useful to identify intracranial abscesses.

Major Findings

CT demonstrates opacification of a pneumatized petrous apex early in the disease course. Generally adjacent middle ear opacification, with or without thickening of the soft tissues of the external auditory canal, and tympanic membrane thickening are also identified due to concurrent otitis media/externa. As the disease progresses, there is bony destruction with soft tissue extension into the intracranial cavity or anteriorly into the nasopharynx (Figs. 33.1 and 33.2) [1–5].

MRI typically demonstrates fluid signal in the petrous air cells (high T2 signal, low T1 signal). With early intracranial extension, there is enhancement of the adjacent dura. Later in the disease process, there may be leptomeningeal enhancement, predominantly affecting the frontal lobes, due to meningitis. Presence of a ring-enhancing lesion with centrally restricted diffusion is consistent with abscess. If intracranial disease progresses, further

Fig. 33.1 (**a**) CT bone windows. There is destruction of the posterior cortex of the opacified petrous apex (*black arrow*). Dehiscence extends into the intracranial cavity posteriorly and into the internal auditory canal medially (*white arrow*). Also note opacification of the mastoid air cells and middle ear. The smooth expansion of the petrous apex suggests that underlying pneumatization was present before the infection. (**b**) CT soft tissue windows. There is destruction and soft tissue opacification of the left petrous apex with dehiscence into the intracranial cavity (*thin black arrows*). At this level, the carotid canal appears to be involved (*thick black arrow*). (**c**) Axial postcontrast T1WI MRI. It demonstrates abnormal enhancement within the left petrous apex. There is also abnormal enhancement of the 7th and 8th nerves bilaterally (*arrows*), consistent with leptomeningeal involvement. The left mastoid also enhances abnormally. (**d**) Axial postcontrast T1WI MRI. More superiorly, there is bilateral leptomeningeal and parenchymal enhancement involving the anterior temporal lobes (*white arrows*) as well as evidence of ventriculitis with abnormal ependymal enhancement (*black arrows*). Similar abnormal enhancement is also seen at the level of the basilar cisterns. (**e**) Axial postcontrast T1WI MRI. In the left superior frontal lobe, there is extensive leptomeningeal and parenchymal enhancement (*white arrows*) consistent with cerebritis (Courtesy of Fernando Boschini, MD and Teerath Tanpitukpongse, MD of Duke University)

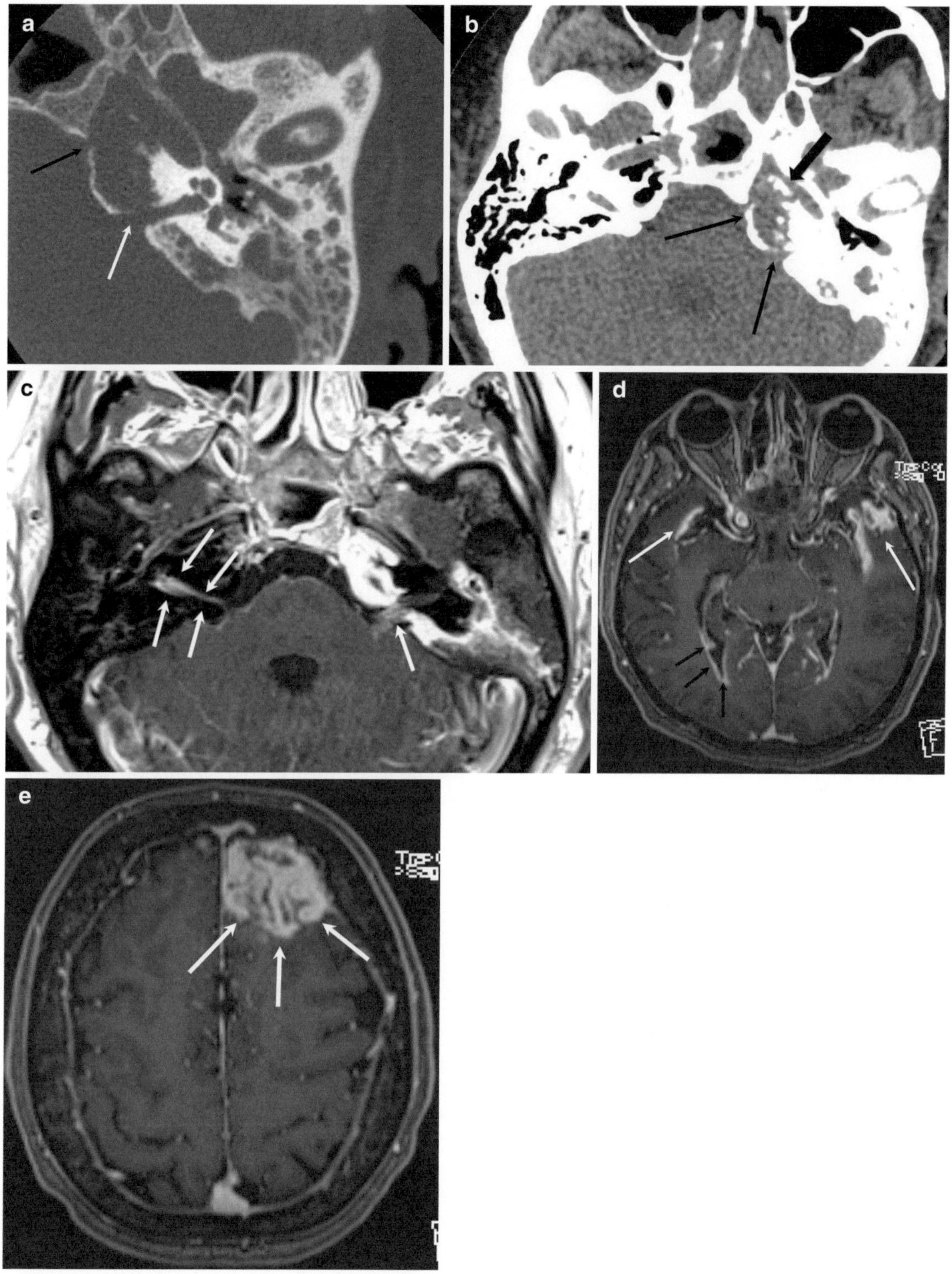
a
b
c
d
e

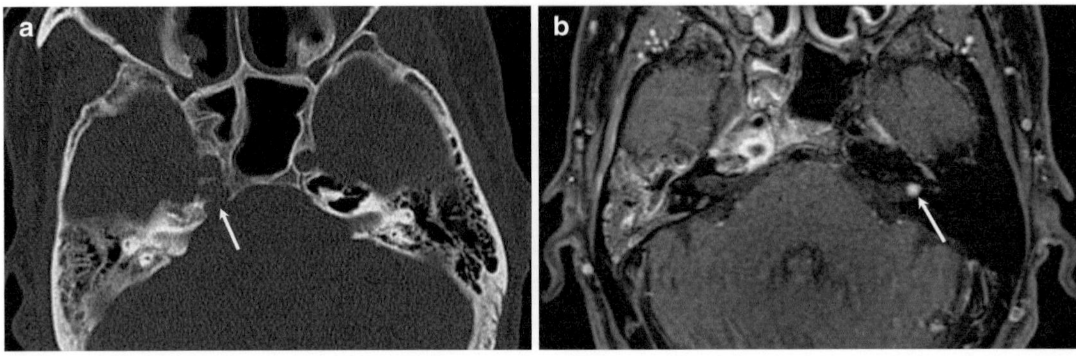

Fig. 33.2 (**a**) Axial CT bone windows. There is opacification of the right petrous apex with dehiscence of its walls (*arrow*). (**b**) Axial postcontrast TIWI MRI. There is expansion and abnormal enhancing right petrous apex with disruption of the posterior wall at the level of the prepontine cistern. Also note the effusion and abnormal enhancement of the mastoid and right sphenoid air cells. Incidental note is made of an enhancing mass in the left internal auditory canal which may represent a schwannoma (*arrow*)

ventriculitis may occur, characterized by periventricular enhancement and increased T2 signal along the ventricles (Figs. 33.1 and 33.2) [1–5].

It is necessary to evaluate the adjacent cranial nerves to assess for spread of infection. Nerves may demonstrate enhancement in this case. Close attention to Meckel's cave and the adjacent dura, along Dorello's canal should be paid.

Remember to evaluate the anterior structures for extension into the nasopharynx and abscess.

Imaging Follow-Up

Follow-up imaging after treatment, usually surgical, is recommended with either CT or MRI. Once the patient is asymptomatic, additional follow-up can be obtained in 2 months. If symptomatic, then imaging follow-up should be prompt to exclude additional complications. If there is intracranial extension on the initial imaging, then follow-up should be done with MRI rather than CT [1].

Main Differential Diagnosis

Petrous apex effusion should not be confused with infection, as it is a benign condition that requires no treatment.

Differential diagnosis of petrous apicitis also includes *inflammatory pseudotumor* and *osteomyelitis* (which can be concurrent with apicitis). It should be noted that osteomyelitis can also be found in a non-pneumatized petrous apex.

Destructive malignant tumors, such as metastases and chondrosarcoma, and lateral chordoma should also be in the differential diagnosis of destructive lesions of the petrous apex [1–5].

Tips

CT

- Provide a clear description of the extent of the inflammation.
- Mention the absence or presence of bony destruction or obliteration of fat planes especially those surrounding blood vessels and cranial nerves at the base of the skull.
- Mention of middle ear opacification and the appearance of the ossicles.
- Brain edema or any other intracranial abnormality should be promptly reported.

MRI

- Make mention of dural enhancement or other signs of leptomeningeal disease.
- Carefully evaluate Meckel's cave and the dura along the clivus to assess for neural involvement.
- Evaluate for intracranial abscess or cerebritis.

References

1. Lemmerling M, De Foer B. Temporal bone imaging. Springer-Verlag Berlin Heildelberg; 2014. p 249–56.
2. Motamed M, Kalan A. Gradenigo's syndrome. Postgrad Med J. 2000;76:559–60.
3. Som P, Curtin H. Head and neck imaging. 5th ed. St Louis: Elsevier; 2011. p. 1188–98.
4. Vazquez E, Castellote A, Piqueras J, et al. Imaging complications of acute mastoiditis in children. Radiographics. 2003;23:359–72.
5. Razek A, Huang B. Lesions of the petrous apex: classification and findings at CT and MR imaging. Radiographics. 2012;32:151–73.

External Malignant Otitis

34

Carlos Toyama

Abstract

External malignant otitis is an invasive infection of the external auditory canal and surrounding tissues and is consider a life-threatening condition. The infection starts as an inflammation in the dermal and epidermal tissues at the junction of the cartilaginous and osseous external auditory canal and spreads adjacent soft tissues and skull base. It more commonly occurs in diabetics and other immunocompromised patients.

Background

External malignant otitis (EMO) is an invasive infection of the external auditory canal (EAC) and a life-threatening condition. The infection begins as an inflammation in the dermal and epidermal tissues at the junction of the cartilaginous and osseous EAC and spreads to adjacent soft tissues and skull base including the temporomandibular joint. It most commonly occurs in diabetics and other immunocompromised patients [1].

C. Toyama, MD
Division of Head and Neck Radiology, Hospital Santa Casa de Misericórdia de São Paulo, Rua Dr. Cesário Motta Junior 112, Vila Buarque, 01221-020 Sao Paulo, SP, Brazil

Division of Neuroradiology, Fleury Medicina e Saúde, Sao Paulo, SP, Brazil
e-mail: carlos.toyama@grupofleury.com.br

Clinical manifestations include severe otalgia accompanied by otorrhea. The pain often extends to the temporomandibular joint and is aggravated by chewing, a clinical clue that should raise the possibility of EMO. As the infection progresses, it may lead to central skull base osteomyelitis, involvement of cranial nerves, meningitis, cerebritis, intracranial empyema, and/or venous sinus thrombosis. Paralysis of the facial nerve is common, followed by involvement of the glossopharyngeal, vagal, spinal accessory, and hypoglossal nerves. The trigeminal and abducens nerves can be also affected when the petrous apex is involved [2].

Treatment is based on management of diabetes, systemic antibiotics, local debridement, and ear surgery in selected patients [3]. The classic diagnostic criteria include clinical manifestations such as persistent severe otalgia and otorrhea, combined with imaging signs of osteomyelitis and/or positive ear secretion culture for *Pseudomonas aeruginosa*, which is positive in more than 90 % of patients. Diabetes is not a

R. Hoffmann Nunes et al. (eds.), *Critical Findings in Neuroradiology*,
DOI 10.1007/978-3-319-27987-9_34

significant prognostic factor by itself. The early diagnosis and treatment is important to prevent the extension of the disease to the skull base or underlying meninges, as well as to the brain parenchyma [4].

Key Points

Etiology

The causative organism is most commonly *Pseudomonas aeruginosa*, although other organisms such as *Staphylococcus sp.*, *Proteus mirabilis*, and *Klebsiella* sp. have been isolated. Classically, EMO occurs in elderly diabetic patients. The disease can also affect other immunocompromised hosts, mainly HIV-infected patients, who are usually younger. Although uncommon, other immunosuppressed individuals may also be affected [1, 2].

Best Imaging Modality

- *Temporal bone computed tomography* (*CT*): CT scan is the first choice for anatomic imaging of the temporal bone. It is ideal to assess bone erosion that follows bone demineralization. CT can show spread to the infratemporal fossa, temporomandibular joint, and nasopharyngeal and masticator space. The CT study should extend from above the petrous ridge through the mastoid tip, and submillimeter images should be reconstructed in different planes using a high-detail bone kernel. Intravenous iodinated contrast is recommended for better evaluation of soft tissue involvement. Assessment of intracranial complications and skull base is limited, but it can be also demonstrated on CT [4–7].
- *Magnetic resonance imaging* (*MRI*): MRI is superior to CT in evaluating soft tissue disease and it is the technique of choice for this purpose due to its superior contrast resolution. Intravenous gadolinium injection is recommended to better demonstrate lesion extension. MRI is indicated to evaluate extension to the retrocondylar fat, infratemporal fossa, masticator space, and nasopharyngeal and parapharyngeal fat. Assessment of the skull base and intracranial complications is better performed by MRI due to its ability to depict bone marrow involvement and meningeal involvement [4–7].
- *Scintigraphy*: Technetium-99 bone scintigraphy can be useful in the initial evaluation of questionable osteomyelitis. A positive scan represents osteoblastic activity. Gallium-67 concentrates in areas of inflammation by binding to bacteria directly, which can be used to assess the response to treatment [8].

Major Findings

- *CT*:
  Early abnormalities in EMO are in the form of nonspecific soft tissue enhancement. Bone erosions are late findings and are the radiographic hallmark of EMO (Fig. 34.1). On postcontrast CT, there is thickening and enhancing soft tissue in the region of the EAC with or without formation of phlegmon/abscess. In cases of abscess, a ring-enhancing collection with a low attenuation (necrotic) center can be observed [4–7].
- *MRI*:
  MRI is able to better evaluate the extension to the adjacent spaces. Assessment of the skull base and intracranial complications is also better demonstrated on MRI as follows [4–7]:
  - Bone marrow changes: T1-weighted hypointensity, T2-weighted hyperintensity, and postcontrast enhancement within the bone marrow are indicative of osteomyelitis (Fig. 34.2).
  - Facial neuritis: Asymmetrical enhancement and thickening of the labyrinthine and tympanic and mastoid segments of the facial nerve correlate with neuritis.
  - Petrous apicitis: Abnormal petrous apex enhancement. The trigeminal and abducens nerves can be involved and also demonstrate nerve enlargement and abnormal enhancement. Complete occlusion of the

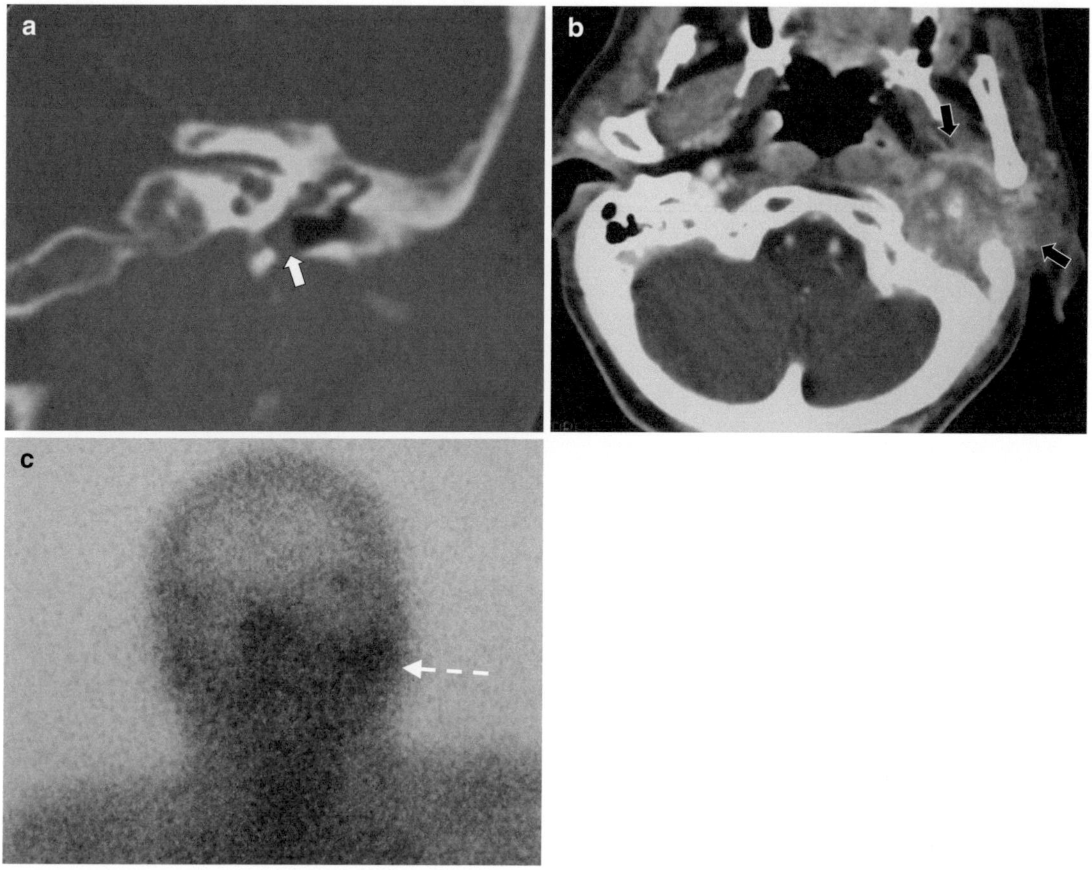

Fig. 34.1 A 62-year-old woman with type 2 diabetes, presenting with otalgia and otorrhea on the left. (**a**) Coronal temporal bone CT image demonstrates soft tissue within the left EAC and middle ear. Discontinuity of the inferior aspect of the EAC, posteromedially close to the temporomandibular joint (*arrow*). (**b**) Axial postcontrast CT image reveals anterior extension with involvement of the parotid gland and parapharyngeal and masticator space (*arrows*). This pattern of spread has probably occurred due to discontinuity of EAC. (**c**) Galium-67 scan shows increase uptake in the left mastoid (*dashed arrow*), indicating active inflammation and/or infection, which confirms the suspicious of underlying osteomyelitis related to external malignant otitis

petrous segment of the internal carotid artery may occur.
  - Intracranial involvement: EOM can lead to the development of meningitis, cerebritis, and abscess formation, as well as venous sinus thrombosis.
- The *local spreading patterns* are anterior, midline, intracranial, and combined as follows [5]:
  - An anterior extension pattern involves the retrocondylar fat, condylar bone marrow, temporomandibular joint, and masticator space (Fig. 34.1). Retrocondylar fat infiltration is reported to be the earliest change in EOM.
  - The medial extension pattern involves the parapharyngeal fat and nasopharyngeal and petrous apex (Fig. 34.2).
  - The midline extension pattern involves preclival soft tissue, clivus, and contralateral nasopharynx.
  - Alternatively the infection can erode the cartilaginous bone of the EAC, resulting in direct intracranial spread, involving the middle and posterior fossa (Fig. 34.2).
  - A combined pattern of extension is a poor prognostic factor.

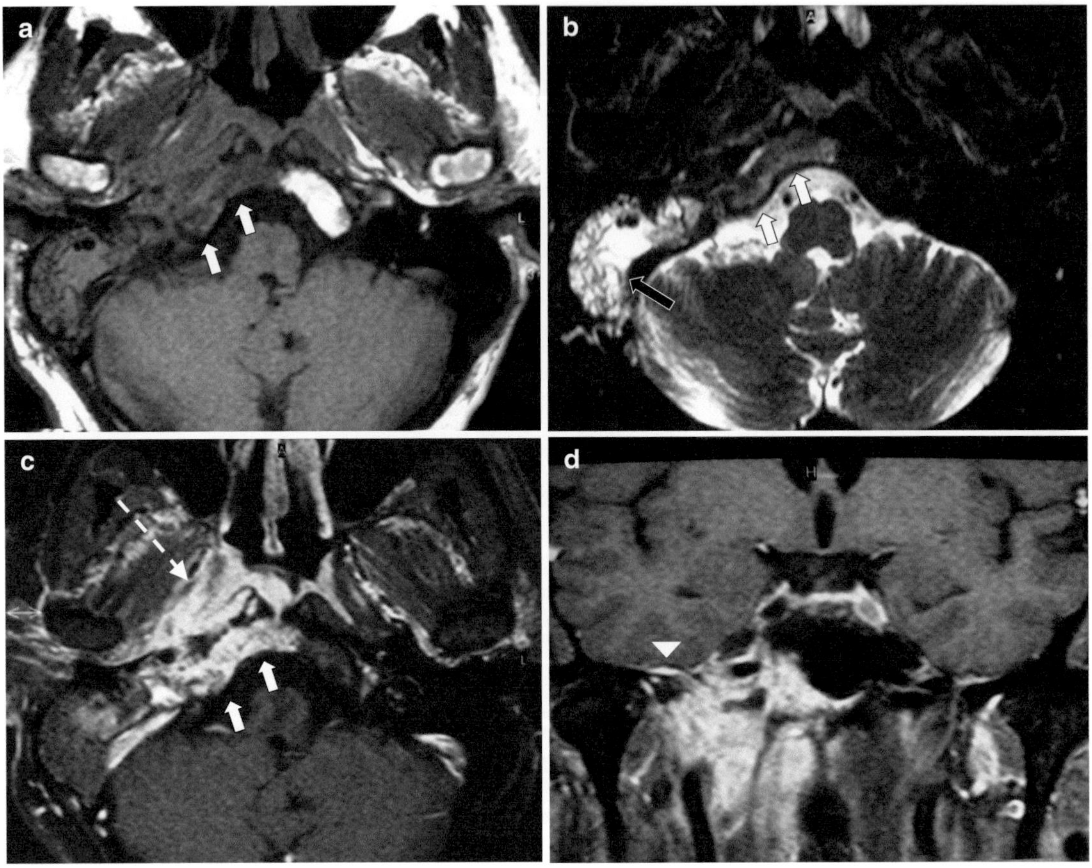

Fig. 34.2 A 52-year-old man with external malignant otitis. (**a**) Axial T1WI shows abnormal signal intensity of the bone marrow of the clivus and right petrous apex (*white arrows*). (**b**) Axial fat-saturated T2WI demonstrates inflammatory secretion fulfilling the right mastoid cells (*black arrow*) and subtle bone marrow hyperintensity involving the right petrous apex and the clivus (*white arrows*). (**c**) Axial postcontrast fat-saturated T1WI depicts abnormal enhancement on the right petrous apex and clivus (*arrows*), extending to the nasopharynx and the masticator space on the same side (*dashed arrow*). These findings are consistent with osteomyelitis related to external malignant otitis. (**d**) Coronal postcontrast fat-saturated T1WI demonstrates extensive abnormal enhancement involving the right nasopharynx, masticator space, and clivus. There is also dural thickening and contrast enhancement adjacent to the roof of the right mastoid (*arrowhead*), indicating intracranial spread

- *Scintigraphy*: Technetium-99 bone can be useful in the initial evaluation of patients with suspected osteomyelitis because its accumulation correlates with osteoblastic activity [8, 9].

Imaging Follow-Up

Imaging findings may help guide treatment. CT is not considered an accurate method to evaluate treatment response; however, bone remineralization which implies healing can be assessed by this method, and even if its absence is considered nonspecific, remineralization indicates a good response to treatment [6]. Changes on MRI, such as resolution of soft tissue and bone marrow changes, are also considered markers of good clinical response [7].

Gallium-67 single-photon emission tomography shows increased uptake in active infections and can be used for monitoring of therapeutic effect (Fig. 34.1) [9].

Main Differential Diagnosis

- *Squamous cell carcinoma* (SCCa) may be synchronous with EMO. A primary skin

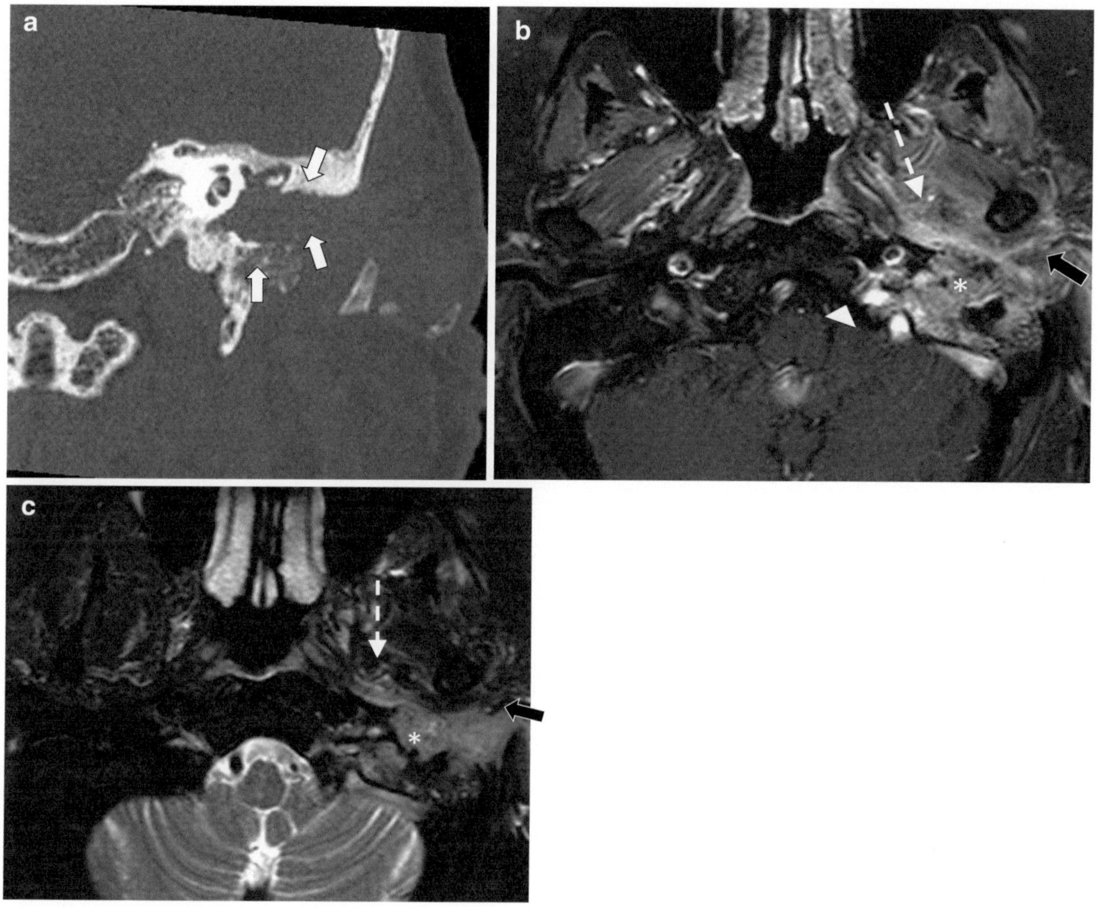

Fig. 34.3 External malignant otitis with underlying squamous cell carcinoma in a 68-year-old man. (**a**) Coronal bone CT image reveals a mass with soft tissue density within the external auditory canal associated with adjacent bone erosions (*arrows*). (**b**, **c**) Axial postcontrast fat-saturated T1WI and fat-saturated T2WI demonstrates extensive involvement of the left mastoid, extending to the middle ear (*star*), retromandibular fat, and parotid space (*black arrow*), as well as to the masticator space (*dashed arrow*). There is also involvement of the left hypoglossal canal (*arrowhead*)

SSCa is more common than primary tumor in the EAC. Isolated CT and MRI findings cannot distinguish EMO from SCCa (Fig. 34.3). When an underlying SCCa is suspected, biopsy is recommended [8]. Repeated infections or lack of response to treatment may be clues of underlying tumor.

- *Cholesteatoma* is characterized by a soft tissue mass associated with a typical pattern of smooth bone erosion. Although restricted diffusion can also be seen in abscess related to ear infections, it is considered a specific finding for cholesteatoma [8].

Tips

The radiology report should also include a detailed description of potential complications, as follows:

- Mention the involvement of neighboring anatomic structures. Presence of a combined or diffuse spreading pattern is a poor prognostic factor [5].
- Nasopharyngeal involvement must be assessed as it is related to poor prognosis, requiring a prolonged treatment, and confers reduced chances of survival

[10]. Once the nasopharynx is involved, base of the skull and intracranial spread may rapidly occur.

- Carefully evaluate the skull base searching for osteomyelitis and cranial nerve involvement as well as intracranial complications. In such cases morbidity and mortality are high and appropriated treatment cannot be delayed [4].
- Remember that isolated imaging findings cannot distinguish EMO from SCCa and sometimes they may have a synchronous presentation [8].

References

1. Verim A, Naiboglu B, Karaca C, Seneldir L, Kulekci S, Oysu C. Clinical outcome parameters for necrotizing otitis externa. Otol Neurotol: Off Publ Am Otol Soc, Am Neurotol Soc, Eur Acad Otol Neurotol. 2014; 35(2):371–6.
2. Rubin Grandis J, Branstetter BF, Yu VL. The changing face of malignant (necrotising) external otitis: clinical, radiological, and anatomic correlations. Lancet Infect Dis. 2004;4(1):34–9.
3. Karaman E, Yilmaz M, Ibrahimov M, Haciyev Y, Enver O. Malignant otitis externa. J Craniofac Surg. 2012;23(6):1748–51.
4. Chen CN, Chen YS, Yeh TH, Hsu CJ, Tseng FY. Outcomes of malignant external otitis: survival vs mortality. Acta Otolaryngol. 2010;130(1):89–94.
5. Lee JE, Song JJ, Oh SH, Chang SO, Kim CH, Lee JH. Prognostic value of extension patterns on follow-up magnetic resonance imaging in patients with necrotizing otitis externa. Arch Otolaryngol Head Neck Surg. 2011;137(7):688–93.
6. Sudhoff H, Rajagopal S, Mani N, Moumoulidis I, Axon PR, Moffat D. Usefulness of CT scans in malignant external otitis: effective tool for the diagnosis, but of limited value in predicting outcome. Eur Arch Otorhinolaryngol. 2008;265(1):53–6.
7. Adams A, Offiah C. Central skull base osteomyelitis as a complication of necrotizing otitis externa: imaging findings, complications, and challenges of diagnosis. Clin Radiol. 2012;67(10):e7–16.
8. Chen YA, Chan KC, Chen CK, Wu CM. Differential diagnosis and treatments of necrotizing otitis externa: a report of 19 cases. Auris Nasus Larynx. 2011; 38(6):666–70.
9. Stokkel MP, Takes RP, van Eck-Smit BL, Baatenburg de Jong RJ. The value of quantitative gallium-67 single-photon emission tomography in the clinical management of malignant external otitis. Eur J Nucl Med. 1997;24(11):1429–32.
10. Al-Noury K, Lotfy A. Computed tomography and magnetic resonance imaging findings before and after treatment of patients with malignant external otitis. Eur Arch Otorhinolaryngol. 2011;268(12):1727–34.

Ludwig's Angina

35

Benjamin Y. Huang

Abstract

Ludwig's angina is a severe, diffuse, rapidly progressive cellulitis of the sublingual and submandibular spaces, which usually develops from a preceding odontogenic infection. Imaging is frequently obtained on patients with the condition in order to assess the extent of the cellulitis, to localize drainable fluid collections and soft tissue gas, and to identify complications such as airway narrowing or mediastinal extension. Although the incidence and mortality associated with Ludwig's angina has declined dramatically with the introduction of antibiotics, it remains a serious and potentially life-threatening condition that requires prompt diagnosis and management to avoid serious morbidity or death.

Background

First described by Wilhelm Frederick von Ludwig in 1836, Ludwig's angina is a severe, diffuse, and rapidly progressing cellulitis of the floor of mouth, usually involving the submandibular, sublingual, and submental spaces which produces a brawny, hard induration of the floor of the mouth and suprahyoid region [1]. The disease is serious and potentially life threatening, as progressive edema of the soft tissues of the oral cavity and pharynx, posterior displacement of the tongue, inflammatory distention of the fascial planes, and associated pain and trismus can lead to severe airway obstruction [1–3].

Diagnosis of Ludwig's angina is made clinically. The traditional criteria proposed by Grodinsky in 1939 includes the following: (1) involvement of the sublingual and submandibular spaces that is almost always bilateral; (2) gangrene or serosanguinous phlegmon with little or no frank pus; (3) involvement of connective tissue, fascia, and muscles but not the glandular structures; and (4) spread by contiguity and not by lymphatics [4]. These features result in a characteristic bilateral woody cellulitis of the suprahyoid neck. Patients typically present with fever, neck and bilateral submandibular swelling, and tongue elevation. Drooling of secretions and

B.Y. Huang, MD, MPH
Department of Radiology,
University of North Carolina,
CB#7510, 101 Manning Drive,
Chapel Hill, NC 27599, USA
e-mail: bhuang@med.unc.edu

R. Hoffmann Nunes et al. (eds.), *Critical Findings in Neuroradiology*,
DOI 10.1007/978-3-319-27987-9_35

dysphonia (sometimes described as a "hot potato" voice) are common. Other symptoms can include toothache, odynophagia, trismus, dysphagia, or difficulty breathing [3]. Frequently, patients will report onset of symptoms within a few days following dental extraction from the lower jaw (usually of the second or third molars). Prior to the antibiotic era, some reports also described complaints of severe chest pain due to spread of infection into the mediastinum [5].

Although Ludwig's angina is still occasionally encountered today, its incidence has declined over the years due to the advent of antibiotics and improved dental care [6]. It occurs most often in young adult patients with dental infections; however, the disorder can develop at any age. Roughly a quarter to a third of cases are diagnosed in children, and cases have been reported in infants as young as 12 days of age [7, 8].

Treatment of Ludwig's angina revolves around the triad of (1) maintaining airway patency, (2) aggressive antibiotic therapy, and (3) decompression of the sublingual, submental, and submandibular spaces [1]. In milder cases, antibiotic therapy and close observation alone may be appropriate, and steroids may be helpful in reducing edema. However, severe cases usually warrant intubation or tracheostomy for airway management and surgical decompression/drainage of the affected sites. Although Ludwig's angina is classically described as demonstrating relatively little to no purulence, the presence of frank pus at surgery has been reported to be as high as 81 % in older series [9].

Prior to the modern antibiotic era, the disease was usually fatal due to airway compromise if left untreated, and even with surgical intervention, mortality rates at the time still exceeded 50 %. In modern practice, with combination antibiotic and surgical therapy, mortality from the disease has been significantly reduced, although it is still reported to be up to 10 % [1].

Key Points

Etiology

Most cases of Ludwig's angina (roughly 90 % in some studies) are odontogenic in origin, with most cases arising from the mandibular molar teeth [1, 3, 10]. The remaining cases may be due to nonodontogenic head and neck infections, sialolithiasis, facial trauma, or oral malignancies [1, 8, 10]. In addition, systemic conditions such as diabetes mellitus, organ transplantation, AIDS, and aplastic anemia may predispose to the condition.

Cultures in cases of Ludwig's angina are often polymicrobial, reflecting normal oral flora, and may include aerobes and anaerobes (most commonly alpha-hemolytic streptococci, staphylococci, and bacteroides species) [1].

Best Imaging Modality

Computed tomography (*CT*). It is the most widely used imaging modality used in the evaluation of patients with Ludwig's angina. However, because airway obstruction can be aggravated in the supine position, CT of the neck should be performed with caution, and patients should be closely monitored for signs of respiratory distress. Any patient who has airway compromise should have control of the airway ensured before any imaging is undertaken [11, 12].

Because the diagnosis of Ludwig's angina is made clinically, the primary role of imaging in the evaluation of patients with the disease is to evaluate the presence and degree of airway narrowing, to localize any drainable abscesses, to identify the presence of air from gas producing organisms, to assess for spread of disease to other areas (such as the retropharyngeal space and mediastinum), and to search for underlying odontogenic sources of infection [12]. CT should be performed with administration of intravenous contrast and should also extend through the upper mediastinum to rule out secondary mediastinitis.

Ultrasound (*US*). It can also be considered for imaging patients with Ludwig's angina, particularly if the patient is unable to undergo CT evaluation. Ultrasound can give a reliable determination of abscess versus cellulitis and can be used to guide percutaneous drainage of abscesses.

Major Findings

On contrast-enhanced CT imaging, Ludwig's angina classically manifests with swelling and inflammatory changes (soft tissue thickening, enhancement, and fat reticulation) in the bilateral submandibular and sublingual spaces [13] (Fig. 35.1). Abscesses will be evident as discrete, peripherally enhancing collections (Fig. 35.2). Miller et al. have reported that contrast-enhanced CT alone has a high sensitivity (95 %) for identifying drainable abscesses in patients with deep neck infections but has low specificity (53 %); however, addition of clinical assessment to CT substantially improves the specificity to 80 % while maintaining 95 % sensitivity. Viewing with bone windows may also be useful to identify associated odontogenic disease, including dental caries, periapical abscesses, and adjacent bone dehiscence.

Critical findings to assess for are the presence of substantial airway narrowing, extension of disease into the mediastinum, and presence of soft tissue gas (Fig. 35.3). Gas within the soft tissues raises concern for a gangrenous infection. Identification of any of these findings merits immediate direct communication with the ordering provider.

Imaging Follow-Up

Follow-up for patients with Ludwig's angina is clinical, and surveillance imaging is generally not indicated unless a patient fails to show an adequate clinical response to therapy or develops progressive symptoms or suspected complications, such as mediastinitis or venous thrombosis.

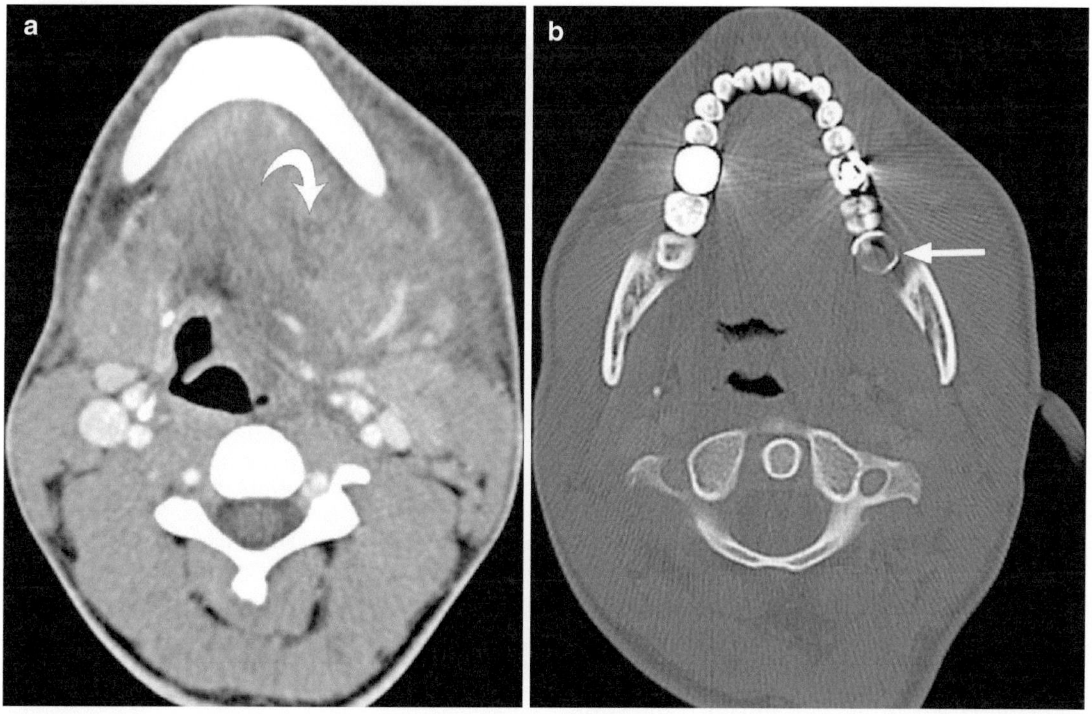

Fig. 35.1 (**a**) Axial contrast-enhanced CT image in a patient with left jaw pain and submandibular swelling demonstrates soft tissue swelling and inflammatory changes (fat stranding, edema, and skin thickening) in the left sublingual and submandibular spaces and to a lesser degree in the right sublingual and submandibular regions. Small low-density focus in the left sublingual region (*curved arrow*) could represent a developing abscess. Note also mass effect on the oropharyngeal airway with effacement of the left vallecular and slight posterior displacement of the left epiglottis. (**b**) Axial image presented in bone windows through the mandibular teeth demonstrates several dental fillings as well as a cavity of the left third molar (*arrow*)

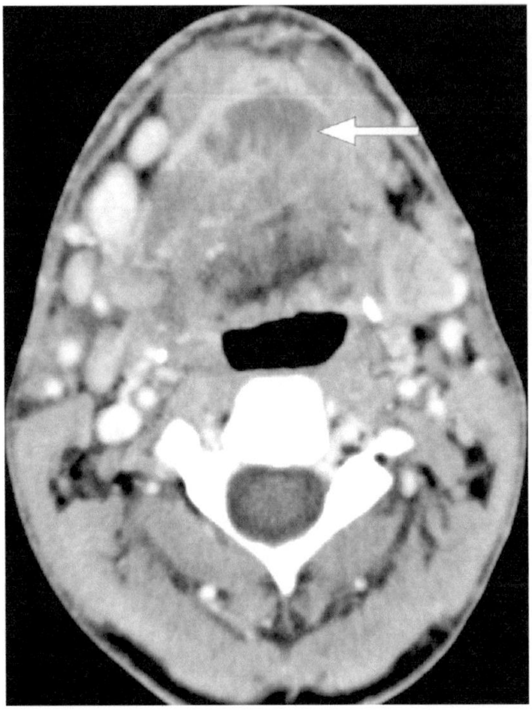

Fig. 35.2 Axial contrast-enhanced CT image in a patient with submandibular and submental swelling demonstrates inflammatory changes in the submandibular and submental regions with a peripherally enhancing fluid collection (*arrow*) in the anterior floor of mouth. There is reactive submandibular lymphadenopathy

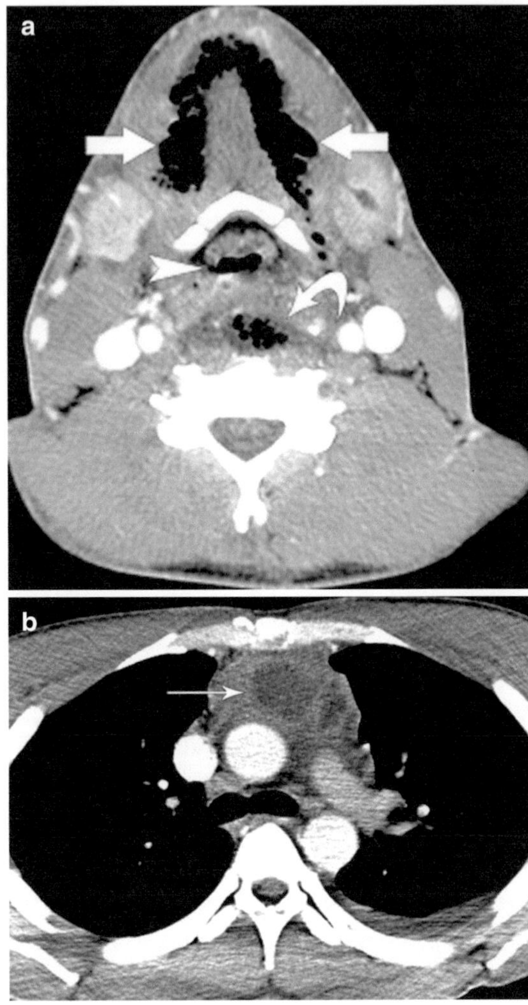

Fig. 35.3 (**a**) Postcontrast axial CT image in a patient with a several days history of tooth pain and neck swelling demonstrates diffuse soft tissue edema with subcutaneous gas in the floor of mouth bilaterally (*large arrows*), raising concern for a gangrenous infection. There is also evidence of spread in the retropharyngeal space, where there is gas and fluid collection (*curved arrow*) that contributes to significant airway narrowing (*arrowhead*). (**b**) Axial CT image through the upper chest in this patient demonstrates inflammatory changes and a peripherally enhancing fluid collection in the anterior mediastinum, indicating mediastinal spread of infection (*arrow*)

Main Differential Diagnosis

The primary differential diagnostic considerations on imaging are other infections including *facial cellulitis* (which may also be related to dental infection) and *submandibular sialadenitis*. These entities both demonstrate more localized inflammatory changes and are usually unilateral.

Other cystic floor of mouth lesions, including ranulas, dermoids and epidermoids, and thyroglossal duct cysts can mimic abscesses, particularly when they are inflamed; however, these entities do not demonstrate the extensive inflammatory change associated with abscesses in Ludwig's angina. Tumors in the anterior floor of mouth can also obstruct and cause dilatation of Wharton's duct and secondary inflammation of the submandibular gland. In these cases, however, the tumors are usually clinically evident.

Tips

- For cases of Ludwig's angina, the radiology report should include:
  - The presence, locations, and extent of inflammatory changes
  - The presence and location of any drainable fluid collections
  - The presence of soft tissue gas
  - The presence and degree of airway compromise (in patients with an unsecured airway)
  - Whether there is extension of disease into the mediastinum (imaging should include the upper mediastinum)
  - Whether there is odontogenic disease which could be the source of infection (look for dental caries, periapical lucencies, or dehiscence of the mandibular cortex)

References

1. Busch RF, Shah D. Ludwig's angina: improved treatment. Otolaryngol Head Neck Surg: Off J Am Acad Otolaryngol Head Neck Surg. 1997;117(6):S172–5.
2. Shockley WW. Ludwig angina: a review of current airway management. Arch Otolaryngol Head Neck Surg. 1999;125(5):600.
3. Srirompotong S, Art-Smart T. Ludwig's angina: a clinical review. Eur Arch Otorhinolaryngol: Off J Eur Fed Otorhinolaryngol Soc. 2003;260(7):401–3.
4. Grodinsky M. Ludwig's angina: an anatomical and clinical study with review of the literature. Surgery. 1939;5:678–96.
5. La'porte SJ, Juttla JK, Lingam RK. Imaging the floor of the mouth and the sublingual space. Radiogr: Rev Publ Radiol Soc N Am Inc. 2011;31(5):1215–30.
6. Parhiscar A, Har-El G. Deep neck abscess: a retrospective review of 210 cases. Ann Otol Rhinol Laryngol. 2001;110(11):1051–4.
7. Hartmann Jr RW. Ludwig's angina in children. Am Fam Physician. 1999;60(1):109–12.
8. Larawin V, Naipao J, Dubey SP. Head and neck space infections. Otolaryngol Head Neck Surg: Off J Am Acad Otolaryngol Head Neck Surg. 2006;135(6):889–93.
9. Finch RG, Snider Jr GE, Sprinkle PM. Ludwig's angina. JAMA. 1980;243(11):1171–3.
10. Derber CJ, Troy SB. Head and neck emergencies: bacterial meningitis, encephalitis, brain abscess, upper airway obstruction, and jugular septic thrombophlebitis. Med Clin North Am. 2012;96(6):1107–26.
11. Osborn TM, Assael LA, Bell RB. Deep space neck infection: principles of surgical management. Oral Maxillofac Surg Clin North Am. 2008;20(3):353–65.
12. Nguyen VD, Potter JL, Hersh-Schick MR. Ludwig angina: an uncommon and potentially lethal neck infection. AJNR Am J Neuroradiol. 1992;13(1):215–9.
13. Hoang JK, Eastwood JD, Glastonbury CM. What's in a name? Eponyms in head and neck imaging. Clin Radiol. 2010;65(3):237–45.

Retropharyngeal Abscess in Children

36

Carlos Jorge da Silva

Abstract

Retropharyngeal space abscess is typically a bacterial infection with a pus collection resulting from suppurative retropharyngeal lymphadenitis. On contrast-enhanced computed tomography images, a retropharyngeal abscess appears as a low-attenuation region expanding the retropharyngeal space, with enhancement along its margins. Complications result from spread to adjacent spaces and structures. The prognosis is generally satisfactory if early diagnosis and aggressive treatment are provided.

Background

Retropharyngeal space abscess is typically a bacterial infection with a collection of pus resulting from suppurative retropharyngeal lymphadenitis associated with tonsillitis, pharyngitis, sinonasal infection, otitis media, dental infection, or trauma to the neck and oropharynx [1, 2].

Historically, a retropharyngeal space abscess was believed to be the ultimate result of efferent spread of infection to the retropharyngeal lymph nodes. The common-source spread included the sinonasal tract, throat, tonsil, oral cavity, and middle ear [1, 2].

A retropharyngeal abscess can also be the result of penetrating trauma to the oropharynx or nasopharynx. These abscesses may also develop from a cervical spine osteomyelitis or discitis or as a complication of spinal surgery [3].

Retropharyngeal space infections were believed to occur almost exclusively in children younger than 6 years of age. However, with the increase size of the immunocompromised patient population, these infections have become frequent also in adults, being more common in males than in females (2:1) [1, 2].

Patients often present with fever, chills, odynophagia, sore throat, dysphagia, nausea, vomiting, respiratory distress, neck pain, and stiffness. Neck pain and stiffness may suggest associated meningitis. On physical examination, patient may be drooling and diaphoretic, with bulging

C.J. da Silva, MD, PhD
Division of Head and Neck Radiology,
Hospital Santa Casa de Misericórdia de São Paulo,
Rua Dr. Cesário Motta Junior 112, Vila Buarque,
Sao Paulo, SP 01221-020, Brazil

Division of Neuroradiology, Fleury Medicina e Saúde,
Sao Paulo, SP, Brazil
e-mail: carlos.silva@grupofleury.com.br

R. Hoffmann Nunes et al. (eds.), *Critical Findings in Neuroradiology*,
DOI 10.1007/978-3-319-27987-9_36

inflamed posterior nasopharyngeal/oropharyngeal wall [1, 2].

Administration of intravenous broad-spectrum antibiotics is essential. Surgical drainage is warranted if the clinical treatment fails or if a large and complex abscess is present, either by intraoral or open procedures, depending on the size of the lesion and the age and clinical stability of the patient [4, 5].

The prognosis is generally excellent if early diagnosis and aggressive treatment are provided. However, complications may result from adjacent space spread [6–8].

Key Points

Etiology

Retropharyngeal space abscess is typically a bacterial infection with a pus collection resulting from suppurative lymphadenitis associated with tonsillitis, pharyngitis, sinonasal infection, otitis media, dental infection, or trauma to the neck and oropharynx. Cultures are often polymicrobial, and the most common related bacteria are *Staphylococcus aureus*, *Streptococcus pyogenes*, and *Haemophilus influenzae* [1, 2].

Best Imaging Modality

The initial diagnostic imaging evaluation of a patient suspected of having a retropharyngeal space infection may consist of a lateral radiograph of the neck, taken during quiet breathing with the head in a neutral position. However, computed tomography (CT) with iodinated contrast is usually performed to better assess the airway and extent of the process. CT is considered the preferred imaging modality because of its high resolution, shorter scan times, lower costs, and overall better evaluation of nodal disease when compared to magnetic resonance imaging (MRI) [9–11].

Even though MRI is able to better characterize the neck soft tissues and estimate the extension of the process, the reduction in scan time with CT is especially advantageous in the pediatric population and may reduce or eliminate the need for sedation in infants and young children. Imaging studies should be performed with caution, and patients should be closely monitored for signs of respiratory distress. Airway control must be ensured before any imaging is undertaken [9–11].

Contrast-enhanced CT scan with slice thickness less than 3 mm from the skull base to the superior mediastinum is the recommended imaging protocol [9–11].

Major Findings

A lateral radiograph of the neck, taken with the head in a neutral position (Fig. 36.1), may show prevertebral swelling causing widened prevertebral distance (in patients older than 15 years old, usually more than one-half of the AP diameter of C4 and in younger patients, more than 1.5 cm thick), loss of the normal cervical lordosis, and air in the prevertebral soft tissues are all findings suggestive of underlying infection. However, radiographs alone usually cannot determine the exact location and extent of the process [9–11].

CT and MRI allow accurate localization of infections involving the deep neck and help distinguish between suppurative retropharyngeal adenitis with associated retropharyngeal space edema and a true retropharyngeal abscess [9–12].

MRI is rarely used in a septic patient, but it may reveal a pus collection that is iso-/hyperintense on T1-weghted imaging and hyperintense on T2-weighted imaging, with restricted diffusion and a thick wall after contrast enhancement [12].

On contrast-enhanced CT images, a retropharyngeal abscess appears as a low-attenuation region expanding the retropharyngeal space, with enhancement along the margins of the space. There is often an associated significant mass effect, and the posterior pharyngeal wall may be displaced ventrally (Figs. 36.1 and 36.2). Air may occasionally be seen within the abscess. Narrowing of the arteries and veins in the neck may also be seen [9–12].

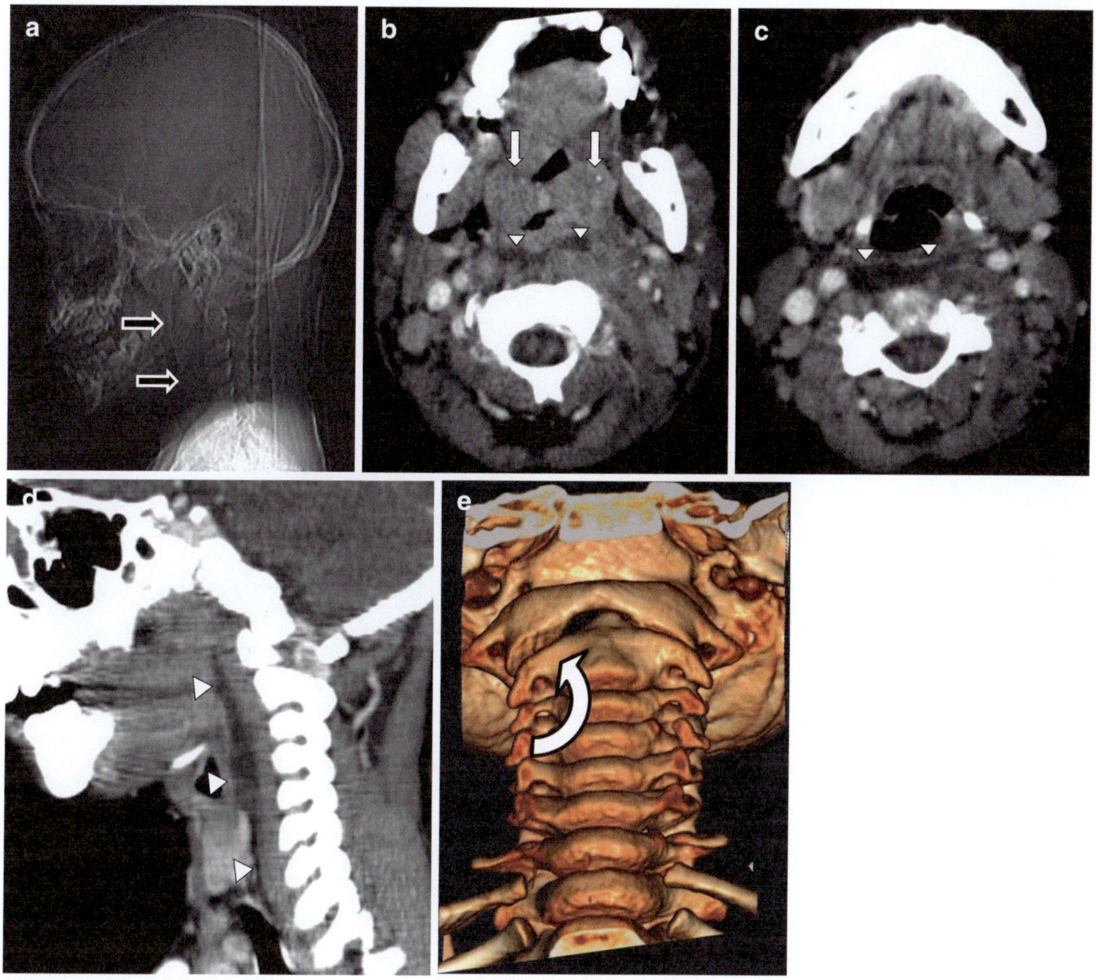

Fig. 36.1 A 6-year-old girl with tonsillitis, fever, and torticollis. (**a**) Lateral radiograph shows marked increase in prevertebral distance with ventral displacement of the pharynx and larynx (*arrows*). (**b**, **c**) Axial contrast-enhanced CT image show signs of bilateral non-suppurative tonsillitis (*arrows*) and a median retropharyngeal abscess (*arrowheads*), displacing the posterior pharyngeal wall ventrally. (**d**) Sagittal contrast-enhanced CT reformatted image shows the full extension of the retropharyngeal abscess (*arrowheads*) displacing the posterior pharyngeal wall ventrally. (**e**) 3D CT reformatted image demonstrates Grisel syndrome (nontraumatic rotational atlantoaxial subluxation), a rare complication (*curved arrow*)

Imaging Follow-Up

Follow-up for patients with retropharyngeal abscess is clinical, and surveillance imaging is generally not indicated unless a patient fails to show an adequate clinical response to therapy or develops progressive symptoms or suspected complications as a result from adjacent space spread: [6–8]

- Infections that involve the retropharyngeal space may enter the danger space and thus extend into the mediastinum.
- Narrowing of pharyngeal lumen may lead to upper airway compromise (Fig. 36.2).
- Carotid space involvement may lead to jugular vein thrombosis or thrombophlebitis, narrowing of internal carotid artery, potential internal carotid artery pseudoaneurysm, and rupture and even cerebral infarctions.
- Aspiration pneumonia.

Grisel syndrome (nontraumatic rotational atlantoaxial subluxation) is a rare complication (Fig. 36.1).

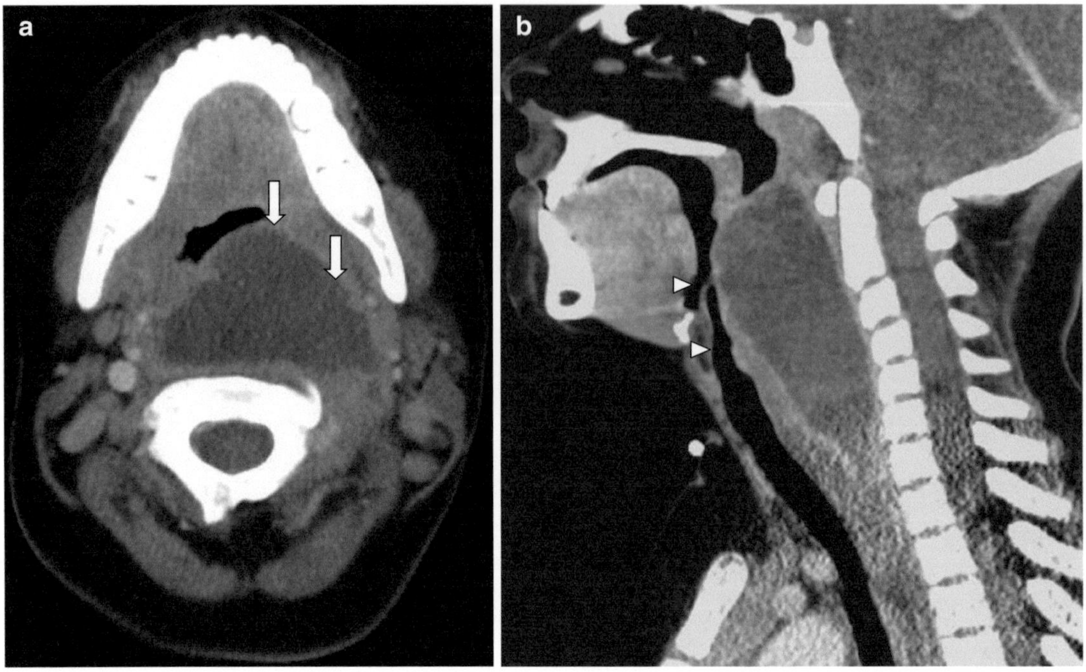

Fig. 36.2 An 8-year-old girl with a 2-week history of sore throat and worsening dysphagia, trismus, and difficulty moving her head. (**a**, **b**) Axial and sagittal contrast-enhanced CT images show a large rim-enhancing collection in the retropharyngeal space (*arrows*) displacing and narrowing the airway (*arrowheads*)

Main Differential Diagnosis

Non-abscess fluid in the retropharyngeal space is commonly seen in internal jugular vein thrombosis, chemotherapy or radiotherapy, pharyngitis, and longus colli tendinitis. On contrast-enhanced CT images, there is no mass effect or wall enhancement, and it does not require drainage [9–12].

Retropharyngeal suppurative lymph node: The patient is typically sick and suspected of having a retropharyngeal abscess. It results from pus formation in a reactive lymph node with intranodal abscess. On postcontrast CT images, there is a cystic-appearing node with ring enhancement in the lateral retropharyngeal space with adjacent cellulitis. It may progress to retropharyngeal space abscess if therapy is inadequate. Its lateral location is typical and serves to separate it from a retropharyngeal abscess [9–12].

Retropharyngeal space invasion from neoplastic process: This is more frequent in older patients with known pharyngeal squamous cell carcinoma and rare in children. Postcontrast CT images show a solid posterior pharyngeal wall enhancing soft tissue mass with necrosis extending to the retropharyngeal space. In these patients, the tumors are usually clinically evident [9–12].

Tips

Radiologists should provide a detailed description of the retropharyngeal space abscess and its relationships with the adjacent structures. Retropharyngeal/danger space abscess is the recommended term to be used as it may be impossible to exclude the extension of the pus collection to the danger space.

The radiology report should also include:

- The presence and location of any drainable fluid collections
- The presence of soft tissue gas
- The presence and degree of airway compromise (in patients with an unsecured airway)
- Whether there is extension of disease into the mediastinum (imaging should include the upper mediastinum)
- Whether there is extension of disease into the prevertebral space
- Compromise of vascular structures if present

References

1. Georget E, Gauthier A, Brugel L, Verlhac S, Remus N, Epaud R, Madhi F. Acute cervical lymphadenitis and infections of the retropharyngeal and parapharyngeal spaces in children. BMC Ear Nose Throat Disord. 2014;14:8. doi:10.1186/1472-6815-14-8.
2. Cheng J, Elden L. Children with deep space neck infections: our experience with 178 children. Otolaryngol Head Neck Surg. 2013;148(6):1037–42. doi:10.1177/0194599813482292.
3. Gianoli GJ, Espinola TE, Guarisco JL, Miller RH. Retropharyngeal space infection: changing trends. Otolaryngol Head Neck Surg. 1991;105(1):92–100.
4. Bolton M, Wang W, Hahn A, Ramilo O, Mejias A, Jaggi P. Predictors for successful treatment of pediatric deep neck infections using antimicrobials alone. Pediatr Infect Dis J. 2013;32(9):1034–6. doi:10.1097/INF.0b013e31829331f2.
5. Schuler PJ, Cohnen M, Greve J, Plettenberg C, Chereath J, Bas M, Koll C, Scheckenbach K, Wagenmann M, Schipper J, Hoffmann TK. Surgical management of retropharyngeal abscesses. Acta Otolaryngol. 2009;129(11):1274–9. doi:10.3109/00016480802642088.
6. Baldassari CM, Howell R, Amorn M, Budacki R, Choi S, Pena M. Complications in pediatric deep neck space abscesses. Otolaryngol Head Neck Surg. 2011;144(4):592–5. doi:10.1177/0194599810393882.
7. Hudgins PA, Dorey JH, Jacobs IN. Internal carotid artery narrowing in children with retropharyngeal lymphadenitis and abscess. AJNR Am J Neuroradiol. 1998;19(10):1841–3.
8. Wang LF, Kuo WR, Tsai SM, Huang KJ. Characterizations of life-threatening deep cervical space infections: a review of one hundred ninety-six cases. Am J Otolaryngol. 2003;24(2):111–7. doi:10.1053/ajot.2003.31.
9. Freling N, Roele E, Schaefer-Prokop C, Fokkens W. Prediction of deep neck abscesses by contrast-enhanced computerized tomography in 76 clinically suspect consecutive patients. Laryngoscope. 2009;119(9): 1745–52. doi:10.1002/lary.20606.
10. Raffaldi I, Le Serre D, Garazzino S, Scolfaro C, Bertaina C, Mignone F, Peradotto F, Tavormina P, Tovo PA. Diagnosis and management of deep neck infections in children: the experience of an Italian paediatric centre. J Infect Chemother. 2015;21(2):110–3. doi:10.1016/j.jiac.2014.10.011.
11. Vural C, Gungor A, Comerci S. Accuracy of computerized tomography in deep neck infections in the pediatric population. Am J Otolaryngol. 2003;24(3): 143–8.
12. Weber AL, Siciliano A. CT and MR imaging evaluation of neck infections with clinical correlations. Radiol Clin North Am. 2000;38(5):941–68. ix.

Lemierre Syndrome

37

Kenny Emmanuel Rentas and Benjamin Y. Huang

Abstract

Lemierre syndrome is a rare disease that is characterized by thrombophlebitis of the internal jugular vein, bacteremia, and septic emboli following a recent oropharyngeal infection. In most instances, anaerobic microorganisms are responsible for the infectious process with *bacterium Fusobacterium necrophorum* being the most common. Often patients present with high fevers and neck pain followed by pulmonary symptoms from septic emboli. Contrast-enhanced CT is the study of choice to confirm the diagnosis as it enables visualization of occluded thrombophlebitic veins as well as surrounding structures. Growth of anaerobic bacteria on blood culture is also part of the diagnosis. Early detection is crucial as the disease carries a high mortality rate if left untreated. Treatment includes drainage of any abscess and use of antibiotics targeted to the specific pathogen's susceptibility. Although controversial, some authors advocate for the use of anticoagulation agents.

Background

First discussed in a case series by André-Alfred Lemierre in the early 1900s, Lemierre syndrome (LS) is a rare and potentially lethal disease that was once common before the advent of antibiotic therapy [1]. The syndrome describes a specific subset of septic thrombophlebitis that is characterized by internal jugular vein (IJV) thrombosis and anaerobic bacteremia following a primary oropharyngeal infection [2, 3]. Classically, LS occurs in otherwise healthy children, adolescents, or young adults and is associated with distant septic emboli in the majority of cases.

K.E. Rentas, MD (✉) • B.Y. Huang, MD, MPH
Department of Radiology,
University of North Carolina,
101 Manning Dr. Campus, Box 7510,
Chapel Hill, NC 27599-7510, USA
e-mail: Dr.Rentas@gmail.com;
bhuang@med.unc.edu

R. Hoffmann Nunes et al. (eds.), *Critical Findings in Neuroradiology*,
DOI 10.1007/978-3-319-27987-9_37

Septic emboli most commonly affect the lungs, but any other organ can be involved [3]. Before the use of antibiotics, early case series demonstrated mortality rates of 62–90 %, whereas in modern times, mortality rates range from 4 % to 22 % [2, 4]. Several authors have noticed an increase in the number of cases in recent decades with reported incidences in Europe of 3.6 cases per 1 million per year [5–7]. The reason for the increased incidence of LS is unknown, but several theories include increased awareness, better bacteriological detection, and population changes [4–6, 8].

Most LS cases present in the second and third decades of life have no gender predominance and are diagnosed during the late winter and early spring seasons [2, 8, 9]. The most common physical finding is fever followed by pharyngitis or peritonsillar abscess and neck mass. Presenting symptoms also include pleuritic chest pain, dyspnea, dysphagia, neck pain, cough/hemoptysis, ear pain, bone/joint pain, dental pain, and abdominal pain [2]. Given the various clinical presentations, diagnosis is often delayed. Furthermore, imaging findings often precede clinical suspicion and blood culture results; therefore, radiologists play an essential role in early recognition of LS [10]. Treatment includes drainage of any abscess and use of antibiotics targeted to the specific pathogen's susceptibility. Although controversial, some authors advocate for the use of anticoagulation agents to treat patients with LS [3].

Key Points

Etiology

The palatine tonsils and peritonsillar tissue are the primary sources of infection in most cases of LS; however, other sources include the lungs, middle ear, mastoid, teeth, and sinuses [2]. In the vast majority of cases of LS, the microorganism responsible for the infection is *Fusobacterium necrophorum. Fusobacterium necrophorum* is a gram-negative anaerobic rod that is part of the normal flora of the oropharynx [2, 3]. There is no general agreement in the pattern of spread of the organism from the tonsils to the IJV; however, given the low virulence of *F. necrophorum*, hematogenous spread via thrombophlebitis seems most likely and is perhaps facilitated by an alteration in the pharyngeal mucosa by a viral or bacterial pharyngitis [2, 3, 8]. Following septic thrombophlebitis, metastatic infections occur in 63–100 % of patients and are most common to the lungs and major joints [9]. Some authors have also described some LS variants with sources of infection from the teeth, paranasal sinuses, or ear [5].

Best Imaging Modality

Computed tomography (CT): Contrast-enhanced CT is the study of choice as it provides a fast comprehensive assessment and enables visualization of occluded thrombophlebitic veins as well as surrounding structures. CT is also most readily available, is less susceptible to motion artifact, and provides better assessment of the lungs if there is clinical suspicion for septic pulmonary emboli [2].

Magnetic resonance imaging and magnetic resonance venography (MRI/MRV): MRI and MRV can demonstrate vein thrombosis, however, is susceptible to motion, most costly and less available than CT. Furthermore, venous thrombosis can have variable signal on conventional sequences and be difficult to detect. Contrast-enhanced MRI avoids radiation and can assess intracranial complications such as abscess formation, meningitis, and cavernous sinus thrombosis.

Ultrasonography (US): Doppler US can screen for venous thrombosis rapidly without the use of ionizing radiation or intravenous contrast. Evaluation of surrounding structures is limited, and evaluation for intracranial spread of disease and lung involvement is not possible.

Major Findings

The classic radiologic findings of LS are IJV thrombosis and evidence of metastatic infection. IJV thrombosis on postcontrast CT is typically seen as a low-attenuation intraluminal filling defect within a distended vessel with enhancing

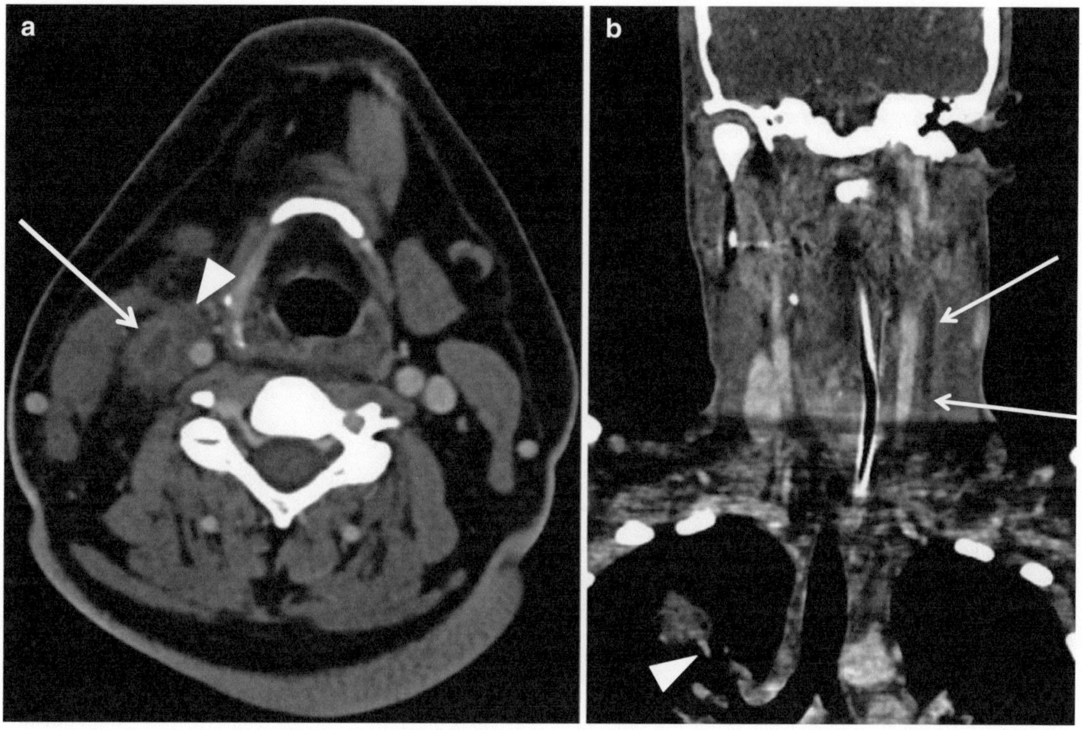

Fig. 37.1 Septic thrombophlebitis of the IJV. (**a**) Axial CECT image shows lack of opacification of the right IJV consistent with thrombosis (*arrow*). The IJV wall enhances and there is surrounding inflammation manifested as stranding of the adjacent fat (*arrowheads*). (**b**) Coronal CECT image on a different patient also shows lack of opacification of the left IJV (*arrows*) as well as an incompletely imaged vessel leading to an ill-defined right upper lobe nodule (*arrowhead*)

walls [11] (Fig. 37.1). Associated findings include surrounding inflammatory changes manifested as fat stranding, edema, adenopathy, and retropharyngeal effusion. Ipsilateral tonsillar fullness, edema, or abscess as well as septic thrombophlebitis of tributary veins may also be seen (Fig. 37.2). Retropharyngeal or tonsillar abscesses often manifest on postcontrast CT as a rim-enhancing hypodense fluid collection within an enlarged and inflamed tonsil or retropharyngeal space (Fig. 37.3). Septic pulmonary emboli usually manifest on CT as multiple, predominately peripheral ill-defined opacities that may be round or wedge-shaped and eventually progress to cavitation (Fig. 37.4). Classically, the opacities are related to a branching vessel, a finding often described as the "feeding vessel sign" (Fig. 37.1b) [4, 8, 10].

On ultrasonography, the vein is non-pulsatile, noncompressible, and usually distended with intraluminal echoes reflecting thrombus [11]. Sonographic evaluation of the IJV cephalad to the level of the mandible is not possible as it is obscured by the overlying osseous structures.

Imaging Follow-Up

There are no clear guidelines for imaging follow-up; however, repeat imaging is often considered when there is no clinical improvement or worsening despite optimal medical treatment. Follow-up imaging may reveal an abscess that may require surgical drainage.

Main Differential Diagnosis

Aseptic internal jugular vein thrombosis is secondary to indwelling catheter, tumor compression/invasion, or hypercoagulable state. This may lack

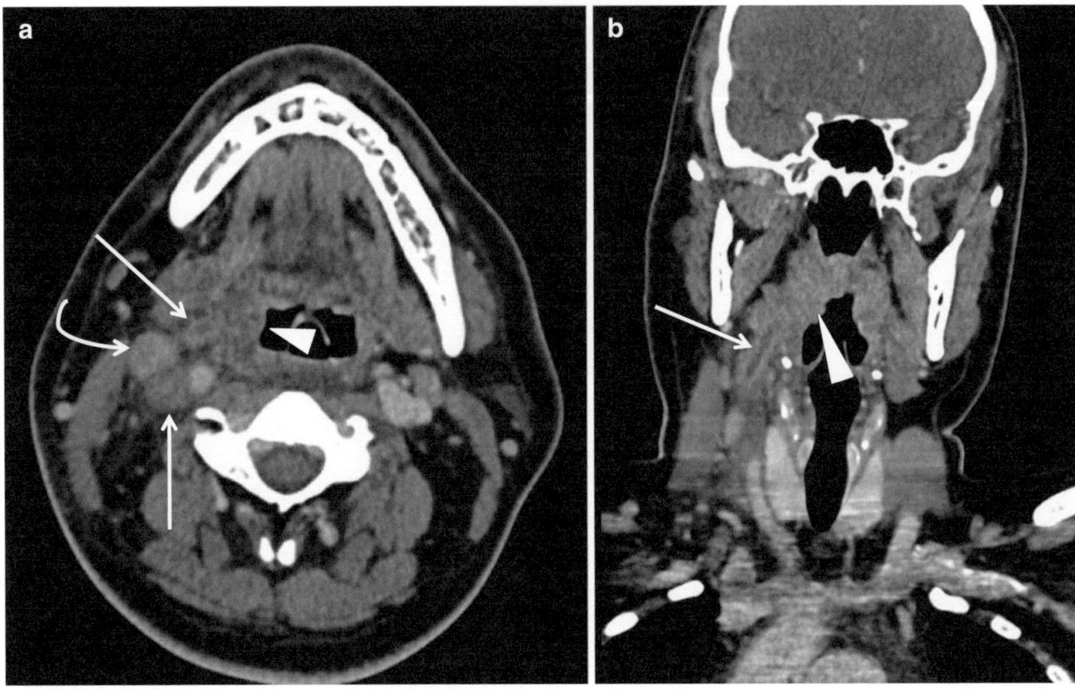

Fig. 37.2 Tonsillar enlargement and septic thrombophlebitis. Axial (**a**) and coronal (**b**) CECT images showing right tonsillar edema (*arrowhead*) and occluded right tributary and internal jugular veins (*arrows*). Inflammation of the surrounding fat is also noted as well as enlarged cervical lymph nodes (*curved arrow*)

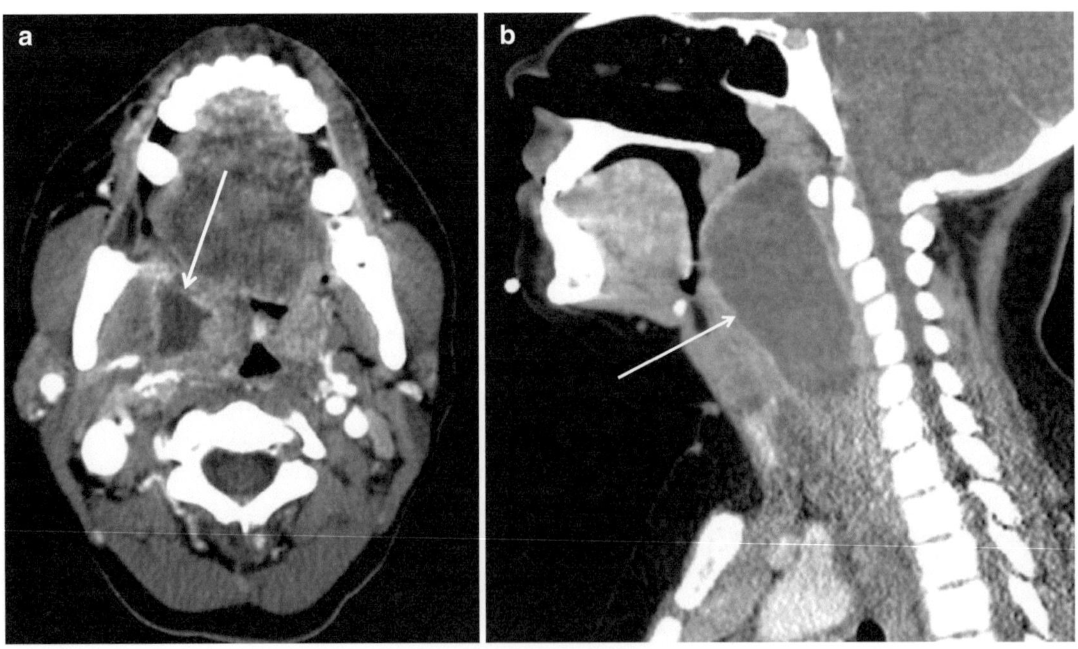

Fig. 37.3 Tonsillar and retropharyngeal abscesses. (**a**) Axial CECT image shows right tonsillar edema and rim-enhancing fluid collection consistent with a tonsillar abscess (*arrow*). (**b**) Sagittal CECT shows a large rim-enhancing fluid collection in the retropharyngeal space resulting in marked airway narrowing (*arrow*)

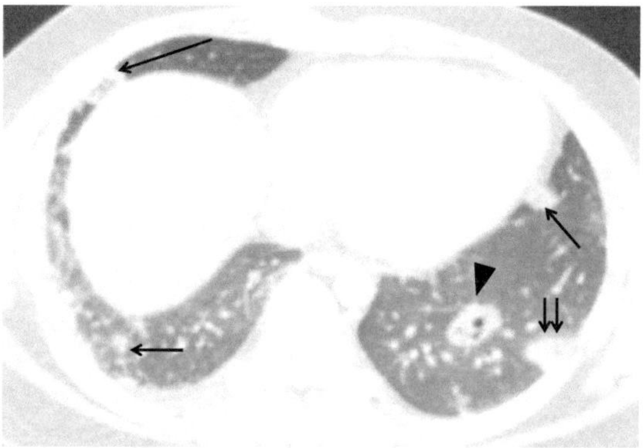

Fig. 37.4 Septic pulmonary emboli in a patient with Lemierre syndrome. Axial CT image through the lung bases shows multiple ill-defined peripherally located pulmonary nodules (*arrows*). Cavitary (*arrowhead*) and wedge-shaped (*double arrows*) nodules are noted in the left lower lobe

significant surrounding inflammatory changes; however, edema and abnormal vessel wall enhancement can be seen depending on the chronicity and extent of disease. The presence of a tonsillar/peritonsillar abscess and ill-defined pulmonary nodules/cavitations in the setting of IJV thrombosis would be more consistent with Lemierre syndrome.

Tips

- Lemierre syndrome should be suspected in young healthy patients with prolonged symptoms of pharyngitis followed by systemic or respiratory symptoms, pharyngitis associated with lateral neck pain and dysphagia, and pharyngitis followed by sepsis or multiple pulmonary abscesses [2, 4].
- Classic imaging presentation includes ipsilateral pharyngeal fullness, IJV thrombosis, and septic pulmonary emboli.
- IJV thrombosis can extend inferiorly into the subclavian vein or superiorly into the sigmoid, transverse, or cavernous sinuses; therefore, brain MRI should be considered for suspected intracranial disease.

References

1. Lemierre A. On certain septicæmias due to anaerobic organisms. Lancet. 1936;227:701–3. doi:10.1016/s0140-6736(00)57035-4.
2. Eilbert W, Singla N. Lemierre's syndrome. Int J Emerg Med. 2013;6:40. doi:10.1186/1865-1380-6-40.
3. O'Brien W, Lattin G, Thompson A. Lemierre syndrome: an all-but-forgotten disease. Am J Roentgenol. 2006;187:W324. doi:10.2214/ajr.06.0096.
4. Wright W, Shiner C, Ribes J. Lemierre syndrome. South Med J. 2012;105:283–8. doi:10.1097/smj.0b013e31825581ef.
5. Hagelskjær Kristensen L, Prag J. Lemierre's syndrome and other disseminated Fusobacterium necrophorum infections in Denmark: a prospective epidemiological and clinical survey. Eur J Clin Microbiol Infect Dis. 2008;27:779–89. doi:10.1007/s10096-008-0496-4.
6. Ramirez S, Hild T, Rudolph C, et al. Increased diagnosis of lemierre syndrome and other fusobacterium necrophorum infections at a Children's Hospital. Pediatrics. 2003;112:e380–5. doi:10.1542/peds.112.5.e380.
7. Brazier JS, Hall V, Yusuf E, Duerden B. Fusobacterium necrophorum infections in England and Wales 1990–2000. J Med Microbiol. 2002;51:269–72.
8. Riordan T. Human infection with fusobacterium necrophorum (necrobacillosis), with a focus on Lemierre's syndrome. Clin Microbiol Rev. 2007;20:622–59. doi:10.1128/cmr.00011-07.
9. Karkos P, Asrani S, Karkos C, et al. Lemierre's syndrome: a systematic review. Laryngoscope. 2009;119:1552–9. doi:10.1002/lary.20542.
10. Screaton N, Ravenel J, Lehner P, et al. Lemierre syndrome: forgotten but not extinct—report of four cases 1. Radiology. 1999;213:369–74. doi:10.1148/radiology.213.2.r99nv09369.
11. De Sena S, Rosenfeld D, Santos S, Keller I. Jugular thrombophlebitis complicating bacterial pharyngitis (Lemierre's syndrome). Pediatr Radiol. 1996;26:141–4. doi:10.1007/bf01372094.

Epiglottitis

38

João Lopes Dias and Pedro Alves

Abstract

Epiglottitis is a life-threatening condition. Despite being traditionally seen as a childhood disease, adults are now primarily affected. Imaging is not usually required for the diagnosis but may be useful if medical treatment is unsuccessful or complications are suspected.

Background

Epiglottitis remains one of the most threatening causes of "sore throat" in children. This potentially lethal condition deserves high clinical suspicion and emergent treatment [1, 2].

The classic presentation of the pediatric patient is fever and signs of "tripod position" which includes drooling, stridor, dyspnea, and tachypnea. These signs highly suggest airway involvement may be absent early in the disease process. Physical examination findings are variable and include enlarged cervical lymph nodes, pharyngeal hyperemia, and excessive salivation [1–4].

In the absence of characteristic physical findings, it may be difficult to identify those patients who are at risk for airway compromise. Older children and adults may have widely varying symptoms, including inability to lay flat, voice changes, odynophagia, and dysphagia. Moreover, patients who have been previously vaccinated typically have more subtle presentations [1, 2].

The treatment of epiglottitis includes intravenous antibiotics, oxygen administration, and airway management. Some authors recommend the use of steroids in acute presentations of epiglottitis, but further research is required [2, 4].

As adults have larger and more rigid airways, their need for intubation is significantly less than it is in children. In the pre-vaccination years, children were primarily affected, and the need for intubation approached 100 %, so early aggressive airway management was recommended. Nowadays, early aggressive intubation is only recommended when respiratory distress and stridor are present [2, 3].

Securing the airway in the emergency department is not recommended, and intubation should be performed in the operating room. For unstable patients, fiber-optic or nasotracheal intubation may be performed. Emergent tracheostomy or

J.L. Dias, MD (✉) • P. Alves, MD
Department of Radiology, Centro Hospitalar Lisboa Central, Rua José António Serrano, Lisboa 1150-199, Portugal
e-mail: Joaolopesdias85@gmail.com; tojais.pedro48@gmail.com

R. Hoffmann Nunes et al. (eds.), *Critical Findings in Neuroradiology*,
DOI 10.1007/978-3-319-27987-9_38

cricothyrotomy should be considered if intubation failed because of airway collapse and severe airway edema [2, 3].

Key Points

Etiology

Epiglottitis used to be a childhood disease mainly caused by *Haemophilus influenzae* type b, a gram-negative, coccobacillary, facultative anaerobic bacterium. However, its epidemiology has significantly shifted over the last decades due to the advent of vaccinations, and the incidence of acute epiglottitis in children has decreased from 4.9 to 0.02 cases/100,000/year [3]. Consequently, epiglottitis is now primarily a disease of adults, who tend to show a more variable and progressive disease with less severe presentations [1, 2, 4].

Epiglottitis produced by *Streptococcus pneumoniae*, a gram-positive bacterium, has increased since the introduction of vaccinations. Other pathogens like *Streptococcus pyogenes*, *Staphylococcus aureus*, *Moraxella catarrhalis*, *Streptococcus viridans*, *Streptococcus agalactiae*, *Neisseria meningitidis*, *Kingella kingae*, *Bacteroides* species, and the herpes simplex virus are now relatively common causes of epiglottitis [2].

Best Imaging Modality

The diagnosis of epiglottitis usually does not require imaging. Direct laryngoscopy may suffice and typically shows diffuse edema and erythema of the epiglottis. Severe presentations often need prompt airway management, and no imaging evaluation is required [1, 3].

Radiographs: Lateral neck radiographs can be useful by demonstrating the typical "thumb print" sign, which represents an enlarged and edematous epiglottis [1, 5]. Frontal radiographs are less useful for the diagnosis of epiglottitis and should always be obtained in combination with the lateral radiograph when foreign body aspiration is a part of the clinical differential diagnosis.

Computed tomography (CT) and magnetic resonance imaging (MRI): Sectional imaging is recommended when the diagnosis of epiglottitis is uncertain or medical treatment is ineffective. CT and MRI can readily exclude abscesses which may require emergent surgical drainage. It should be remembered that the supine position required for CT or MRI increases the risk of acute respiratory distress [1].

Major Findings

Both CT and MRI are able to depict the extent of the inflammation which frequently involves the prevertebral soft tissues, the valleculae, the uvula, base of the tongue, and the soft palate. Both techniques can assess the surrounding structures and may be helpful in excluding other diseases included in the clinical differential diagnosis such as peritonsillar abscess, retropharyngeal abscess, or foreign body aspiration [2].

Thickening of the epiglottis, stranding and obliteration of the pre-epiglottic fat, as well as thickening of the subcutaneous tissues and the pre-laryngeal muscles are commonly seen on CT (Fig. 38.1). If an abscess is present, it may be depicted as a hypoattenuating mass with an enhancing rim [1]. Air bubbles may be seen within or surrounding the epiglottis (Fig. 38.2).

Similarly to CT, MRI has been used to exclude complications and clarify uncertain cases. However, time of acquisition is longer on MRI, and motion and respiratory artifacts may hamper the study. Longer acquisition time also increases the risk of airway complications.

Imaging Follow-Up

Data in the literature are scarce in regard to the imaging follow-up of epiglottitis. In daily practice, no imaging follow-up is usually required unless complications are suspected.

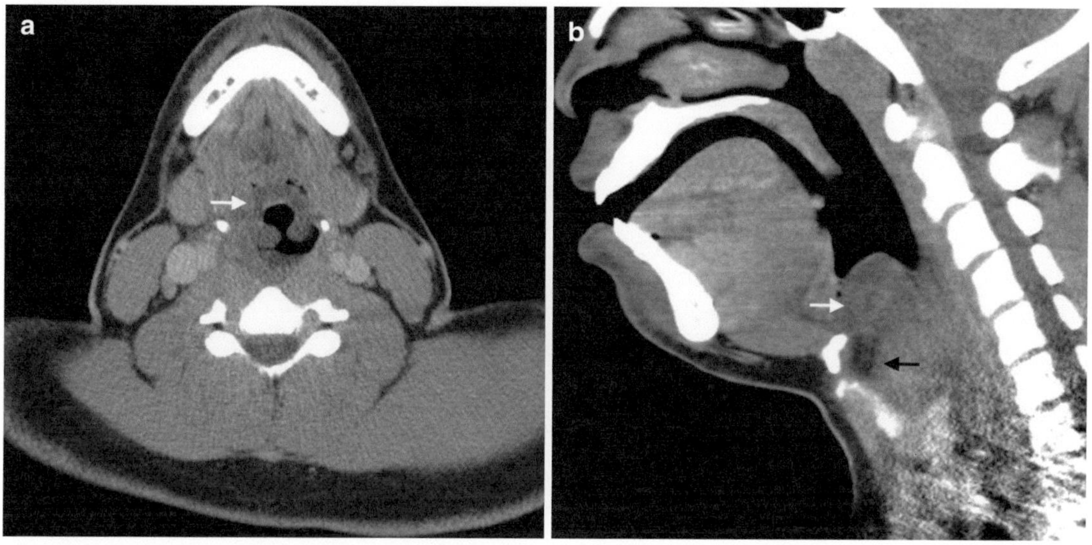

Fig. 38.1 Bacterial epiglottitis in a 5-year-old. Axial (**a**) and sagittal (**b**) contrast-enhanced CT images show edematous thickening of the epiglottis (*white arrows*) and stranding of the pre-epiglottic fat (*black arrow*) (Courtesy of Benjamin Huang, MD. Chapel Hill (NC) – USA)

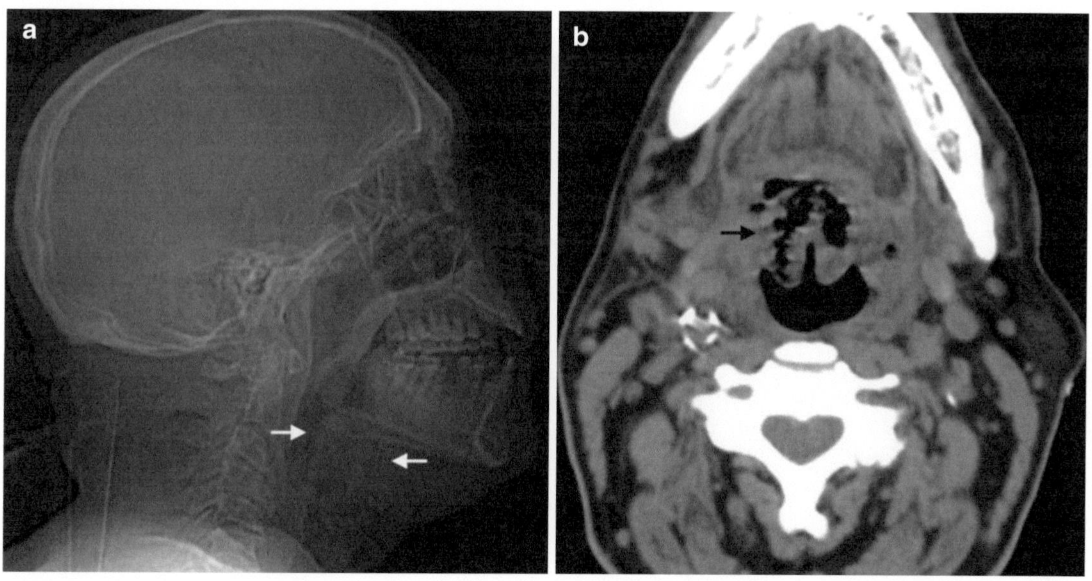

Fig. 38.2 Emphysematous epiglottitis in a 70-year-old man. Lateral CT scout view (**a**) demonstrates the "thumb print" sign (*arrows*) and air bubbles within the epiglottis. Axial (**b**) and sagittal (**c**) non-enhanced CT images show heterogeneous thickening of the epiglottis, which is replaced by an air-filled, ill-defined collection (*arrows*)

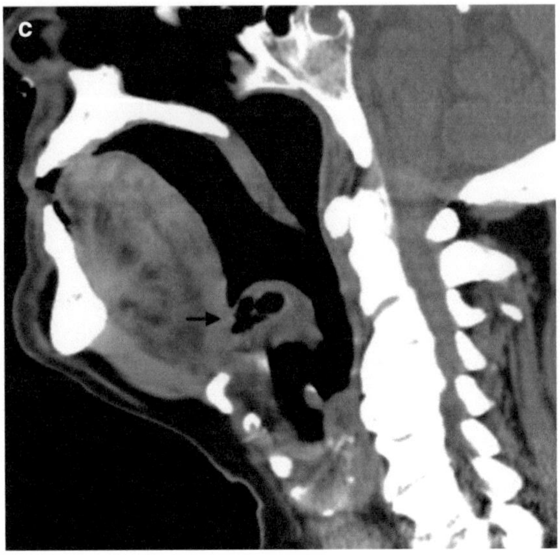

Fig. 38.2 (continued)

Main Differential Diagnosis

Main differential diagnosis includes pharyngitis, laryngitis, peritonsillar abscess, retropharyngeal abscess, or foreign body aspiration.

> **Tips**
> - The "thumb print" sign on lateral neck radiographs is classic of epiglottitis.
> - While performing CT or MRI, besides the thickening of the epiglottis and surrounding tissues, pre-epiglottic fat should be evaluated, and complications like abscesses and airway obstruction have to be excluded.

References

1. Ozanne A, Marsot-Dupuch K, Ducreux D, Meyer B, Lasjaunias P. Acute epiglottitis: MRI. Neuroradiology. 2004;46(2):153–5. doi:10.1007/s00234-003-1094-x.
2. Cirilli AR. Emergency evaluation and management of the sore throat. Emerg Med Clin North Am. 2013;31(2):501–15. doi:10.1016/j.emc.2013.01.002.
3. Reilly BK, Reddy SK, Verghese ST. Acute epiglottitis in the era of post-Haemophilus influenzae type B (HIB) vaccine. J Anesth. 2013;27(2):316–7. doi:10.1007/s00540-012-1500-9.
4. Hindy J, Novoa R, Slovik Y, Puterman M, Joshua B-Z. Epiglottic abscess as a complication of acute epiglottitis. Am J Otolaryngol. 2013;34(4):362–5. doi:10.1016/j.amjoto.2013.01.003.
5. Grover C. Images in clinical medicine. "Thumb sign" of epiglottitis. N Engl J Med. 2011;365(5):447. doi:10.1056/NEJMicm1009990.

Orbital Trauma

39

Prashant Vijay Shankar

Abstract

Orbital trauma accounts for a significant portion of emergency department visits and is most frequently seen in conjunction with multiple trauma. Trauma is a significant source of monocular blindness in the United States. Multidetector CT is the best imaging modality for evaluating orbital trauma.

Background

Orbital trauma accounts for 3 % of all emergency department visits in the United States and is most commonly seen in patients with multiple trauma [1]. Up to 40 % of cases of monocular blindness in the United States are secondary to trauma [2], underscoring the importance of recognizing these injuries. An understanding of orbital anatomy and recognition of common orbital injuries are essential skills that all radiologists should possess. Computed tomography is the imaging modality of choice in the evaluation of acute orbital trauma.

P.V. Shankar, MD
Department of Radiology,
University of North Carolina at Chapel Hill,
101 Manning Drive, Chapel Hill, NC 27514, USA
e-mail: pshankar@unch.unc.edu

Key Points

Etiology

These injuries are most frequently encountered in young males (up to 81 %) and are most commonly due to sports injuries. In older males and adults, these injuries are often the result of assault and motor vehicle accidents [1].

Best Imaging Modality

Computed tomography (*CT*): CT is the imaging modality of choice in the evaluation of acute orbital trauma due to its widespread availability, ease of image acquisition, speed, and superior characterization of the bony anatomy as well as clear depiction of orbital soft tissue structures.

Face radiographs: They are rarely obtained in the setting of emergent trauma. Although the sensitivity for detection of acute fractures has been reported as high as 78 % [3], their sensitivity for

R. Hoffmann Nunes et al. (eds.), *Critical Findings in Neuroradiology*,
DOI 10.1007/978-3-319-27987-9_39

accompanying soft tissue injury is extremely low. The orbital contents cannot be assessed with radiography.

Magnetic resonance imaging (*MRI*): MRI is often contraindicated in the setting of acute trauma, particularly if retained metallic projectiles preclude entry into the MRI suite. CT generally provides all information required for acute management. Patients with unexplained vision loss, proptosis, and/or cranial nerve palsies may need MRI.

Ultrasonography (*US*): It can be useful for assessing orbital contents but is contraindicated in the setting of globe rupture. US during the acute period has very limited benefits.

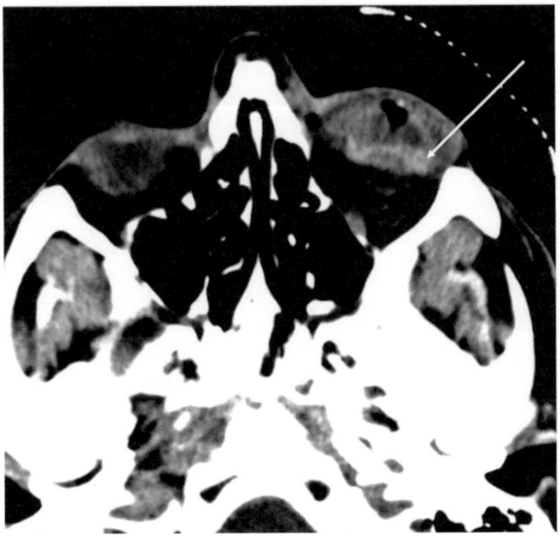

Fig. 39.1 Ruptured globe. Axial non-contrast CT in soft tissue window. There is marked deformity and volume loss of the left globe with blood seen in the posterior chamber (*arrow*). Air is also seen within the globe. Findings are consistent with left globe rupture

Major Findings

Ruptured globe: A ruptured globe or open globe injury should be treated nearly immediately in any victim of orbital trauma as it is a common cause of blindness. Ruptures are most common at the insertions of the extraocular muscles where the sclera is thinnest [4]. The diagnosis of ruptured globe can be made clinically if intraocular contents are present on examination; otherwise, CT is the next step in evaluating these injuries. CT findings of an open globe injury include a change in globe contour, volume loss, hemorrhage within the globe, scleral discontinuity, and intraocular air/foreign bodies (Figs. 39.1 and 39.2).

Hematomas of soft tissues: Hematoma in the periorbital or retro-orbital soft tissues can also produce a deformity of the globe even if there is no frank open globe injury (Fig. 39.3). Compression by hematomas may injure the globe and/or optic nerve. A hematoma at the scleral insertion of the optic nerve portrays a poor prognosis.

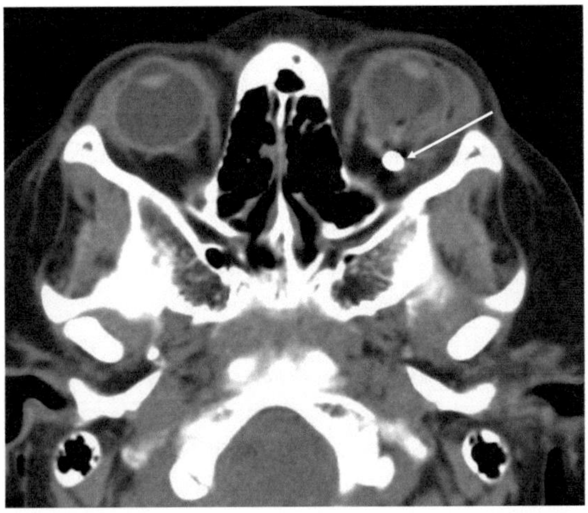

Fig. 39.2 Ruptured left globe secondary to a gunshot wound. Axial non-contrast CT of the face in soft tissue window shows a deformed and small left globe and blood in the vitreous humor. Note the retained projectile in the retrobulbar soft tissues (*arrow*)

Orbital blowout fracture: An orbital blowout fracture is a traumatic deformity involving the orbital floor or medial wall (lamina papyracea) resulting from the impact of a blunt object larger than the orbital aperture. Orbital fractures can occur in isolation or with fractures. Close attention should be paid to the shape and position of the inferior and medial rectus muscles. If the muscle remains flattened and appears in the correct position, it is likely intact. However, if the muscle is enlarged and round (intramuscular hematoma), if there is accompanying perimuscular stranding, or if there is evidence of inferior or medial displacement, clinical correlation for entrapment should be requested. Remember that entrapment is a clinical and not an imaging diagnosis. Medial orbital wall fractures are strongly associated with diplopia due to loss of the posterior-medial bulge of the orbit and mechanical entrapment of the medial rectus muscle (Figs. 39.4 and 39.5) [5].

Zygomaticomaxillary complex fracture: The zygomaticomaxillary complex refers to the temporal bone, maxilla, frontal bone, and skull base. Displaced zygomaticomaxillary complex fractures often increase orbital volume by angulation of the lateral orbital wall at the zygomaticosphenoid suture or blowout of the orbital floor. The zygomatic arch maintains facial width and profile, so fractures of it produce loss of cheek projection with increased facial width. The fracture line may traverse the infraorbital foramen and produce nerve damage, resulting in impaired sensation of the cheek/upper lip. Close attention should be paid to the lateral orbital wall, the orbital floor, the anterior maxilla, and the zygomatic arch. A frequently missed zygomaticomaxillary complex fracture is at the temporal bone portion of the upper transverse maxillary buttress [6]. Zygomaticomaxillary complex fractures most commonly occur after a

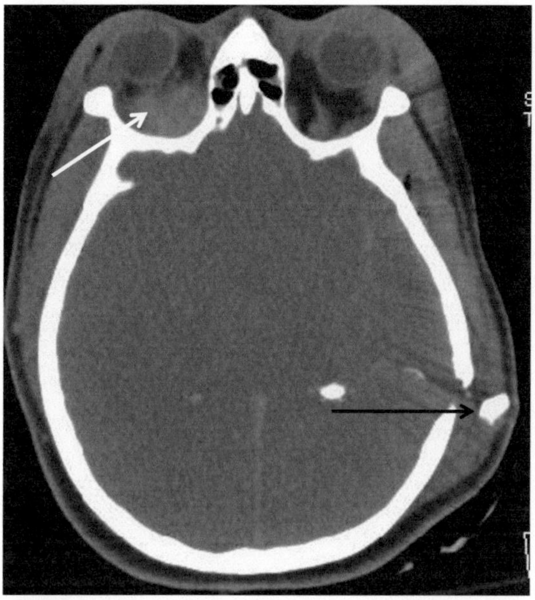

Fig. 39.3 Retrobulbar hematoma secondary of gunshot wound. Axial non-contrast head CT. There is a right retro-orbital hematoma (*white arrow*). A left temporal skull fracture with a retained projectile foreign body in the adjacent scalp is seen (*black arrow*)

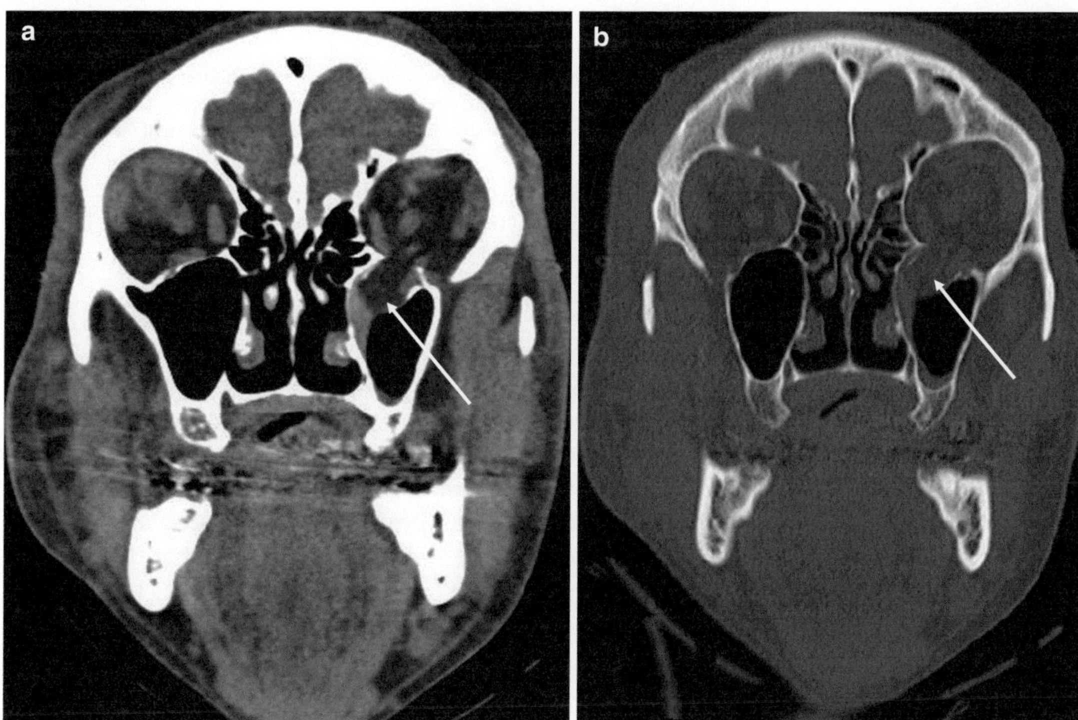

Fig. 39.4 Inferior blowout fracture. Coronal face CT in soft tissue (**a**) and bone (**b**) windows. There is a blowout fracture of the left orbital floor. Fat and the left inferior rectus muscle are seen herniating through the defect (*arrows*). In (**b**) the osseous defect is demonstrated

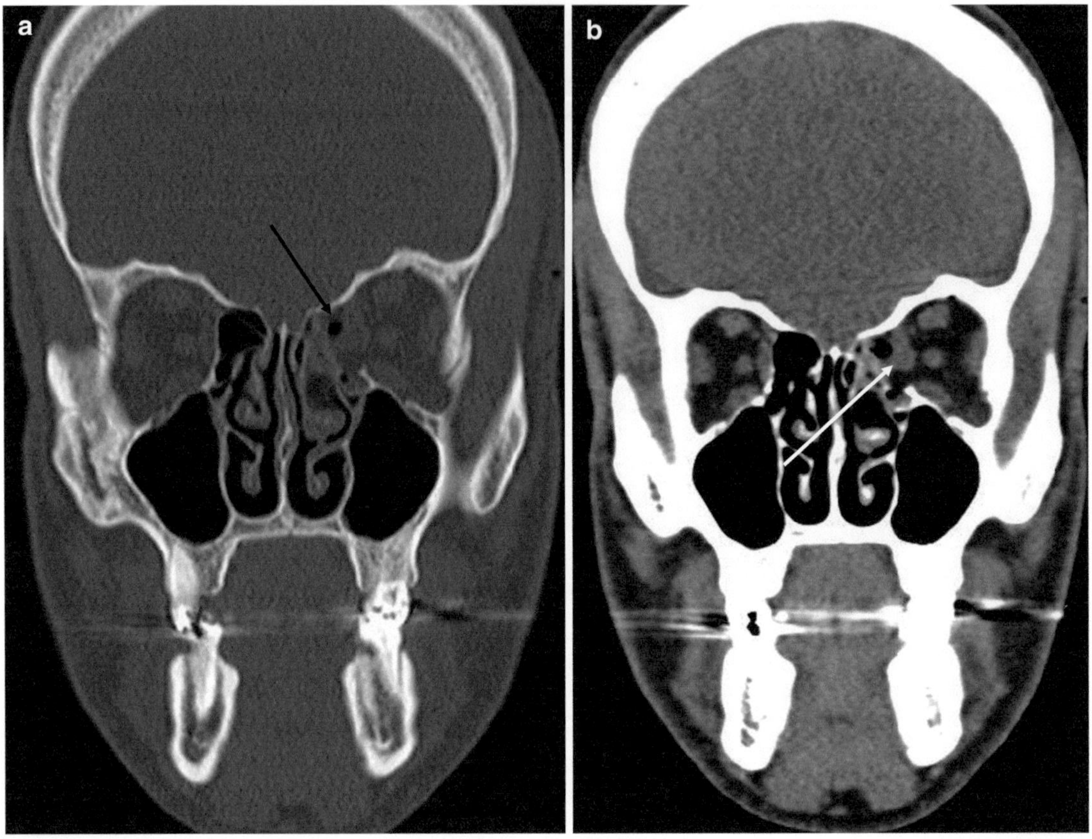

Fig. 39.5 Medial blowout fracture. Coronal face CT in bone (**a**) and soft tissue (**b**) windows. There is a defect of the medial wall of the left orbit. Gas is present within the orbit (*black arrow*), likely originating from the ethmoid sinuses. The left medial rectus muscle is thickened along its posteromedial aspect due to entrapment (*white arrow*)

direct blow to the cheek (malar eminence) during assault. Teenagers and young males are most frequently affected (Fig. 39.6).

Naso-orbital-ethmoidal complex fracture. A naso-orbital-ethmoidal complex fracture is a complex upper midface fracture involving the confluence of the medial and upper maxillary buttresses and their posterior extensions. These fractures are the result of force being transmitted through the nasal bones with extension into the ethmoid sinuses and medial orbital walls. These fractures are stratified according to the Manson classification as follows [7]:

Type I: The medial canthal tendon remains attached to a large osseous fragment.
Type II: The medial canthal tendon is attached to a small osseous fragment.
Type III: The medial canthal tendon is completely avulsed.

The radiologist should comment on the degree of comminution of the medial vertical maxillary buttresses, specifically in the region of the lacrimal fossa, where the medial canthus attaches. It is also useful to describe the degree of comminution of the ethmoid sinus in the region of the nasofrontal ducts, as disruption of these ducts can predispose patients to mucocele formation (Fig. 39.7) [8].

Imaging Follow-Up

Patients with facial trauma are best assessed in the emergency setting with CT. Postoperative imaging is usually only obtained on a clinical

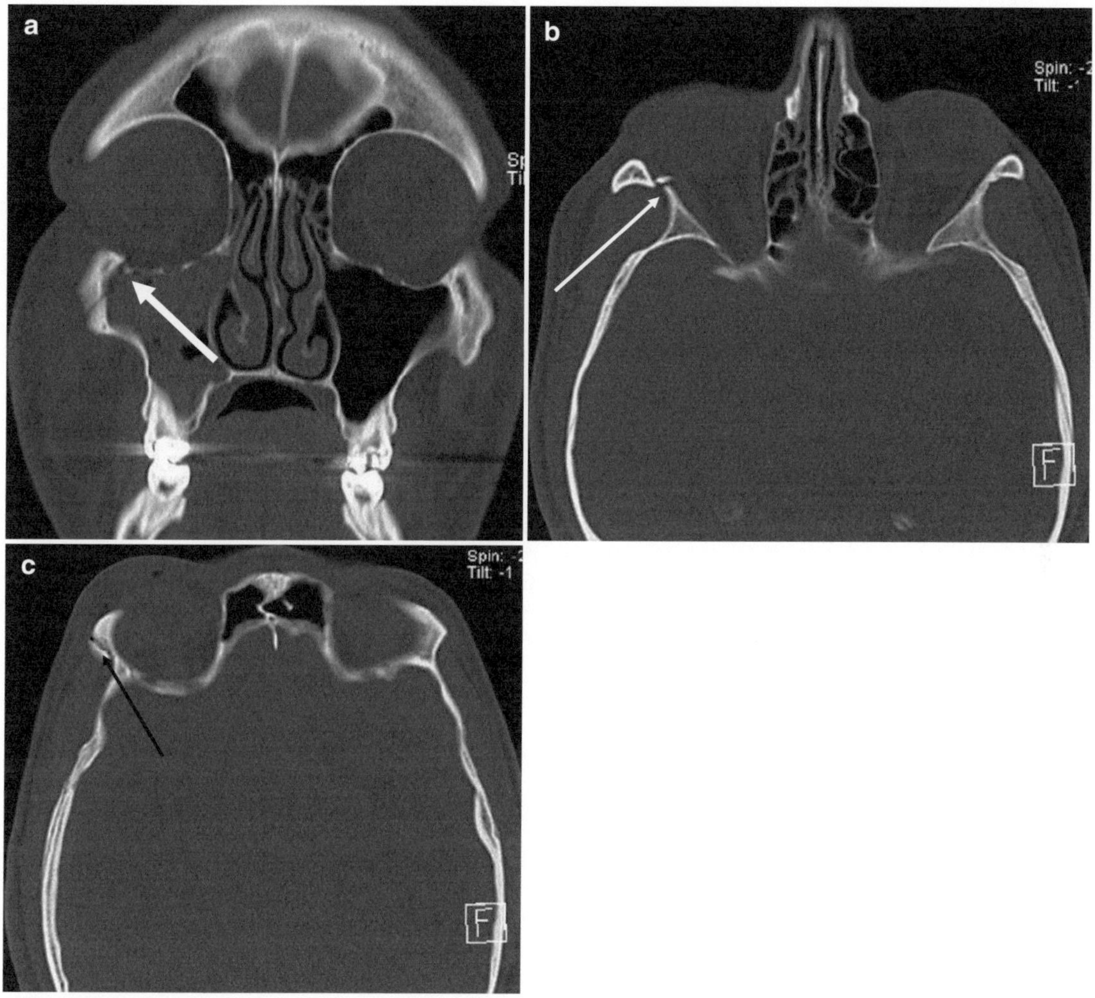

Fig. 39.6 Zygomaticomaxillary complex fracture. (**a**) Coronal CT of the face in bone window shows zygomaticomaxillary complex fracture. Note the fracture through the anterolateral wall of the right maxillary sinus extending into the right orbital floor (*white thick arrow*). (**b**, **c**) Axial CT in bone window at different levels depict a displaced fracture of the right lateral orbital wall, and an osseous fragment projects into the orbit impinging upon the right lateral rectus muscle (*white thin arrow*) superior continuation of the fracture, involving the right superior orbital rim (*black thin arrow*)

basis. CT remains the best imaging modality in the postoperative setting.

Main Differential Diagnoses

Alternate diagnoses are rarely considered in the setting of orbital trauma, as the patient almost always presents with a history and examination consistent with trauma. Nonetheless, there are other radiographic entities which should be considered.

Globe Rupture

- *Phthisis bulbi* is a shrunken and scarred globe which reflects an old injury or a series of multiple ocular insults.
- *Coloboma* is a congenital anomaly in which there forms a gap in the posterior pole of the globe, resulting in a posterior outpouching continuous with the vitreous chamber.
- *Staphyloma* is an acquired defect which produces a stretched or ectatic appearance of the eye.

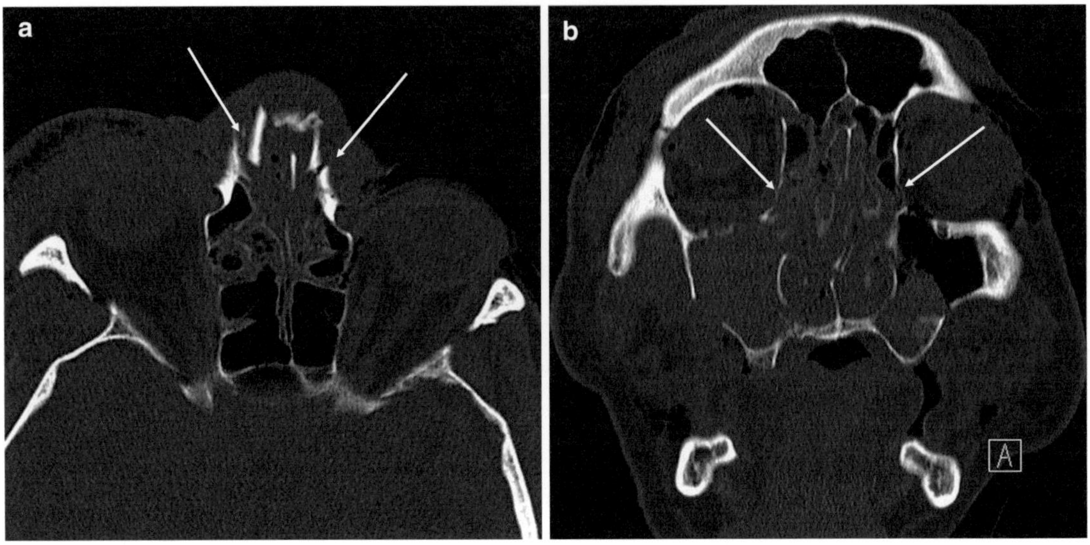

Fig. 39.7 Naso-orbital-ethmoidal complex fracture. Axial (**a**) and coronal (**b**) CT of the face in bone window shows fractures of the medial orbital walls and ethmoid sinuses and disruption of the medial canthal regions (*arrows*). In the coronal plane, the findings in (**a**) are remonstrated, and there are extensive bilateral medial wall fractures. Also there is extensive subcutaneous gas. *Arrows* point to fractures involving the lacrimal fossae

- *Buphthalmos* refers to a diffusely enlarged globe generally seen in patients with neurofibromatosis type 1 or chronic glaucoma.

Orbital Blowout Fracture

- *Dehiscent lamina papyracea* may be an acquired post-traumatic deformity, congenital, or the result of erosive sinus disease. The medial rectus and fat may herniate through the defect into the ethmoid labyrinth.
- *Orbital decompression surgery* is often performed in patients with thyroid ophthalmopathy, and the postsurgical distortion of the orbital walls can mimic an orbital blowout fracture. Correlation with medical/surgical history is important in these cases.

Zygomaticomaxillary Complex and Naso-Orbital-Ethmoidal Fractures

- One should consider complex midface fractures (i.e., "Le Fort" fractures) in patients presenting with these fractures. Close attention should be paid to the pterygomaxillary junction and the maxillary buttresses to exclude a complex midface injury.

Tips

- Ruptured globe is a surgical emergency, and this finding should be communicated to the referring provider in a timely fashion. The radiologist should comment on the presence of retained projectiles or foreign bodies.
- Orbital blowout fractures may produce extraocular muscle entrapment. Entrapment is a clinical diagnosis, but imaging findings of extraocular muscles contour abnormality, herniation, or perimuscular stranding should be included in the report if present.
- Disruption of the nasofronal ducts may be present in naso-orbital-ethmoidal fractures and can later result in mucocele formation. It is important to evaluate for this finding.

References

1. Kubal W. Imaging of orbital trauma. Radiographics. 2008;28:1729–39.
2. Kuhn F, Morris R, Mester V, et al. Epidemiology and socioeconomics. Ophthalmol Clin North Am. 2002; 15:145–51.
3. Iinuma T, Hirota Y, Ishio K. Orbital wall fractures: conventional views and CT. Rhinology. 1994;32:81–3.
4. Bord SP, Linden J. Trauma to the globe and orbit. Emerg Med Clin North Am. 2008;26:97–123.
5. Hopper R, Salmey S, Sze R. Diagnosis of midface fractures with CT: what the surgeon needs to know. Radiographics. 2006;26:783–93.
6. Laine FJ, Conway WF, Laskin DM. Radiology of maxillofacial trauma. Curr Probl Diagn Radiol. 1993;22(4):145–88.
7. Markowitz BL, Manson PN, Sargent L, et al. Management of the medial canthal tendon in nasoethmoid orbital fractures: the importance of the central fragment in classification and treatment. Plast Reconstr Surg. 1991;87(5):843–53.
8. Gassner R, Tuli T, Hachl O, Rudisch A, Ulmer H. Cranio-maxillofacial trauma: a 10 year review of 9,543 cases with 21,067 injuries. J Craniomaxillofac Surg. 2003;31(1):51–61.

Temporal Bone Fractures

40

Benjamin Y. Huang

Abstract

Temporal bone fractures occur in up to 20 % of patients presenting with significant closed head injuries and can be associated with complications including hearing loss, facial paralysis, and CSF fistula. Traditionally, fractures of the temporal bone have been classified as longitudinal or transverse depending on their orientation relative to the long axis of the petrous bone, but in reality, most temporal bone fractures are oblique or have overlapping features. The role of imaging in temporal bone trauma is not only to identify the fracture but also to assess for involvement of important structures such as the otic capsule, ossicular chain, facial nerve, and carotid artery.

Background

Fractures of the temporal bones occur in 10–20 % of patients presenting with significant closed head injuries and account for approximately 20 % of skull fractures, with between 8 % and 29 % being bilateral [1–3]. While these fractures may be observed at any age, roughly 70 % occur during the second through fourth decades of life, with males being predominantly affected at a ratio of approximately 3:1.

B.Y. Huang, MD, MPH
Department of Radiology, University of North Carolina, CB#7510, 101 Manning Drive, Chapel Hill, NC 27599, USA
e-mail: bhuang@med.unc.edu

Traditionally, temporal bone fractures are classified as either longitudinal or transverse, depending on their course relative to the long axis of the petrous pyramid. *Longitudinal fractures* extend parallel to the long axis of the petrous pyramid, whereas transverse fractures are oriented perpendicular to this axis [2]. Longitudinal fractures (Fig. 40.1) typically course along the long axis of the petrous bone with the vector extending through the middle ear cavity, the malleoincudal joint, and the anterior genu of the facial nerve. As a result, these fractures are often associated with ossicular fractures or subluxations, and facial nerve injury (usually along the tympanic portion) occurs in roughly 25 % of cases [4]. Classic exam findings in patients with longitudinal fractures include hemotympanum, perforation of the tympanic membrane, and blood in the EAC.

R. Hoffmann Nunes et al. (eds.), *Critical Findings in Neuroradiology*,
DOI 10.1007/978-3-319-27987-9_40

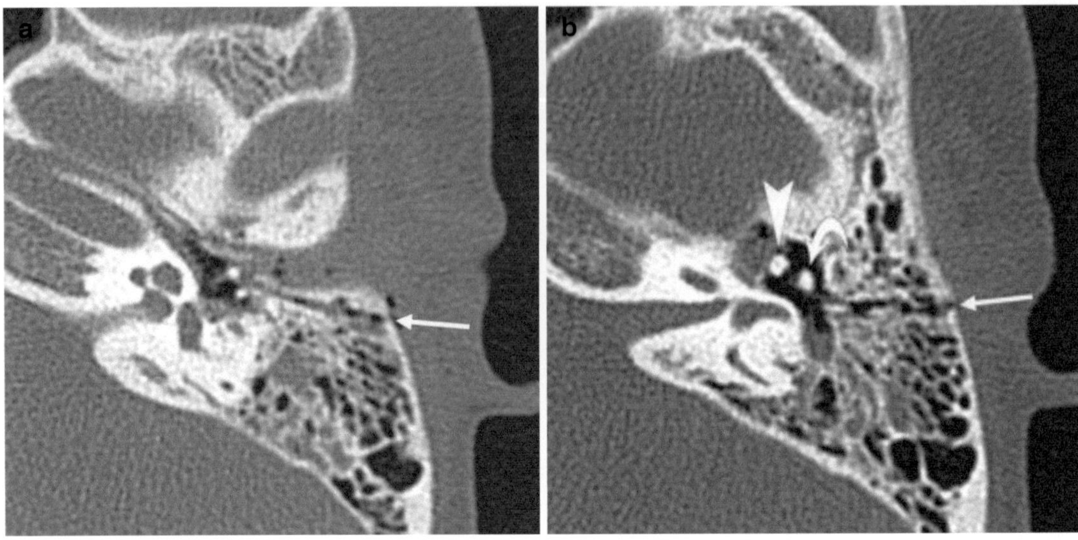

Fig. 40.1 Longitudinal temporal bone fracture. (**a**) Axial unenhanced CT image through the left temporal bone at the level of the EAC demonstrates a fracture line (*arrow*) oriented along the long axis of the petrous bone. The fracture extends through the mastoids and the medial aspect of the posterior wall of the EAC. (**b**) Slightly more cephalad axial image through the epitympanum again demonstrates the fracture line (*arrow*) extending into middle ear. There is malleoincudal separation, evident as a gap between the head of the malleus (*arrowhead*) and the body of the incus (*curved arrow*)

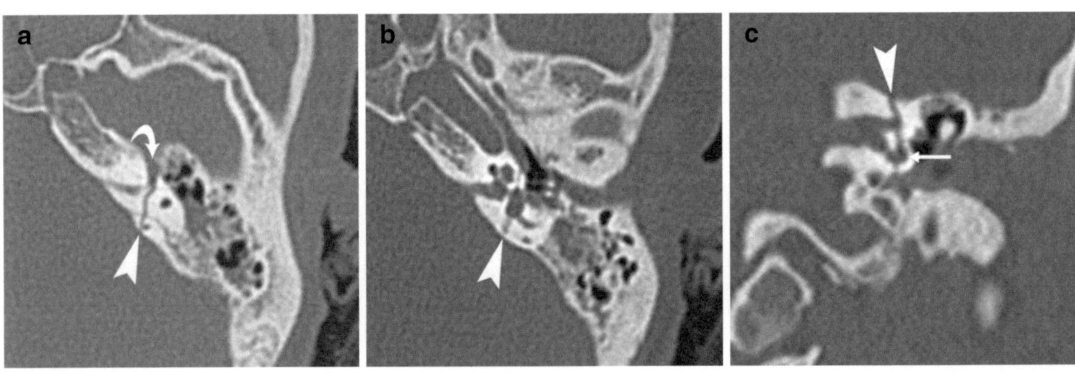

Fig. 40.2 Transverse temporal bone fracture. (**a**) Axial non-contrast CT image of the left temporal bone demonstrates a fracture line (*arrowhead*) which traverses the petrous temporal bone roughly perpendicular to the long axis of the bone. The fracture extends into the fossa for the geniculate ganglion (*curved arrow*). (**b**) Axial image slightly inferior to (**a**) demonstrates the fracture line (*arrowhead*) to extend through the vestibule. (**c**) Coronal non-contrast left temporal bone image in the same patient demonstrates the fracture (*arrowhead*) to traverse the fundus of the IAC and the basal turn of the cochlea (*arrow*)

Transverse fractures (Fig. 40.2) frequently begin in the region of foramen magnum or the jugular foramen and course perpendicular to the long axis of the petrous triangle. These fractures may extend through the IAC or across the cochlea and vestibule, so they often cause sensorineural hearing loss and/or vertigo. Approximately 50 % of patients with transverse fractures also suffer some degree of facial nerve injury [4]. Bleeding from the EAC, hemotympanum, and perforation of the tympanic membrane are less commonly associated with transverse fractures than longitudinal fractures.

Based on the above classification system, roughly 80 % of temporal bone fractures are characterized as longitudinal in orientation, with the remainder being considered transverse [4]. In truth, most temporal bone fractures more accurately described oblique or complex in nature [5, 6]. For this reason, it may be more useful to classify these fractures based on whether they involve or spare the otic capsule, because fractures disrupting the otic capsule almost always produce sensorineural hearing loss and are associated with a higher incidence of facial nerve paralysis compared to otic capsule sparing fractures [7, 8]. Using this method of classification, up to 6 % of temporal bone fractures would fall into the category of involving the otic capsule.

As alluded to above, complications of temporal bone fractures include hearing loss (due to either disruption of the ossicular chain or otic capsule), facial nerve injury, cerebrospinal fluid (CSF) fistula, perilymph fistula, and carotid artery injury. Hearing loss may be conductive, sensorineural, or mixed, and most patients with temporal bone fractures present acutely with some conductive hearing loss due to hemotympanum. In 80 % of cases, the conductive hearing loss will resolve spontaneously with the hemotympanum. Continued conductive hearing loss following resolution of hemotympanum suggests ossicular fracture or discontinuity.

A variety of ossicular abnormalities (Fig. 40.1), ranging from mild subluxation to complete fractures, can result from a temporal bone fracture. Subluxation of the incudostapedial joint is the most commonly reported post-traumatic derangement, occurring in roughly 80 % of cases, followed by dislocation of the incus (60 %) and fracture of the stapes crura (30 %). Most stapes fractures are associated with incus dislocations [1, 9]. Conductive hearing loss of more than 30 dB that lasts for more than 2 months after injury is treated with ossicular reconstruction.

Roughly 7 % of temporal bone fractures cause some degree facial nerve paralysis, and a quarter of these manifest with complete paralysis [7]. The vast majority of traumatic facial nerve palsies resolve spontaneously; however, patients presenting with immediate-onset paralysis associated with a temporal bone fracture are much less likely to recover complete facial nerve function. This subset of patients may therefore benefit from exploration and potential decompression, particularly if the nerve is suspected of being severed, crushed, or impaled with bone fragments or if there is loss of nerve stimulability [1].

CSF fistulae develop in 17 % of temporal bone fractures and can predispose to the development of meningitis. These fistulae may be evident clinically when there is clear watery drainage from the ear canal or the nose [1]. Most post-traumatic CSF fistulae close spontaneously or with placement of a lumbar drain. For fistulae that persist for more than 7–10 days, surgical closure is recommended.

Key Points

Etiology

The most common cause of temporal bone fractures is automobile accidents, which account for approximately 30 % [7]. Other common causes include assaults, falls, motorcycle and bicycle accidents, and gunshot wounds. Longitudinal fractures are classically caused by a blow to the side of the head in the temporoparietal region, while transverse fractures usually develop as a result of severe trauma to the frontal or occipital regions [4]. The anteroposterior direction of the force in these impacts produces a fracture that begins in the region of the foramen magnum or jugular foramen and courses perpendicular to the long axis of the temporal bone.

Best Imaging Modality

Non-enhanced computed tomography (CT): CT imaging is the preferred examination for evaluation of the temporal bone, and a dedicated thin section CT of the region should be performed whenever a temporal bone fracture is suspected. The scan should extend from above the petrous ridge through the mastoid tip, and submillimeter images should be reconstructed using a high detail bone kernel in multiple planes (axial and coronal at a minimum) for viewing. If a fracture is seen extending into the petrous carotid canal, dedicated imaging of the carotid artery with either computed tomography angiography (CTA) or magnetic resonance angiography (MRA) should be considered to rule out injury to the vessel. MRI is not otherwise generally indicated in the acute setting to specifically evaluate temporal bone trauma; however, brain MRI may be performed to assess for concomitant brain abnormalities, as injuries of sufficient force to cause a temporal bone fracture are often associated with significant intracranial injuries.

Major Findings

Longitudinal fractures typically involve squamosal portion of the temporal bone and the posterosuperior wall of the EAC and extend through the mastoid and middle ear cavity with disruption of the tegmen mastoideum and tegmen tympani and frequently involve the ossicular chain (Fig. 40.1). Transverse fractures often begin in the region of foramen magnum or the jugular foramen and course perpendicular to the long axis of the temporal bone. These fractures may extend through the IAC or across the otic capsule (Fig. 40.2).

The majority of temporal bone fractures are associated with ipsilateral opacification of the mastoid air cells, and patients who present with signs of a basilar skull fracture and an opacified mastoid without an obvious fracture by CT should be assumed to have an occult temporal bone fracture. Reversible causes of facial nerve palsy such as hematomas or bone fragments impinging on the facial nerve should be identified, as decompressive surgery or intravenous steroid administration may be warranted in certain instances in order to preserve facial nerve function.

The radiology report should therefore provide information regarding the orientation and course of the fracture and the structures involved, including the IAC, otic capsule, facial nerve canal, ossicular chain, and the carotid canal, as well as findings suggesting CSF fistula (Fig. 40.3) or perilymph fistulae (Fig. 40.4). Pneumocephalus or pneumolabyrinth in the setting of head trauma implies the presence of a fracture, even if a clear fracture line is not evident. In addition, the presence of significant comminution, displacement, or distraction of the fracture should be commented on.

The ossicular chain should be closely scrutinized for signs of discontinuity, although the presence of significant hemotympanum may make assessment difficult. Malleoincudal dislocations, which are the most commonly detected ossicular

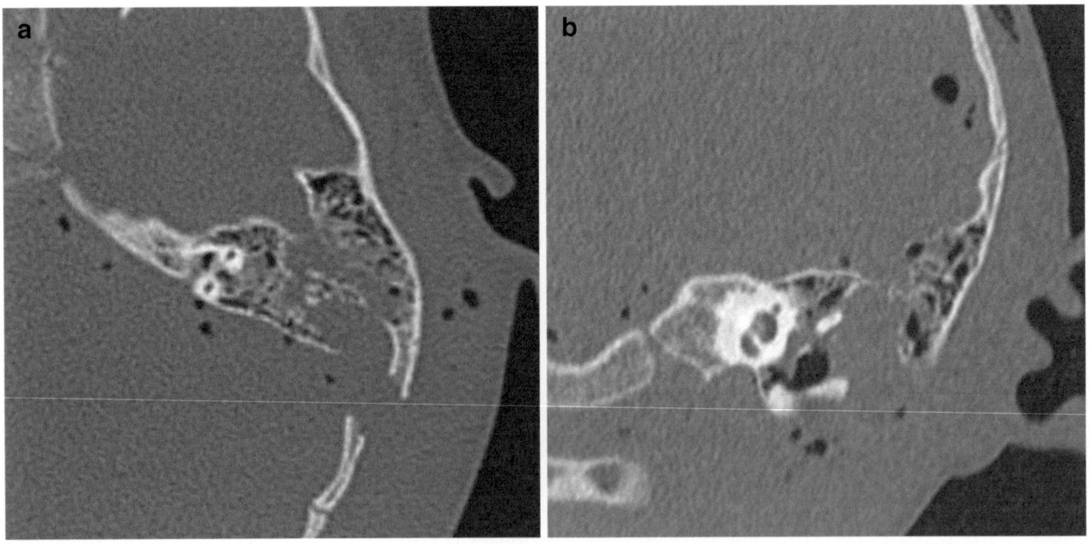

Fig. 40.3 Comminuted temporal bone fracture. (**a**) Axial and (**b**) coronal non-contrast CT image through the left temporal bone in a child demonstrates a severely comminuted and distracted left temporal bone fracture. The fracture can be seen to extend through the sigmoid plate on (**a**) and through the tegmen mastoideum on (**b**). There is pneumocephalus, which indicates violation of the dura with a CSF fistula

chain injuries on CT [9], can be diagnosed when there is derangement of the normal "ice cream cone" configuration of the joint on axial images through the epitympanum (Fig. 40.1).

In all cases, the status of the tegmen tympani and tegmen mastoideum should also be determined, as fracture extension through these areas places patients at higher risk for CSF leak (Fig. 40.3). In children, extensive longitudinal fractures may completely separate the petrous apex from the other portions of the temporal bone. This is termed a "floating cochlea" and is associated with acute conductive hearing loss and paralysis of the abducens and facial nerves [10].

Imaging Follow-Up

For uncomplicated temporal bone fractures, follow-up imaging is not generally indicated. However, repeat CT imaging of the temporal bone may be warranted if conductive hearing loss persists after resolution of hemotympanum to identify ossicular chain injuries which may not have been evident in the acute setting. Imaging may also be required if there is concern for a persistent CSF fistula, in order to identify potential sites of leak or a post-traumatic encephalocele. CT is preferred for assessing the fine bony details, while MRI may be superior for diagnosing an encephalocele.

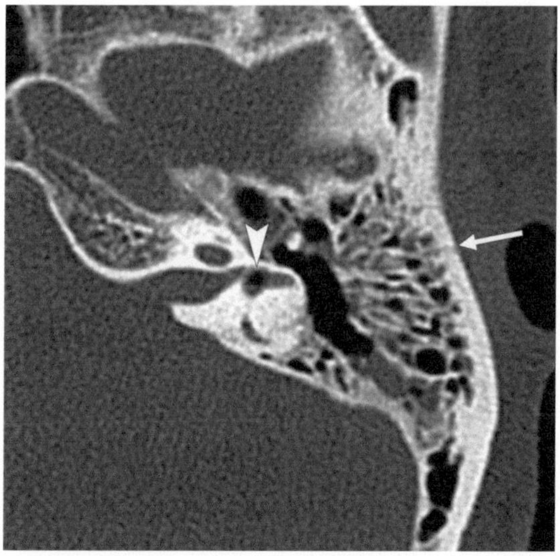

Fig. 40.4 Perilymph fistula. Axial non-contrast CT image through the left temporal bone demonstrates a subtle fracture line (*arrow*) oriented slightly obliquely relative to the long axis of the petrous bone extending through the mastoid cortex into the epitympanum. A small collection of gas is noted in the vestibule (*arrowhead*), which indicates the presence of a perilymph fistula

Main Differential Diagnosis

There is really no differential for temporal bone fractures in the setting of traumatic head injury. Occasionally, normal anatomic structures can be mistaken for fracture lines on CT. These include various sutures and fissures, such as the tympanosquamous, petrotympanic, tympanomastoid, and petrosquamous fissures and occipitomastoid suture; emissary vein canals; the subarcuate canal, which courses between the two limbs of the superior semicircular canal; the cochlear and vestibular aqueducts; and the singular canal [11]. Familiarity with these structures will prevent one from misinterpreting them as fractures.

Tips

- In patients with temporal bone fractures, the report should include:
  - The orientation of the fracture (while they have traditionally been classified as longitudinal or transverse in orientation, in reality most are oblique or more complex)
  - Whether the otic capsule is involved or spared
  - The integrity of the ossicular chain
  - Involvement of the facial nerve and whether there is evidence of bone fragments encroaching on the nerve
  - Status of the tegmen tympani and tegmen mastoideum
  - Involvement of the petrous carotid canal
- In patients with blunt head trauma, the presence of fluid in the mastoid, pneumocephalus near the temporal bone, or pneumolabyrinth should prompt a search for a subtle temporal bone fracture.

References

1. Brodie HA. Management of temporal bone trauma. In: Flint PW, Haughey BH, Lund VJ, et al., editors. Cummings otolaryngology head & neck surgery. 5th ed. Philadelphia: Mosby; 2010. p. 2036–48.
2. Cannon CR, Jahrsdoerfer RA. Temporal bone fractures. Review of 90 cases. Arch Otolaryngol. 1983;109(5):285–8.
3. Nageris B, Hansen MC, Lavelle WG, Van Pelt FA. Temporal bone fractures. Am J Emerg Med. 1995;13(2):211–4.
4. Parisier SC, Fayad JN, McGuirt WF. Injuries of the ear and temporal bone. In: Bluestone CD, Stool SE, Alper CM, et al., editors. Pediatric otolaryngology, vol. 1. 4th ed. Philadelphia: Saunders; 2003. p. 829–60.
5. Aguilar 3rd EA, Yeakley JW, Ghorayeb BY, Hauser M, Cabrera J, Jahrsdoerfer RA. High resolution CT scan of temporal bone fractures: association of facial nerve paralysis with temporal bone fractures. Head Neck Surg. 1987;9(3):162–6.
6. Williams WT, Ghorayeb BY, Yeakley JW. Pediatric temporal bone fractures. Laryngoscope. 1992; 102(6):600–3.
7. Brodie HA, Thompson TC. Management of complications from 820 temporal bone fractures. Am J Otol. 1997;18(2):188–97.
8. Dahiya R, Keller JD, Litofsky NS, Bankey PE, Bonassar LJ, Megerian CA. Temporal bone fractures: otic capsule sparing versus otic capsule violating clinical and radiographic considerations. J Trauma. 1999;47(6):1079–83.
9. Meriot P, Veillon F, Garcia JF, et al. CT appearances of ossicular injuries. Radiographics. 1997;17(6): 1445–54.
10. Merwin W, May M, Curtin HD. Floating petrous bone fracture. Otolaryngol Head Neck Surg. 1989;100(1): 69–73.
11. Connor SE, Tan G, Fernando R, Chaudhury N. Computed tomography pseudofractures of the mid face and skull base. Clin Radiol. 2005;60(12): 1268–79.

Penetrating Neck Trauma

41

Prashant Vijay Shankar

Abstract

Penetrating neck trauma is a significant source of morbidity and mortality and has been reported in between 5 and 10 % of all trauma cases presenting to the emergency department. As such, it is critical for the radiologist to be familiar with the sequelae of penetrating neck injuries, the gravest of which are catastrophic arterial and spinal cord injuries. The use of multidetector CT has grown rapidly over the past decade and has allowed clinicians to reserve diagnostic angiography surgical and exploration only for the most serious cases. Percutaneous embolizations of actively bleeding patients have also decreased the numbers of patients undergoing surgery.

Background

Penetrating neck trauma is a significant source of morbidity and mortality (ranging from 2 to 10 %) because of the high concentration of vital structures that are densely packed within this relatively small anatomic region [1, 2]. The injuries are often the result of low- or high-velocity projectiles. Patients with signs and symptoms of penetrating neck injury may present with dysphagia, hoarseness, bleeding/hypotension (if the degree of hemorrhage is severe), respiratory distress/stridor, and possibly neurological deficits if cerebrovascular flow is impaired [3]. In the setting of multiple trauma, it is critical to evaluate for possible penetrating neck injuries, as they may be missed on the primary survey [4].

P.V. Shankar, MD
Department of Radiology,
University of North Carolina at Chapel Hill,
101 Manning Drive, Chapel Hill, NC 27514, USA
e-mail: pshankar@unch.unc.edu

Key Points

Etiology

Penetrating neck injuries can be classified as high-energy or low-energy injuries. Low-energy injuries are the result of sharp object penetration (knives, glass, etc.), while high-energy injuries are the result of bullets or other projectiles from high-energy sources such as guns and rifles. These latter injuries produce greater tissue damage due to higher kinetic energy transference and tissue cavitation. Because so many vital structures are so densely packed in a tight anatomic

R. Hoffmann Nunes et al. (eds.), *Critical Findings in Neuroradiology*,
DOI 10.1007/978-3-319-27987-9_41

space within the neck, damage may be severe in the setting of high-energy injuries even when there is no direct impact between the projectile and the affected tissue.

Blunt force trauma sustained during motor vehicle accidents may also produce imaging findings of neck soft tissue injury, including cartilage fractures and vascular injury. Seatbelts may also damage neck soft tissues including the vascular structures.

Best Imaging Modality

While penetrating neck injuries were classically managed with surgical exploration, recent advances in diagnostic imaging – multidetector computed tomography (CT) and computed tomography angiography (CTA) – have allowed for a more selective approach. Clinically stable patients can be evaluated with non-emergent conventional angiography, endoscopy, or esophagoscopy. Esophageal injury is difficult to assess in the immediate post-traumatic setting, particularly with CT, and necessitates barium fluoroscopic studies when patients are stable [5].

Computed tomography: CT is the preferred modality in the initial evaluation of penetrating neck injuries due to its ubiquitous use in the emergency setting, speed of image acquisition, and superiority in characterizing large anatomic regions with high spatial resolution. CT allows one to identify signs of active hemorrhage or airway compromise and assess tracheolaryngeal and pharyngeal injuries [5]. CT also provides information about skeletal structures, the mediastinum, and, most importantly, the neck vasculature. It is an excellent modality for demonstrating the full extent of the wound track and can often identify injuries that are not clinically apparent [6].

CT angiography: CTA with multiplanar reconstructions is useful allowing characterization of the vasculature and identifying injuries that require immediate surgical (extravasations) or endovascular repair (pseudoaneurysms, occlusions).

Limitations in CT and CTA imaging of penetrating neck trauma are largely due to artifacts from retained projectile fragments and poor imaging technique. For example, poor timing of the contrast bolus may produce artifactual occlusion of the arteries or severe venous contamination. Patients with large or obese body habitus may have poor images, particularly in the region of the shoulders and lower neck, secondary to photon starvation artifact.

Magnetic resonance imaging (MRI) and magnetic resonance angiography (MRA): While blunt carotid/vertebral artery injuries can be assessed with MRI and MRA, they have limited use in the setting of acute penetrating neck injury. Many acutely retained projectile fragments serve as a contraindication to entry into the MRI suite [6].

Digital subtraction angiography (DSA): In spite of advances in CT, DSA remains the gold standard in the diagnosis and treatment of acute vascular injury in the neck. However, DSA does not provide nearly as comprehensive an evaluation as multidetector CT/CTA and can be accompanied by rare but clinically significant risks (including puncture site hematoma, dissection, distal embolization, vasospasm, etc.).

Major Findings

Vascular injuries: Up to 25 % of penetrating neck injuries may result in arterial injuries. Signs of arterial injury on CT include partial or complete occlusion, active extravasation, pseudoaneurysm, fistulas, and/or dissection [7]. CTA is the preferred modality when evaluating vascular injuries, although image quality is predicated on proper technique and bolus timing. If an arterial injury is identified, the ordering clinician should be contacted, as surgical or endovascular therapy may be required (Figs. 41.1, 41.2 and 41.3) [8].

An arteriovenous fistula may arise as a complication of trauma, due to carotid or vertebral artery pseudoaneurysm rupture into adjacent venous structures. Close attention should be paid to the adjacent veins, as abnormal venous dilatation may suggest the presence of a fistula.

Spinal injuries: Penetrating injuries to the cervical spine account for up to 14 % of all spine injuries [9]. Fractures are usually readily apparent

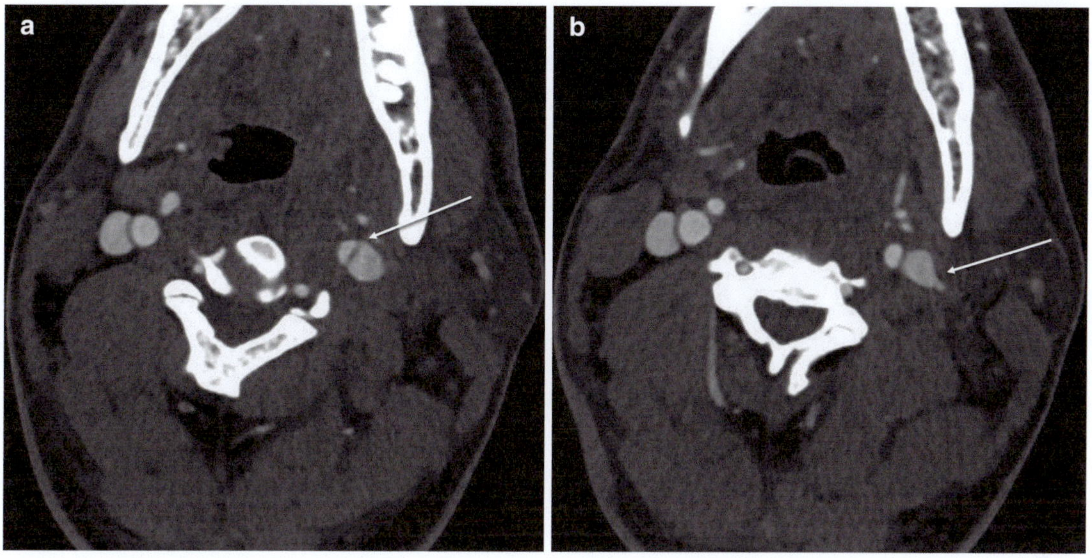

Fig. 41.1 (**a**, **b**) Neck CTA in two different levels in a patient victim of penetrating trauma. (**a**) There is a dissection flap in the left internal carotid artery (*arrow*). In (**b**) note the irregular contour of the lateral wall of the left internal carotid artery (*arrow*). These findings are consistent with a dissecting pseudoaneurysm

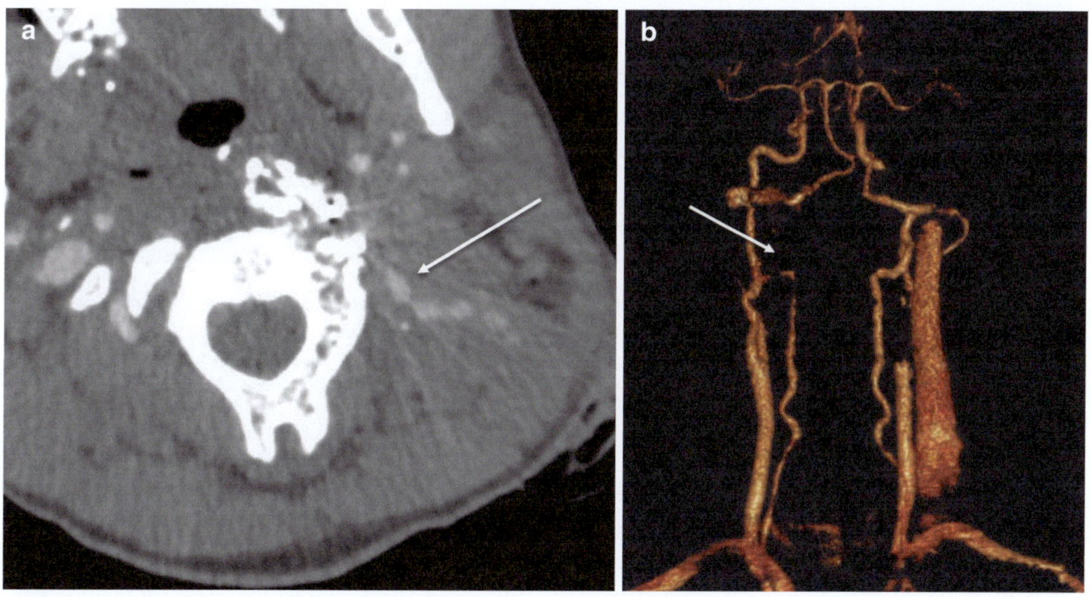

Fig. 41.2 Vascular injury in a patient victim of a gunshot wound to the neck. (**a**) Axial CTA at the C1–C2 level shows contrast extravasation from the left vertebral artery consistent with active arterial bleeding (*arrow*). (**b**) 3D CTA reconstruction depicts clear occlusion of the left vertebral artery at the level of the gunshot wound (*arrow*)

on CT and should be described in the report and mentioned in its impression. In the setting of clear neurologic deficits, MRI of the cervical spine should be performed to assess for cord/nerve injuries provided there are no contraindications.

Laryngeal injuries: Tracheolaryngeal injuries are present in approximately 1–7 % of patients with penetrating neck injuries [10]. Although rare, these injuries carry the potential for fatal airway compromise. Imaging can aid in identifica-

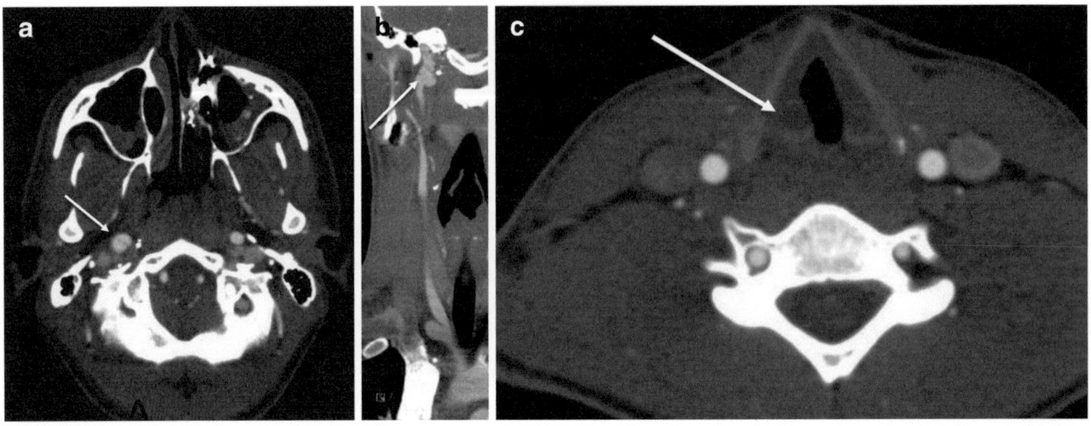

Fig. 41.3 Gunshot wound victim with vascular injury. (**a**) Axial CTA at the nasopharynx level shows a dissection flap in the right internal carotid artery. There is shrapnel in the left maxillary sinus. (**b**) Coronal CTA showing a dissecting pseudoaneurysm of the right internal carotid artery (*arrow*). (**c**) Axial CTA at a level inferior to (**a**) depicts a paralyzed and medialized right vocal cord (*arrow*) due to vagal nerve injury/impingement in the suprahyoid carotid space either due to direct trauma from the gunshot or due to the carotid pseudoaneurysm

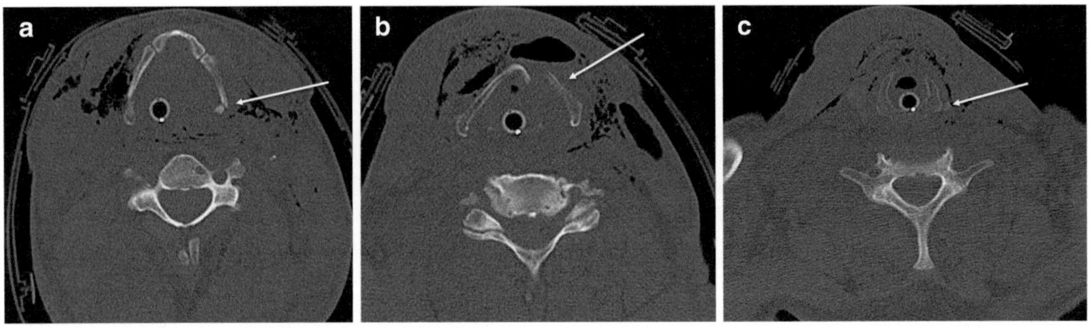

Fig. 41.4 Neck axial CT in bone window in different levels in a patient with penetrating and blunt neck injury due motor vehicle collision. (**a**) There is a medially displaced fracture of the left posterior hyoid bone (*arrow*). (**b**) At a more inferior level, an anterolaterally displaced fracture of the left ala of the thyroid cartilage is seen (*arrow*). (**c**) There is a minimally displaced fracture of the posterior aspect of the left cricoid cartilage (*arrow*). Note the extensive subcutaneous emphysema secondary to the airway compromise

tion of a penetrating injury and is useful for surgical planning. CT is the preferred imaging modality. Endoscopy and bronchoscopy remain the gold standard for evaluating such injuries, however, particularly if CT findings are indeterminate. The cricoid is the most commonly injured cartilaginous structure in the larynx, as it provides circumferential ring support (Fig. 41.4) (Please see chapter on Laryngeal Fractures).

Esophageal injuries: Esophageal injuries are poorly characterized on CT. If pneumomediastinum is present, esophageal injury should be suspected in the setting of high-impact or penetrating trauma, as mortality is high in the setting of penetrating esophageal injuries [10]. These injuries are best characterized on esophagoscopy or contrast esophagography.

Imaging Follow-Up

CT is the preferred modality to follow patients with penetrating neck trauma and is usually obtained on a clinical and not a routine basis.

Main Differential Diagnosis

Although patients with penetrating neck trauma usually present with a clinical history of trauma and show physical evidence of injury, other differential diagnoses should be considered when appropriate:

Dissecting aneurysm: This is the result of intramural hematoma from rupture of the vasa vasorum which dilates and weakens the vessel wall. An intimal flap can be seen between the true and false lumens. Although trauma is probably the most common cause, it can also be seen in the setting of atherosclerosis, fibromuscular dysplasia, or collagen vascular disease.

Fibromuscular dysplasia: This has a classic appearance of multifocal stenoses and dilatations and usually involves the mid and upper cervical internal carotid artery segment. While it is usually bilateral, unilateral forms may also be present. The carotid and vertebral arteries may be involved.

Vocal cord paralysis: Vocal cord paralysis is most commonly a problem due to injuries of the recurrent laryngeal nerve (which innervates all of the muscles in the larynx except the cricothyroid muscle). It presents with displacement of the arytenoid cartilage anteromedially which may mimic a cartilage fracture/dislocation. The principal causes include neoplasms and surgical iatrogenic injuries.

Radiation laryngitis: This may present with sclerosis and fragmentation of cartilages which can mimic fractures. Generally, there is evidence of radiation to the adjacent tissues.

Tips

- "Active extravasation" implies arterial bleeding and thus a life-threatening situation. Look carefully at the arteries and follow their course to evaluate for potential dissections and/or pseudoaneurysms. Active arterial bleeding is an emergency that requires immediate surgical or endovascular treatment. An urgent phone call should be made to the referring clinician in this setting.
- Evaluate the osseous anatomy carefully. Unstable cervical spinal fractures can be seen not only in the setting of blunt trauma but also with high-energy projectile injuries. MRI may be needed for cord assessment.
- Displaced bone fragments may act as "internal projectiles" and cause surrounding soft tissue/vascular injuries. It is important to include these in the impression of the radiology report, as surgical management may be necessary in certain cases.
- Evaluate for skull base fractures. The cranial vault is often overlooked in the neck CT/CTA report.
- Evaluate for airway cartilage injuries (thyroid/cricoid cartilage fractures).

References

1. Steenburg SD, Sliker CW, Kathirkamanathan S, et al. Imaging evaluation of penetrating neck injuries. Radiographics. 2010;30:869–86.
2. Múnera F, Soto JA, Nuñez D. Penetrating injuries of the neck and the increasing role of CTA. Emerg Radiol. 2004;10(6):303–9.
3. LeBlang SD, Nunez Jr DB. Noninvasive imaging of cervical vascular injuries. AJR Am J Roentgenol. 2000;174(5):1269–78.
4. Woo K, Magner DP, Wilson MT, Margulies DR. CT angiography in penetrating neck trauma reduces the need for operative neck exploration. Am Surg. 2005;71(9):754–8.
5. Kendall JL, Anglin D, Demetriades D. Penetrating neck trauma. Emerg Med Clin North Am. 1998;16(1):85–105.
6. MacFarlane C, Benn CA. Penetrating neck injury: a review. Trauma. 2002;4(2):79–90.
7. Bell RB, Osborn T, Dierks EJ, Potter BE, Long WB. Management of penetrating neck injuries: a new paradigm for civilian trauma. J Oral Maxillofac Surg. 2007;65(4):691–705.
8. Múnera F, Soto JA, Palacio DM, et al. Penetrating neck injuries: helical CT angiography for initial evaluation. Radiology. 2002;224(2):366–72.
9. Inaba K, Muñera F, McKenney M, et al. Prospective evaluation of screening multislice helical computed tomographic angiography in the initial evaluation of penetrating neck injuries. J Trauma. 2006;61(1):144–9.
10. LeBlang SD, Nunez Jr DB. Helical CT of cervical spine and soft tissue injuries of the neck. Radiol Clin North Am. 1999;37:515–32.

Laryngeal Fractures 42

Carlos Toyama

Abstract

External laryngeal trauma is a rare but potentially life-threatening situation in the acutely injured patient. Trauma mechanism and intensity as well as patient's age influence the spectrum of injuries. The correct diagnosis and management are paramount in order to avoid patient death or long-term airway compromise, swallowing, and speaking disabilities. Computed tomography and magnetic resonance imaging findings are important for the noninvasive evaluation of laryngeal injuries and treatment planning.

Background

A laryngeal fracture can occur following trauma and is a potentially life-threatening situation in the acutely injured patient. The incidence of laryngeal trauma varies between 1:5000 and 1:137,000 trauma patients [1]. Complications have been estimated to be as high as 15–17 % and mainly due to chronic airway obstruction [2]. The mortality of laryngeal trauma is directly related to the subsequent capacity to maintain the airway patent. Nonetheless, once the airway is secured and the laryngeal injury is assessed, the mortality significantly decreases. Patients with a suspected laryngeal fracture must be treated in an emergent manner [1].

The clinical manifestations vary considerably and include dysphonia, aphonia, hoarseness, anterior neck pain, dyspnea, stridor, dysphasia, odynophagia, as well as some clinical signs, such as ecchymosis, hematoma, and cracking upon palpation [1].

Key Points

Etiology

Laryngeal injury can be categorized as penetrating or blunt trauma and as external or internal based on the trauma mechanisms. The most

C. Toyama, MD
Division of Head and Neck Radiology, Hospital Santa Casa de Misericórdia de São Paulo, Sao Paulo, SP, Brazil

Division of Neuroradiology, Fleury Medicina e Saúde, Sao Paulo, SP, Brazil
e-mail: carlos.toyama@grupofleury.com.br

R. Hoffmann Nunes et al. (eds.), *Critical Findings in Neuroradiology*,
DOI 10.1007/978-3-319-27987-9_42

common cause is external and is typically secondary to motor vehicle collisions and less often to sport injuries, hanging, strangulation, and gunshot injuries. Internal trauma is often iatrogenic typically following intubation or rarely sneezing. In children, neck injuries are most commonly due to blunt external trauma and are often associated with multiple organ injuries. These occur predominantly secondary to bicycle, snowmobile, and vehicle collisions [1–4].

Laryngeal fractures are associated with other life-threatening injuries in 45 % of patients and are isolated in 55 % of them. The trauma mechanisms of isolated laryngeal fractures are related to direct neck injuries, such as falls, direct blows, stabbing, motor vehicle accidents, and sneezing [1–4].

Patients with suspected laryngeal trauma are evaluated clinically, endoscopically, and with imaging to confirm the clinically suspected lesion and to precisely assess its extent prior to treatment. The Schaefer and Fuhrman classification [3, 4] is used to categorize the severity of the injury guiding initial treatment and predicting outcome (Table 42.1). This system is based on presence, absence, and number of fractures that are demonstrated by CT and/or MRI. Hematoma and mucosal lacerations are better detected by endoscopy.

Table 42.1 Classification of blunt laryngotracheal injuries

Classification	Injury
I	No airway compromise. Minor endolaryngeal hematomas or lacerations without detectable fractures
II	Varying degrees of airway compromise. More severe edema, hematoma, minor mucosal disruption without exposed cartilage, or non-displaced fractures
III	Airway compromise. Massive edema, large mucosal lacerations, exposed cartilage, displaced fractures, or vocal cord immobility
IV	Same as group 3, but more severe, with at least two or more fracture lines or massive mucosal edema. Disruption of anterior larynx, unstable fractures, or severe mucosal injuries may also be seen
V	Total laryngotracheal separation

Modified from Schaefer et al. [3] and Furhrman et al. [4]

Laryngeal fractures may also be divided based on the site of injury as supraglottic, glottic, subglottic, or a combination of all three. Hyoid bone, thyroid cartilage, cricoid cartilage, and arytenoids must be evaluated [1].

Best Imaging Modality

After a secure airway is established, the cervical spine is secured and the patient remains stable; imaging is indicated to determine presence and extent of damage to the laryngeal framework. Computed tomography (CT) plays a major role in the diagnosis, management, and therapeutic choices, whereas magnetic resonance imaging (MRI) may be used as a second line approach [1].

- *Non-contrast CT*: It is the first imaging choice for the diagnosis of fractures of ossified cartilages. Due to the rapid acquisition of CT with high anatomic detail and the possibility to perform two-dimensional multiplanar reconstructions (2D MPR), three-dimensional volume rendering (3D VR) and virtual endoscopy, noninvasive evaluation, and treatment planning are facilitated [1]. Most laryngeal fractures can be identified on axial CT images, except for horizontal fractures. MPRs enhance diagnostic accuracy of horizontal fractures of thyroid and hyoid and arytenoid subluxations and dislocations. 3D VR increases detection of mucosal lacerations and laryngotracheal narrowing [5].
- *MRI*: It is infrequently used for the assessment of the traumatized larynx. MRI may be considered in young patients with non-ossified cartilages and when laryngeal fractures are suspected clinically and CT normal [1].

The imaging protocol includes:

CT [1]

- Thin slices (1–1.2 mm reconstructed with 50 % overlap) are recommended.
- 2D MPR improve diagnosis of fractures, especially horizontal ones. Axial 2D MPR

should be obtained perpendicular to long axis of the airway and coronal 2D MPR parallel to it. Head tilting renders interpretation more difficult.

- Soft tissue and bone window evaluation are mandatory.
- Intravenous iodinated contrast material is recommended whenever associated vascular injuries are suspected while its routine use is not necessary.
- The use of 3D VR aids in the assessment of laryngotracheal narrowing.

MRI [1]

- High-resolution MRI with surface coils.
- Patients without airway impairment should be observed or monitored carefully, and the duration of the examination should be kept to a minimum to avoid unnecessary risks related to secondary airway compromise due to acute soft tissue swelling.
- High-resolution images are recommended in order to visualize fracture lines within non-ossified cartilages; therefore, the field of view should be small and the matrix high (512×512). The slice thickness should not exceed 3 mm.
- The protocol includes axial T2-weighted imaging (T2WI) and fat-saturated T1-weighted imaging (T1WI). If the clinical situation permits, additional planes may be acquired.
- Postcontrast fat-saturated T1WI is indicated, because traumatized soft tissue enhances following contrast administration, while fracture lines in cartilages remain hypointense.

Major Findings

Hyoid bone: Fractures of the hyoid are relatively common in sporting injuries such as baseball, jet skiing, and karate [6] and are also related to strangulation and hanging. Hyoid bone fractures are most commonly reported with increased age due to increased ossification and diminished elasticity. Fractures typically occur in the body or the greater cornua of the hyoid and most often unilateral (Fig. 42.1) [1, 2, 5]. An abnormally low position of the hyoid bone has been reported in cases of strangulation; due to the action of the infrahyoid muscles, the hyoid bone is pulled downwards. An abnormally high position of the hyoid bone (above the third cervical vertebra) has been reported in tracheal transection due ruptured the infrahyoid muscles and as consequence the suprahyoid muscles pull the hyoid upwards [1, 2, 5].

Thyroid cartilage: The thyroid cartilage is the most often fractured part of the airway and the injury may be unilateral or bilateral (Fig. 42.2). Vertical fractures result when the thyroid cartilage is pressed against the spine. Horizontal

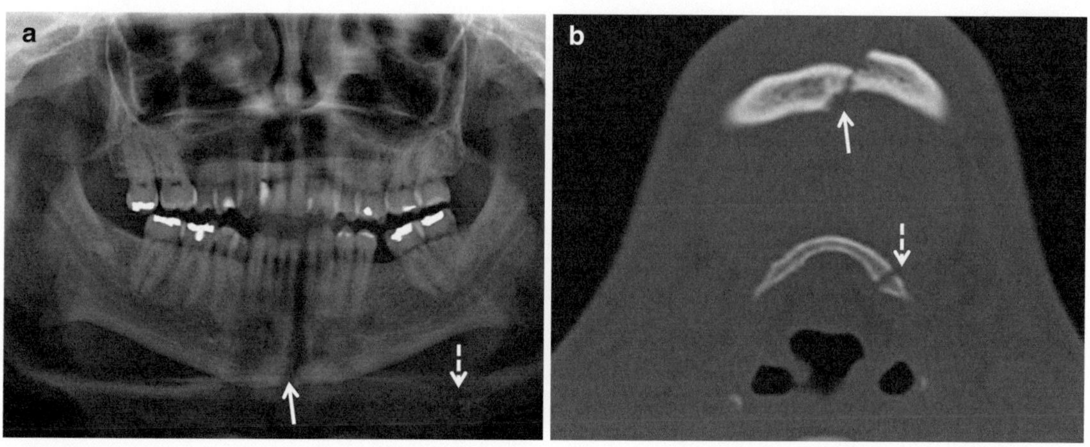

Fig. 42.1 Hyoid fracture. (**a**, **b**) Panoramic radiograph and bone-windowed neck CT images show fractures of the mandible symphysis (*arrows*) and left body of the hyoid (*dashed arrow*)

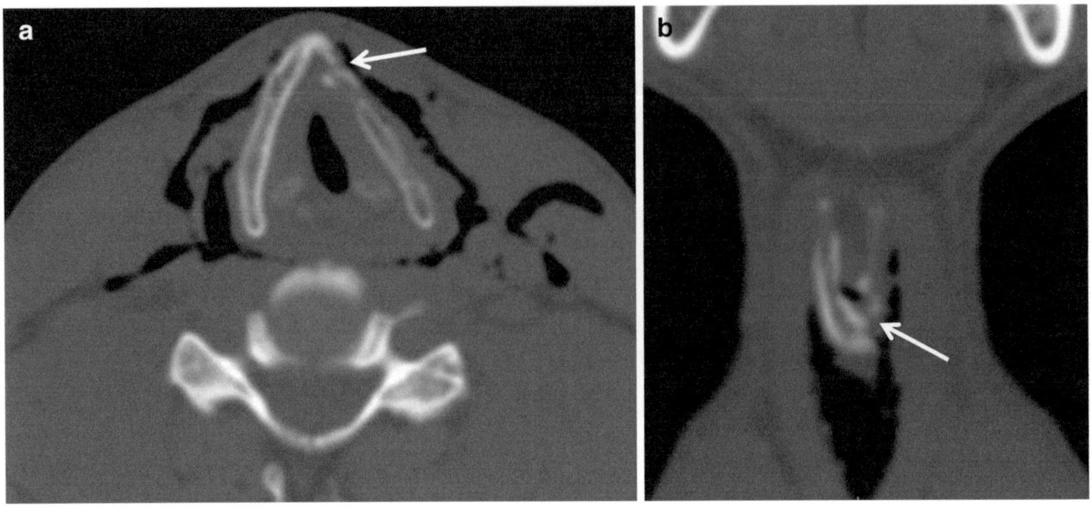

Fig. 42.2 Glottic fracture. (**a**, **b**) Axial (**a**) and coronal (**b**) show a left thyroid fracture (*arrows*) and medial dislocation of a small fragment. There is also extensive cervical emphysema

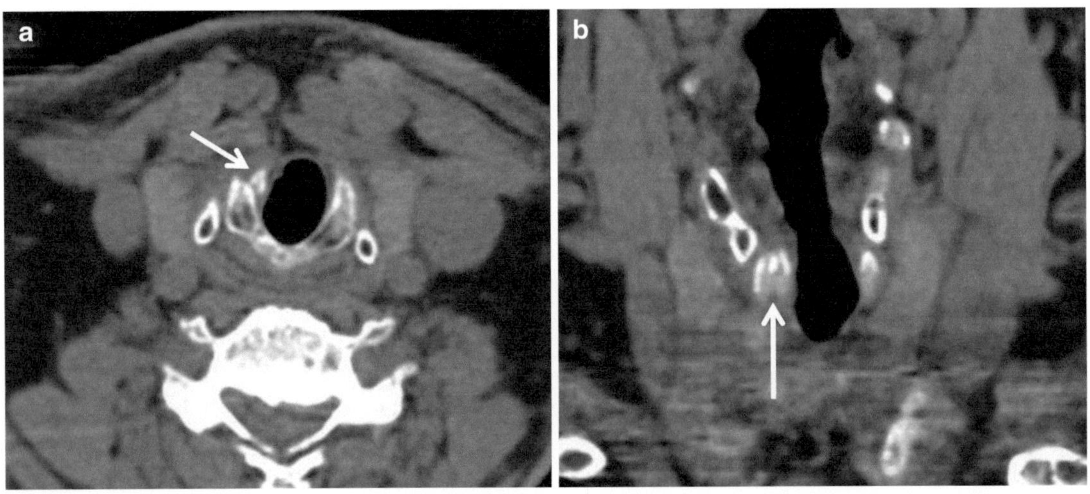

Fig. 42.3 Subglottic fracture. (**a**, **b**) Axial and coronal neck CT images demonstrate a right cricoid fracture (*arrows*) and medial dislocation of a bone fragment, narrowing the airway

fractures often cross the midline and may be difficult to demonstrate on axial images. They are classically described in strangulation and can involve the superior border of the thyroid laminae and the superior horns of the thyroid cartilage. Coronal and sagittal 2D MPR are useful for diagnosis [1, 2, 5].

Cricoid cartilage: Fractures of the cricoid cartilage (Fig. 42.3) are often bilateral resulting in anterior and posterior fragments and a risk for collapse into the airway resulting in airway obstruction. Isolated cricoid fractures are rare. Any contour deformity or tissue in the thin mucosa overlying the cricoid may indicate hematoma or edema [1, 2, 5].

Arytenoid cartilages: Arytenoid fractures often occur in association with fractures of the thyroid and cricoid cartilages. Isolated arytenoid dislocation is rare and is often a complication of upper aerodigestive tract instrumentation; however, it may occur with external laryngeal trauma. It is diagnosed when the cricothyroid space is widened and whenever the arytenoid is dislocated anteromedially or posterolaterally. Quantitative analysis of dislocation and rotation of the arytenoid and position and elongation of the vocal fold may be evaluated by 3D VR [7].

Cricotracheal junction: The separation between the cricoid and trachea is an uncommon injury best seen in coronal or sagittal CT planes that shows widening of cricotracheal distance due to retraction of the trachea. It is most lethal form of laryngeal trauma and is often associated with cricoid fractures and bilateral recurrent laryngeal nerve palsies [8].

Imaging Follow-Up

MRI should be used in those patients in whom laryngeal fractures are suspected clinically and when CT findings do not clearly show the injury [1].

For uncomplicated laryngeal fractures, follow-up imaging is not generally indicated. Follow-up is usually clinical and surveillance imaging is indicated when a patient fails to show adequate response to clinical or surgical therapies or develops progressive symptoms or suspected complications [1, 2, 5].

Imaging can also be valuable for assessing long-term sequelae, such as post-traumatic cartilage deformation, pseudarthrosis, nodular chondrometaplasia, cricoarytenoid ankylosis, subglottic stenosis, and post-traumatic granulomas [1].

Main Differential Diagnosis

There is no differential for temporal bone fractures in the setting of traumatic head injury. Occasionally, normal anatomic structures can be mistaken for fracture lines on CT. Familiarity with the normal ossification centers will prevent one from misinterpreting them as fractures [1].

Tips

- *Always search* for laryngeal fractures in neck and spine CT in the setting of trauma. Soft tissue window may be valuable to evaluate the fractures in poorly ossified cartilage.
- *Identify and describe all the displaced cartilaginous fractures*, since they are related to the prognosis and are essential to guide the treatment.
- *Identify and describe the presence of hematoma* because it can be use to classify the injury and may also be a clue as to the location of a fracture or dislocation.
- *Describe the injury site*: Supraglottic larynx (epiglottic hematoma or avulsion, hyoid bone fracture, thyroid cartilage fracture, arytenoid dislocation), glottic (thyroid cartilage fractures, vocal cord edema), and subglottic (cricoid cartilage and trachea).

References

1. Becker M, Leuchter I, Platon A, Becker CD, Dulguerov P, Varoquaux A. Imaging of laryngeal trauma. Eur J Radiol. 2014;83(1):142–54.
2. Jewett BS, Shockley WW, Rutledge R. External laryngeal trauma analysis of 392 patients. Arch Otolaryngol Head Neck Surg. 1999;125(8):877–80.
3. Schaefer SD. The acute management of external laryngeal trauma. A 27-year experience. Arch Otolaryngol Head Neck Surg. 1992;118(6):598–604.
4. Fuhrman GM, Stieg 3rd FH, Buerk CA. Blunt laryngeal trauma: classification and management protocol. J Trauma. 1990;30(1):87–92.
5. Becker M, Duboe PO, Platon A, Kohler R, Tasu JP, Becker CD, et al. MDCT in the assessment of laryngeal trauma: value of 2D multiplanar and 3D reconstructions. AJR Am J Roentgenol. 2013;201(4):W639–47.
6. Bell RB, Verschueren DS, Dierks EJ. Management of laryngeal trauma. Oral Maxillofac Surg Clin North Am. 2008;20(3):415–30.
7. Hiramatsu H, Tokashiki R, Kitamura M, Motohashi R, Tsukahara K, Suzuki M. New approach to diagnose arytenoid dislocation and subluxation using three-dimensional computed tomography. Eur Arch Otorhinolaryngol. 2010;267(12):1893–903.
8. McCrystal DJ, Bond C. Cricotracheal separation: a review and a case with bilateral recovery of recurrent laryngeal nerve function. J Laryngol Otol. 2006;120(6):497–501.

Extracranial Artery Dissections

43

Kenny Emmanuel Rentas and Benjamin Y. Huang

Abstract

Extracranial arterial dissections are a leading cause of strokes in young adults resulting in increased neurologic morbidity and mortality. Dissections can occur in the setting of trauma or spontaneously with a history of insignificant trauma elicited in a minority of cases. Clinical diagnosis is often challenging as most patients do not show the classic clinical triad of head, facial, or neck pain accompanied by Horner syndrome and cerebral or retinal ischemia. Imaging studies are essential in the diagnosis and traditionally conventional arteriography has been considered the gold standard. However, noninvasive imaging modalities such as computed tomography angiography and magnetic resonance angiography have replaced conventional angiography in many institutions. Cross-sectional noninvasive imaging techniques can demonstrate intramural hematomas as well as the vessel lumen and the presence of an intimal flap. Treatment usually consists of antithrombotic medication to prevent thromboembolic complications. Endovascular stenting is a treatment option in selected cases.

Background

Extracranial arterial dissections (EAD) are a significant source of neurologic morbidity and mortality. An arterial dissection is defined by either a tear in the vessel's inner lining known as the tunica intima or a rupture of the vasa vasorum. The intimal tear or ruptured vasa vasorum allows for the formation of an intramural hematoma, thus leading to arterial stenosis or occlusion. The intimal defect also exposes circulating blood to intrinsic clotting factors, leading to acute thrombosis and a risk of thromboembolism. Involvement of the

K.E. Rentas, MD (✉) • B.Y. Huang, MD, MPH
Department of Radiology,
University of North Carolina at Chapel Hill,
101 Manning Dr. Campus, Box 7510,
Chapel Hill, NC 27599-7510, USA
e-mail: Dr.Rentas@gmail.com;
bhuang@med.unc.edu

R. Hoffmann Nunes et al. (eds.), *Critical Findings in Neuroradiology*,
DOI 10.1007/978-3-319-27987-9_43

outer layers of the vessel wall may result in formation of a pseudoaneurysm. Extracranial internal carotid artery (ICA) dissections comprise 70–80 % of all craniocervical artery dissections and account for 5–22 % of strokes in patients younger than 45 years old [1, 2]. Extracranial vertebral artery (VA) dissections account for 15 % of all craniocervical artery dissections [1]. The annual incidence of ICA dissections is 2.5–3 cases per 100,000, whereas that of VA dissections is 1–1.5/100,000 [2, 3]. Approximately 60 % of extracranial dissections are spontaneous with the remainder resulting from blunt or penetrating injuries [4].

Classically, the clinical presentation consists of a triad of unilateral head, facial, or neck pain accompanied by Horner syndrome and cerebral or retinal ischemia. However, the clinical diagnosis is often challenging as only a minority of patients present with this triad and up to 5 % of carotid artery dissections are asymptomatic or only have minor symptoms [1, 2]. Headaches and neck pain are the most common clinical presentation, but patients can also present with cerebral or retinal ischemic symptoms as well as lower cranial nerve palsies and pulsatile tinnitus [2, 4]. In addition to headaches and neck pain, patients with VA dissections can present with cerebellar, brainstem, or spinal cord ischemic symptoms [1, 2, 5].

Distal ischemia is most commonly the result of emboli released from the injury site rather than hypoperfusion from focal stenosis or occlusion at the site of dissection [5]. Therefore, treatment is typically aimed at limiting neurological deficits by preventing thromboembolic complications via the use of antithrombotic medication. Endovascular stenting is a treatment option in selected cases. Overall, neurological outcome is good or excellent as the majority of stenoses and occlusions induced by EAD spontaneously resolve or recanalize on their own [5]. The risk of recurrent dissection is low and reported as 2 % in the first year and 1 % per year thereafter. Recurrences after the first year tend to occur in a different vessel than the one originally involved [2, 4]. Mortality rates associated with spontaneous extracranial cerebrovascular dissection range from 3 to 7 %; however, they are higher for those induced by trauma. The higher mortality associated with trauma-induced dissections may relate to other coexisting injuries [5, 6].

Key Points

Etiology

Trauma: Traumatic EAD occur in approximately 1–2 % of patients with direct or blunt trauma to the neck. The majority of dissections caused by blunt trauma result from motor vehicle accidents with the most common mechanisms of injury being rapid deceleration or hyperflexion with subsequent stretching of the involved vessel [2, 5]. Additional physiological mechanisms include extreme hyperextension/rotation, direct vascular blow, intraoral trauma, or direct laceration from bony fracture fragments [6]. The majority of vertebral artery injuries are caused by subluxations and vertebral fractures that extend into a foramen transversarium [5]. Iatrogenic dissections are uncommon and may occur from direct mechanical trauma during catheter cerebral angiography or other interventional procedures. Extracranial carotid artery injuries most often occur in the distal cervical ICA, particularly at the level of C1–C3 vertebrae (Fig. 43.1) [5]. In contrast, VA dissections most commonly occur in the V2 or V3 segments as the vessel travels through the transverse foramina or as it emerges from the transverse process of C2 and sweeps laterally to pass by C1 vertebra prior to piercing the dural membrane (Fig. 43.2) [5–7]. Traumatic pseudoaneurysms are present in a minority of cases of traumatic cerebrovascular incidents and usually occur in the middle or distal cervical parts of the vessel (Fig. 43.3) [5]. Extracranial arteriovenous fistulae involving the ICA and vertebral arteries most often result from penetrating trauma and can also involve branches of the external carotid artery [5].

Spontaneous: The term spontaneous EAD is usually reserved for dissections that occur in the absence of significant blunt or penetrating trauma; however, often times spontaneous dissections follow a precipitating trivial event such as neck

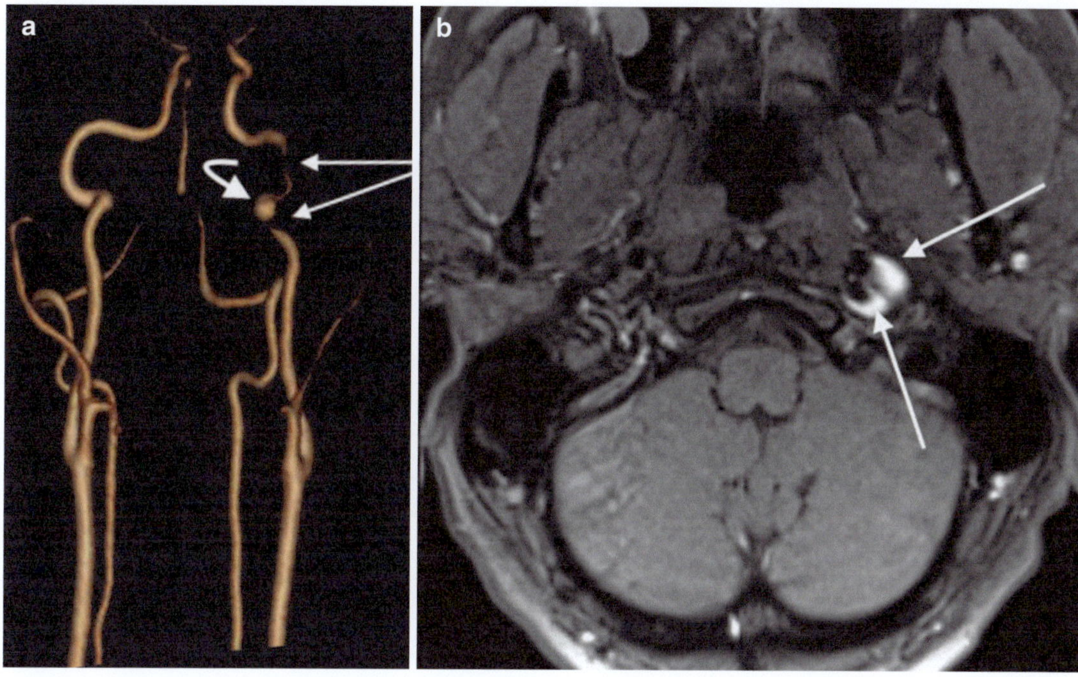

Fig. 43.1 Carotid artery dissection and pseudoaneurysm in a 40-year-old male with left-sided neck pain and tongue swelling. (**a**) Three-dimensional contrast-enhanced MRA coronal MIP reconstruction showing tapered narrowing of the distal left ICA (*arrows*) with a small dissecting pseudoaneurysm (*curved arrow*). (**b**) Axial fat-saturated T1WI showing a crescent-shaped hyperintense intramural hematoma (*arrows*)

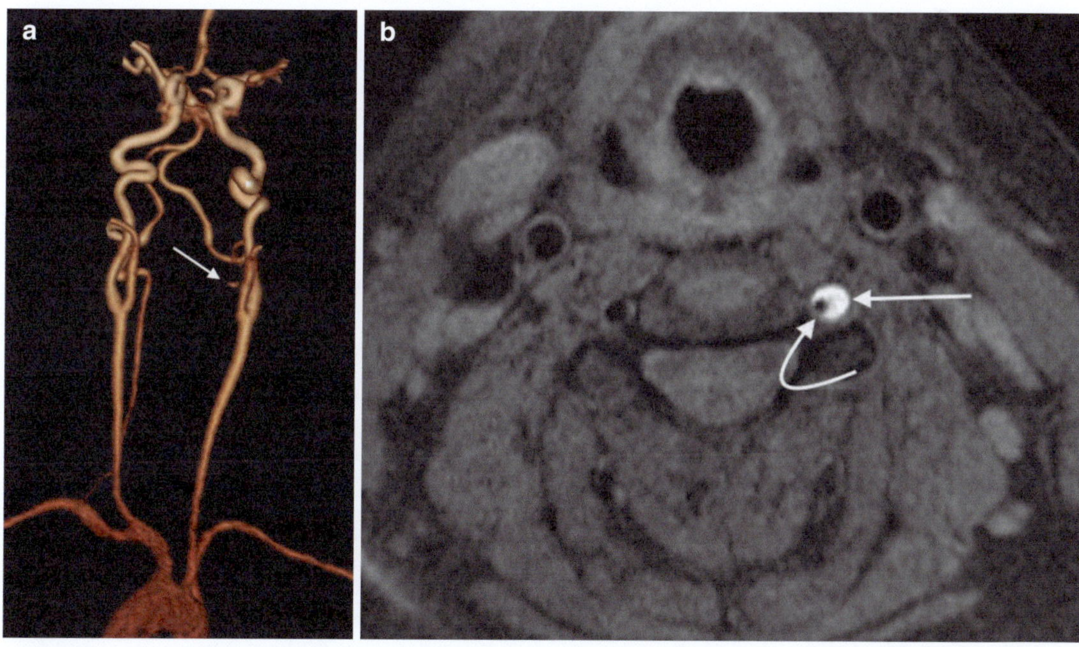

Fig. 43.2 Vertebral artery dissection in a 29-year-old female with diffuse weakness, paresthesias, syncopal episodes, nausea, vomiting, diplopia, and neck pain after a minor fall. (**a**) Three-dimensional contrast-enhanced MRA coronal MIP reconstruction showing no appreciable flow in the proximal left vertebral artery. (**b**) Axial fat-saturated T1WI showing an enlarged vessel diameter and a crescent-shaped hyperintense intramural hematoma in the left vertebral artery (*arrow*), adjacent to the eccentric lumen (*curved arrow*)

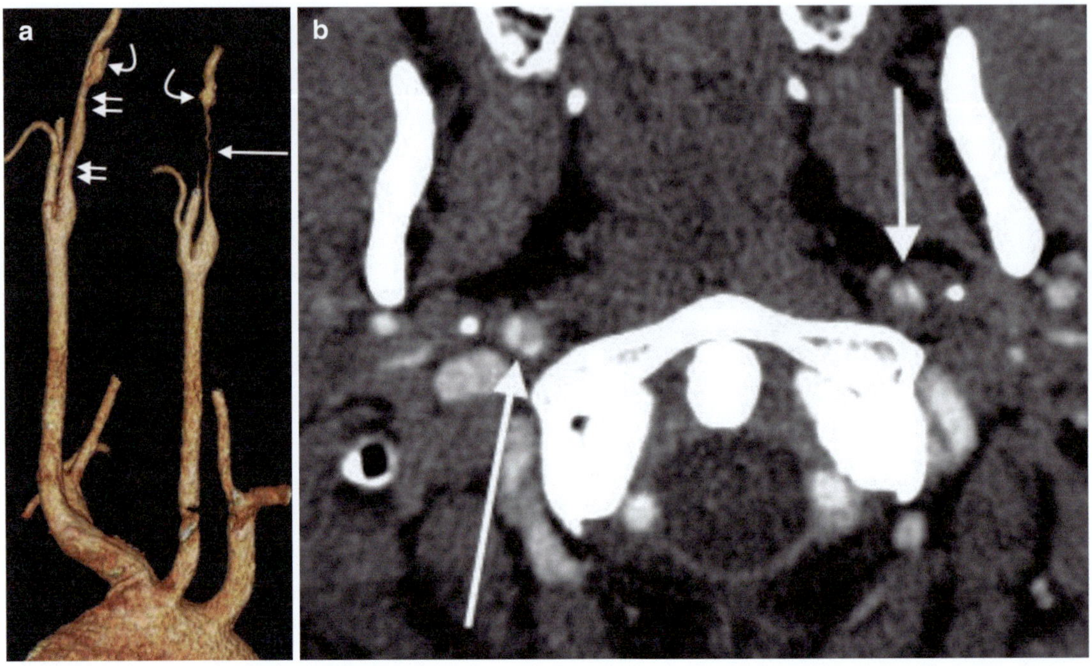

Fig. 43.3 Traumatic bilateral internal carotid artery dissections and pseudoaneurysms in a 27-year-old male status post-motorcycle accident. (**a**) Volume-rendered image from CTA showing a long-segment high-grade stenosis (string sign) at the left ICA (*long arrow*), multifocal stenosis at the right ICA (*double short arrows*), and bilateral ICA pseudoaneurysms (*curved arrows*). (**b**) Axial CTA image showing bilateral intimal flaps (*arrows*)

rotation, coughing, or vomiting [4]. Therefore, it is currently believed that spontaneous dissections may result from a combination of environmental and intrinsic factors [2]. This theory is supported by the observation that spontaneous arterial dissections are sometimes associated with various connective tissue disorders, such as Ehlers–Danlos syndrome type IV, Marfan syndrome, cystic medial necrosis, polycystic kidney disease, osteogenesis imperfecta, and fibromuscular dysplasia (FMD). While only a minority of patients show clinical manifestations of an underlying connective tissue disorder, skin biopsy specimens have shown underlying ultrastructural connective tissue abnormalities in many of them [2, 4]. Spontaneous dissections have also been associated with some infectious or inflammatory processes [4].

Best Imaging Modality

Magnetic resonance angiography (MRA): Combined with magnetic resonance imaging (MRI), MRA is replacing conventional catheter angiography as the standard for diagnosing EAD, particularly in the case of carotid artery dissections. MRA allows for the visualization of the intramural hematoma as well as the vessel lumen [8]. Visualization of the intimal flap is also more readily evident on cross-sectional MRI compared with conventional catheter angiography [2]. Cross-sectional MRI can also provide complementary information about ischemic injury to the brain (Fig. 43.4).

Computed tomography angiography (CTA): Similar to MRA, CTA with postprocessing multiplanar 2D and 3D reformatted images provide high-resolution and high-contrast images of the arterial lumen and wall including intramural hematomas. CTA is usually preferred in the setting of suspected traumatic dissection over other imaging modalities as it better demonstrates the relationship of arterial injury to adjacent fractures or dislocation [2]. CTA may be superior to MRI/MRA in diagnosing vertebral dissections [2, 8].

Digital subtraction catheter angiography (DSA): Commonly regarded as the gold standard procedure for diagnosing EAD, DSA shows the

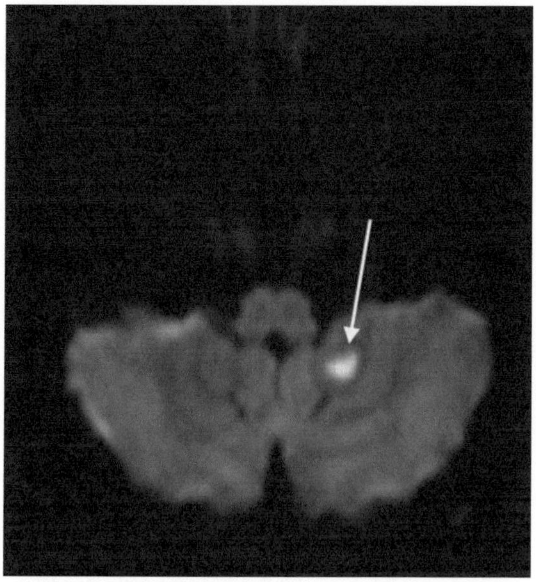

Fig. 43.4 Cerebellar infarct secondary to a left vertebral artery dissection. Diffusion-weighted MR image shows an inferomedial left cerebellar hemisphere infarct on the same patient as in Fig. 43.2 (*arrow*)

arterial lumen and associated vessel wall irregularities, such as fibromuscular dysplasia (FMD) [9]. DSA also provides great accuracy in identifying the intraluminal thrombus and assessing collateral circulation in cases of hemodynamically significant stenosis or occlusion [5]. Disadvantages of DSA include the inability to demonstrate abnormalities associated with the arterial wall such as intramural hematomas or thrombi in false lumens and complications inherent to the procedure [9].

Ultrasonography (*US*): US is the most limited imaging technique in terms of usefulness in the setting of EAD [5]. Nevertheless, US may provide hemodynamic information, direct visualization of vessel wall abnormalities, and evaluation of lumen patency [9]. US may be most useful for serial imaging of a dissection and to monitor for possible recanalization or progression [2, 5].

The optimal imaging protocol will depend on the clinical scenario such as history of trauma, chronicity, and the presence of neurological deficits and other comorbidities. MRI protocols usually include cross-sectional fat-saturated T1WI, three-dimensional contrast-enhanced, and TOF MRA. Axial T1WI and T2WI may demonstrate acute dissections. CTA with multiplanar reformations may be superior in the setting of trauma and vertebral dissections [8, 10].

Major Findings

General features: Typical findings of EAD dissection include a narrow eccentric lumen that can range from mild stenosis to diffuse luminal narrowing ("string" sign) or complete occlusion (Fig. 43.3a) [2]. Extracranial carotid artery dissections usually spare the carotid bifurcation and intracranial part of the ICA and are most commonly located 2–3 cm distal to the carotid bulb [2, 8]. Characteristic signs of EAD, such as an intimal flap or double lumen, are seen only in a minority of cases on cross-sectional imaging (Fig. 43.3b) [2]. Additional findings of EAD include a dissecting aneurysm and an intraluminal thrombus (Figs. 43.1a and 43.3a) [5].

CT: Unenhanced CT may show a crescent-shaped hyperdense focus corresponding to an intramural hematoma [8]. Less conspicuous and often undetectable on CTA, these intramural hematomas appear isodense to intraluminal contents and surrounding structures and may mimic atherosclerotic thickening or thrombus [8].

MRI: A common finding seen with carotid dissections on cross-sectional MRA imaging is an enlarged external diameter of the involved artery despite luminal narrowing [2, 8]. The intensity of the intramural hematoma on MRI depends on its chronicity. In the early and chronic stages, intramural hematomas are usually isointense to the surrounding structures, whereas from 1 to 9 weeks, they tend to be hyperintense on T1WI [2, 8]. An acute intramural hematoma can be easily missed on T2WI and T1WI as they tend to be hypointense and therefore difficult to delineate from an area of flow void [9]. Usually a subacute intramural hematoma presents as a crescentic hyperintensity surrounding an eccentrically located flow void on T1WI and T1 fat-saturated sequences (Fig. 43.2b). Time-of-flight (TOF) MRA also allows for the visualization of a subacute intramural hematoma which can be easily overlooked on contrast-enhanced MRA as its

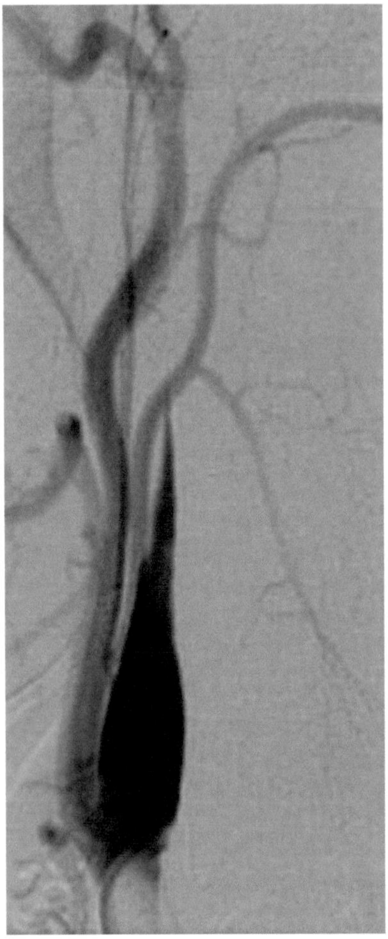

Fig. 43.5 Flame sign. Digital subtraction angiography image showing a tapered occlusion of the left internal carotid artery that spares the carotid bulb

signal becomes inseparable from that of slower moving blood [2, 8]. Contrast-enhanced MRA, on the other hand, is less time consuming, less susceptible to motion and flow artifacts, and better demonstrates luminal irregularities as well as stenoses. Contrast-enhanced MRA may also be superior at demonstrating dissecting aneurysms and vertebral artery dissections.

DSA: DSA may also show the string sign; however, the thickness and configuration of the arterial wall cannot be assessed. Additional signs include the "string and pearl" sign which consists of a tapered stenosis proximal to a dissecting aneurysm. The "flame" sign describes a tapered occlusion that spares the carotid bulb (Fig. 43.5) [8].

Imaging Follow-Up

No clear guidelines for imaging follow-up of EAD exist. However, given that the majority of stenoses and occlusions caused by EAD resolve in 3–12 months after the acute event, most authors advocate treating dissections with at least 3 months of antiplatelet therapy. Therefore, it would be reasonable to reassess for luminal recovery at least after 3 months of treatment [11].

Main Differential Diagnosis

Fibromuscular dysplasia: FMD is an arterial disease of unknown etiology affecting medium- and large-sized arteries. The characteristic findings are alternating stenoses and dilatations often described as a "string of beads." A common complication of FMD is dissection and when only a single artery is involved, the underlying imaging features of FMD can be overlooked. In the setting of multiple arterial dissections, other craniocervical vessels should be carefully evaluated for features suggestive of FMD, as bilateral and multifocal involvement is more common with FMD than spontaneous EAD (Fig. 43.6) [12].

Atherosclerosis: This usually occurs in the elderly, affects multiple vessels, and commonly involves the vessel origin, carotid bifurcation, and carotid bulb. On the contrary, EAD usually spare the vessel origin, carotid bifurcation, and carotid bulb. Furthermore, EAD are usually solitary except in the setting of underlying vasculopathy or extensive trauma [4, 8].

Post-radiation changes: Diffuse concentric narrowing of the internal carotid artery may be seen in patients who received radiation therapy to the neck.

Tips

- Always carefully assess flow void involving the upper portions of the ICA and vertebral arteries on brain MRI sequences.

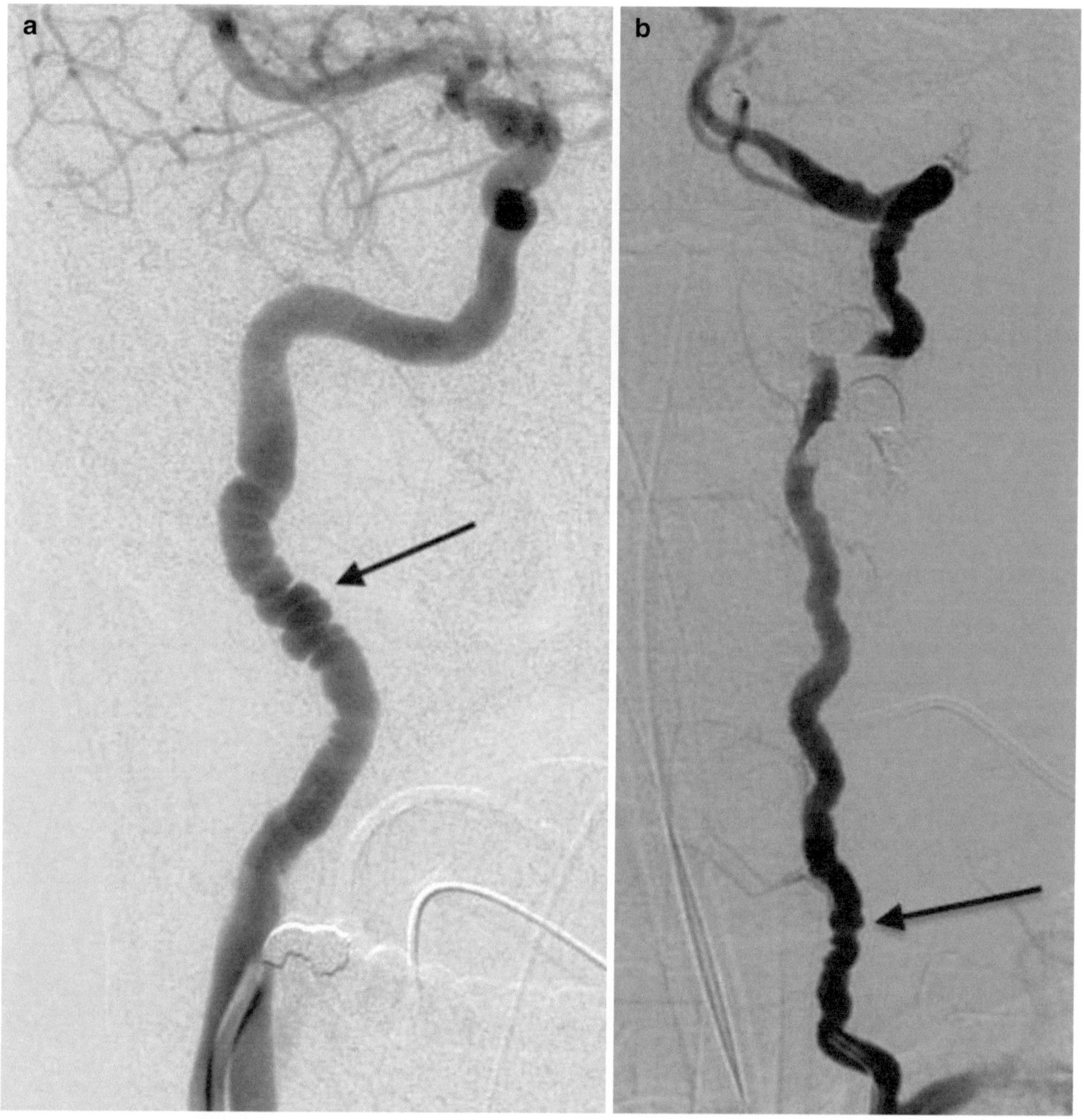

Fig. 43.6 Fibromuscular dysplasia. Anteroposterior DSA view of a right ICA (**a**) and left vertebral artery (**b**) showing alternating regions of mural dilatation and focal stenoses consistent with the string-of-beads appearance of FMD (*arrows*)

- Consider VA dissection in a young- to middle-aged adult with posterior circulation stroke.
- In the setting of trauma, assess for cervical fractures that involve the transverse foramen and result in VA dissection.
- Use T1 fat-saturated images to look for an eccentric hyperintense hematoma and avoid mistaking periarterial fat for an intramural hematoma (Fig. 43.2b).

- Take into account artifacts such as entry slice phenomenon when flow-related enhancement is seen at the extreme of an imaging volume on MRI [13].
- Asymmetry of the bilateral vertebral arteries is very common and may be secondary to developmental hypoplasia (right > left), whereas hypoplasia or dysplasia of the ICA is much more rare (Fig. 43.7a) [8, 14].

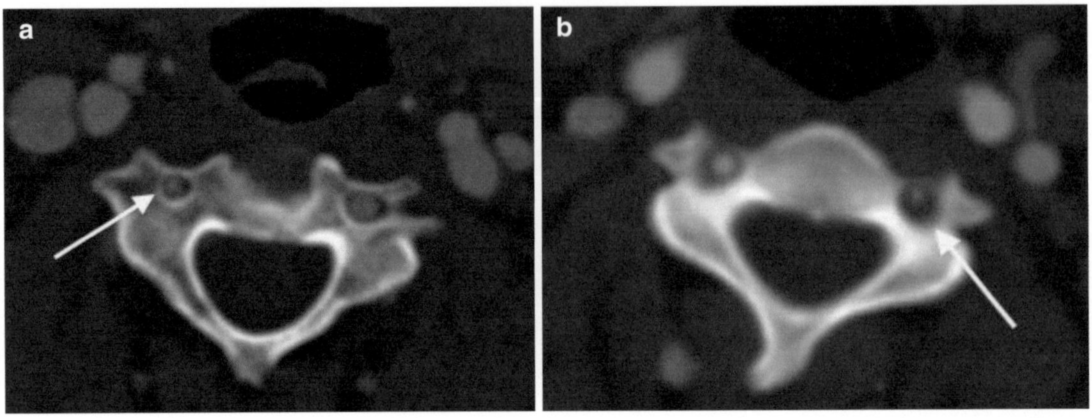

Fig. 43.7 Vertebral artery hypoplasia. (**a**) Axial CTA image shows asymmetric size of the bilateral vertebral arteries with a small vertebral artery noted on the right accompanied by a small transverse foramen (*arrow*). (**b**) Axial CTA image showing a small left vertebral artery within a larger transverse foramen suggesting an arterial dissection (*arrow*). Findings were confirmed by MRI (see Fig. 43.2)

- A diffusely small VA artery within a small transverse foramen is highly suggestive of developmental hypoplasia, whereas a diffusely narrowed VA within a larger transverse foramen suggests pathology (Fig. 43.7b) [15].

References

1. Thanvi B, Munshi SK, Dawson SL, et al. Carotid and vertebral artery dissection syndromes. Postgrad Med J. 2005;81:383–8. doi:10.1136/pgmj.2003.016774.
2. Patel R, Adam R, Maldjian C, et al. Cervical carotid artery dissection. Cardiol Rev. 2012;20:145–52. doi:10.1097/crd.0b013e318247cd15.
3. Ali MS, Amenta PS, Starke RM, et al. Intracranial vertebral artery dissections: evolving perspectives. Interv Neuroradiol. 2012;18:469–83.
4. Osborn A. Osborn's brain. In: Vasculopathy. 1st ed. Salt Lake City: Amirsys Pub; 2013. p. 263–7.
5. Fusco M, Harrigan M. Cerebrovascular dissections—a review part I: spontaneous dissections. Neurosurgery. 2011;68:242–57. doi:10.1227/neu.0b013e3182012323.
6. Fusco M, Harrigan M. Cerebrovascular dissections: a review. Part II: blunt cerebrovascular injury. Neurosurgery. 2011;68:517–30. doi:10.1227/neu.0b013e3181fe2fda.
7. Morris P. Practical neuroangiography. In: The extradural vertebral arteries. 3rd ed. Lippincott Williams & Wilkins, Philadelphia; 2013. p. 200–4.
8. Rodallec M, Marteau V, Gerber S, et al. Craniocervical arterial dissection: spectrum of imaging findings and differential diagnosis. RadioGraphics. 2008;28:1711–28. doi:10.1148/rg.286085512.
9. Flis C, Jäger H, Sidhu P. Carotid and vertebral artery dissections: clinical aspects, imaging features and endovascular treatment. Eur Radiol. 2006;17:820–34. doi:10.1007/s00330-006-0346-7.
10. Vertinsky A, Schwartz N, Fischbein N, et al. Comparison of multidetector CT angiography and MR imaging of cervical artery dissection. Am J Neuroradiol. 2008;29:1753–60. doi:10.3174/ajnr.a1189.
11. Rao A, Makaroun M, Marone L, et al. Long-term outcomes of internal carotid artery dissection. J Vasc Surg. 2011;54:370–5. doi:10.1016/j.jvs.2011.02.059.
12. Furie D, Tien R. Fibromuscular dysplasia of arteries of the head and neck: imaging findings. Am J Roentgenol. 1994;162:1205–9. doi:10.2214/ajr.162.5.8166011.
13. Provenzale J, Sarikaya B, Hacein-Bey L, Wintermark M. Causes of misinterpretation of cross-sectional imaging studies for dissection of the craniocervical arteries. Am J Roentgenol. 2011;196:45–52. doi:10.2214/ajr.10.5384.
14. Katsanos A, Kosmidou M, Kyritsis A, Giannopoulos S. Is vertebral artery hypoplasia a predisposing factor for posterior circulation cerebral ischemic events? A comprehensive review. Eur Neurol. 2013;70:78–83. doi:10.1159/000351786.
15. Kim C, Lee S, Park S, et al. A quantitative comparison of the vertebral artery and transverse foramen using CT angiography. J Clin Neurol. 2012;8:259. doi:10.3988/jcn.2012.8.4.259.

Part III

Spine

Nontraumatic Vertebral Collapse

44

Ana Lorena Abello

Abstract

Nontraumatic vertebral collapse or compression fractures refer to acute body vertebral fractures caused by osteoporosis or metastatic infiltration. Benign osteoporotic and malignant fractures are commonly encountered without a corresponding history of an acute traumatic episode. In some cases of vertebral collapse, it is difficult to differentiate between benign and malignant etiologies. The aim of this chapter is to discuss the specific findings of each fracture type which help to differentiate them.

Background

Nontraumatic vertebral collapse or compression fracture refers to a fracture in a vertebral body affected by osteoporosis or metastatic infiltration. Many times, benign osteoporotic and malignant fractures are commonly encountered without a corresponding history of an acute traumatic episode [1]. In some cases of vertebral collapse, it is difficult to differentiate between benign and malignant etiologies.

Osteoporosis is the most common primary bone disease in humans and represents a major public health problem. This condition affects an enormous number of people, of both sexes and all races, and its prevalence increases as the population ages. In osteoporotic compression fractures, patients may present with localized back pain that develops gradually over weeks or acutely during normal daily activities. In some cases, fractures are detected incidentally during the routine screening of patients with no known primary malignancies. Mortality is increased following vertebral fractures, which cause significant complications including back pain, height loss, and kyphosis [2].

Metastatic disease involves the axial skeleton and may result in pathologic fractures if excessive trabecular bone has been destroyed. Nearly 40 % of all bone metastases are located in the spine [2]. In patients with known malignancies, however, one-third of vertebral compression fractures are estimated to be benign and due to associated osteoporosis [3].

A.L. Abello, MD
Department of Radiology,
University of North Carolina, Chapel Hill, NC, USA
e-mail: anaabellop@hotmail.com

R. Hoffmann Nunes et al. (eds.), *Critical Findings in Neuroradiology*,
DOI 10.1007/978-3-319-27987-9_44

Appropriate staging and treatment planning requires the differentiation between benign and malignant collapse. Accurate diagnosis of benign compression fracture avoids the risk of biopsy and the cost of unnecessary additional imaging studies.

Key Points

Etiology

Benign compression fractures: occur because bone substance itself has been lost or weakened. Vertebral osteoporosis results in varying degrees of cortical and trabecular bone thinning, but the hematopoietic tissue remains relatively constant. With softening of the bone, vertebral fat content increases and spontaneous pathological fractures occur [4].

Pathological compression fractures: Metastases are the most frequent source of bone tumors; skeletal metastases arise mainly from carcinomas of the breast, prostate, kidney, and thyroid, in order of decreasing frequency. They occur mostly in middle-aged and elderly patients. The spine is a common site of metastatic disease, accounting for up to 39 % of all bone metastases. When cortical involvement occurs or there is sufficient osteolysis, metastases result in pathological compression fractures. Commonly, metastatic compression fractures show total or partial replacement of the normal bone marrow of the vertebral body. Most vertebral metastases do not result in compression fractures until the entire body is infiltrated by tumor causing structural bone weakening from destruction of trabeculae and cortex [4].

Best Imaging Modality

Computed tomography (*CT*): Several CT features may be helpful in the evaluation of nontraumatic acute vertebral collapse [5]. Although CT is useful in demonstrating cortical destruction, it is less valuable in characterizing trabecular infiltration. Since bone marrow evaluation is critical in vertebral collapse, CT images may lead to diagnostic uncertainty.

Magnetic resonance imaging (*MRI*): MRI is the modality of choice for detection and characterization of bone marrow abnormalities. Sagittal imaging plane is critical for the morphologic characterization of vertebral collapse and in the identification of signal intensity features that allow differentiation between benign and malignant etiologies. Therefore, MRI is more sensitive and specific in the demonstration of metastases, including extraosseous extension into the paraspinal and/or epidural soft tissues [6, 7]. In the evaluation of vertebral collapse, the protocol should include pre- and postcontrast T1-weighted (T1WI) (the latter especially with fat suppression), T2-weighted images (T2WI), and short tau inversion recovery (STIR) sequence. In last years, several studies have shown that diffusion-weighted images (DWI) may improve accuracy in the diagnosis of malignant spinal fractures specifically when quantitative estimation of diffusion and values of apparent diffusion coefficient (ADC) are calculated [8, 9]. Perfusion imaging has also been used, but it is difficult to implement in clinical practice.

Positron emission tomography with fluorine-18 deoxyglucose–computed tomography (*PET-CT*): FDG-PET does not accumulate in acute benign fractures but shows increased uptake in tumors and infections, and thus it may help to distinguish between vertebral fractures due to osteoporosis and those due to malignant or inflammatory processes. PET–CT shows similar sensitivity and specificity in the differentiation of osteoporotic and malignant vertebral fractures when compared to MRI; nevertheless for clinical use, the high costs of PET must be considered. In patients with indeterminate MRI findings and those suspected of having systemic metastatic disease, a PET investigation may be justified. PET may also add important information in postmenopausal women and those with breast cancer by showing additional lesions [10].

Major Findings

Preservation of normal bone marrow signal in the fractured vertebrae. Osteoporotic compression fracture poses no diagnostic difficulty since

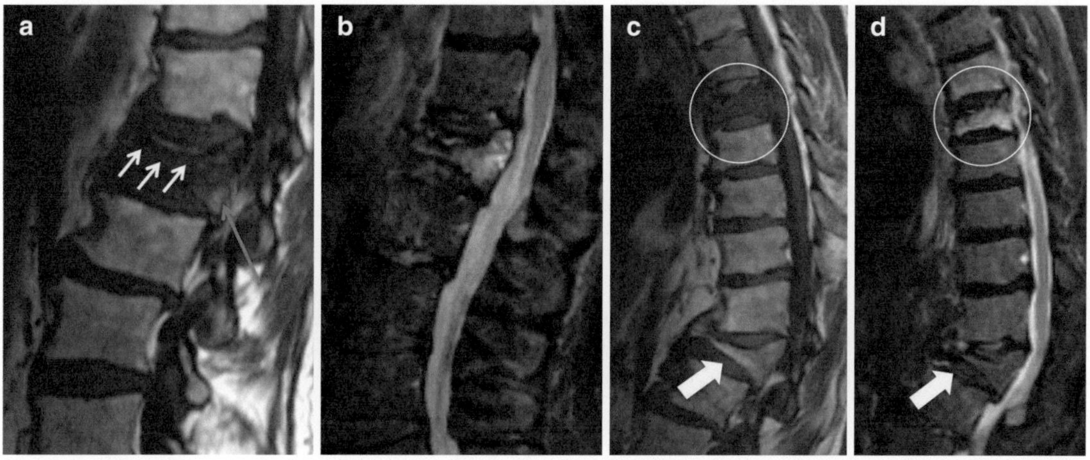

Fig. 44.1 Benign compression fracture in a 70-year-old male. (**a**) Sagittal T1WI shows an L1 vertebral collapse with preservation of fat marrow signal in the posterior vertebral body (*blue arrow*). A linear fracture plane that parallels the superior end plate of L1 is demonstrated (*white arrows*). (**b**) Sagittal STIR shows edema on the vertebral body that allows a better visualization of the linear fracture. (**c**, **d**) Sagittal T1WI and sagittal STIR 2 years later. L1 is almost totally collapsed. The bone marrow is similar to the other vertebral bodies and the edema has disappeared suggesting an old osteoporotic compression fracture (*thick arrow*). A new benign fracture is seen at T8 level (*circles*)

T1WI shows identical signal intensities in the collapsed and adjacent normal vertebral bodies. Typically, this signal intensity is similar to fat, conclusively excluding neoplastic involvement (Figs. 44.1 and 44.3) [11]. Even though in the presence of severe reactive marrow edema with diffusely marrow signal, this MRI criterion for distinguishing benign from malignant collapse is not definitive [3].

Fracture line: A critical difference between benign and malignant collapse is the development of a linear fracture plane in the affected vertebral body. In osteoporotic compression, this fracture line becomes visible due to trabecular compaction and/or reactive bone formation. The trabecular scaffolding structurally weakened due to quantitative loss of bone mass retains its capability for healing. In contrast, malignant collapse occurs because the trabecular architecture is partially or completely destroyed and replaced with neoplastic cells. The linear fracture plane in benign collapse parallels an end plate, usually the superior end plate [12, 13]. On T2WI images, the fracture plane usually becomes visible because it remains low in signal intensity, whereas the surrounding marrow edema increases in signal intensity (Figs. 44.1, 44.2, and 44.3).

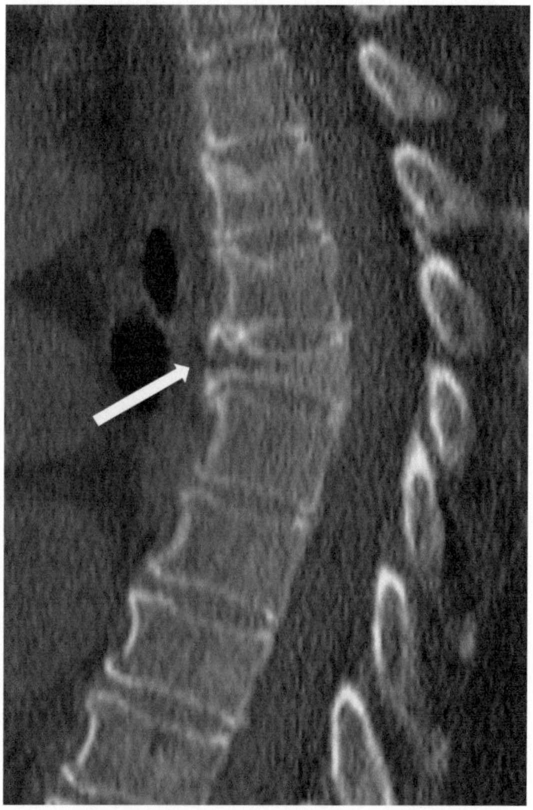

Fig. 44.2 Line fracture. Thoracic spinal CT in a 68-year-old woman shows an osteoporotic fracture at T7 with a fracture seen in the anterior vertebral body (*arrow*)

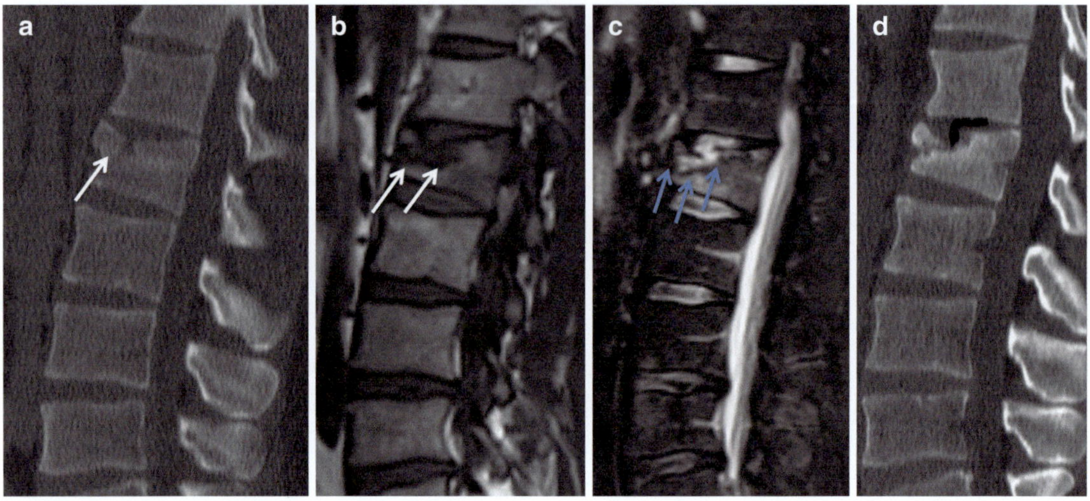

Fig. 44.3 Fluid in the vertebral body in a benign compression fracture. (**a**) Sagittal CT and (**b**) sagittal T1WI showing a T10 vertebral collapse with a fracture line (*arrows*) and preserved fat bone marrow in the affected vertebral body. In a follow up study 2 years later, a sagittal T2WI shows fluid (*blue arrows*) (**c**). Four years later, a sagittal CT shows air in the cleft confirming the benign nature of the fracture (**d**)

Intravertebral fluid collection: A highly specific sign of benign compression fracture is the presence of fluid in a collapsed vertebral body. Intravertebral fluid often demonstrates the same signal characteristics as cerebrospinal fluid (CSF). Therefore, T2WI shows a sharply defined region of homogeneously increased signal intensity that does not enhance following gadolinium administration. The etiology of fluid accumulation is unknown. One proposed hypothesis is fracture nonunion due to repetitive shearing forces that occur during daily activities or ambulation and cause constant micromotion across the fracture plane preventing bony bridging. As the bony margins become sclerotic and remodel to form a pseudoarthrosis, fluid accumulates in that space (Fig. 44.3) [14–16].

Extraosseous soft tissue mass. One of the most specific findings in malignant collapse is extraosseous extension of soft tissue from the vertebral body into the adjacent epidural ("curtain sign") or paraspinal spaces. Whenever an epidural soft tissue mass is identified, a pathologic fracture can be diagnosed with nearly a 100 % confidence. The sensitivity of this finding is much lower, however, ranging from 16 % to 80 %. In acute osteoporotic compression, edema and hemorrhage can surround a vertebral body and simulate a solid extraosseous mass even though in malignancy the soft tissue abnormality represents only a relatively small component of a larger lesion that appears centered in the vertebral body. Its peripheral contour is sharply marginated and usually shows focal nodularity and irregularity [12, 17, 18].

Contrast enhancement features are less helpful in the differentiation. Following intravenous contrast administration, paravertebral soft tissue enhancement may reflect either viable neoplasm or reactive inflammation (Fig. 44.4).

Pedicle abnormality: In the majority of spine metastases, MRI demonstrates tumor spread to at least one pedicle in the absence of either cortical destruction or vertebral collapse [19]. In patients who have malignant collapse, pedicle involvement has been reported in 70–88 % of cases, compared to 6–30 % of cases in patients with benign collapse [18, 20].

Vertebral morphology: In malignancy, morphologic changes reflect the presence of noncompressible tumor within the vertebral body. During collapse, peripheral cortical displacement results from the random, centrifugal dissipation of axial forces throughout the tumor. Thus, a bulging,

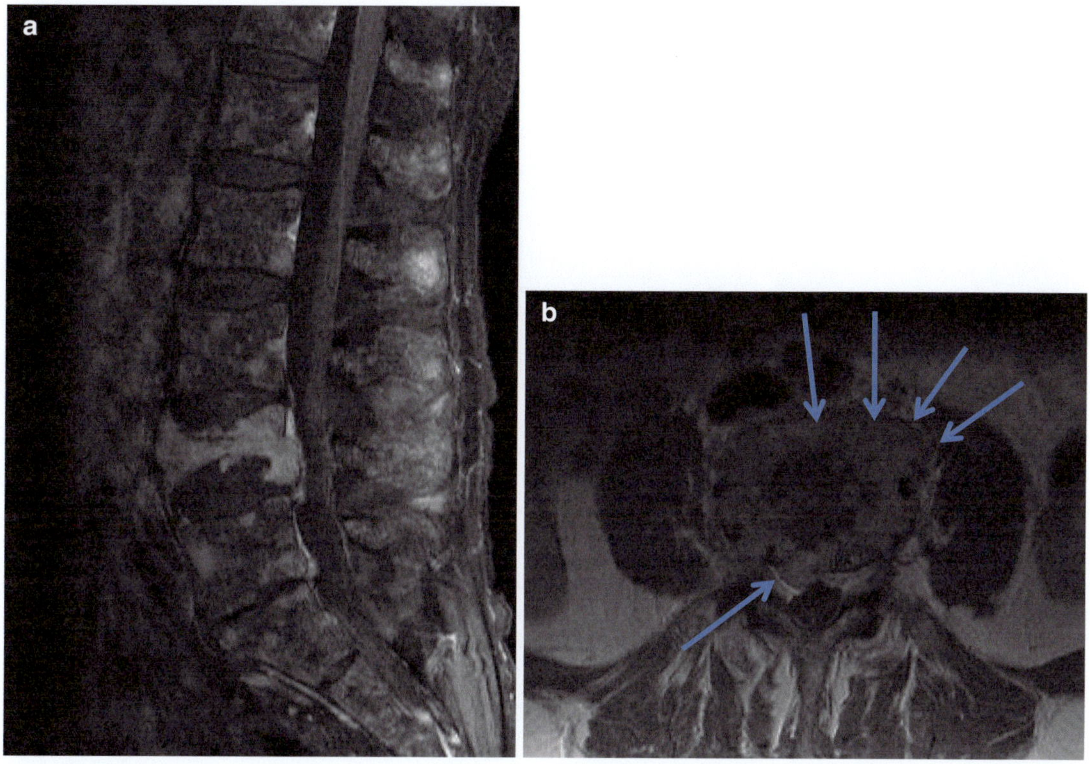

Fig. 44.4 Extraosseous soft tissue mass. A 69-year-old man with metastases from prostatic cancer. (**a**) Sagittal postcontrast T1WI shows metastatic lesions with enhancement and a malignant vertebral collapse in L4. (**b**) Axial postcontrast T1W1 shows extraosseous soft tissues extending anteriorly of the L4 vertebral body and posteriorly into the spinal canal (*blue arrows*)

diffusely convex contour suggests malignancy (Fig. 44.5) [20]. Malignant collapse tends to cause equal loss of anterior and posterior cortical heights, whereas benign compression usually causes greater loss of anterior height, resulting in the classical wedge-shaped vertebral body. Posterior retropulsion of a bone fragment into the spinal canal is considered to be specific for benign vertebral collapse (Fig. 44.6) [17].

Contrast enhancement: Contrast enhancement patterns are extremely complex in both benign and malignant collapses. Generally, they cannot be relied upon to distinguish osteoporotic from metastatic fractures due to overlapping MRI features. Some metastases demonstrate dense, diffuse contrast enhancement. In other lesions, patchy, heterogeneous enhancement reflects tumor necrosis and uneven blood supply. Peritumoral edema often enhances more densely than the actual metastasis. In benign collapse, enhancement may be diffuse and homogeneous, or markedly heterogeneous due to osteonecrosis. The degree of contrast enhancement depends on the extent of reactive marrow inflammation and often is as dense as that seen in neoplasm (Fig. 44.7) [17].

Imaging characteristics of adjacent vertebrae: Secondary findings in the spine are sometimes helpful to distinguish benign from malignant collapses. The majority of malignant fractures (68–88 %) are associated with focal metastases at other vertebral levels. These metastases may involve the vertebral body or posterior elements, usually demonstrating a rounded shape that is sharply marginated against the surrounding marrow fat (Fig. 44.5). In osteoporotic compression, low-signal foci in adjacent vertebrae are less common (19 %) and usually represent Schmorl's nodes or other benign fractures [17].

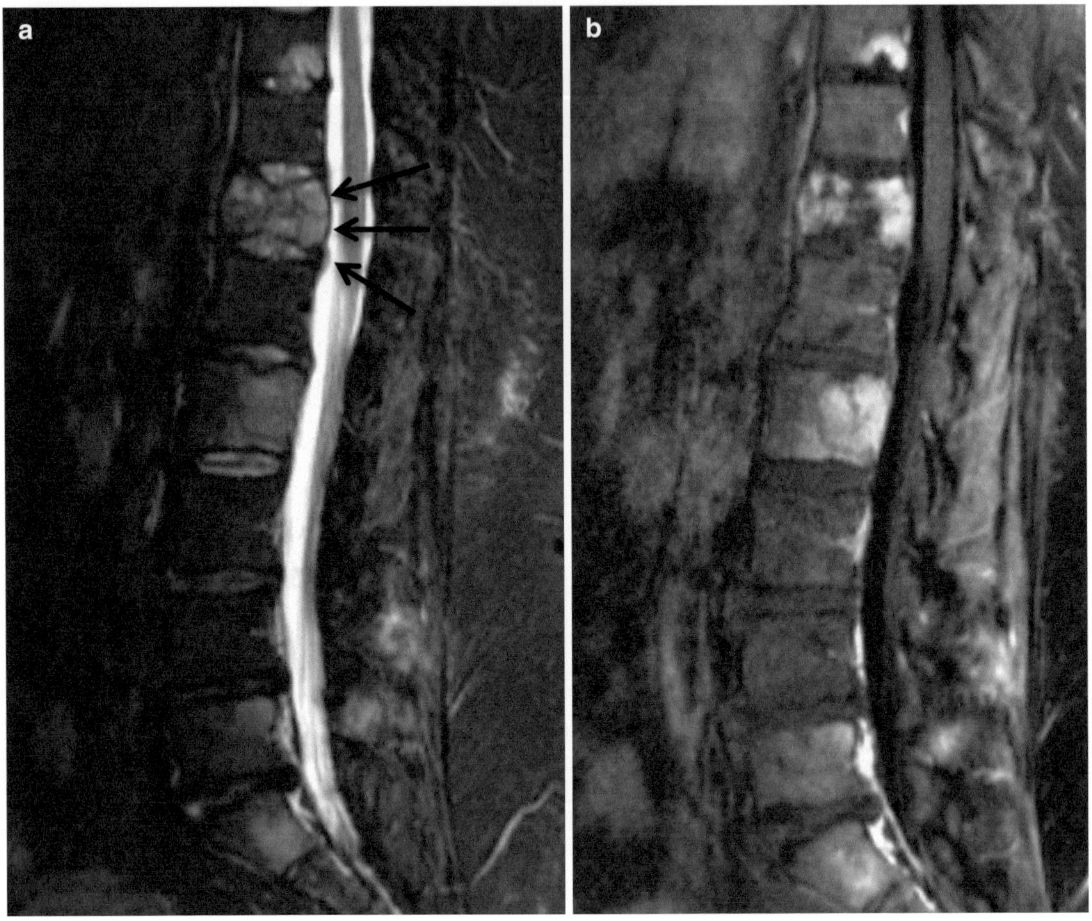

Fig. 44.5 Malignant vertebral collapse in a patient with breast cancer metastases. (**a**) Sagittal STIR shows several hyperintense focal lesions and a slightly vertebral collapse of T12 with a posterior convex contour (*black arrows*). (**b**) Sagittal postcontrast T1WI shows the lesions to have intense and heterogeneous enhancement in the collapsed vertebral body and elsewhere

Restricted diffusion: Malignant compression fractures show restricted diffusion due to the fact that metastases have high cellularity therefore lower ADC and higher signal intensity on DWI than benign fractures where the increased interstitial space associated with edema in the acute phase leads higher ADC (Fig. 44.8) [21]. The affected vertebral body should be compared with the adjacent ones that are not involved. Although many sequences have been used to image the spine with diffusion, one can use the same sequence as used for the brain lowering the B value to about 500–700 to increase signal to noise. Unfortunately, the results are variable with severely distorted images produced in some MRI units.

A summary of the above mentioned findings can be found in Table 44.1.

Imaging Follow-Up

When MRI cannot distinguish between benign and malignant vertebral fractures especially in a setting of patient with cancer, the best complementary study is PET-CT. However, in some patients, it is not diagnostic, and histopathological confirmation is necessary.

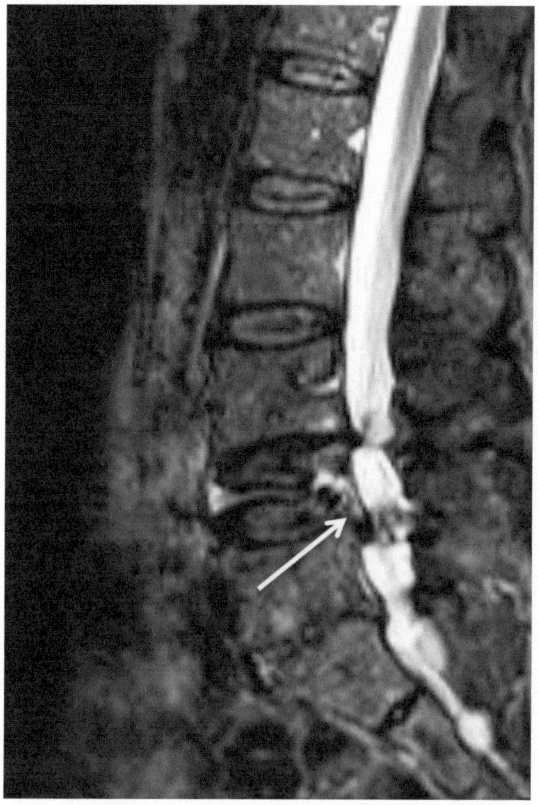

Fig. 44.6 Posterior retropulsion of a bone fragment in a benign acute osteoporotic compression fracture. Sagittal STIR shows high signal in an L4 collapsed vertebral body and posterior retropulsion of a bone fragment into the spinal canal *(arrow)*

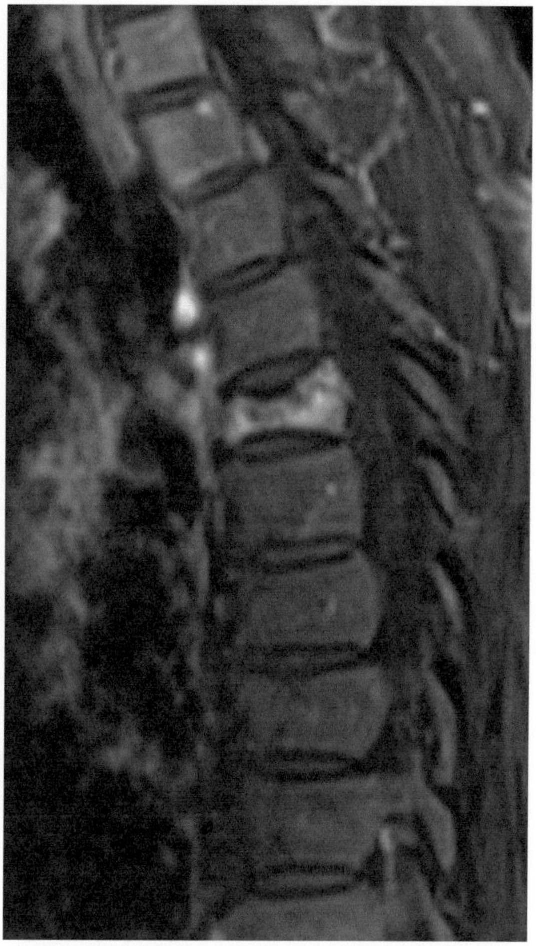

Fig. 44.7 Acute benign compression fracture in the thoracic spine. Sagittal postcontrast fat suppressed T1WI shows intense enhancement in the vertebral body in which a fracture line is also seen

No general consensus exists on the optimal imaging algorithm for monitoring the response of malignant bone involvement to therapy. Follow-up protocols may vary for different malignancies [22].

Main Differential Diagnosis

Pathologic fractures can also be due to *primary malignant bone tumors* such as myeloma [1] and sarcomas [23].

Rarely, primary spinal *hemangiomas* may have an aggressive presentation and become symptomatic producing a pathological burst fracture [24].

Paget disease is a chronic metabolic bone disorder. The spine is the second most commonly involved site. Pathologic fractures may result from it [25].

Tuberculous spondylitis: Approximately 50 % of skeletal tuberculosis involves the spine. Infection usually begins in the anterior part of the vertebral body adjacent to the end plate. These end plate changes allow the spread of infection to the adjacent intervertebral disk. The loose internal structure of the disk allows the infection to disseminate into additional spinal segments resulting in the classic pattern of involvement of more than one vertebral body with little disk involvement. If left untreated, the infection even-

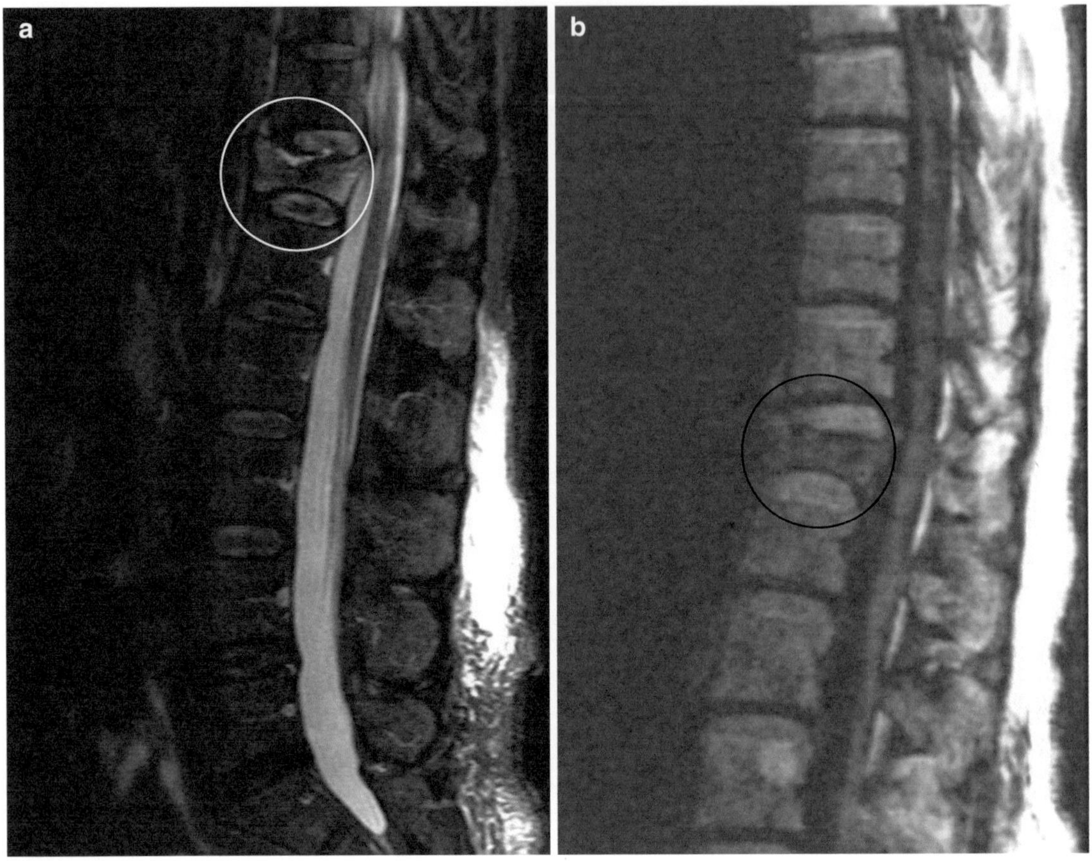

Fig. 44.8 Acute osteoporotic compression fracture with facilitated diffusion. (**a**) Sagittal STIR shows homogeneous hyperintensity in an entire vertebral body (*circle*). (**b**) Sagittal DWI shows low signal intensity which on the ADC map (not shown) demonstrated no restricted diffusion

Table 44.1 Benign osteoporotic versus malignant compression fractures

Findings	Benign osteoporotic compression fractures	Malignant compression fractures
Bone marrow signal	Bone marrow signal intensity is preserved	Bone marrow signal intensity is abnormal
Fracture line	Can be present	Absent
Intravertebral fluid collection	Can be present	Absent
Extraosseous soft tissue mass	If it is present, it tends to form a circumferential rim around the vertebral body	Sharply marginated and usually shows focal nodularity ("curtain sign") in ventral epidural space
Pedicle	Rarely compromised	Commonly compromised
Vertebral morphology	Retropulsion of a bone fragment into the spinal canal	Convex posterior contour (bulging)
Contrast enhancement	Diffuse and homogeneous or heterogeneous due to osteonecrosis	Intense, diffuse, or heterogeneous due to tumor necrosis
Imaging characteristics of adjacent vertebrae	Schmorl's nodes or other benign fractures	Focal metastases
ADC maps	Facilitated diffusion	Restricted diffusion

tually results in vertebral collapse and anterior wedging, leading to kyphosis and gibbus formation [26].

Tips

- If T1WI shows identical signal intensities in the collapsed and adjacent vertebral bodies, osteoporotic fracture diagnosis is likely.
- Fracture line sometimes is better visualized in T2WI and postcontrast T1WI, and this sign has also high specificity for benign vertebral collapse.
- A specific finding in malignant vertebral collapse is extraosseous extension of soft tissues from the affected vertebral body into the adjacent epidural or paraspinal spaces ("curtain sign").
- Both acute benign and malignant vertebral fractures may show avid contrast enhancement, and therefore this finding is nonspecific.
- An abnormal appearance of other vertebral bodies can be key in differentiating benign from pathology vertebral collapses.

References

1. Kang HS, Lee JW, Kwon JW, SpringerLink (Online service). Radiology illustrated: spine. Berlin/Heidelberg: Springer Berlin Heidelberg: Imprint: Springer; 2014. Available from: http://VB3LK7EB4T.search.serialssolutions.com/?V=1.0&L=VB3LK7EB4T&S=JCs&C=TC0001187485&T=marc.
2. National Osteoporosis Foundation. Clinician's guide to prevention and treatment of osteoporosis. Washington, DC: National Osteoporosis Foundation; 2010.
3. Fornasier VL, Czitrom AA. Collapsed vertebrae: a review of 659 autopsies. Clin Orthop Relat Res. 1978;131:261–5.
4. Cicala D, Briganti F, Casale L, Rossi C, Cagini L, Cesarano E, et al. Atraumatic vertebral compression fractures: differential diagnosis between benign osteoporotic and malignant fractures by MRI. Musculoskelet Surg. 2013;97 Suppl 2:S169–79.
5. Laredo JD, Lakhdari K, Bellaiche L, Hamze B, Janklewicz P, Tubiana JM. Acute vertebral collapse: CT findings in benign and malignant nontraumatic cases. Radiology. 1995;194(1):41–8.
6. Daffner RH, Lupetin AR, Dash N, Deeb ZL, Sefczek RJ, Schapiro RL. MRI in the detection of malignant infiltration of bone marrow. AJR Am J Roentgenol. 1986;146(2):353–8.
7. Modic MT, Masaryk T, Paushter D. Magnetic resonance imaging of the spine. Radiol Clin North Am. 1986;24(2):229–45.
8. Herneth AM, Philipp MO, Naude J, Funovics M, Beichel RR, Bammer R, et al. Vertebral metastases: assessment with apparent diffusion coefficient. Radiology. 2002;225(3):889–94.
9. Balliu E, Vilanova JC, Pelaez I, Puig J, Remollo S, Barcelo C, et al. Diagnostic value of apparent diffusion coefficients to differentiate benign from malignant vertebral bone marrow lesions. Eur J Radiol. 2009;69(3):560–6.
10. Schmitz A, Risse JH, Textor J, Zander D, Biersack HJ, Schmitt O, et al. FDG-PET findings of vertebral compression fractures in osteoporosis: preliminary results. Osteoporos Int: J Established Result Cooperation Between Eur Found Osteoporos Natl Osteoporos Found USA. 2002;13(9):755–61.
11. Baker LL, Goodman SB, Perkash I, Lane B, Enzmann DR. Benign versus pathologic compression fractures of vertebral bodies: assessment with conventional spin-echo, chemical-shift, and STIR MR imaging. Radiology. 1990;174(2):495–502.
12. Yuh WT, Zachar CK, Barloon TJ, Sato Y, Sickels WJ, Hawes DR. Vertebral compression fractures: distinction between benign and malignant causes with MR imaging. Radiology. 1989;172(1):215–8.
13. Palmer WE, Suri R, Kattapuram SV. Benign versus malignant vertebral collapse: value of a fracture line on MR images. Radiology. 1999;213:93.
14. Naul LG, Peet GJ, Maupin WB. Avascular necrosis of the vertebral body: MR imaging. Radiology. 1989;172(1):219–22.
15. Malghem J, Maldague B, Labaisse MA, Dooms G, Duprez T, Devogelaer JP, et al. Intravertebral vacuum cleft: changes in content after supine positioning. Radiology. 1993;187(2):483–7.
16. Dupuy DE, Palmer WE, Rosenthal DI. Vertebral fluid collection associated with vertebral collapse. AJR Am J Roentgenol. 1996;167(6):1535–8.
17. Cuenod CA, Laredo JD, Chevret S, Hamze B, Naouri JF, Chapaux X, et al. Acute vertebral collapse due to osteoporosis or malignancy: appearance on unenhanced and gadolinium-enhanced MR images. Radiology. 1996;199(2):541–9.
18. Shih TT, Huang KM, Li YW. Solitary vertebral collapse: distinction between benign and malignant causes using MR patterns. J Magn Reson Imaging: JMRI. 1999;9(5):635–42.
19. Blomlie V, Lien HH, Iversen T, Winderen M, Tvera K. Radiation-induced insufficiency fractures of the sacrum: evaluation with MR imaging. Radiology. 1993;188(1):241–4.
20. Jung HS, Jee WH, McCauley TR, Ha KY, Choi KH. Discrimination of metastatic from acute osteoporotic compression spinal fractures with MR imaging. Radiographics: Rev Publ Radiol Soc N Am Inc. 2003;23(1):179–87.

21. Zhou XJ, Leeds NE, McKinnon GC, Kumar AJ. Characterization of benign and metastatic vertebral compression fractures with quantitative diffusion MR imaging. AJNR Am J Neuroradiol. 2002;23(1):165–70.
22. Even-Sapir E. Imaging of malignant bone involvement by morphologic, scintigraphic, and hybrid modalities. J Nucl Med: Off Publ Soc Nucl Med. 2005;46(8):1356–67.
23. Ilaslan H, Sundaram M, Unni KK, Shives TC. Primary vertebral osteosarcoma: imaging findings. Radiology. 2004;230(3):697–702.
24. Vinay S, Khan SK, Braybrooke JR. Lumbar vertebral haemangioma causing pathological fracture, epidural haemorrhage, and cord compression: a case report and review of literature. J Spinal Cord Med. 2011;34(3):335–9.
25. Pedicelli A, Papacci F, Leone A, De Simone C, Meglio M, Bonomo L, et al. Vertebroplasty for symptomatic monostotic Paget disease. J Vasc Interv Radiol: JVIR. 2011;22(3):400–3.
26. Burrill J, Williams CJ, Bain G, Conder G, Hine AL, Misra RR. Tuberculosis: a radiologic review. Radiographics: Rev Publ Radiol Soc N Am Inc. 2007;27(5):1255–73.

Spinal Cord Compression

45

Ana Lorena Abello and Florencia Álamos

Abstract

Spinal cord compression refers to an inward displacement of the dural sac and/or its contents by a lesion arising outside of the spinal cord. It is caused by metastatic or primary spine tumors, disk herniations, vertebral fractures, cysts, spinal epidural abscesses and hematomas, and degenerative disease most commonly. MRI is the study of choice in patients suspected of having cord compression.

Background

Spinal cord compression refers to an inward displacement of the dural sac and/or its contents by a lesion arising outside of the spinal cord. Prompt diagnosis of acute spinal cord compression is critical because patient outcomes are based on early treatment. Spinal cord and cauda equina compression may be caused by metastatic or primary spine tumors, disk herniations, vertebral fractures, cysts, spinal epidural abscesses and hematomas, and degenerative disease among other causes (Table 45.1) [1]. This chapter focuses on disk herniations, degenerative changes, trauma, as well as metastatic and primary spine bone tumors and cystic lesions as causes of cord compression. Epidural abscess and hematomas causing cord compression are discussed separately in this book.

Clinical findings. Back, radicular, or central pain, motor and sensory deficits, ataxia, abnormal gait, impotence, and bowel and bladder dysfunctions are the most common signs and symptoms of spinal cord compression regardless its etiology [1, 2]. Most patients with symptomatic cervical disk herniations report severe neck and arm pain, reflex changes, and motor weakness of the upper extremity [3]. The most common symptom of disk herniation in lumbar spine after low back pain is sciatica [4]. One of the common clinical presentations in

A.L. Abello, MD (✉)
Department of Radiology,
University of North Carolina, Chapel Hill, NC, USA
e-mail: anaabellop@hotmail.com

F. Álamos, MD
Department of Neuroscience, School of Medicine
Universidad Católica de Chile, Luz Larrain,
3946 Lo Barnechea, Santiago, Chile
e-mail: flopi1987@yahoo.com

R. Hoffmann Nunes et al. (eds.), *Critical Findings in Neuroradiology*,
DOI 10.1007/978-3-319-27987-9_45

Table 45.1 Causes of spinal cord compression

Disk herniation
Degenerative disease
Spondylosis
OLLP
Trauma
Tumors
Intradural–extramedullary
Nerve sheath tumors
Schwannoma
Neurofibroma
Meningioma
Lipoma
Epidermoid/dermoid
Hemangiopericytoma
Paraganglioma
Extradural–extramedullary
Primary vertebral tumors
Metastases
Cystic lesions
Epidural abscess
Epidural hematoma

compressive myelopathy secondary to trauma is the central cord syndrome, which consists of acute motor and sensory impairment. Central cord syndrome is most commonly seen with lesions in the cervical spine, and, therefore, the symptoms are most pronounced in the upper extremities [5]. In children, intradural tumors may be associated with skeletal deformities such as kyphoscoliosis [6]. Extramedullary cysts of the spinal canal usually produce a slowly progressive myelopathy, myeloradiculopathy, or radiculopathy, and less frequently, these lesions may cause acute symptomatic spinal cord compression [7].

Epidemiology. Radhakrishnan et al. reported an annual incidence of cervical disk herniations of 18.6 per 100,000 with its peak in the sixth decade of life [8].

Spondylosis and ossification of the posterior longitudinal ligament (OPLL) usually occur in older patients and are very rare under age 40 years at least in the Western world [9]. In the East, younger patients may be affected.

Traumatic spinal cord injury occurs in all countries throughout the world with an annual incidence of 15–40 cases per million with the causes of these injuries ranging from motor vehicle accidents and community violence to recreational activities and workplace-related injuries [10].

Spinal tumors are divided into extradural, intradural–extramedullary, and intramedullary. Extradural tumors make up 50 % of all spinal tumors, while intradural–extramedullary tumors account for 40 %, and intramedullary tumors account for 5–10 % [11]. In patients under 30 years of age, bone tumors of the spine (extradural tumors) are uncommon and are generally benign except for Ewing sarcoma and osteosarcoma. In patients over 30 years of age, most bone tumors are malignant and metastases are the most common lesions [12].

Key Points

Etiology

Disk Herniation

It is broadly defined as a localized or focal displacement of disk material beyond the limits of the intervertebral disk space and thus beyond the annulus fibrosus. The disk material may be nucleus, cartilage, fragmented apophyseal bone, annular tissue, or any combination thereof [13].

A herniated disk can compress spinal nerve roots and occasionally the spinal cord itself. In the cervical region, the levels most commonly affected are the C5–C7 segments. In the lumbar area, most disk protrusions occur at L4–L5 and L5–S1 [14, 15]. The etiology of cervical spine disk herniations is multifactorial, and proposed risk factors include male gender, cigarette smoking, heavy lifting, and frequent diving [3].

Degenerative Disease

Spondylosis: It is the more common cause of cord compression in the cervical spine. Cervical spondylotic myelopathy is a condition in which degenerative changes result in myelopathy. The common mechanical compressive factors contributing to cervical spondylotic myelopathy include bulging disks, anterior and posterior osteophyte formation, and buckling of the ligamentum flavum. These mechanical compressive factors directly injure neural tissue and initiate secondary ischemia, inflammation, and apoptosis [9].

OPLL: Ossification of the posterior longitudinal ligament is a pathologic condition whose etiology is unclear. The posterior longitudinal ligament of the cervical (C2–C5) or thoracic (T4–T7) spine is ossified and thickened and may even form bone marrow. OPLL may be located at the vertebral body levels without involvement of disk levels (segmental type), or it may continuously extend over several levels (continuous type). Continuous OPLL is significantly thicker, and the degree of spinal cord compression it produces is more severe than that associated with the segmental type [9].

Trauma

Cord compression following trauma may be due to the presence of associated spinal fractures, subluxation, ligamentous injury, prevertebral swelling, and hematomas [5].

Spinal Tumors (Diagram 45.1)

Intradural–Extramedullary Tumors

The most common intradural extramedullary lesions are the nerve sheath tumors (schwannomas and neurofibromas) followed by meningiomas.

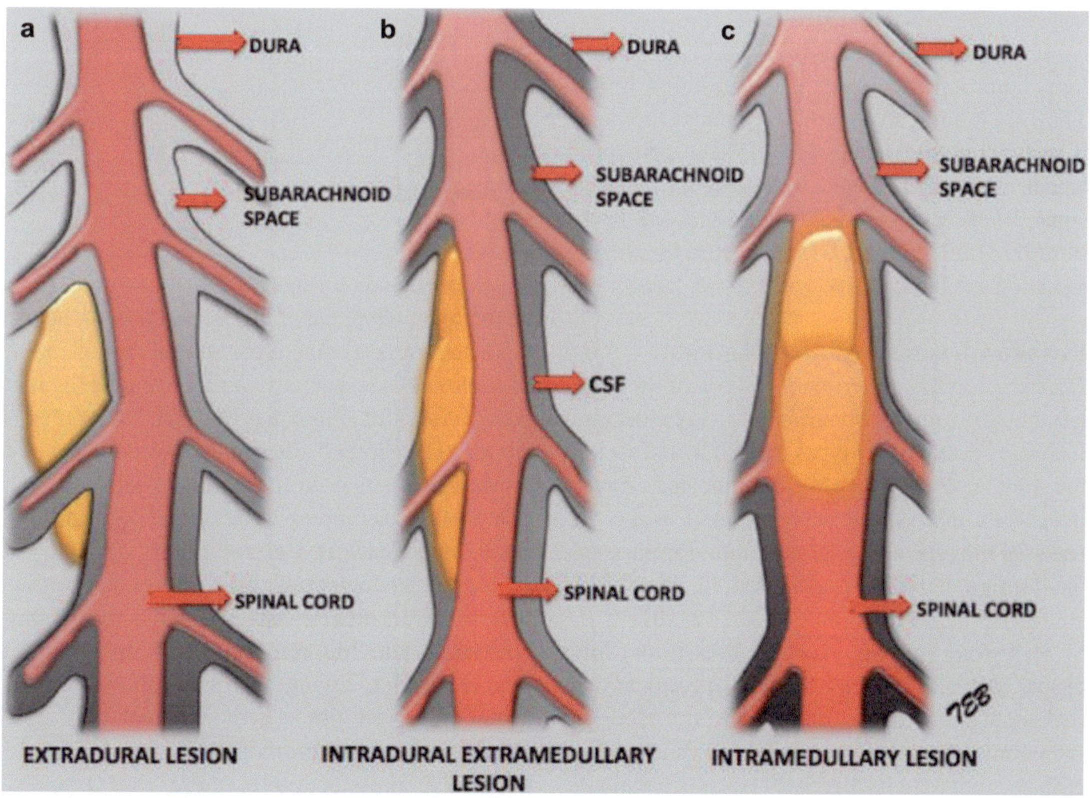

Diagram 45.1 Spinal lesions. (**a**) Extradural lesion displaces the spinal cord to the opposite side and collapses the subarachnoid spaces on both sides. A cap of epidural fat is seen above and below the lesion. (**b**) Intradural–extramedullary lesion displaces the cord to the opposite side and expands the subarachnoid space at the poles of the lesion, leaving a cap of CSF above and below the lesion. (**c**) Intramedullary lesion expands the spinal cord and collapses the subarachnoid spaces around the cord

Less common lesions include paragangliomas, metastases, lipomas, spinal nerve sheath myxomas (neurothekeoma), sarcomas, and vascular tumors [6, 16, 17].

Nerve sheath tumors: Nerve sheath tumors are classified as either neurofibromas or schwannomas. Neurofibromas are benign neoplasms composed of thin fibroblastic-type cells. These lesions infiltrate nerve fascicles. Neurofibromas may be associated with neurofibromatosis type 1 (NF1), especially the plexiform type. In the setting of NF1, these lesions are typically multiple. Schwannomas are benign neoplasms of myelin-producing Schwann cells. They are composed of two cells types, Antoni A and Antoni B, which contribute to their imaging characteristics. They are encapsulated and do not infiltrate nerve fascicles. Schwannomas rarely occur in children and are typically solitary. However, multiple schwannomas are common in the setting of neurofibromatosis type 2 (NF2) [17].

Meningiomas: Meningiomas are the second most common extramedullary–intradural tumor. They are benign slow-growing tumors that arise from arachnoid cap cells [11]. Fifteen percent of spinal cord meningiomas occur in the cervical spine, 81 % in the thoracic spine, and 4 % in the lumbar spine. NF2 and prior exposure to ionizing radiation are the only recognized risk factors [2].

Extradural–Extramedullary Tumors

Primary neoplasms: Primary tumors of the spine are thought to be uncommon. However, because there are several tissue types located in and around the spinal column, there is a complicated array of neoplasms that should be considered in the differential diagnosis of a spinal tumor. Primary spinal tumors must be considered in cases of a solitary spinal lesion (Table 45.2) [12, 18].

Table 45.2 Classification of primary spinal tumors by tissue of origin [12]

Origin	Tumors
Osteogenic	Osteoid osteoma
	Osteoblastoma
	Osteosarcoma
Chondrogenic	Osteochondroma
	Chondroblastoma
	Chondrosarcoma
Fibrogenic	Fibrous dysplasia
	Benign fibrous histiocytoma[a]
	Malignant fibrous histiocytoma[a]
Vascular	Hemangioma
	Paraganglioma[a]
	Hemangiosarcoma[a]
	Hemangiopericytoma[a]
Hematopoietic, reticuloendothelial, lymphatic	Histiocytosis
	Plasmocytoma
	Multiple myeloma
	Lymphoma
	Leukemia
	Ewing sarcoma
Notochordal	Chordoma
Unknown	Aneurysmal bone cyst (ABC)
	Giant cell tumor

[a]Extremely rare in the spine

Metastatic lesions: Prostate, breast, and lung cancer each account for 15–20 % of patients with malignant spinal cord compression. Non-Hodgkin lymphoma, multiple myeloma, and renal cancer each account for a further 5–10 % of such patients. Colorectal cancer, tumors of unknown primary origin (most of which orginate from unrecognized lung or gastrointestinal primary tumors), and sarcomas are other common ones. Although the valveless Batson's venous plexus was thought to be the route of spread of metastatic disease, newer evidence suggests that direct arterial embolization of tumor cells, especially of clonogenic cells that have affinity for spinal marrow, is the main mechanism. This spread results in a vertebral body mass that enlarges to impinge on the thecal sac anteriorly and compresses the spinal cord and epidural venous plexus. Destruction of cortical bone by tumor can compound this compression by vertebral body collapse and retropulsion of bony fragments into the epidural space. In children, neuroblastoma, Ewing sarcoma, Wilms' tumor, lymphoma, soft tissue sarcoma, and bone sarcoma are the most common tumor types that lead to cord compression. Furthermore, cord compression is more likely to be caused by paravertebral masses that impinge on the spinal cord directly, rather than by involvement of bony elements in the spine [19].

Table 45.3 Classification of spinal meningeal cyst [21]

I. Extradural meningeal cyst without spinal nerve root fiber
IA. Extradural meningeal cyst (extradural arachnoid cyst)
IB. Sacral meningocele
II. Extradural meningeal cyst with spinal nerve root fibers (Tarlov's perineural cyst and spinal nerve root diverticulum)
III. Spinal intradural meningeal cyst (intradural arachnoid cyst)

Arachnoid Cystic Lesions

Arachnoid–dural cysts may be congenital or acquired abnormalities and be extradural or intradural. The extradural type may result from a congenital or acquired dural defect allowing the arachnoid membrane and cerebrospinal fluid (CSF) to herniate through the dural layer. The intradural type may also be congenital or can result from adhesions caused by spinal trauma, infection, or interventions [20]. According to the classification described by Nabors et al., the spinal meningeal extramedullary cysts can be divided into three main groups (Table 45.3) [21].

Best Imaging Modality

Computed tomography (CT) and magnetic resonance imaging (MRI) are complementary to each other in diagnosis of compressive myelopathy although if only one examination is to be performed, MRI should be chosen. Bony changes such as osteophytes and uncovertebral hypertrophy and spinal bone tumors are better seen on CT, whereas MRI is superior to image soft tissues, disk herniations, tumors, and cysts and for evaluation of the spinal cord [5].

Magnetic resonance imaging: MRI is the modality of choice to assess spinal cord integrity. Cord signal intensity is best assessed on T2-weighted images (T2WI). Cord signal changes on MRI depend on the duration of the compression. In acute to subacute stages where the changes are predominately due to cord edema, T2WI will show bright signal intensity while T1-weighted images (T1WI) show the affected region to be isointense to normal cord. If the cord compression is present over a long period of time, irreversible changes such as gliosis and myelomalacia develop within the cord. These changes present as focal areas of increased signal intensity in the cord on T2WI with corresponding hypointensity on T1WI [5].

Gradient-recalled echo (GRE) is a very sensitive MRI sequence to distinguish osteophytes from disk herniations because osteophytes show low signal intensity relative to higher signal intensity disk material [5]. This sequence is also useful to detect spinal cord hemorrhagic lesions in the setting of trauma and spontaneous hemorrhage (hematomyelia).

Contrast enhancement with gadolinium assists in characterizing and defining the extent of neoplasms and in identifying regions of blood–brain barrier breakdown. Short-time inversion recovery (STIR) sequence is excellent for evaluating the spinal cord as well as bone marrow and soft tissues, and postcontrast fat-suppressed T1WI is ideal as it suppresses the normal high-signal intensity from fatty bone marrow which at times may become indistinguishable from enhancing lesions after contrast administration [6, 11].

Computed tomography: In bone tumors of the spine, CT is the most accurate method for evaluating the extent of osseous involvement and the degree of cancellous and cortical bone loss. CT helps evaluate the risk for vertebral body collapse and is helpful in planning surgery [12]. In medullary spinal cord compression due to metastatic lesions, CT is useful for the planning of radiotherapy since CT can generate a dose plan and is needed for 3D and conformal radiotherapy even if MRI was used for the initial diagnosis [19].

CT myelography: CT myelography is especially helpful in establishing communication of the arachnoid cysts with the subarachnoid space [7]. Communicating cysts usually opacify with contrast, and therefore, CT myelography can help differentiate an arachnoid cyst causing spinal cord compression from other lesions with cystic degeneration or from lesions mimicking cysts in the spinal canal. CT myelography is only used for cord compression when MRI cannot be done and the upper and lower limits of the compression cannot be determined by any other imaging method.

Radiography. The role of radiographs is debatable; however, in clinical practice, radiographs often remain the first investigation performed. In the assessment of degenerative disease, a routine radiograph series may consist of up to six images: anterior–posterior (AP), lateral, lateral with flexion and extension, and both oblique views.

In spinal bone tumors, initial imaging is usually radiography which is not sensitive enough to make a diagnosis. Radiography may, however, help the surgeon in making a decision regarding overall spinal balance and the need for stabilization [9].

The nerve sheath tumors very often cause neural foramen remodeling, which can be easily visualized in lateral radiographs.

Major Findings

Disk Herniation

MRI is the most sensitive and specific study for spinal cord compression associated to disk herniations. In a herniation in which the base is wider than its length and involves less than 25 % of the disk circumference, the term "protrusion" is applied. When the length of the herniated disk is longer than the width of its base, the term "extrusion" is recommended [13]. On T2WI axial images, the relationship of the posterior margin of the intervertebral disks with the dural sac and nerve roots should be carefully defined to identify a herniated disk [9].

In the cervical spine, it is not easy to differentiate a disk herniation from end-plate osteophytes on MRI, and CT sometimes is necessary to make the differentiation. On MRI, sagittal T1WI may provide a clue in identifying disk herniation as it is isointense and in continuity with the parent disk in contrast to posterior osteophytes which have low signal intensity similar to that of the vertebral body cortex (Fig. 45.1) [9].

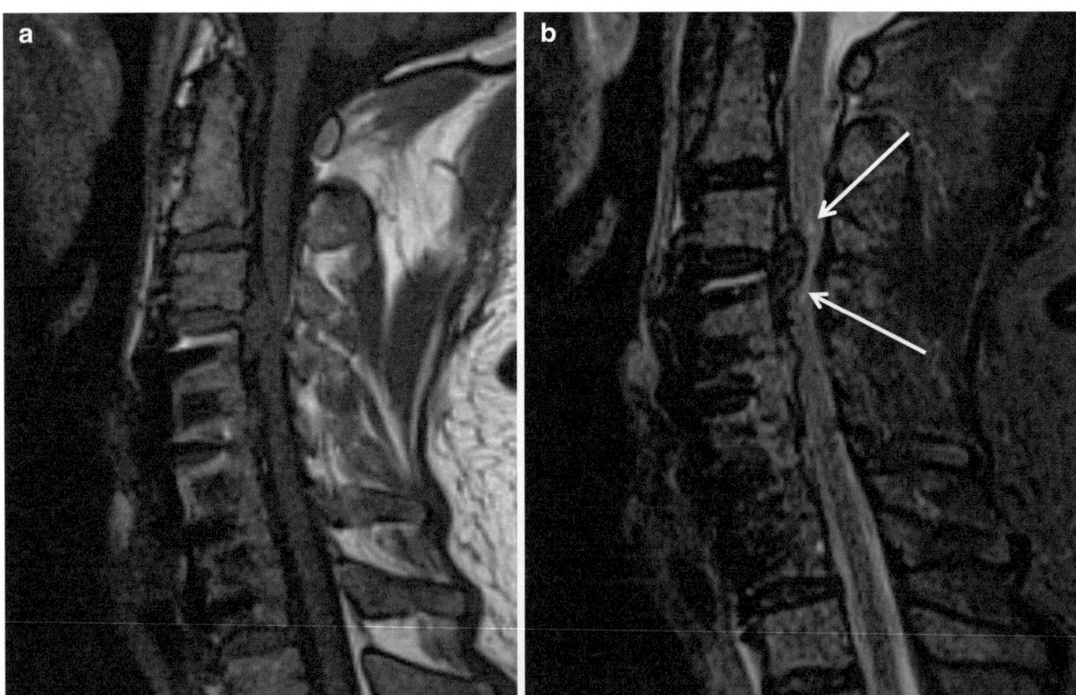

Fig. 45.1 Disk herniation in the cervical spine in a patient with a previous C4–C7 fusion. Sagittal T1WI (**a**) and sagittal STIR (**b**) depict a disk herniation at C3–C4 level causing severe spinal cord compression and abnormal signal of the spinal cord indicating myelopathy (*arrows* in **b**). Notice that in (**a**) the herniated disk is isointense and is in contiguity with the parent disk. This is an example of adjacent level degenerative changes commonly found in previously fused patients

Degenerative Disease

Spondylosis: In spondylosis, spinal canal narrowing can be assessed on lateral radiographs of the cervical spine by measuring the distance from the most posterior aspect of one vertebral body to the closest spinolaminar line. Measurements less than 13 mm are associated with an increased risk for myelopathy, and severe stenosis is defined as a measurement less than 10 mm [5].

Using MRI, the diagnosis of cervical central canal stenosis and grading of its severity can be aided by assessing the degree of CSF obliteration around the spinal cord, spinal cord deformity, and intramedullary T2 high-signal change. In grade 1 central canal stenosis, there is central canal narrowing resulting in more than 50 % obliteration of the subarachnoid space around the spinal cord anteriorly and/or posteriorly without spinal cord deformity. Central canal narrowing with deformity of the spinal cord is defined as grade 2 central canal stenosis, and central canal narrowing with intramedullary T2 high-signal change is defined as grade 3 central canal stenosis [9].

OPLL: This entity is well demonstrated by radiographs or CT as ossification immediately posterior to the vertebral bodies leading to narrowing of the spinal canal. T1WI provides useful information about the degree and extent of spinal cord compression as well as the nature of the ossification. T2WI sequences are most effective to evaluate both spinal cord compression due to the ossification and also document abnormal signal intensity of the spinal cord (Fig. 45.2) [5].

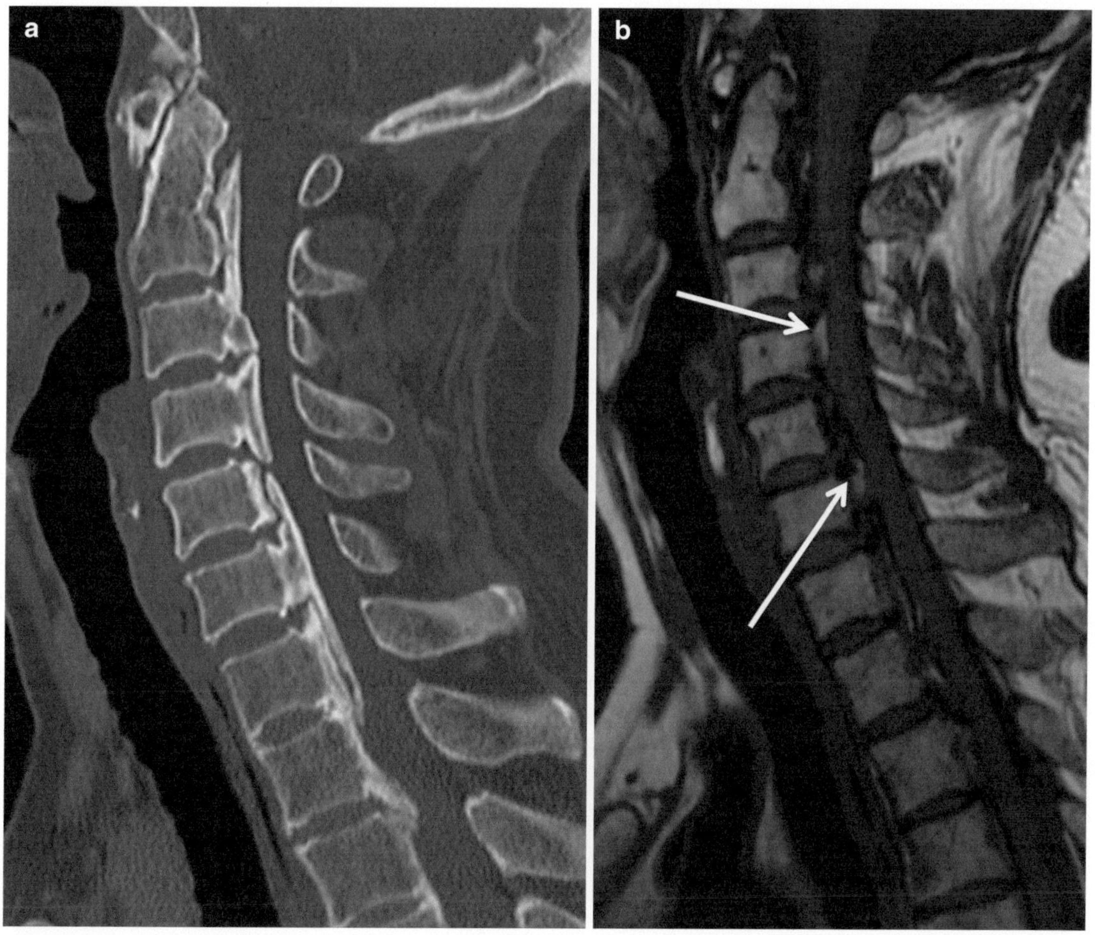

Fig. 45.2 OPLL. (**a**) Sagittal CT shows segmental and contiguous ossification of the posterior longitudinal ligament in the cervical spine. (**b**) Sagittal T1WI depicts high signal (*arrows*) indicating fatty marrow formation. There is a moderate degree of spinal cord compression

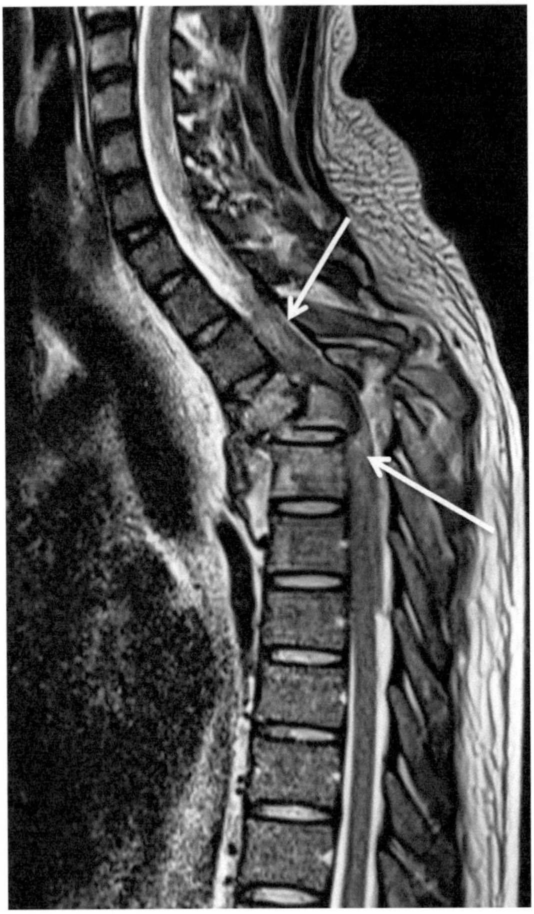

Fig. 45.3 Burst fracture/dislocation causing cord compression. Sagittal T2WI depicts a thoracic vertebral fracture with kyphotic deformity of the spine. There is posterior displacement of the inferior fracture fragment into the spinal canal resulting in severe spinal cord compression. High signal is seen in the spinal cord superiorly and inferiorly to the level of the compression indicating edema (*arrows*) (Case courtesy by Daniel Varón, MD. Cali, Colombia)

Trauma

CT and MRI may show bone fracture fragments, subluxations, extradural or subdural hematomas causing severe canal compromise, and cord compression. MRI is more sensitive than any other imaging technique in identifying cord injuries. MRI may show mild to diffuse cord swelling, focal or diffuse edema, intramedullary hemorrhage, and cord compression. Cord edema is seen as focal or diffuse hyperintensity on T2WI. Intramedullary hemorrhage is seen as foci of low signal intensities within cord edema, on T2WI, and on GRE (Fig. 45.3) [5]. Suspected post-trauma infarctions may be documented with diffusion-weighted imaging (DWI).

Spinal Tumors

Intradural–Extramedullary Tumors

Nerve sheath tumors: Neurofibromas and schwannomas can be difficult to differentiate by imaging and perhaps to do so is not critical. Both tumors may widen the neuroforamina, erode bone, and cause posterior vertebral body scalloping all readily detected on CT [17]. On MRI, most nerve sheath tumors are isointense to the spinal cord on T1WI and hyperintense to it on the T2WI. The most characteristic pattern on the postcontrast and T2WI sequences is the "target sign" which corresponds to the pathologic anatomy of the lesion. The decreased signal centrally represents fibrous Antoni A tissue, while the increased signal in the periphery represents myxomatous Antoni B tissue. This MRI appearance is unique to nerve sheath tumors. *Neurofibromas* typically have a classic "dumbbell shape" (intra- and extradural configuration). They are typically more homogeneous on MRI when compared with schwannomas [11]. MRI shows *schwannomas* as solid tumors in the dorsal root regions with displacement of the spinal cord, conus medullaris, and/or filum terminale. They are isointense on T1WI and hyperintense on T2WI/FLAIR. Contrast enhancement varies from intense homogeneous to faint, and cystic components may be present (Fig. 45.4) [2, 6, 16].

Meningiomas: On CT, they are iso- to hyperattenuating. The hyperattenuation reflects the cellular nature of these lesions, but the presence of calcification also contributes to this appearance. Hyperostosis may be seen but is not as common as in intracranial meningiomas. Meningiomas are commonly isointense on both T1WI and T2WI. Some may be hyperintense on T2WI and flow voids may be seen. If they are densely calcified, they will show low signal on both T1WI and T2WI. Meningiomas prominently enhance on contrast-enhanced imaging and a dural tail may be seen (Fig. 45.5) [2, 6, 16, 17].

Extradural–Extramedullary Tumors

Primary neoplasms: In the assessment of solitary spinal bone tumors, it is necessary to evaluate several characteristics that allow an

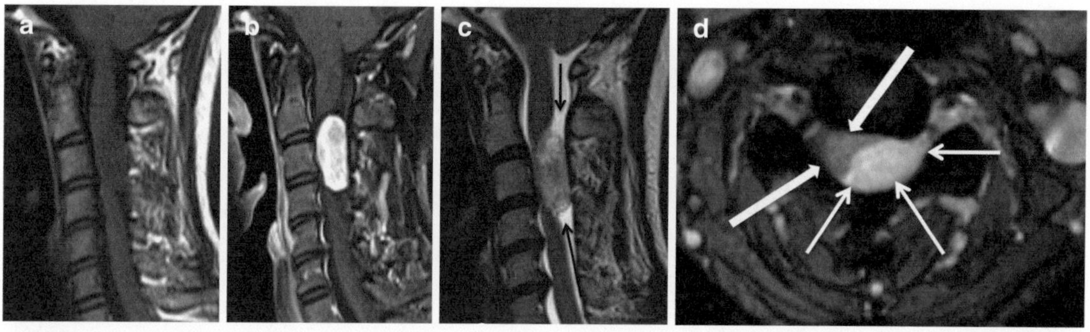

Fig. 45.4 Schwannoma of the cervical spine. (**a**, **b**) Sagittal T1WI pre- and postcontrast show an eccentric intradural–extramedullary tumor with homogeneous and intense enhancement causing compression of the spinal cord. (**c**) Sagittal T2WI shows the tumor to have a central hypointensity and increased signal in the periphery compatible with a "target sign." There is expansion of the subarachnoid space leaving a cap of CSF above and below the lesion (*arrows*) characteristic of intradural–extramedullary lesions. (**d**) Axial T2WI depicts the mass (*thin arrows*) displacing the cord to the opposite side (*arrow*). There is abnormal increased signal intensity in the spinal cord indicating myelopathy

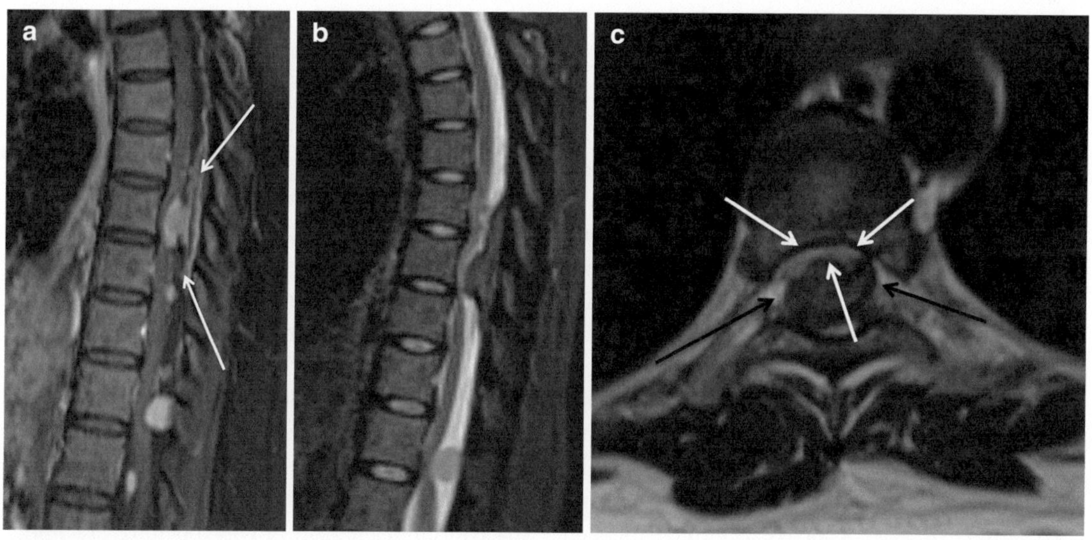

Fig. 45.5 Multiple spinal meningiomas in a patient with NF2. (**a**) Postcontrast sagittal T1WI shows multiple intradural–extramedullary masses causing compression at different levels in the thoracic and upper lumbar spinal cord. All meningiomas show avid contrast enhancement and some of them have a dural tail (*arrows*). (**b**) Sagittal STIR depicts the low signal of the meningiomas and abnormal increased signal in the spinal cord. (**c**) Axial T2WI at T8–T9 level shows the dark lesion (*black arrows*) causing severe displacement and compression of the spinal cord (*white arrows*). Multiple schwannomas are also present

accurate diagnosis (location, type of matrix, margins, limits, and extension). The matrix of osteoblastic tumors most often appears amorphous or cloudlike on radiographs and CT because it is less dense than normal bone and lacks its organized trabecular pattern. The amount and degree of matrix mineralization is widely variable; thus, the radiographic appearance of osteoblastic tumors may range from densely blastic to nearly completely lytic. Dense osteoblastic lesions display low T1WI–T2WI intensities on MRI. Cartilage-forming tumors typically exhibit punctate comma-like or annular calcifications on radiographs and CT. These calcifications appear as low signal intensity foci in all MRI sequences.

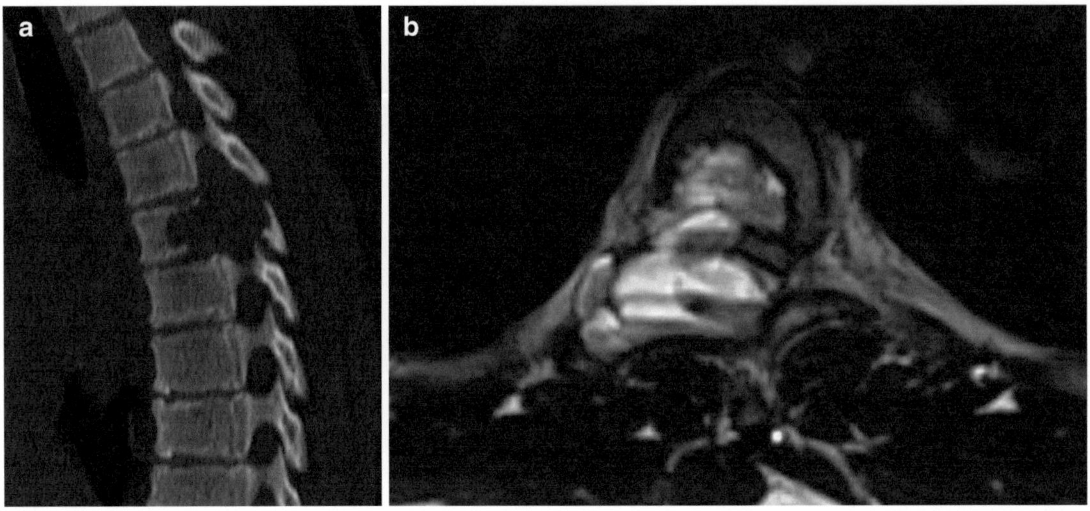

Fig. 45.6 Aneurysmal bone cyst. (**a**) Sagittal CT shows a lytic lesion in the vertebral body and posterior elements of at least two levels of the thoracic spine. (**b**) Axial T2WI depicts the lesion to have the classic appearance of fluid–fluid levels characteristic of ABC. The lesion invades the spinal canal and the spinal cord is compressed

Benign tumors usually exhibit geographic bone destruction and sclerotic margins without soft tissue extension. Conversely, malignant tumors usually exhibit poorly defined margins, permeative bone destruction, and a soft tissue mass. Fluid–fluid levels help to make the diagnosis of intratumoral hemorrhage. The imaging finding of prominent fluid-filled hemorrhagic spaces in a vertebral lesion is suggestive of aneurysmal bone cyst (ABC) (Table 45.2) (Fig. 45.6) [12].

Metastases: On radiography, around 50 % of the bone has to be destroyed before lesions become visible. Radiographs show only bony changes and cannot determine the type of soft tissue impingement on the thecal sac or spinal cord [22]. CT shows bone destruction and can demonstrate spinal canal invasion but lacks sensitivity in evaluating the spinal cord. On MRI, bony metastases are seen as hypointense foci within normal high-signal fatty marrow on T1WI. Patterns of osseous neoplastic involvement tend to be similar for STIR and T2WI, and the appearance is variable but lesions are more often hyperintense. Contrast enhancement provides additional information for cases of dural or pial involvement [23]. Lesser amounts of tumor extension into the epidural space may not be evident without contrast administration. The invasion of the spinal canal and the integrity of the spinal cord are better depicted in T2WI and STIR where the acute myelopathy changes will appear hyperintense (Fig. 45.7).

Arachnoid Cystic Lesions

Intradural arachnoid cysts can be difficult to identify because focal displacement and compression may be the only findings at MRI and conventional CT or CT myelography. An imaging finding of diminished or increased CSF flow artifact in a widened dorsal subarachnoid space may suggest an intradural–extramedullary cystic space-occupying lesion. Depending on the type and location and whether they communicate with the subarachnoid space through a narrow or wide opening, arachnoid cysts will fill with intrathecal contrast material during CT myelography. MRI allows characterization of the cyst's nature and extent and associated abnormalities such as a syrinx. Types I (extradural) and II arachnoid cysts typically are iso- to hyperintense to CSF on T1WI and T2WI, but variability in signal intensity may result from the pulsatility of the CSF and/or higher protein contents in the cyst. Type II arachnoid cysts contain neural elements such as nerve roots. Type III cysts have signal intensity similar to those of type I and II cysts but are intradural. Mass effect may be seen with a possible spinal cord signal intensity abnormality if the cyst is sufficiently large. Arachnoid cysts are

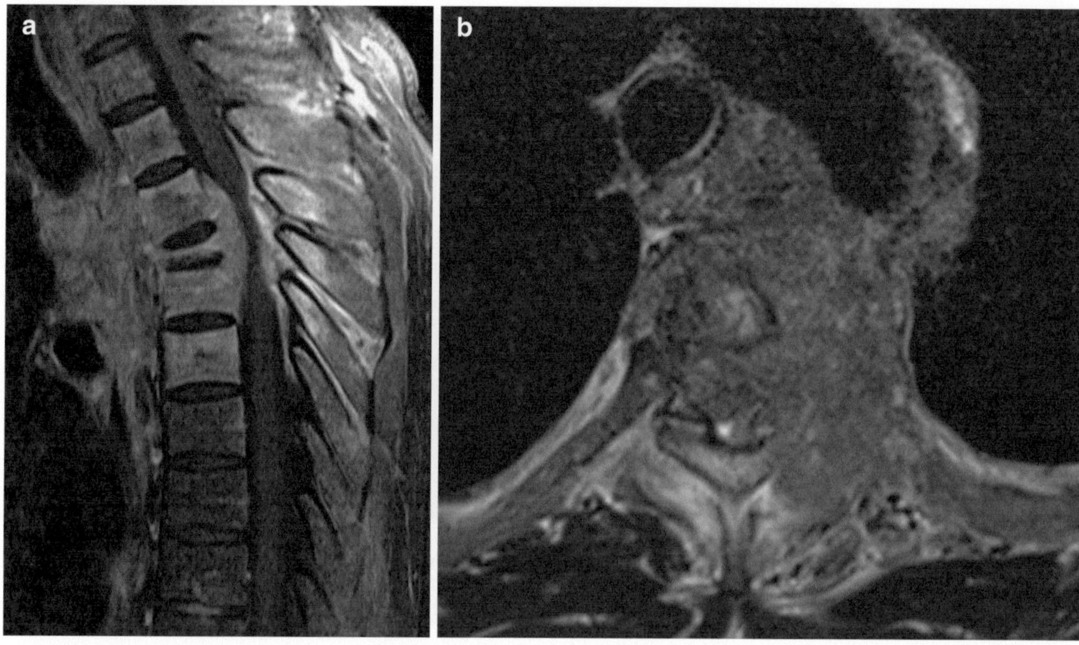

Fig. 45.7 Vertebral metastases from lung carcinoma. (**a**) Sagittal postcontrast TIWI with fat suppression shows soft tissue mass with intense enhancement involving several thoracic vertebral bodies and extending to the prevertebral and epidural spaces anteriorly and posteriorly, respectively, causing spinal cord compression. (**b**) Axial non contrast T1WI demonstrates extensive involvement with invasion of the spinal canal and compromise of the posterior elements of the vertebral bodies, ribs, and paraspinal soft tissues

non-enhancing and do not demonstrate restricted diffusion at DWI (Fig. 45.8) [7, 20, 24].

Imaging Follow-Up

MRI is the modality of choice for evaluating the integrity of the spinal cord regardless of the underlying disease causing cord compression. There is no evidence of the optimal time for follow-up in patients treated conservatively. Worsening of symptomatology is an indication for emergency spinal MRI. Most patients treated surgically receive a short-term MRI examination after their treatment and sooner if complications are suspected.

Main Differential Diagnosis

Idiopathic spinal cord herniation: This is a relatively uncommon disease in which the spinal cord is displaced through a defect in the anterior or lateral dura mater and may be confused with a cyst displacing the cord. The exact cause of spinal cord herniation is unknown but occult or repetitive trauma is a possible cause. Findings on MRI and CT myelography demonstrate obliteration of the CSF space ventral to the cord and a widened dorsal CSF space with no solid or cystic masses posterior to the cord. On MRI, continuous normal CSF pulsation artifact in the widened CSF space is an important diagnostic finding that implies unimpeded flow of CSF and argues against an obstructing lesion such as a cyst. At CT myelography, free flow of contrast material immediately after intrathecal contrast agent injection supports the diagnosis of spinal cord herniation but cannot completely exclude a space-occupying lesion such as a wide-neck communicating arachnoid cyst because such space-occupying lesions can show immediate contrast agent filling (Fig. 45.9) [24].

Hirayama disease: Also known as nonprogressive juvenile spinal muscular atrophy, it is characterized by the insidious onset of unilateral

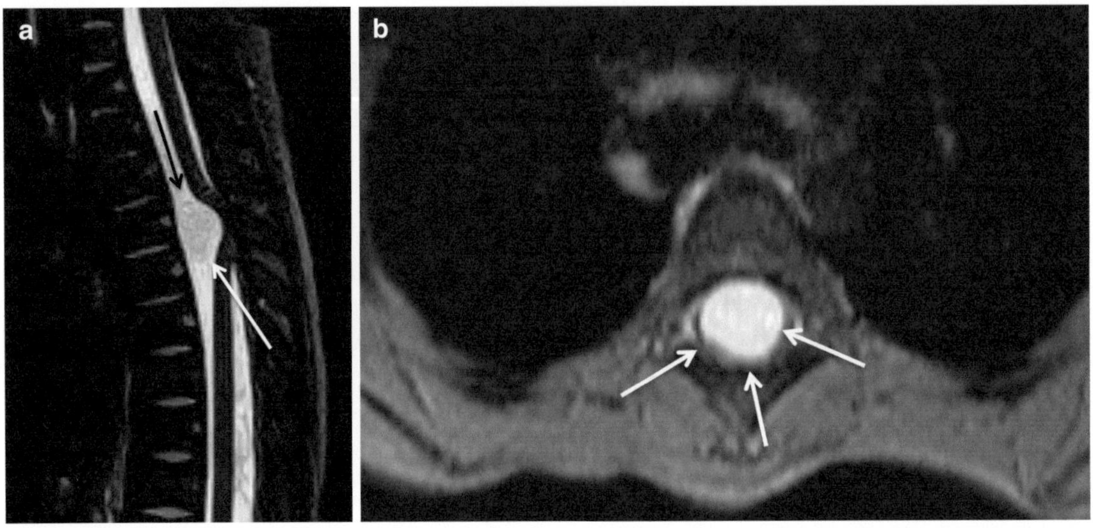

Fig. 45.8 Intradural arachnoid cyst (type III – Nabors classification) in the thoracic spine. (**a**) Sagittal STIR shows an intradural rounded cyst displacing the spinal cord posteriorly with slightly lower signal intensity compared to CSF (*arrows*). (**b**) On an axial T2WI, the cyst is isointense with CSF, and absence of fluid voids in the subarachnoid space suggests a true lesion with mass effect. The spinal cord (*arrows*) is compressed posteriorly and shows high-signal intensity indicating myelopathy

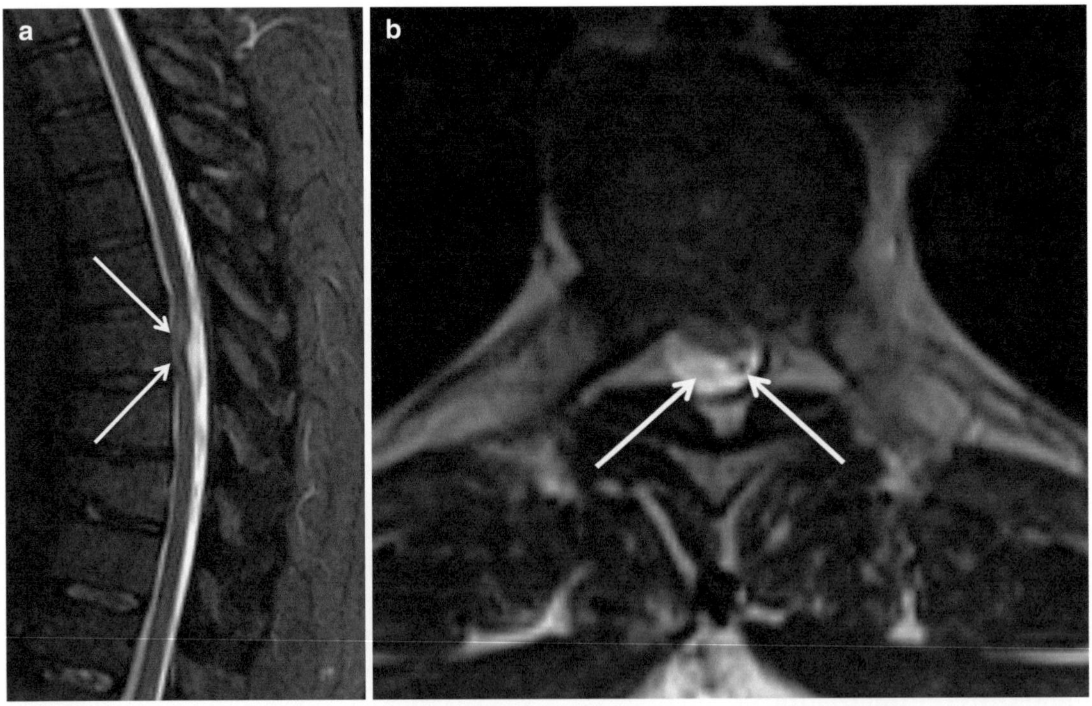

Fig. 45.9 Spinal cord herniation. (**a**) Sagittal STIR image shows ventral displacement and posterior indentation of the thoracic cord with widening of the dorsal subarachnoid space. There is an abnormal hyperintensity of the spinal cord due to myelopathy (*arrows*). (**b**) Axial T2WI depicts CSF pulsation artifacts in the widened CSF space (*arrows*) that rule out occupying space lesion

or asymmetric oblique amyotrophy originating from the cervical spine. It occurs most frequently in young men. MRI of the spine reveals localized cord atrophy (C5–C7) and a kyphotic cervical curvature, abnormal cord flattening with a pear-shaped cord on axial images, and loss of attachment of the posterior dural sac and subjacent lamina on neutral position imaging. Images in flexion show anterior displacement of the dorsal dura and a crescent-shaped epidural mass isointense to the cord on T1WI and hyperintense on T2WI with strong homogeneous enhancement, that should not be misdiagnosed as an epidural neoplasia [25].

Spinal arachnoid webs: Arachnoid webs are intradural–extramedullary bands of arachnoid tissue that can extend to the pial surface of the spinal cord causing a focal dorsal indentation of the cord. These webs tend to occur in the upper thoracic spine and may produce a characteristic deformity of the cord called the "scalpel sign" because of the resemblance on sagittal MRI and CT myelographic images to a scalpel with its blade pointing posteriorly. Spinal webs are associated with syringomyelia above or below the level of cord indentation. This entity should be differentiated from intradural arachnoid cysts [26].

Tips

- MRI is the study of choice in spinal cord compression regardless the etiology, and T2WI and STIR are the most sensitive sequences to evaluate the integrity of the spinal cord. Whenever possible, fat-suppressed postcontrast T1WI are also very helpful.
- In the cervical spine, it is important to differentiate cord compression secondary to disk herniation from degenerative disease; therefore, the CT and MRI are complementary.
- Nerve sheath tumors are the most common intradural–extramedullary neoplastic lesions. The "target sign" is an imaging feature of both neurofibromas and schwannomas and useful to diagnose them on MRI.
- An intradural arachnoid cyst should be differentiated from a spinal cord herniation, arachnoid web, and focal spinal cord atrophy. The absence of CSF pulsation artifacts sometimes is the only sign that can be used to suggest the diagnosis of an arachnoid cyst.

References

1. Dugas AF, Lucas JM, Edlow JA. Diagnosis of spinal cord compression in nontrauma patients in the emergency department. Acad Emerg Med: Off J Soc Acad Emerg Med. 2011;18(7):719–25.
2. Chamberlain MC, Tredway TL. Adult primary intradural spinal cord tumors: a review. Curr Neurol Neurosci Rep. 2011;11(3):320–8.
3. Wong JJ, Cote P, Quesnele JJ, Stern PJ, Mior SA. The course and prognostic factors of symptomatic cervical disc herniation with radiculopathy: a systematic review of the literature. Spine J: Off J N Am Spine Soc. 2014;14(8):1781–9.
4. Suthar P, Patel R, Mehta C, Patel N. MRI evaluation of lumbar disc degenerative disease. J Clin Diagn Res: JCDR. 2015;9(4):TC04–9.
5. Grayev AM, Kissane J, Kanekar S. Imaging approach to the cord T2 hyperintensity (myelopathy). Radiol Clin N Am. 2014;52(2):427–46.
6. Abul-Kasim K, Thurnher MM, McKeever P, Sundgren PC. Intradural spinal tumors: current classification and MRI features. Neuroradiology. 2008; 50(4):301–14.
7. Khosla A, Wippold 2nd FJ. CT myelography and MR imaging of extramedullary cysts of the spinal canal in adult and pediatric patients. AJR Am J Roentgenol. 2002;178(1):201–7.
8. Radhakrishnan K, Litchy WJ, O'Fallon WM, Kurland LT. Epidemiology of cervical radiculopathy. A population-based study from Rochester, Minnesota, 1976 through 1990. Brain: J Neurol. 1994; 117(Pt 2):325–35.
9. Kang HS, Kwon JW, Lee JW, SpringerLink (Online service). Radiology illustrated: spine. Berlin/Heidelberg: Springer Berlin Heidelberg: Imprint: Springer; 2014. Available from: http://VB3LK7EB4T.search.serialssolutions.com/?V=1.0&L=VB3LK7EB4T&S=JCs&C=TC0001187485&T=marc.

10. Sekhon LH, Fehlings MG. Epidemiology, demographics, and pathophysiology of acute spinal cord injury. Spine. 2001;26(24 Suppl):S2–12.
11. Beall DP, Googe DJ, Emery RL, Thompson DB, Campbell SE, Ly JQ, et al. Extramedullary intradural spinal tumors: a pictorial review. Curr Probl Diagn Radiol. 2007;36(5):185–98.
12. Rodallec MH, Feydy A, Larousserie F, Anract P, Campagna R, Babinet A, et al. Diagnostic imaging of solitary tumors of the spine: what to do and say. Radiograph: Rev Publ Radiol Soc N Am Inc. 2008;28(4):1019–41.
13. Fardon DF, Williams AL, Dohring EJ, Murtagh FR, Gabriel Rothman SL, Sze GK. Lumbar disc nomenclature: version 2.0: recommendations of the combined task forces of the North American Spine Society, the American Society of Spine Radiology and the American Society of Neuroradiology. Spine J: Off J N Am Spine Soc. 2014;14(11):2525–45.
14. Allam GJ, Baker RA, Jones HR, Netter FH, Srinivasan J. Netter's neurology. Philadelphia: Elsevier Saunders; 2012. Available from: http://VB3LK7EB4T.search.serialssolutions.com/?V=1.0&L=VB3LK7EB4T&S=JCs&C=TC0000578855&T=marc.
15. Rowland LP, Pedley TA, Merritt HH. Merritt's neurology. Philadelphia: Lippincott Williams & Wilkins; 2010. Available from: http://libproxy.lib.unc.edu/login?url=http://ovidsp.ovid.com/ovidweb.cgi?T=JS&NEWS=N&PAGE=booktext&D=books&SC=01412541.
16. Traul DE, Shaffrey ME, Schiff D. Part I: spinal-cord neoplasms-intradural neoplasms. Lancet Oncol. 2007; 8(1):35–45.
17. Soderlund KA, Smith AB, Rushing EJ, Smirniotopolous JG. Radiologic-pathologic correlation of pediatric and adolescent spinal neoplasms: part 2, intradural extramedullary spinal neoplasms. AJR Am J Roentgenol. 2012;198(1):44–51.
18. Sansur CA, Pouratian N, Dumont AS, Schiff D, Shaffrey CI, Shaffrey ME. Part II: spinal-cord neoplasms – primary tumours of the bony spine and adjacent soft tissues. Lancet Oncol. 2007;8(2):137–47.
19. Prasad D, Schiff D. Malignant spinal-cord compression. Lancet Oncol. 2005;6(1):15–24.
20. Samir E, Noujaim KLM, Daniel L. Noujaim. Cystic lesions in spinal imaging: a pictorial review and classification. Neurographics. 2013;3:14–27.
21. Nabors MW, Pait TG, Byrd EB, Karim NO, Davis DO, Kobrine AI, et al. Updated assessment and current classification of spinal meningeal cysts. J Neurosurg. 1988;68(3):366–77.
22. Schiff D. Spinal cord compression. Neurol Clin. 2003;21(1):67–86. viii.
23. Johnson AJ, Ying J, El Gammal T, Timmerman RD, Kim RY, Littenberg B. Which MR imaging sequences are necessary in determining the need for radiation therapy for cord compression? A prospective study. AJNR Am J Neuroradiol. 2007;28(1):32–7.
24. Haber MD, Nguyen DD, Li S. Differentiation of idiopathic spinal cord herniation from CSF-isointense intraspinal extramedullary lesions displacing the cord. Radiograph: Rev Publ Radiol Soc N Am Inc. 2014;34(2):313–29.
25. Raval M, Kumari R, Dung AA, Guglani B, Gupta N, Gupta R. MRI findings in Hirayama disease. Indian J Radiol Imaging. 2010;20(4):245–9.
26. Reardon MA, Raghavan P, Carpenter-Bailey K, Mukherjee S, Smith JS, Matsumoto JA, et al. Dorsal thoracic arachnoid web and the "scalpel sign": a distinct clinical-radiologic entity. AJNR Am J Neuroradiol. 2013;34(5):1104–10.

Spinal Hemorrhage in Adults: Extramedullary, Extradural, and Intramedullary

46

Lázaro Luís Faria do Amaral,
Anderson Benine Belezia,
and Samuel Brighenti Bergamaschi

Abstract

Intraspinal hemorrhage is a rare and severe condition with possible devastating consequences. It is defined by the presence of blood in any of the following compartments of the spine: intramedullary; intradural extramedullary, which includes subarachnoid and subdural spinal hemorrhages; and extradural or epidural bleeds. Each compartment has unique predisposing factors leading to the hemorrhage, mechanisms of hemorrhage, and preferred locations. Epidural spinal hemorrhages are the most common type (75 %) followed by subarachnoid (about 16 %) and subdural spinal hemorrhages (4 %). Intramedullary hematoma or hematomyelia is very rare and is usually related to trauma or presence of intramedullary tumors or vascular malformations. Hematomas involving more than one spinal compartment can occur. Magnetic resonance imaging is the modality of choice for spinal hemorrhages and is able to evaluate the location, extent, and age of the hemorrhage as well as identify the possible cause of bleeding.

Background

Intraspinal hemorrhage is a rare and severe condition with possible devastating consequences. It is defined by the presence of blood in any of the following compartments of the spine: intramedullary (also known as hematomyelia), intradural extramedullary including subarachnoid and subdural hemorrhages, and extradural or epidural ones. Each compartment has its unique predisposing factors, mechanisms of hemorrhage, and common locations [1].

Three mechanisms for the development of epidural spinal hematomas (ESHs) have been

L.L.F. do Amaral, MD (✉)
Division of Neuroradiology, Medimagem – Hospital Beneficência Portuguesa de São Paulo, Sao Paulo, SP, Brazil

Division of Neuroradiology, Hospital Santa Casa de Misericórdia de São Paulo, Rua Dr. Cesário Motta Junior 112, Vila Buarque, Sao Paulo, SP 01221-020, Brazil
e-mail: lazden@terra.com.br

A.B. Belezia, MD • S.B. Bergamaschi, MD
Radiology Department, Medimagem – Hospital Beneficência Portuguesa de São Paulo, Sao Paulo, SP, Brazil
e-mail: abelezia@gmail.com; samuel.brighentibergamaschi@gmail.com

R. Hoffmann Nunes et al. (eds.), *Critical Findings in Neuroradiology*,
DOI 10.1007/978-3-319-27987-9_46

proposed and include rupture of epidural veins (most accepted explanation), rupture of epidural arteries, and hemorrhage from vascular abnormalities. Similarly, subdural spinal hematomas (SDHs) may originate during sudden intra-abdominal or intrathoracic increases in pressure leading to rupture of veins. The hemorrhage occurs first into the cerebrospinal fluid (CSF) with secondary extension into the subdural space. Subarachnoid spinal hemorrhage (SAH) is thought to originate by injury to radicular blood vessels [2].

ESHs are the most common type of bleed (75 %), followed by SAH (about 16 %), and lastly SDH (4 %). Intramedullary hematoma or hematomyelia is very rare and usually related to trauma, intramedullary tumors, or vascular malformations. Hematomas involving more than one spine compartment can also be observed [2, 3].

Most of ESH are spontaneous, but other causes include trauma, disk herniations, tumors, vascular malformations including arteriovenous malformations (AVMs) and arteriovenous fistulas (AVFs), and coagulopathies. The first peak age is between the ages of 20 and 45 years of age and the second peak is between 50 and 80 years. These hematomas are usually located dorsal in the spinal canal because the epidural space is broader dorsally than ventrally. Most idiopathic ESHs are thought to occur in the cervicothoracic and thoracolumbar regions explained by the fact that weak points of the epidural venous plexus are located there [2].

SDH may be related to intracranial or spine surgery, lumbar puncture, coagulopathies, tumors, and also vascular malformations. They do not show a predilection for any particular age. Signs and symptoms are similar to those of ESH and are nonspecific making the clinical diagnosis challenging. They can be acute (more common), subacute, or chronic. Usually, the first symptom is back pain, followed by extremity weakness, sensory loss, and autonomic dysfunction with bowel and bladder incontinence depending on the size and location of the hematoma [2, 4].

Spinal SAH accounts for less than 1 % of all subarachnoid hemorrhages [5] usually affecting young patients; however, instances occurring in patients between 55 and 70 years old have been reported. Initially, the bleeding happens into the subarachnoid space which causes severe local pain and is followed by radiating pain and signs of meningeal irritation (spinal rigidity ranging up to opisthotonos). If the hemorrhage extends into the cerebral subarachnoid space, then headache, vomiting, optic disk edema, impaired consciousness, and seizures may ensue. If the hemorrhage affects the cervical region, cerebral symptoms develop quickly and make it difficult to reach a correct diagnosis [2]. The most common associated causes are tumors within the spinal canal and coagulopathies including use of anticoagulants, arteriovenous malformations (AVFs and AVMs), spinal artery aneurysms, lumbar puncture, and trauma [2, 6].

The most frequent locations of hematomyelia in adults are the low cervical and thoracolumbar cord which are different from children where the C5–T1 levels are the most frequent location. Spinal vascular malformations are the most common cause of nontraumatic hematomyelia, and it usually presents more acutely than epidural hematomas and with less pain. Paralysis commonly occurs at the same time as pain [1, 2].

Key Points

Etiology

Trauma: Traumatic spinal hemorrhage is usually associated with fractures of the spine due to high-energy trauma and can involve any compartment of the spine but is more commonly seen as epidural hemorrhage. Traumatic ESH is more frequent in patients with underlying diseases like ankylosing spondylitis. Traumatic hematomyelia usually affects in the central gray matter of the cord at the point of maximal mechanical impact following the trauma [2, 7].

Iatrogenic: Several procedures may result in spinal hemorrhages. Myelography [8], lumbar puncture for anesthesia, and spinal surgery are the most common ones. Iatrogenic etiologies result in epidural, subdural, or subarachnoid hemorrhages and only in rare cases in hematomyelia [2].

Spontaneous: When it is not possible to define a causative factor, a spinal hemorrhage is classified as spontaneous. Hemorrhages for which there is no identifiable triggering factor (idiopathic hematomas) are the most common of spinal hematomas. They can involve any compartment and account for the majority of ESH [3, 6, 9–11]. If spontaneous hematomas (i.e., hematomas associated with trivial trauma, coughing, defecation, or activities of daily living such as lifting or sexual intercourse) are included in this group, it account for 38.2 % of cases [2].

Vascular Lesions

Cavernomas of the spinal cord are rare lesions representing about 5 % of all intramedullary lesions. Females are affected more than men. More than one-half of spinal cavernomas are found in the thoracic region. Cavernomas usually present with repetitive microhemorrhages that can be associated with episodes of clinical deterioration. AVFs are the most common spinal vascular malformations. They are acquired lesions that usually result in a chronic congestive myelopathy. Hemorrhages as consequence of AVFs are rare and result in SAH. Hematomyelia is extremely rare with just few reported cases [12]. AVMs constitute about 20 % of all vascular malformations of the spine. Thoracic lesions usually present with subarachnoid or intramedullary hemorrhages. Spinal artery aneurysms associated with arteriovenous malformations are more numerous than isolated spinal artery aneurysms and usually present with SAH [13, 14].

Tumors: Tumor hemorrhages are the most common cause of SAH and are associated with ependymomas, Schwann cell tumors (neurofibroma, schwannoma), hemangioblastomas, glial tumors (astrocytoma and glioblastoma), and meningioma [2]. Ependymomas are the most common intramedullary tumor in adults and can be found anywhere along the spinal cord but most commonly in the cervical spine and almost one-third of them are associated with hemorrhage. The second most common tumor is the astrocytoma, and unlike ependymomas, hemorrhage is very uncommon with them. Hemangioblastomas causing spinal hemorrhage are rare and usually lead to SAH. About 25 % of them are associated with the Von Hippel–Lindau syndrome [15, 16].

Other causes: There are few reports of intracranial subarachnoid hemorrhage and intracranial subdural hematoma migrating to the spine [17]. Coagulopathies such as hemophilia and medications that interfere with coagulation, as clopidogrel [18] and warfarin [19] are considered to be the second most common causes of spinal hemorrhages [2]. Radiotherapy of the spine is another extremely rare condition that may result in hematomyelia [1]. There is at least one case reported of vasculitis resulting in spinal subdural hemorrhage [20] and some reports of endometriosis of the conus medullaris resulting in hematomyelia [21, 22].

Best Imaging Modality

Myelography is contraindicated in patients with coagulopathies, and it does not play any role identifying spinal hematomas [2].

Magnetic resonance imaging (MRI) is the modality of choice in spinal hemorrhages being able to evaluate the location, extent, and age of the hemorrhage, as well as the possible cause of bleeding. As in the brain, signal from the blood varies over time helping define the age of the hematoma. The protocol usually includes axial and/or sagittal T1- and T2-weighted imaging (T2WI) spin-echo sequences as well as axial gradient-echo T2*. Gadolinium administration is also recommended. When a spinal hemorrhage is detected, it is also important to extend the study to the craniocaudal region to determine the extent of the lesion [4]. Susceptibility-weighted imaging (SWI) sequence is very sensitive for blood products and is considered very useful in detecting small hemorrhages also in the spine but are difficult to obtain in most clinical MRI units [23].

Computed tomography (CT) may be helpful in the acute scenario especially in trauma patients. Non-collaborative patients may benefit from CT, but it is to be remembered that the ability of CT to detect hematomas decreases with time as they become isodense [1].

Digital angiography can be performed when there is high suspicion for vascular malformations, traumatic pseudoaneurysms, or aneurysms [2, 4].

Major Findings

A spinal fluid collection in the epidural, subdural, or intramedullary space may be hemorrhagic in origin if shows T1 hyperintensity. In the hyperacute stage, a hematoma is isointense on T1WI and mildly hyperintense on T2WI relatively to the spinal cord. Acute hematomas are characterized by hypointense signal on T1WI and marked hypointensity on T2WI. From 3 to 5 days and after the formation of methemoglobin, the hematoma progressively becomes hyperintense on T1WI (Fig. 46.1) until chronic phase when it becomes hypointense in both T1WI and T2WI due to presence of hemosiderin and ferritin. On gradient-echo T2* and SWI acute spinal blood collections commonly display low signal intensity due to presence of deoxyhemoglobin. On CT, spinal hemorrhagic collections are usually hyperdense lesions of blood-equivalent density, and after 1 week they become inhomogeneous and of variable densities [4, 23].

On CT, an ESH appears as a sharply demarcated, biconvex-shaped mass that closely approximates the bony confines of the spinal canal and displaces and compresses the less dense-appearing thecal sac and the spinal cord. On MRI, their appearance is similar as they present most commonly in a dorsolateral location (Fig. 46.2) and have a typical well-demarcated biconvex shape with superiorly and inferiorly tapering margins usually extending for two to three vertebral bodies [4, 18].

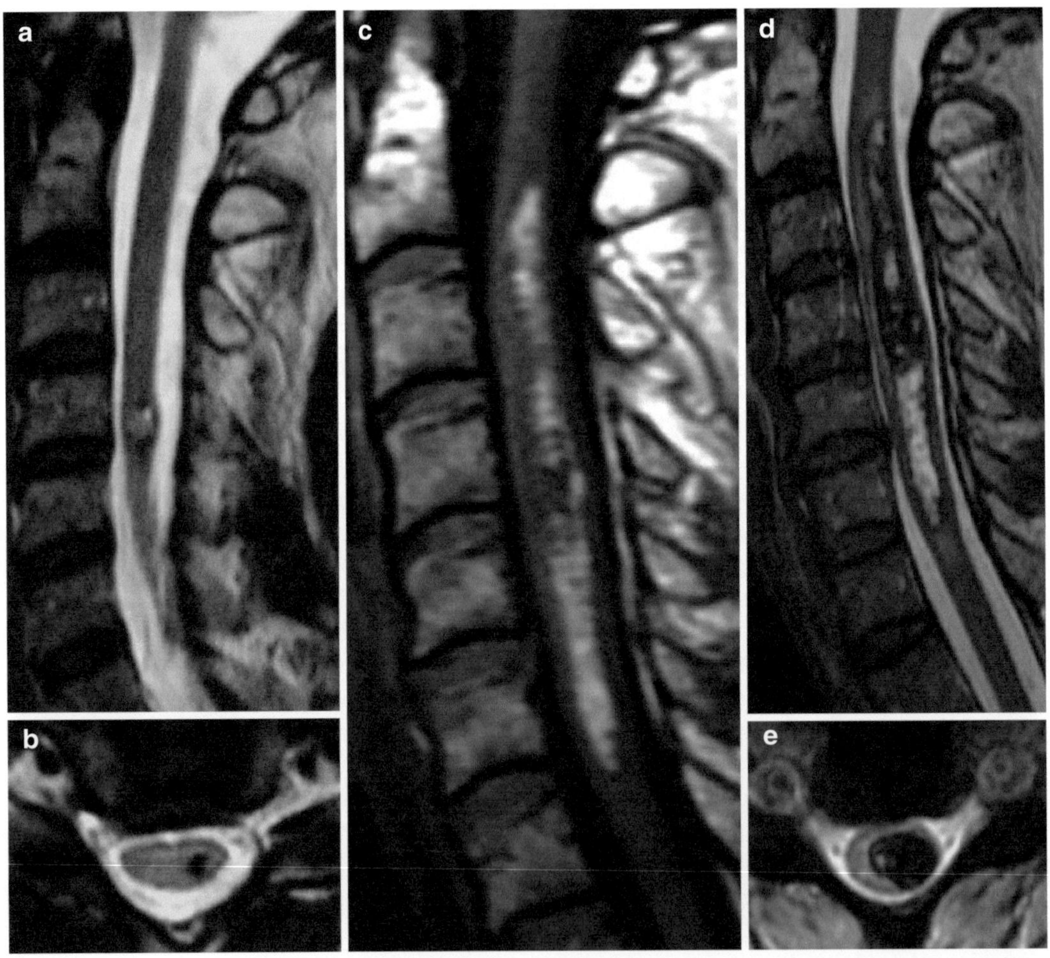

Fig. 46.1 Spinal cord cavernoma and subacute hematomyelia. A 50-year-old male with diagnosis of a spinal cord cavernous malformation. Sagittal (**a**) and axial T2* (**b**) show a round hypointensity in the left cervical cord. After a rapid onset of upper and lower limb paresthesia and paresis, another MRI scan was obtained. Sagittal T1WI (**c**) and T2WI (**d**) show an extensive heterogeneous hyperintense material within the cervical cord compatible with subacute hematomyelia. Sagittal T2WI (**d**) and axial T2* (**e**) demonstrate a marked hypointense nodular area within the lesion corresponding to the cavernoma

Neuroradiological diagnosis of SDH is extremely difficult, and many cases are diagnosed on the basis of surgical or autopsy findings. SDH usually presents as more extensive lesions than ESH extending for over six to seven vertebral bodies and displaying a typical crescent shape on CT and MR axial images. As opposed to acute epidural hematomas which are intermingled with epidural fat, subdural hematomas are located within the thecal sac, separate from the adjacent extradural fat and separate from the adjacent osseous structures (Fig. 46.3). In the distal lumbar subdural space, a subdural hematoma gives rise to the "inverted Mercedes–Benz sign" (Fig. 46.2). The blood signal time change in SDH is usually similar to ESH [4, 19, 20].

SAHs are usually diffuse and on the acute or subacute stages and are seen as non-localized areas of increased stages and or low signal on T2WI surrounding the spinal cord (Fig. 46.4). In later

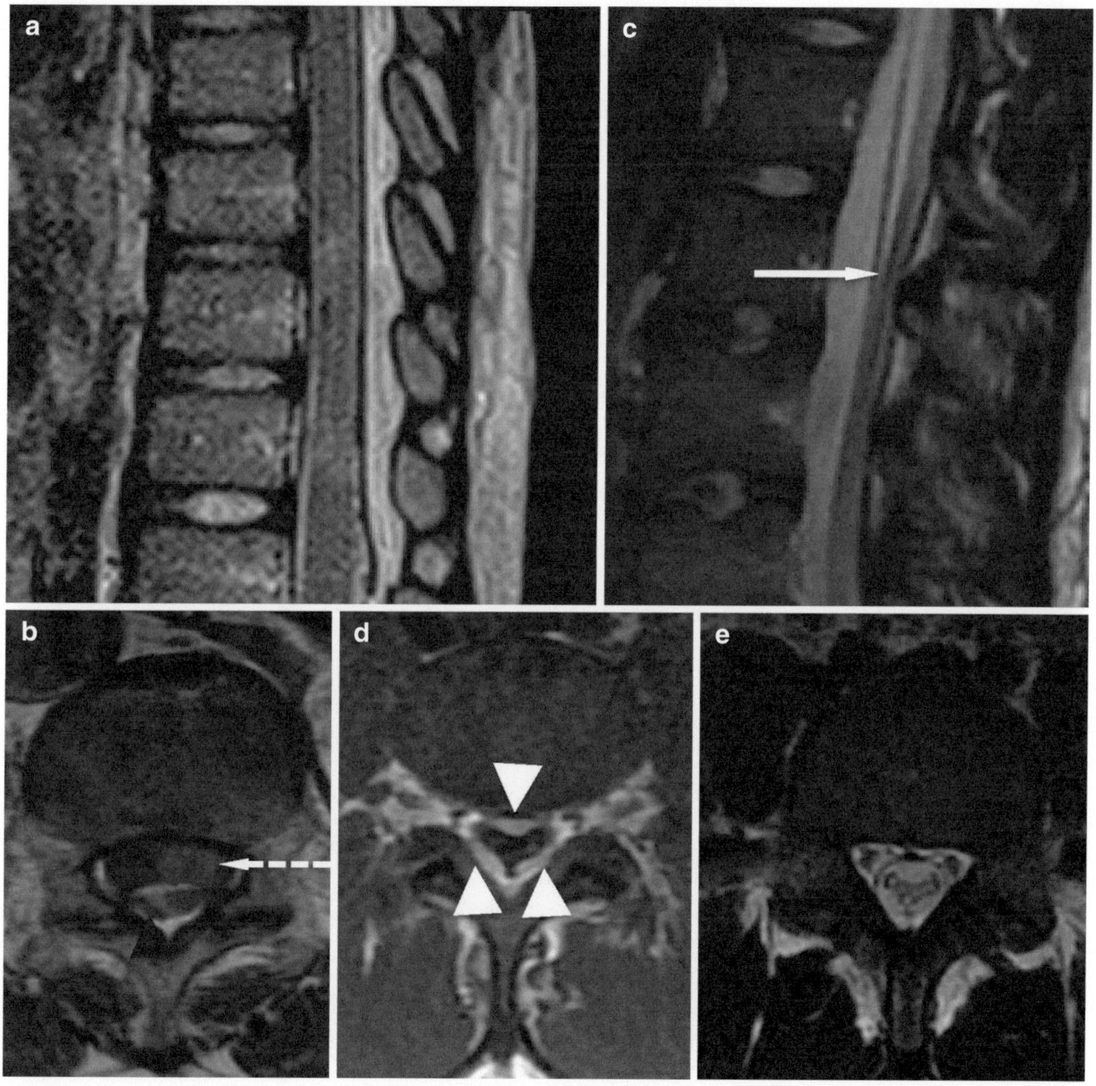

Fig. 46.2 Spinal epidural hematoma and subdural hematoma. A 21-year-old male presents with back pain and subacute lower limb numbness and weakness. (**a**, **b**) Sagittal (**a**) and axial T1WI (**b**) display a large mass located dorsolaterally within the epidural space (*black arrowhead*) displacing the spinal cord contralaterally (*dashed arrow*). A 28-year-old man suffering from sudden onset back pain and sensorimotor paralysis. (**c–e**) Sagittal (**c**) and axial T1WI (**d**) and T2WI (**e**) show a subdural collection which is hyperintense on T1WI and T2WI, compatible with subacute subdural hematoma. (**c**, **e**) Anterior and posterior to the nerve roots have a clumped appearance ("cap sign") (*arrow*). The "Mercedes–Benz" sign is well seen (*white arrowheads*)

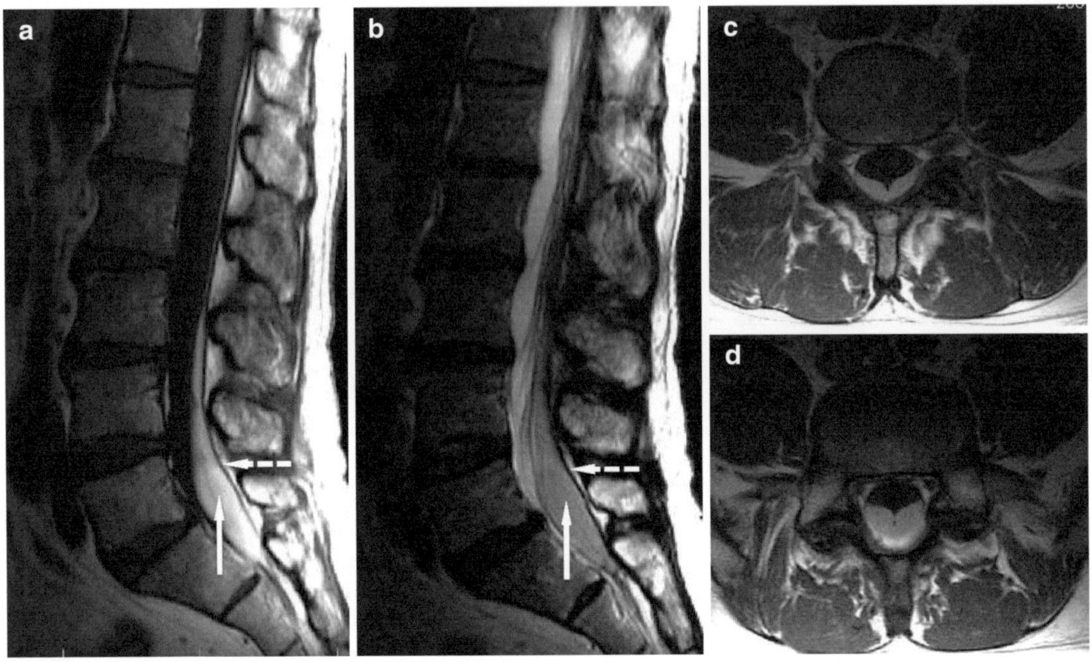

Fig. 46.3 Spinal subdural hematoma. A 56-year-old woman with acute-onset back pain while working in a construction yard. Sagittal T1WI (**a**) shows a large hyperintense posterior collection in the dural sac which is hypointense on a T2WI (**b**). Notice that a *black line* (dura) separates the subdural hematoma (*solid arrows*) from the posterior epidural fat (*dashed arrows*). (**c**, **d**) Axial T1WI at different levels reveals a V-shaped hematoma posterior to the dural sac

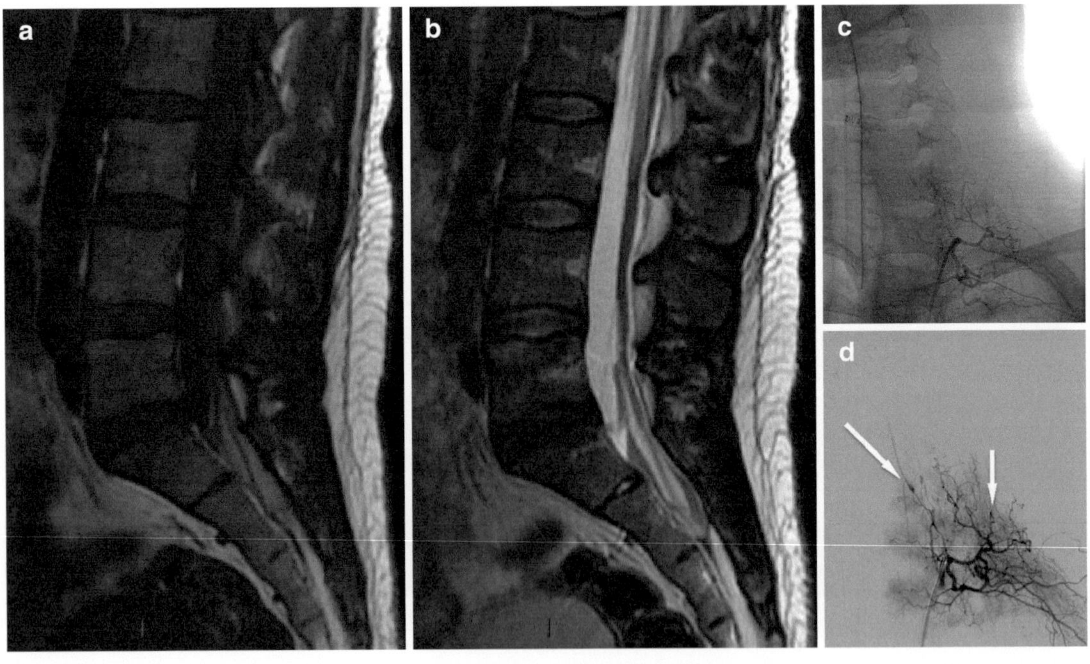

Fig. 46.4 Spinal subarachnoid hemorrhage. A 36-year-old man victim of a motor vehicle collision presenting with back pain. Sagittal T1WI (**a**) and sagittal T2WI (**b**) show a hyperintense collection in the posterior and inferior aspect of the dural sac surrounding the cauda equina which is relatively hypointense to the CSF on T2WI and slightly hyperintense on T1WI compatible with subacute subarachnoid hemorrhage. (**c**, **d**) DSA show multiple traumatic pseudoaneurysms (*arrows*)

stages (Fig. 46.5), a significant finding of SAH is a filling defect called "capping" representing subarachnoid clots or hematomas surrounded by CSF [4, 13, 14].

Hematomyelia appears in MRI as a T1WI hyperintense intramedullary spinal cord collection with mass effect and adjacent edema. SWI and gradient-echo T2* show marked low signal intensity corresponding to the hematoma (Fig. 46.6) [4, 21, 22].

Acute complications from hemorrhages such as canal stenosis and spinal cord compression are common. Abnormally dilated vessels surrounding the spinal canal and cord (Figs. 46.5 and 46.6) are suggestive of a vascular malformation, and digital angiography is recommended. A mass-like lesion with abnormal contrast enhancement may indicate a neoplasm. Almost one-third of ependymomas are associated with hemorrhage that may result in the "cap sign" (Fig. 46.7) [2, 4, 13–16].

Imaging Follow-Up

Patients may be treated conservatively or surgically. In the first, close follow-up MRI allows confirmation that the hematoma is not increasing in size a situation that may indicate surgical management. In patients that had surgical evacuation of a hematoma, serial MRI should be performed to evaluate the resolution of the collection, the presence of any residual spinal cord alterations, and postoperative complications. Follow-up may

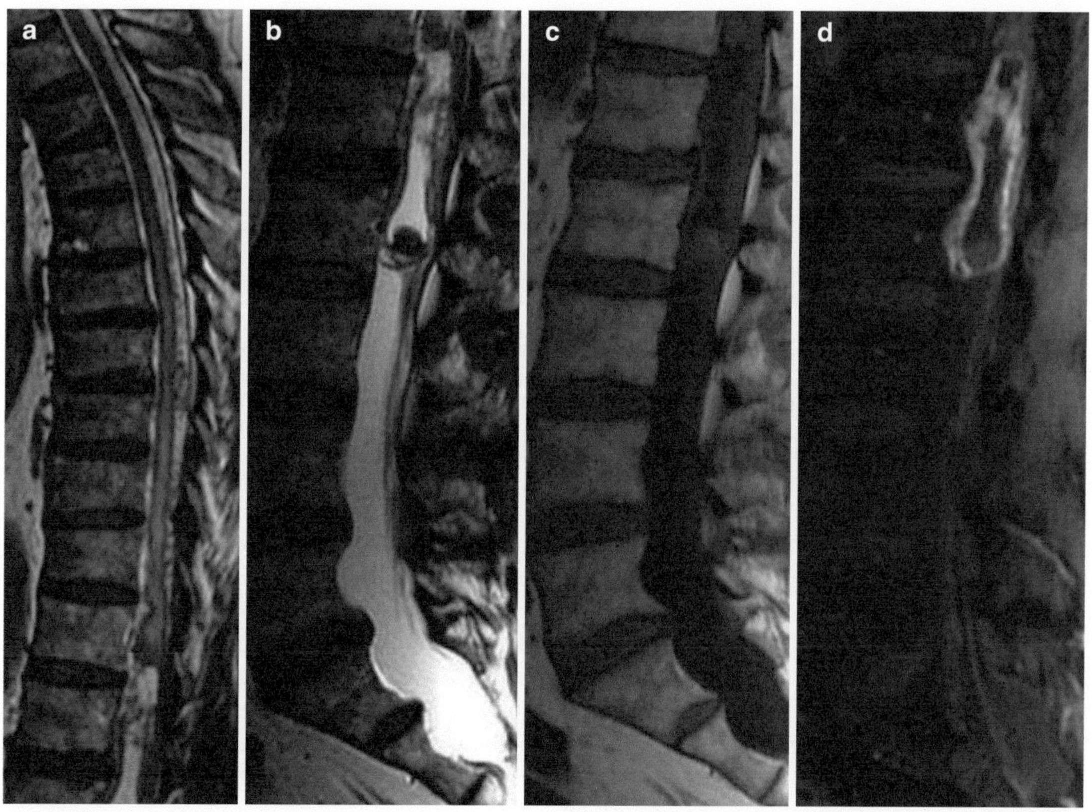

Fig. 46.5 Intradural hematoma. A 39-year-old man patient presenting with progressive lower limb paraparesis for 2 years. (**a**) Sagittal T2WI shows that the lower spinal cord/conus medullaris appears edematous. There are surrounding prominent serpiginous intradural extramedullary flow voids (dilated perimedullary vessels) extending from the lower cord to the filum terminale suggestive of arteriovenous fistula. Sagittal T2WI (**b**) demonstrates a hypointense mass that is hyperintense on T1WI (**c**) in the subarachnoid space compatible with blood products. (**d**) Postcontrast fat-saturated sagittal T1WI reveals peripheral enhancement in the subacute subarachnoid hematoma

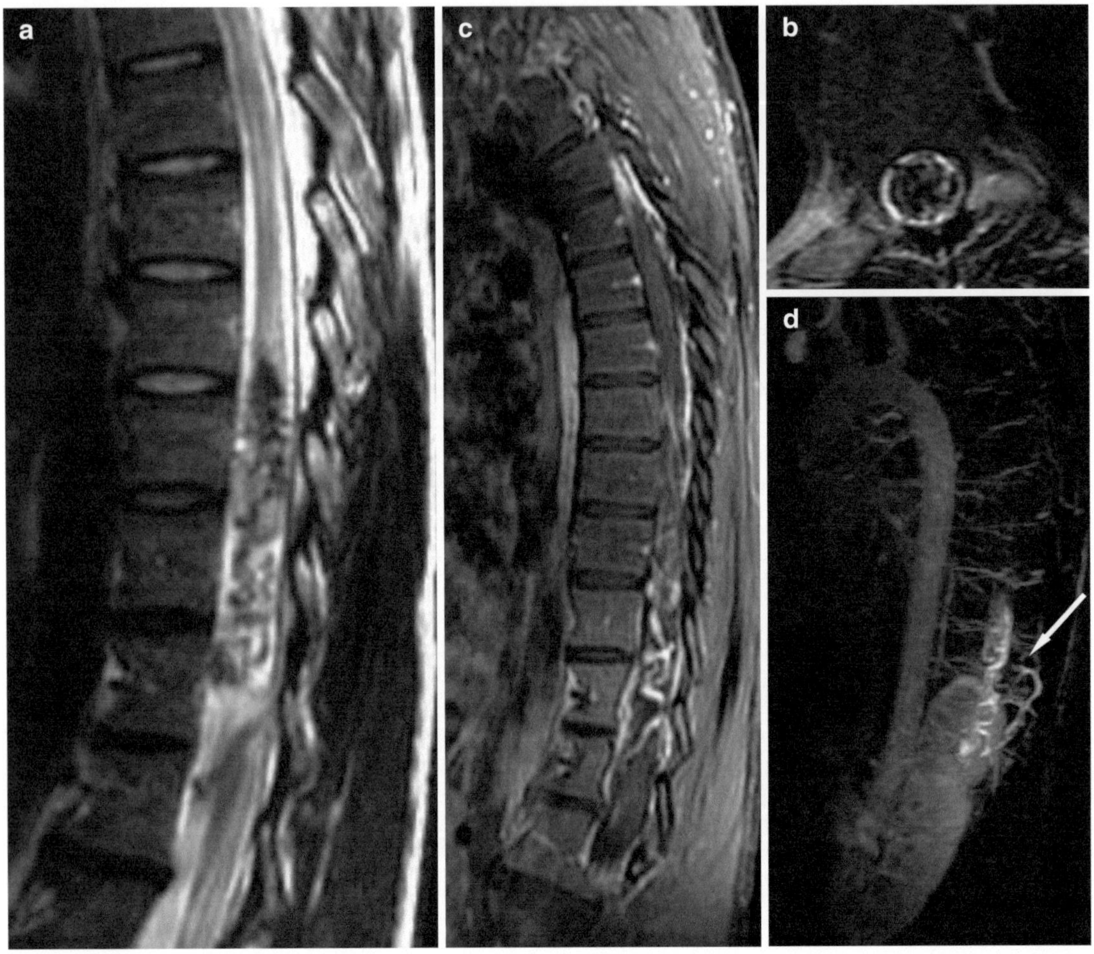

Fig. 46.6 Hematomyelia. A 39-year-old man under investigation for recurrent acute episodes of lower limb numbness and paraparesis. Sagittal T2WI (**a**) and axial T2WI (**b**) demonstrate multiple mid-thoracic serpiginous intra- and extramedullary flow voids and foci of hypointensity related to previous hemorrhages suggestive of hematomyelia and a complex spinal AVM involving the spinal cord. Postcontrast sagittal T1WI (**c**) reveals abnormal enhancement around the intramedullary hemorrhagic area, and sagittal MRA 4-D during the arterial phase (**d**) better demonstrates the lesion (*arrow*)

also reveal possible etiologic factors previously obscured by blood products in the acute setting, especially in hematomyelia [4].

Main Differential Diagnosis

The main differential diagnosis varies according to the location of the hemorrhage.

A spinal epidural abscess represents a rare but important emergency requiring immediate action. It usually presents as a suppurative process localized between the spinal dura mater and the vertebral periosteum in the spinal epidural space. In the phlegmonous stage, it presents with homogeneous enhancement. In later stages, it shows varying degrees of peripheral enhancement with gadolinium. Presence of restricted diffusion and absence of low signal on T2WI and on SWI are characteristic [4].

Spinal subdural empyema is also a rare lesion that may present as an extra-axial, fluidlike isodensity or hyperdense lesion on CT displaying the "cap sign" and the "Mercedes–Benz sign." However, like

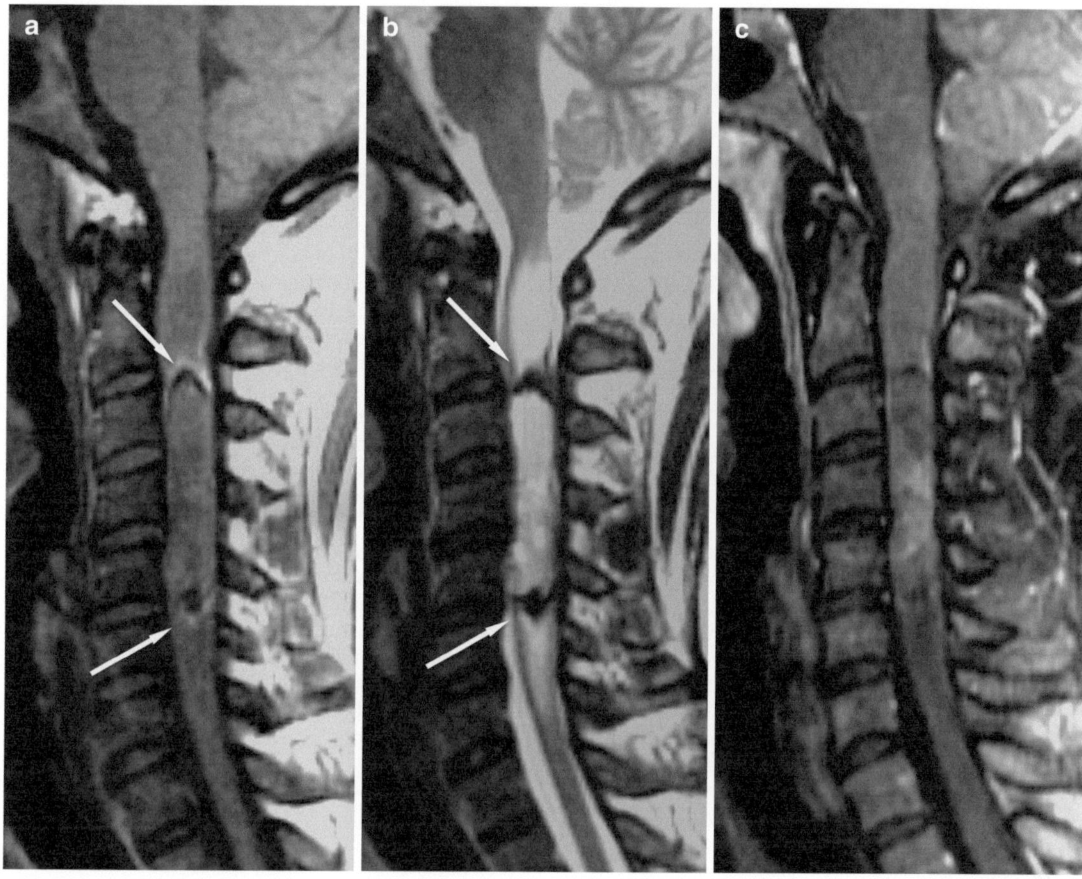

Fig. 46.7 "Cap sign" demonstrated in a 55-year-old man with spinal cord ependymoma. Sagittal T1WI (**a**) and T2WI (**b**) demonstrate a heterogeneous cervical cord mass with hemosiderin deposits peripherally located (*arrows*), which are a common finding in ependymomas. (**c**) Postcontrast fat-saturated T1WI reveals abnormal internal enhancement within the lesion, compatible tumor. The "cap sign" refers to the U-shaped area of chronic hemorrhage at either end of the tumor

other pyogenic infections, the presence of restricted diffusion and absence of low signal on T2WI and on SWI help reaching the correct diagnosis [4].

Tumors, such as lymphoma, metastasis, hemangioma, or angiomyolipoma, may be considered a differential diagnosis of extradural hemorrhagic spinal lesions. However, different from hematomas that present peripheral contrast enhancement, neoplastic lesions usually display solid or heterogeneous enhancement [4].

Spinal cord cavernomas are rare lesions that may cause hematomyelia. They show minimal cord expansion and edema unless there has been a recent hemorrhage. They typically display hypointense "blooming" on gradient-echo T2* and SWI, and the popcorn-like appearance of cavernous malformation is not seen in other causes of hematomyelia [4].

Tips

- As they are a potential cause for severe neurologic compromise, spinal collections should be reported to the emergency room, especially in cases of spinal cord compression as early surgical treatment may prevent death and improve neurological outcomes.

- Report the location, craniocaudal extent, diameter, and degree of medullary compression.
- Axial imaging is helpful in differentiating ESH from SDH, as the former tends to have biconvex shape and the latter crescent shape.
- Sometimes, more than one location is affected and SDH and SAH may be associated.

References

1. Agarwal A, Kanekar S, Thamburaj K, Vijay K. Radiation-induced spinal cord hemorrhage (hematomyelia). Neurol Int. 2014;6(4):1–4.
2. Kreppel D, Antoniadis G, Seeling W. Spinal hematoma: a literature survey with meta-analysis of 613 patients. Neurosurg Rev. 2003;26(1):1–49.
3. Dziedzic T, Kunert P, Krych P, Marchel A. Management and neurological outcome of spontaneous spinal epidural hematoma. J Clin Neurosci. 2015; 22(4):726–9. doi: 10.1016/j.jocn.2014.11.010.
4. Naidich TP, Castillo M, Cha S, Raybaud CA, Smirniotopoulos JG, Kollias SS. Imaging of the spine. Elsevier Health Sciences Philadelphia, PA. 2011; p.211–6 and 253–79.
5. Kappler SB, Davis JE. An uncommon cause of acute back pain: spinal subarachnoid hemorrhage progressing to spinal cord compression. J Emerg Med. 2015;48(4):432–5. doi: 10.1016/j.jemermed.2014.11.009.
6. Kim J-S, Lee S-H. Spontaneous spinal subarachnoid hemorrhage with spontaneous resolution. J Kor Neurosurg Soc. 2009;45(4):253–5.
7. Song J-Y, Chen Y-H, Hung K-C, Chang T-S. Traumatic subdural hematoma in the lumbar spine. Kaohsiung J Med Sci. 2011;27(10):473–6.
8. Sather MD, Gibson MD, Treves JS. Spinal subarachnoid hematoma resulting from lumbar myelography. Am J Neuroradiol. 2007;28(2):220–1.
9. Lee DH, Choi YH. Spontaneous intramedullary hematoma initially mimicking myocardial infarction. Am J Emerg Med. 2014;32(10):1294.e3–4.
10. Chao C-H, Tsai T-H, Huang T-Y, Lee K-S, Hwang S-L. Idiopathic spontaneous intraspinal intramedullary hemorrhage: a report of two cases and literature review. Clin Neurol Neurosurg. 2013;115(7):1134–6.
11. Sasaji T, Shinagawa K, Matsuya S. Spontaneous thoracic spinal subarachnoid hemorrhage diagnosed with brain computed tomography. Tohoku J Exp Med. 2013;231(2):139–44.
12. Hamdan A, Padmanabhan R. Intramedullary hemorrhage from a thoracolumbar dural arteriovenous fistula. Spine J. 2015;15(2):e9–16.
13. Massand MG, Wallace RC, Gonzalez LF, Zabramski JM, Spetzler RF. Subarachnoid hemorrhage due to isolated spinal artery aneurysm in four patients. Am J Neuroradiol. 2005;26(9):2415–9.
14. Seizeur R, Ahmed SS, Simon A, Besson G, Forlodou P. Acute non-traumatic spinal subdural haematoma: an unusual aetiology. J Clin Neurosci. 2009;16(6): 842–3.
15. Koda M, Mannoji C, Itabashi T, Kita T, Murakami M, Yamazaki M, et al. Intramedullary hemorrhage caused by spinal cord hemangioblastoma: a case report. BMC Res Notes. 2014;7(1):823.
16. Yamamoto J, Takahashi M, Akiba D, Soejima Y, Nakano Y, Aoyama Y, et al. Intrasyrinx hemorrhage associated with hemangioblastoma in epiconus. Spine J. 2009;9(5):e10–3.
17. Gilad R, Fatterpekar GM, Johnson DM, Patel AB. Migrating subdural hematoma without subarachnoid hemorrhage in the case of a patient with a ruptured aneurysm in the intrasellar anterior communicating artery. Am J Neuroradiol. 2007;28(10): 2014–6.
18. Morales Ciancio RA, Drain O, Rillardon L, Guigui P. Acute spontaneous spinal epidural hematoma: an important differential diagnosis in patients under clopidogrel therapy. Spine J. 2008;8(3):544–7.
19. Bruce-Brand RA, Colleran GC, Broderick JM, Lui DF, Smith EM, Kavanagh EC, et al. Acute nontraumatic spinal intradural hematoma in a patient on warfarin. J Emerg Med. 2013;45(5):695–7.
20. Fu M, Omay SB, Morgan J, Kelley B, Abbed K, Bulsara KR. Primary central nervous system vasculitis presenting as spinal subdural hematoma. WNEU. 2012;78(1–2):192.e5–8.
21. Steinberg JA, Gonda DD, Muller K, Ciacci JD. Endometriosis of the conus medullaris causing cyclic radiculopathy. J Neurosurg Spine. 2014;21(5): 799–804.
22. Agrawal A, Shetty BJP, Makannavar JH, Shetty L, Shetty J, Shetty V. Intramedullary endometriosis of the conus medullaris: case report. Neurosurgery. 2006;59(2):E428; discussion E428.
23. Wang M, Dai Y, Han Y, Haacke EM, Dai J, Shi D. Susceptibility weighted imaging in detecting hemorrhage in acute cervical spinal cord injury. Magn Reson Imaging. 2011;29(3):365–73.

Spinal Hemorrhage in Children: Extramedullary, Extradural, and Intramedullary

47

Lázaro Luís Faria do Amaral,
Anderson Benine Belezia,
and Samuel Brighenti Bergamaschi

Abstract

Spinal hemorrhages are uncommon but serious conditions. They are rare and have different presentations, locations, etiologies, and outcomes in children when compared to adults. The clinical diagnosis may be difficult, as younger children generally have nonspecific presentations, characterized by crying, irritability, and torticollis. Neurological symptoms may be mild and appear late. Spinal hemorrhages are classified as traumatic or nontraumatic. A causative factor is found in 61.8 % of spinal hematomas, and in 38.2 %, their etiology remains unknown, and thus they are categorized as spontaneous.

Background

Spinal hemorrhages are uncommon and serious conditions. In children, they are rare and have different presentations, locations, etiologies, and outcomes when compared to adults. A clinical diagnosis is often difficult as younger children have completely nonspecific initial presentations with crying, irritability, and torticollis being the main symptoms. Discreet neurological symptoms may be mild and appear late [1]. In this setting, imaging plays a crucial role in their diagnosis.

In children, epidural spinal hematomas (ESHs) are most common type (75 %) followed by subarachnoid hemorrhages (SAHs) and subdural spinal hematomas (SDHs). Intramedullary hematoma (hematomyelia) is very rare and is usually related to trauma [2]. Three mechanisms

L.L.F. do Amaral, MD (✉)
Division of Neuroradiology, Medimagem – Hospital Beneficência Portuguesa de São Paulo, Sao Paulo, SP, Brazil

Division of Neuroradiology, Hospital Santa Casa de Misericórdia de São Paulo, Rua Dr. Cesário Motta Junior 112, Vila Buarque, Sao Paulo, SP 01221-020, Brazil
e-mail: lazden@terra.com.br

A.B. Belezia, MD • S.B. Bergamaschi, MD
Radiology Department, Medimagem – Hospital Beneficência Portuguesa de São Paulo, Sao Paulo, SP, Brazil
e-mail: abelezia@gmail.com; samuel.brighentibergamaschi@gmail.com

R. Hoffmann Nunes et al. (eds.), *Critical Findings in Neuroradiology*,
DOI 10.1007/978-3-319-27987-9_47

for the development of ESH have been proposed and include rupture of epidural veins (the most accepted explanation), rupture of epidural arteries, and hemorrhage from vascular abnormalities. Similarly, SDH may originate during sudden intra-abdominal or intrathoracic increases in pressure leading to rupture of veins. Generally, the hemorrhage occurs first into the cerebrospinal fluid (CSF) with secondary extension into the subdural space. Subarachnoid spinal hemorrhage (SAH) is thought to originate by injury to the radicular blood vessels [2].

Spinal hemorrhages can be classified as traumatic or nontraumatic. A causative factor is found in 61.8 % of spinal hematomas, and in 38.2 %, the etiology remains unknown, and it is called spontaneous. Several causative factors have been identified, more commonly bleeding diathesis, tumors, vascular malformations, iatrogenic, and others. In younger patients, vascular malformations are responsible for 15.6 % of spinal hemorrhages. Different from adults, spinal hematomas that occur in children and young adults and primarily occur in the cervical and superior thoracic regions [2].

Key Points

Etiology

Trauma: The spine in younger patients has unique structural and biomechanical characteristics as muscles and ligaments are more flexible than in adults [3]. Traumatic hemorrhages in children tend to occur in the cervical spine, unlike adults, in whom they usually affect the thoracic and lumbar spine. Younger children are more likely to develop upper cervical bleeds. Non-accidental trauma is also a causative factor and usually results in SDH. Motor vehicle accidents are responsible for 25–60 % of spinal hematomas under 8 years of age. Sports-related hemorrhages occur in older children [4, 5].

Vascular malformations: Spinal arteriovenous malformations (AVMs) are a rare cause of spinal bleeds in children. In a review of 267 patients presenting with spinal AVM, 22 % were found under 18 years of age [6]. They are more common in the youngest especially when associated with syndromes as hereditary hemorrhagic telangiectasia, neurofibromatosis type I, Klippel–Trénaunay–Weber syndrome, and Cobb syndrome. Sudden onset of pain and neurologic deficits are the main presentations of spinal AVMs in children producing intramedullary hemorrhage or SAH [6, 7]. Spinal cavernous malformations are very rare in the pediatric population. They are more commonly located in the thoracic and upper lumbar spinal cord, and unlike adults, they tend to present with severe and acute neurologic deficits caused by intramedullary bleeding [8, 9].

Tumors: Several different tumors may cause spinal hemorrhages in children. Intramedullary tumors represent 35 % of spine neoplasms in the pediatric population and are more commonly associated with spinal hemorrhages than in adults [10]. Astrocytomas predominate in younger children contrary to adults where ependymomas are the predominant type. Usually, a hemorrhage is either intramedullary or in the subarachnoid space, [11];however, tumors affecting the epidural space (usually originating from bone) are relatively common in children and may lead to EDH [12].

Coagulopathies: Although a rare manifestation, hemophilic patients may present with spinal hematomas. EDH and SDH are the most common types and may involve multiple segments and compartments simultaneously. A timely diagnosis is useful to start administration of factor VIII to avoid progression of hematomas [13]. Iatrogenic coagulopathies may also cause spinal hemorrhages although they are not common in children.

Iatrogenic: Lumbar punctures and/or epidural anesthesia may be complicated by hematomas and may be related to the intrinsic technical difficulties related to the highly vascular epidural space in children [14].

Surgery: Children undergoing surgery for scoliosis and other related spine malformations may develop hemorrhages usually EDH [14].

Spontaneous spinal epidural hematomas are rare in children and are seldom reported in the literature. They usually occur in the cervical spine although thoracic and lumbar instances have been reported. The clinical presentation is usually unspecific and consists mostly of acute back pain [1].

Best Imaging Modality

Like in adults, magnetic resonance imaging (MRI) is the modality of choice for suspected spinal hemorrhages in the pediatric population. This technique is able to evaluate the location, extent, and age of the hemorrhage, as well as the possible cause of bleeding.

As in the brain, signal from the blood varies over time helping to estimate the age of the hematoma. The imaging protocol should include axial and/or sagittal T1- and T2-weighted imaging (T1WI and T2WI), spin echo sequences, as well as axial gradient-echo T2*. Gadolinium administration is also recommended and helps in determining a possible etiology for the hemorrhage. When a spinal hemorrhage is detected, it is also important to determine the complete extension of the lesion [4]. Susceptibility-weighted imaging (SWI) sequence is sensitive for blood products and is considered very useful in detecting small hemorrhages also in the spine but are difficult to obtain in most clinical MRI units [15]. A disadvantage of MRI is the long time of the examination which usually requires sedation in children.

Computed tomography (CT) may be helpful in the acute scenario especially in trauma patients. As stated above, children may not be collaborative, and thus CT may be an option to avoid sedation. One should always remember that radiation exposure is best avoided in children and that the diagnostic ability of CT to detect spinal hematomas is limited [16].

Digital angiography may be performed when there is high index of suspicion for underlying vascular malformations and lesions [6].

Major Findings

As in adults, a spinal fluid collection in the epidural, subdural, or intramedullary space may be hemorrhagic if it shows pre-contrast T1 hyperintensity. In the hyperacute stage, a hematoma is isointense-to-dark on T1WI and hyperintense on T2WI relatively to the spinal cord. Acute hematomas are characterized by hypointense signal on T1WI and marked hypointensity on T2WI. From 3 to 5 days, formation of methemoglobin begins and a hematoma becomes hyperintense on T1WI and thereafter T2WI until its chronic phase when it becomes hypointense in T1WI and T2WI due to presence of hemosiderin and ferritin [17]. On gradient-echo T2* and SWI, acute spinal blood collections commonly display low signal intensity due to presence of deoxyhemoglobin [15]. On CT, spinal hemorrhagic collections are usually hyperdense lesions, and after one week they become inhomogeneous and of variable densities [17].

On CT, ESH appear as a sharply demarcated, biconvex-shaped mass that closely approximates the bony confines of the spinal canal and displaces and compresses the less dense-appearing thecal sac and the spinal cord. On MRI, their appearance is similar and most are found in a dorsolateral location and have a typical well-demarcated biconvex shape with superiorly and inferiorly tapering margins usually extending for two to three vertebral bodies. Different from adults, ESH in children and young adults occurs primarily in the cervical and superior thoracic regions (Figs. 47.1 and 47.2) [17].

SDHs usually presents as more extensive lesions than ESHs extending for over six to seven vertebral bodies and displaying a typical crescent shape on CT and MR axial images. As opposed to acute ESH which are intermingled with epidural fat, SDHs are located within the thecal sac and separate from the adjacent extradural fat and the adjacent osseous structures (Fig. 47.3). The blood signal time change in SDH is usually similar to that of ESH [17].

SAHs are usually diffuse and during the acute or subacute stages seen as non-localized areas of increased density or low signal on T2WI surrounding the spinal cord and/or nerve roots [17].

Hematomyelia appears in MRI as a T1WI hyperintense intramedullary spinal cord lesion with mass effect and adjacent edema. SWI and gradient-echo T2* show marked low signal intensity corresponding to the hematoma (Figs. 47.4 and 47.5) [17].

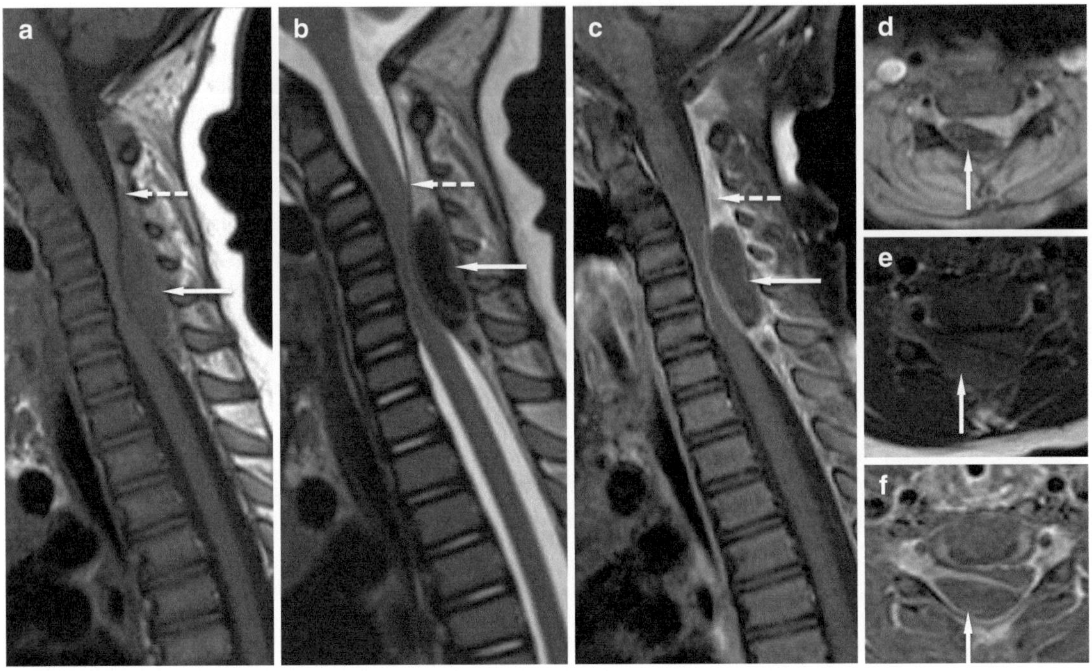

Fig. 47.1 Spontaneous spinal epidural hematoma in a 6-year-old girl presenting with severe neck pain and acute left-side hemiparesis with no history of trauma. Sagittal T1WI (**a**), T2WI (**b**), and postcontrast TWI (**c**) demonstrate a large slightly hyperintensity on T1WI space-occupying lesion extending from the level of C1 to C7, displacing anteriorly the spinal cord. The epidural hematoma is hypointense on T2WI (**b**) and has smooth peripheral enhancement (**c**). Notice that the dura contains both the epidural hematoma (*solid arrows*) and the posterior epidural fat (*dashed arrows*). (**d–f**) Axial T2* (**d**) at the same level of pre- (**e**) and postcontrast (**f**) axial T1WI confirms the location of the hematoma (*arrows*) within the epidural space and the characteristic low signal intensity on T2* (**d**) (Courtesy of Leonardo Furtado de Freitas, MD)

Complications from hemorrhages such as canal stenosis and spinal cord compression are common. Abnormally dilated blood vessels surrounding the spinal cord are suggestive of a vascular malformation, and DSA is recommended. It is important to remember that in children vascular malformations are responsible for 15.6 % of spinal hemorrhages (Figs. 47.4 and 47.5). Different from adults, spinal hematomas in children and young adults involve primarily the cervical and superior thoracic regions. A mass-like lesion with abnormal contrast enhancement may indicate an underlying neoplasm [17].

Imaging Follow-Up

Similar to adults, patients may be treated conservatively or surgically. In the former, close follow-up MRI allows confirmation that the hematoma is not increasing in size a situation that may indicate emergent surgical management. In patients that had surgical evacuation of a hematoma, serial MRI may be performed to evaluate its resolution, presence of any residual spinal cord abnormalities, and postoperative complications. Follow-up may also reveal possible etiologic factors previously obscured by blood products in the acute setting [17]. It is also important to remember that non-accidental trauma is a major cause of spinal hemorrhage in children, and a search for other imaging and clinical signs that confirm that diagnosis is strongly recommended [4, 5].

Main Differential Diagnosis

The main differential diagnosis varies according to the location of the hemorrhages. A spinal epi-

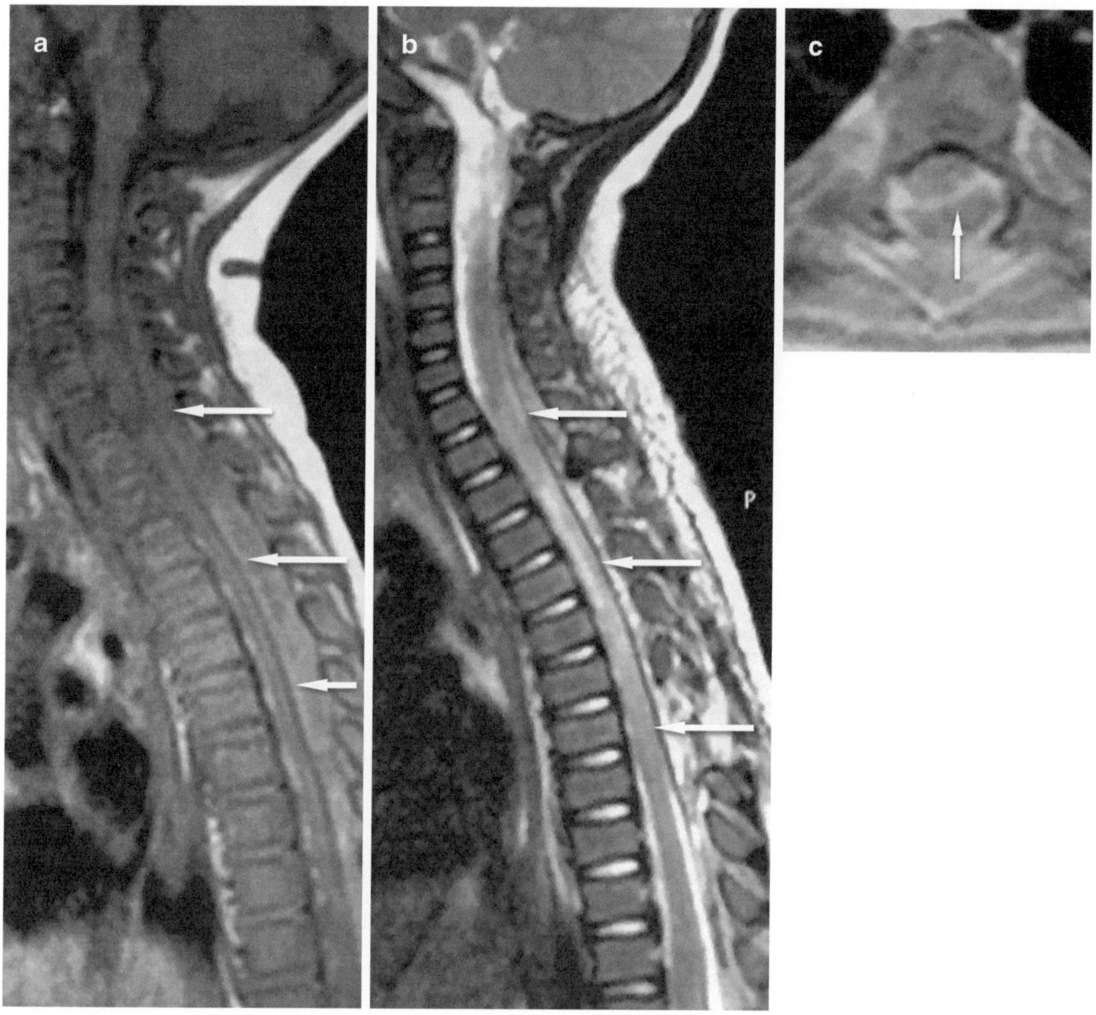

Fig. 47.2 Spinal epidural hematoma. A 1-year-old boy presents with tetraparesis after minor trauma. Sagittal T1WI (**a**) and T2WI (**b**) and axial postcontrast T1WI show an extensive blood collection located dorsolaterally to the cord within the epidural space (*arrows*) displacing the spinal cord contralateral to it (**c**) and compatible with an epidural hematoma

dural abscess presents as an extradural lesion with varying degrees of peripheral enhancement and presence of central restricted diffusion on DWI. Spinal subdural empyema presents as an extra-axial, fluidlike isodensity or hyperdense lesion on CT with characteristic restricted diffusion on MRI. Different from hematomas that present peripheral contrast enhancement, neoplastic lesions usually display solid or heterogeneous enhancement [4]. Caution is advised as many hematomas may also show restricted diffusion, but in these cases the clinical presentation is helpful to differentiate both entities.

Spinal cord cavernomas are rare lesions that may cause hematomyelia. They show minimal cord expansion and edema unless there has been a recent hemorrhage. Although they typically display hypointense "blooming" on gradient-echo T2* and SWI, the popcorn-like appearance of cavernous malformations in other parts of the nervous system may not be seen in cases of hematomyelia (Fig. 47.5) [4].

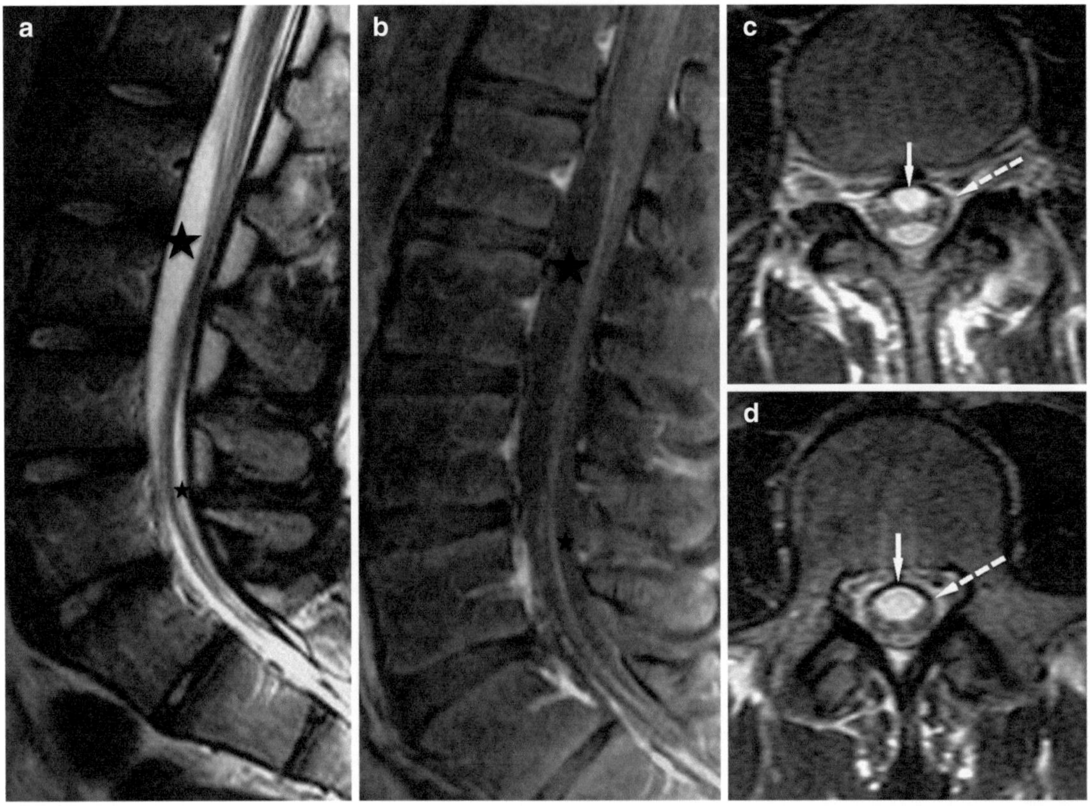

Fig. 47.3 Spinal subdural hematoma. A 12-year-old boy with history of motor vehicle accident 4 months previously presents with lumbar pain, right foot weakness, and gait disturbance. Sagittal T2WI (**a**) and postcontrast fat-saturated T1WI (**b**) reveal a large fluid collection in the lumbar spine occupying the subdural space anteriorly and posteriorly compatible with subdural hematoma (*stars*). Axial T2WIs (**c**, **d**) at different levels show that the dura separates the subdural hematoma (*solid arrows*) from the posterior epidural fat (*dashed arrows*) confirming its location

Tips

- Because spinal hemorrhages may cause rapid and severe neurologic compromise, they should be immediately reported to the emergency room especially in presence of spinal cord compression as early surgical treatment may prevent death and improve neurological outcomes. Report their location, craniocaudal extent, diameter, and degree of medullary compression.
- In young children, non-accidental trauma should be considered as a cause of spinal hemorrhages particularly of SDH.
- In younger patients, vascular malformations are responsible for 15.6 % of spinal hemorrhages.
- Spinal hemorrhages due to AVMs are more common with syndromes, such as hereditary hemorrhagic telangiectasia, neurofibromatosis type I, Klippel–Trénaunay–Weber syndrome, and Cobb syndrome.
- Different from adults, spinal hematomas occur in children and young adults and primarily occur in the cervical and superior thoracic regions.
- Axial imaging is helpful in differentiating ESHs from SDHs, as the former tend to have biconvex shape and the latter are crescent shaped.

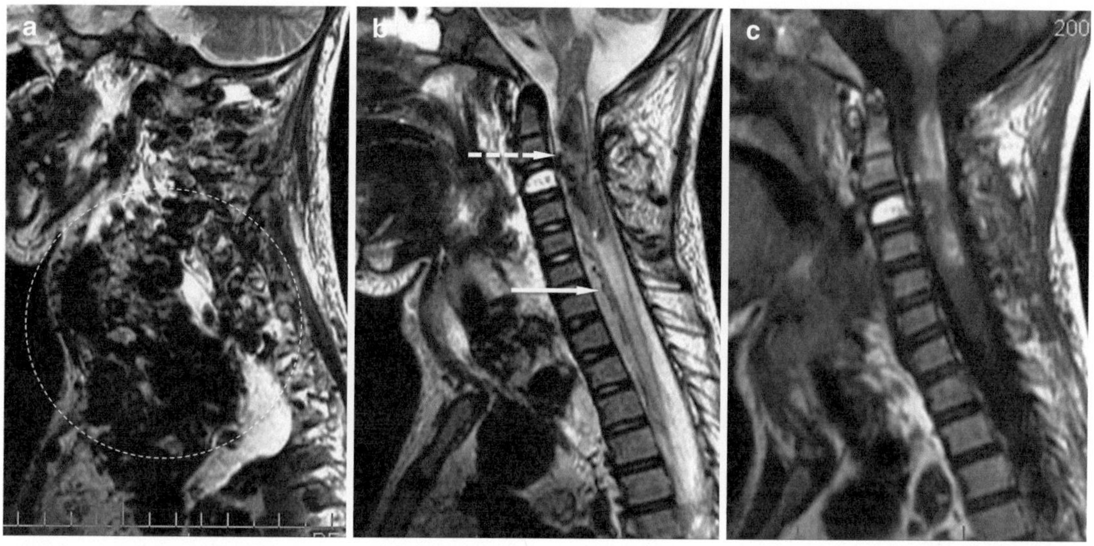

Fig. 47.4 Intramedullary hemorrhage associated with AVM. A 7-year-old boy with neck presents with acute paraplegia. Sagittal T2WI (**a**) shows extensive flow voids in the neck (*circle*) compatible with abnormally dilated vessels. Sagittal T2WI (**b**) reveals subacute blood and surrounding edema in the cervical spinal cord compatible with an intramedullary hematoma associated with a vascular nidus (*dashed arrow*). Tortuous vessels on the cord surface (*solid arrow*) and a hemangioma in C3 are also seen suggesting a metameric vascular syndrome. Postcontrast T1WI (**c**) shows abnormal enhancement in the spinal cord surrounding the hematoma compatible with congestive myelopathy

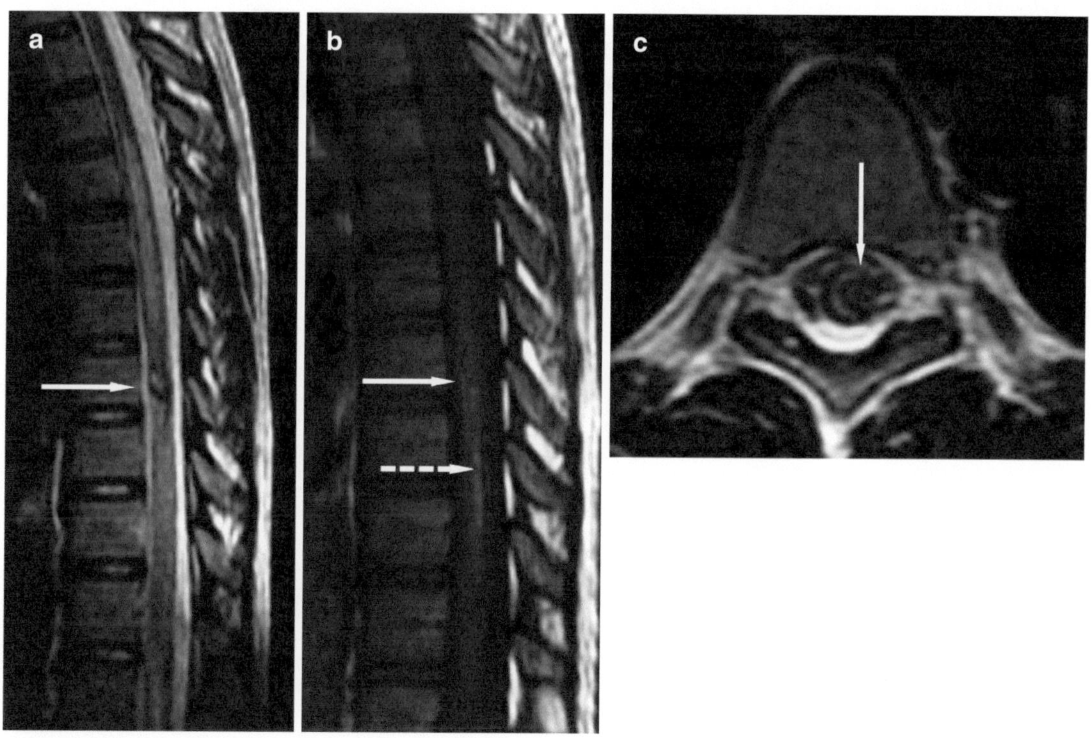

Fig. 47.5 Intramedullary hemorrhage associated with spinal cord cavernoma. A 12-year-old girl presenting with acute onset of paraparesis. Sagittal T2WI (**a**) and T1WI (**b**) demonstrate a round hypointensity (*solid arrow*) in the mid-thoracic spinal cord with edema surrounding it. A subtle linear hyperintensity in the central cord is also seen (*dashed arrow* on **b**) compatible with hematomyelia. Axial T2* (**c**) confirms a hypointense nodular area (*arrow*) in the left thoracic cord compatible with a cavernoma (Courtesy of Cesar Alves, MD)

References

1. Schoonjans A-S, De Dooy J, Kenis S, Menovsky T, Verhulst S, Hellinckx J, et al. Spontaneous spinal epidural hematoma in infancy: review of the literature and the "seventh" case report. Eur J Paediatr Neurol. 2013;17(6):537–42.
2. Kreppel D, Antoniadis G, Seeling W. Spinal hematoma: a literature survey with meta-analysis of 613 patients. Neurosurg Rev. 2003;26(1):1–49.
3. Lustrin ES, Karakas SP, Ortiz AO, Cinnamon J, Castillo M, Vaheesan K, et al. Pediatric cervical spine: normal anatomy, variants, and trauma. Radiographics. 2003;23(3):539–60.
4. Baker C, Kadish H, Schunk JE. Evaluation of pediatric cervical spine injuries. Am J Emerg Med. 1999;17(3):230–4.
5. Hall DE, Boydston W. Pediatric neck injuries. Pediatr Rev. 1999;20(1):13–9; quiz 20.
6. Song D, Garton HJL, Fahim DK, Maher CO. Spinal cord vascular malformations in children. Neurosurg Clin N Am. 2010;21(3):503–10.
7. Saliou G, Tej A, Theaudin M, Tardieu M, Ozanne A, Sachet M, et al. Risk factors of hematomyelia recurrence and clinical outcome in children with intradural spinal cord arteriovenous malformations. Am J Neuroradiol. 2014;35(7):1440–6.
8. Labauge P, Bouly S, Parker F, Gallas S, Emery E, Loiseau H, et al. Outcome in 53 patients with spinal cord cavernomas. Surg Neurol. 2008;70(2):176–81.
9. Cornips EMJ, Vinken PACP, Ter Laak-Poort M, Beuls EAM, Weber J, Vles JSH. Intramedullary cavernoma presenting with hematomyelia: report of two girls. Childs Nerv Syst. 2010;26(3):391–8.
10. Duong LM, McCarthy BJ, McLendon RE, Dolecek TA, Kruchko C, Douglas LL, et al. Descriptive epidemiology of malignant and nonmalignant primary spinal cord, spinal meninges, and cauda equina tumors, United States, 2004–2007. Cancer. 2012;118(17):4220–7.
11. Mohindra S, Rane S, Gupta SK. Symptomatic apoplexy in intramedullary ependymoma: a report of a pediatric patient. Pediatr Neurosurg. 2011;47(5):369–71.
12. Mechtler LL, Nandigam K. Spinal cord tumors: new views and future directions. Neurol Clin N Am. 2013;31(1):241–68.
13. Aulakh R, Panigrahi I, Naranje K, Sharda S, Marwaha RK. Spontaneous hematomyelia in a child with hemophilia A: a case report. J Pediatr Hematol Oncol. 2009;31(10):766–7.
14. Tubbs RS, Smyth MD, Wellons JC, Oakes WJ. Intramedullary hemorrhage in a neonate after lumbar puncture resulting in paraplegia: a case report. Pediatrics. 2004;113(5):1403–5.
15. Wang M, Dai Y, Han Y, Haacke EM, Dai J, Shi D. Susceptibility weighted imaging in detecting hemorrhage in acute cervical spinal cord injury. Magn Reson Imaging. 2011;29(3):365–73.
16. Agarwal A, Kanekar S, Thamburaj K, Vijay K. Radiation-induced spinal cord hemorrhage (hematomyelia). Neurol Int. 2014;6(4):1–4.
17. Naidich TP, Castillo M, Cha S, Raybaud C, Smirniotopoulos JG, Kollias S, et al. Imaging of the spine. Philadelphia, PA: Elsevier Health Sciences; 2011; p.211–6 and 253–79.

Spinal Cord Infarction

48

César Augusto Pinheiro Alves,
Antônio José da Rocha,
and Renato Hoffmann Nunes

Abstract

Spinal cord ischemia is an uncommon disease, varying in its presentation, severity, and outcome. Spinal cord ischemia accounts for approximately 14 % of all acute myelopathies and approximately 1–2 % of all vascular neurologic diseases. The severity of the injury depends on several factors including acute hemodynamic instability and poor perfusion, oxygen delivery and demand, local metabolic rate, and the patients' baseline collateral circulation. Spinal cord ischemia can cause a variety of symptoms and neurological deficits which depend on the affected spinal cord level and artery involved. It is characterized generally by an acute onset which is often preceded by sudden and severe back pain typically at the level of the lesion. Magnetic resonance imaging is the modality of choice for the diagnosis.

Background

Spinal cord ischemia (SCI) is an uncommon disease, varying in its presentation, severity, and outcome, significantly threatening health in some patients. SCI accounts for approximately 14 % of all acute myelopathies and approximately 1–2 % of all vascular neurologic diseases [1, 2]. It may affect the anterior or posterior spinal artery territories and sometimes both arterial and venous territories [3]. The thoracic level is the most frequently affected [4]. The severity of SCI depends on several factors including acute hemodynamic instability and poor perfusion, oxygen delivery and demand, local metabolic rate, and a patients' baseline collateral circulation [5].

C.A.P. Alves, MD (✉) • A.J. da Rocha, MD, PhD
Division of Neuroradiology, Hospital Santa Casa de Misericórdia de São Paulo, Rua Dr. Cesário Motta Junior 112, Vila Buarque, Sao Paulo, SP 01221-020, Brazil

Division of Neuroradiology, Grupo Fleury, Sao Paulo, SP, Brazil
e-mail: cesar.alves@grupofleury.com.br; antonio.rocha@grupofleury.com.br

R. Hoffmann Nunes, MD
Division of Neuroradiology, Santa Casa de São Paulo, São Paulo, Brazil
e-mail: renatohn@hotmail.com

R. Hoffmann Nunes et al. (eds.), *Critical Findings in Neuroradiology*,
DOI 10.1007/978-3-319-27987-9_48

This chapter focuses on nontraumatic arterial ischemic lesions which are the major cause of SCI.

Spinal Cord Arteries

The spinal cord (SC) vascularization (Fig. 48.1) is grossly divided in anterior and posterior territories. The anterior spinal artery (ASA) distributes blood to the anterior two-thirds of the SC via central and pial branches, supplying the anterior horns and the anterior part of the lateral columns at each level [6, 7]. This artery runs along the anterior surface of the SC, located in the anterior median sulcus and descending vertically from the top of the cervical SC [8].

The posterior spinal arteries (PSAs) are usually paired, located on the posterolateral surface of the SC along its entire length, and may occasionally be discontinuous [9]. PSAs are responsible for supplying the SC peripheral structures, including the posterior columns and the apices of the dorsal horns.

Some radicular arteries contribute to the SC blood supply. They can form anterior branches named radiculomedullary arteries and posterior branches named radiculopial arteries, which contribute to the ASA and PSAs, respectively (Fig. 48.1).

In general, the SC longitudinal vascularization is divided into three regions according to the origin of the arterial supply:

1. The first region (superior) corresponds to the level of C1 to the level of T3, and it is supplied by the vertebral arteries from their V4 segments and from the cervical ascending arteries [6, 7, 10].
2. The second region (middle) is located from the level of T3 to T7, and it is relatively poorly vascularized; it is usually supplied by only one radicular artery [11].
3. The third region (inferior) extends from T8 to the conus medullaris and receives blood mainly from the artery of Adamkiewicz (AKA) also knows as the *radicularis magna* artery, the largest and most important supplier of the thoracolumbar SC [12]. In approximately 70 % of cases, the AKA originates from an intercostal or lumbar artery on the left side of the spine and most frequently between the levels of T8 and L1 (Fig. 48.1) [13].

Clinical Presentation

SCI can cause a variety of symptoms and neurological deficits as a consequence of the affected SC level and involved artery. SCI is characterized generally by an acute onset (minutes to a few hours) often preceded by sudden and severe back pain typically at the level of the lesion [14, 15].

In approximately two-thirds of patients, the ASA is involved, and the most common clinical presentation is called the "ASA syndrome" which is characterized by a bilateral loss of motor function (acute paraplegia or quadriplegia) and spinothalamic sensory and pain/temperature sensory abnormalities with relative sparing of proprioception and vibratory senses below the level of the lesion. The acute stages are characterized by flaccidity and loss of deep tendon reflexes, and autonomic dysfunction may also occur [14, 15].

When ischemia compromises the territory of the central or sulcocomissural artery (SSA) and only affects the cervical SC, it presents as "SSA syndrome." This syndrome is characterized by ipsilateral flaccid paresis and spastic (hemi)paresis below the level of infarction as well as contralateral dissociated sensory deficits [4]. If the lesion is in the rostral cervical cord, respiratory function may be compromised [8].

PSA territory infarctions which comprise <3 % of cases result in alterations of posterior column function, usually unilateral, leading to loss of proprioception and vibratory senses below the injury level and associated anesthesia at the level of the injury [3, 14, 16].

Spinal transient ischemic attacks have been described in many clinical settings usually manifesting as transient symptoms that last few minutes to several hours preceding SCI [14, 15].

Watershed Infarcts

Spinal watershed infarcts develop in the border zones between the arterial systems [17]. Due to local or global hypoperfusion, hemodynamic

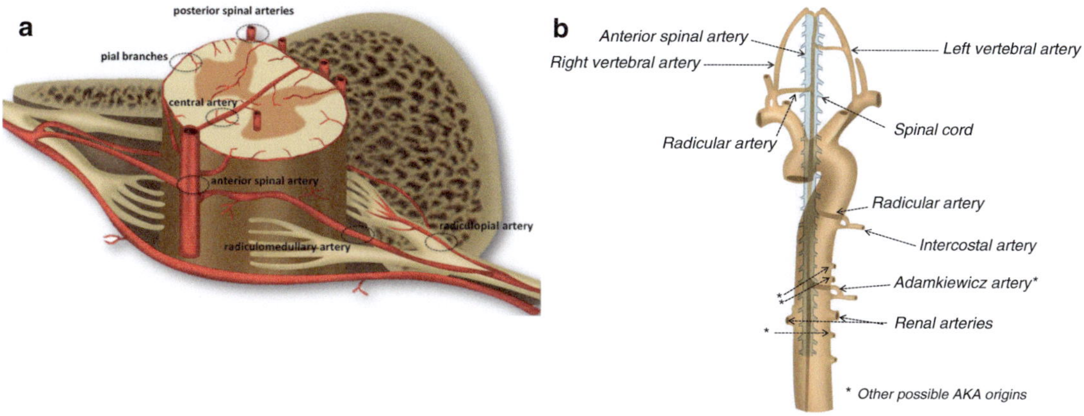

Fig. 48.1 Spinal cord arterial supply anatomy. (**a**) The anterior spinal artery is located in the anterior median sulcus and distributes blood to the anterior two-thirds of the spinal cord tissue by central and pial branches. The posterior spinal arteries are usually paired, located on the posterolateral surface of the spinal cord along the paramedial sulci. Radicular arteries form anterior branches named radiculomedullary arteries and posterior branches named radiculopial arteries contribute to the anterior and posterior spinal arteries, respectively. (**b**) The anterior spinal artery is formed by two small branches arising from the fourth segment of the vertebral arteries and other contributors arising from the vertebral arteries; the ascending cervical artery; the inferior thyroid artery; the intercostal arteries; the lumbar artery, the iliolumbar artery, and lateral sacral arteries; and especially by the artery of Adamkiewicz. The latter generally arises on the left side of the aorta between the T8 and L1 to anastomose with the anterior spinal artery and supply the lower two-thirds of the spinal cord (conus medullaris)

infarcts most often involve the anterior horns because the gray matter has a much higher vulnerability to anoxia [18]. A characteristic clinical finding caused by cervical watershed infarcts is the "man-in-the-barrel syndrome" characterized by atonic proximal paresis of the upper limbs and normal motor function in the lower body [17, 19–21]. Since this particular type of ischemia is often from lesions at the levels C3–C6 and the anterior horns of C7 and C8 are usually spared, the hand motor function is not affected [20].

Other neurologic manifestations include complete SC transection and the Brown–Séquard syndrome which is an incomplete SC lesion characterized by clinical manifestations of SC hemisection [22].

Key Points

Etiology

Even though the etiology of spinal cord infarcts is not well established (28, 74 %) [4, 15, 23], the main causes are atherosclerosis of the aorta and of the vertebral arteries (23,6 %), aortic surgery or interventional aneurysm repair (11 %), and aortic and vertebral artery dissections (11 %) [4, 23]. Other unusual causes are hypovolemic shock [24], fibrocartilaginous emboli that originate from the intervertebral disk and Schmorl's nodes [25–27], sickle cell disease [28], lumbar transforaminal epidural steroid injection [29], vasculitis, antiphospholipid antibody syndrome, and neurosyphilis [15, 30, 31].

An additional cause of SCI without spinal traumatic injury that has been recently reported is surfers' myelopathy which is characterized by a vascular phenomenon that involves dynamic compression, vasospasm, or thrombotic infarction of the great anterior radicular artery of Adamkiewicz. It should be recognized for its epidemiological peculiarity and it usually occurs during recreational activities especially long periods of stretching and lordosis over surfing boards [32].

Best Imaging Modality

Magnetic resonance imaging (MRI) is the modality of choice for the diagnosis of SCI, allowing assessment of the structures inside the vertebral canal even in the hyperacute stage. Besides, MRI should also be obtained to exclude other potential treatable causes of cord dysfunction (e.g., SC acute compression) [15, 20, 33]. Diffusion-weighted imaging (DWI) is a key sequence for the diagnosis [33, 34] revealing signal abnormalities within 3 h after the ictus [30, 35] and much earlier than other MRI sequences.

Applying DWI to SC imaging is challenging for many reasons including the small size of the SC, pulsations of the cord and surrounding CSF, and the extreme field inhomogeneity because of the bone surrounding it. Traditionally, single-shot EPI (SS-EPI) schemes have been used to perform DWI [36], but recently other advanced techniques have been proposed to address this issue such as diffusion tensor imaging.

Currently, the recommended MRI protocol is [8, 37]:

- Sagittal T1-weighted imaging (T1WI)
- Sagittal (and axial) T2-weighted imaging (T2WI)
- Axial T2*
- Axial T1WI
- Postcontrast sagittal and axial T1WI
- Sagittal DWI – a lower *b* value than used in the head which is recommended to improve signal while maintaining diffusion sensitivity ($b = 500–700$)

Vertebral and paravertebral regions should be carefully evaluated in order to detect the source of a possible fibrocartilaginous emboli or artery dissection (aorta and vertebral arteries). MR angiography (MRA) can be useful to evaluate for thrombus or dissection in the aorta. Postcontrast 3D high-spatial-resolution steady-state MRA sequences are recommended since they allow visualization of the AKA in around 81 % of patients despite some difficulties related to the field inhomogeneity caused by surrounding bones [38, 39]. Computed tomography angiography (CTA) may help to assess the blood supply to the SC allowing visualization of the AKA in most patients. Spinal digital subtraction angiography (DSA) is the gold standard for direct visualization the AKA [40, 41].

Major Findings

MRI may be unremarkable in the hyperacute stage (less than 3 h). Later, areas of acute SCI show restricted diffusion. SC swelling and T2 abnormalities can be expected only after 24 h after the ictus (Fig. 48.2) [37]. Contrast enhancement is usually absent at early stages and if detected suggests inflammatory, neoplastic, or infectious diseases [8].

In later stages, it is possible to find central or confluent gadolinium enhancement in the SC (Fig. 48.3). Contrast enhancement of the anterior nerve roots related to the ischemic area can also be seen [4, 30, 42]. In the late acute to early subacute phase, SCI lesions usually demonstrate hypointense signal on T1WI. Nevertheless, around 10 % of patients may show slight hyperintense spinal cord signal changes on this sequence possibly due to hemorrhagic transformation (Fig. 48.4) [4]. Both axial and sagittal T2WI sequences are useful to demonstrate the areas of abnormal increased signal. On the sagittal plane, the lesion can present a typical "pencil-like" appearance on T2WI (Fig. 48.5) [20].

The lesion's distribution in the transverse axis of the cord varies and depends on the compromised vascular region [8]. The most common type is bilateral or unilateral ASA infarcts seen as a linear hyperintense intramedullary lesion on T2WI and DWI confined to the anterior horns and the adjacent white matter displaying the typical "owl eye" or "snake eye" appearance [43, 44]. The second most common finding is central and transverse infarcts due to extensive SC hypoperfusion and arteriopathy [45].

Six different imaging patterns of SCI may occur as follows (Table 48.1) [14]:

1. Limited abnormality in the anterior horns and the surrounding white matter (Figs. 48.5 and 48.6)
2. Unilateral involvement of the anterior horn (Fig. 48.7)
3. Bilateral posterolateral infarcts
4. Posterior unilateral infarct
5. Central infarct
6. Transverse infarct

Other useful signs of SCI include vascular or bone marrow abnormalities (Fig. 48.7) [42, 46]. The common vascularization of the vertebral body, disk, and SC may result in concomitant SC and vertebral body infarcts particularly in adults which are seen as areas of abnormal increased signal on T2WI with or without contrast

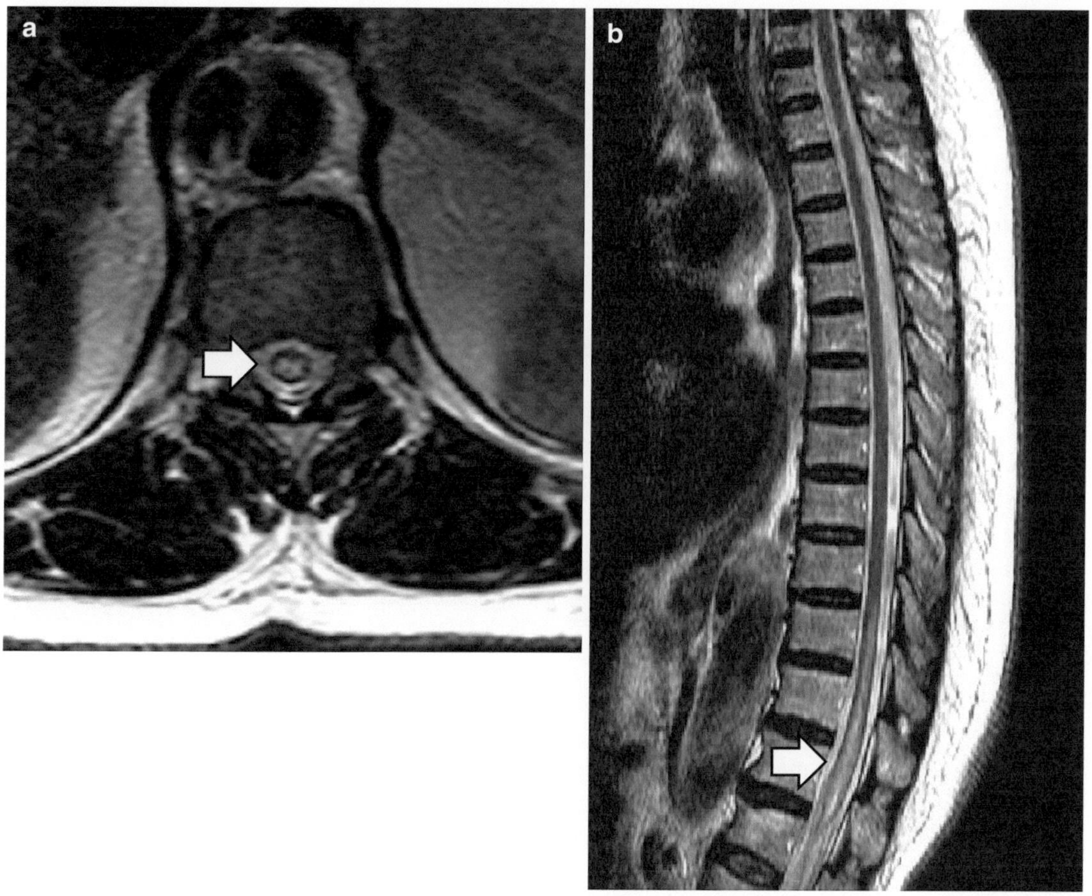

Fig. 48.2 Spinal cord infarction after aorta dissection. (**a**, **b**) Axial and sagittal T2WI show a hyperintense lesion in the distal spinal cord and conus medullaris (*arrows*). The increased signal intensity is located centrally, displaying the classic configuration of the swollen spinal cord gray matter on the axial plane. (**c**) DWI demonstrates pronounced hyperintensity in the affected regions. (**d**) 3D MRA reconstruction reveals an aorta dissection (*arrow*) that can also be seen on axial T2WI (**a**)

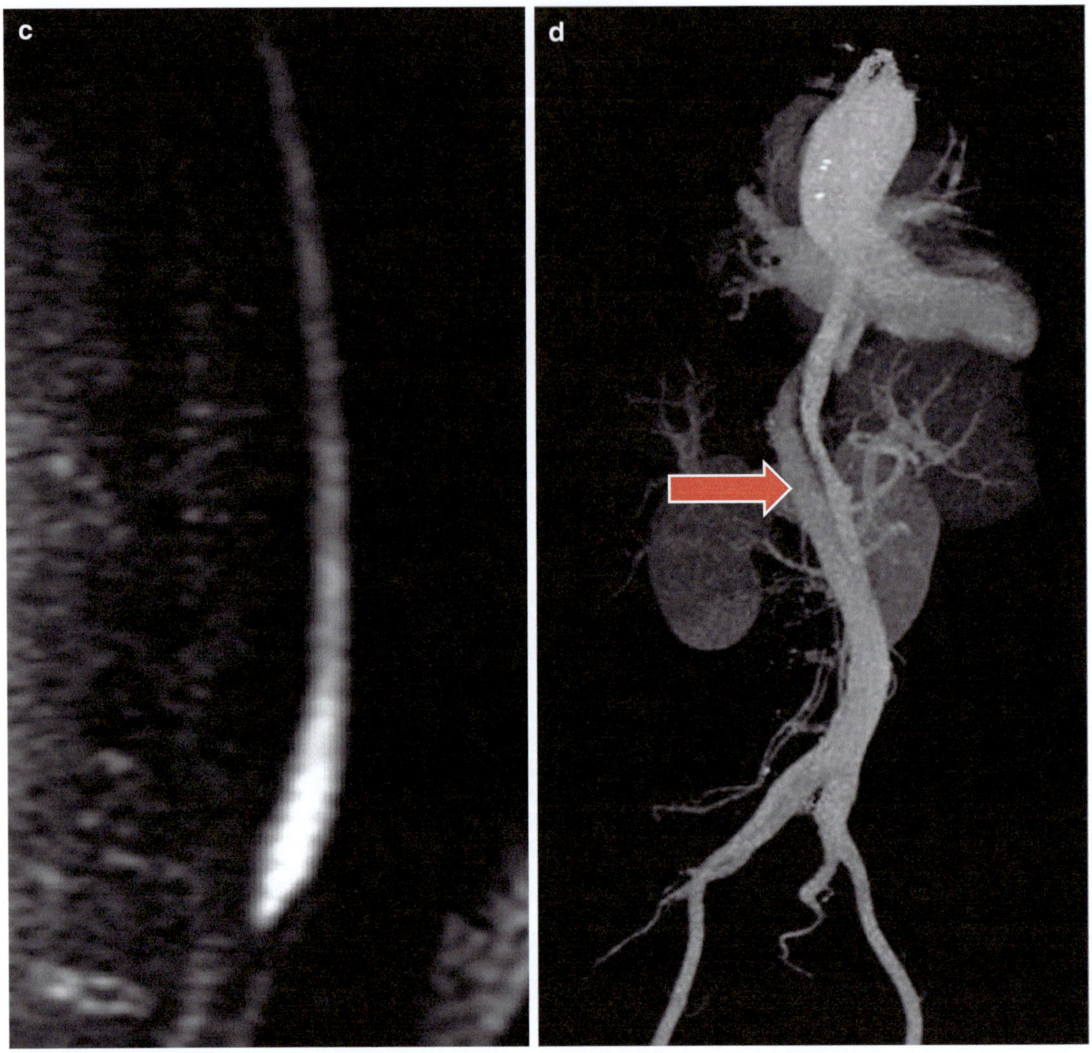

Fig. 48.2 (continued)

enhancement on T1WI in the adjacent intervertebral disk [8, 47]. Bone marrow abnormalities, extensive SC signal changes, and cord hemorrhagic necrosis are findings that have been associated to fibrocartilaginous embolization to the cord [48].

Imaging Follow-Up

The follow-up depends on the patient's clinical status. Imaging may demonstrate persistent gadolinium enhancement, lasting for several months, generally in the gray matter. In chronic stages, the findings are nonspecific and usually characterized by myelomalacia (cord atrophy and T2WI hyperintensity) [33].

Main Differential Diagnosis

There is a broad list of differential diagnoses, including myelopathy from many different etiologies, which can present overlapping clinical and imaging findings. One should consider the most often as follows:

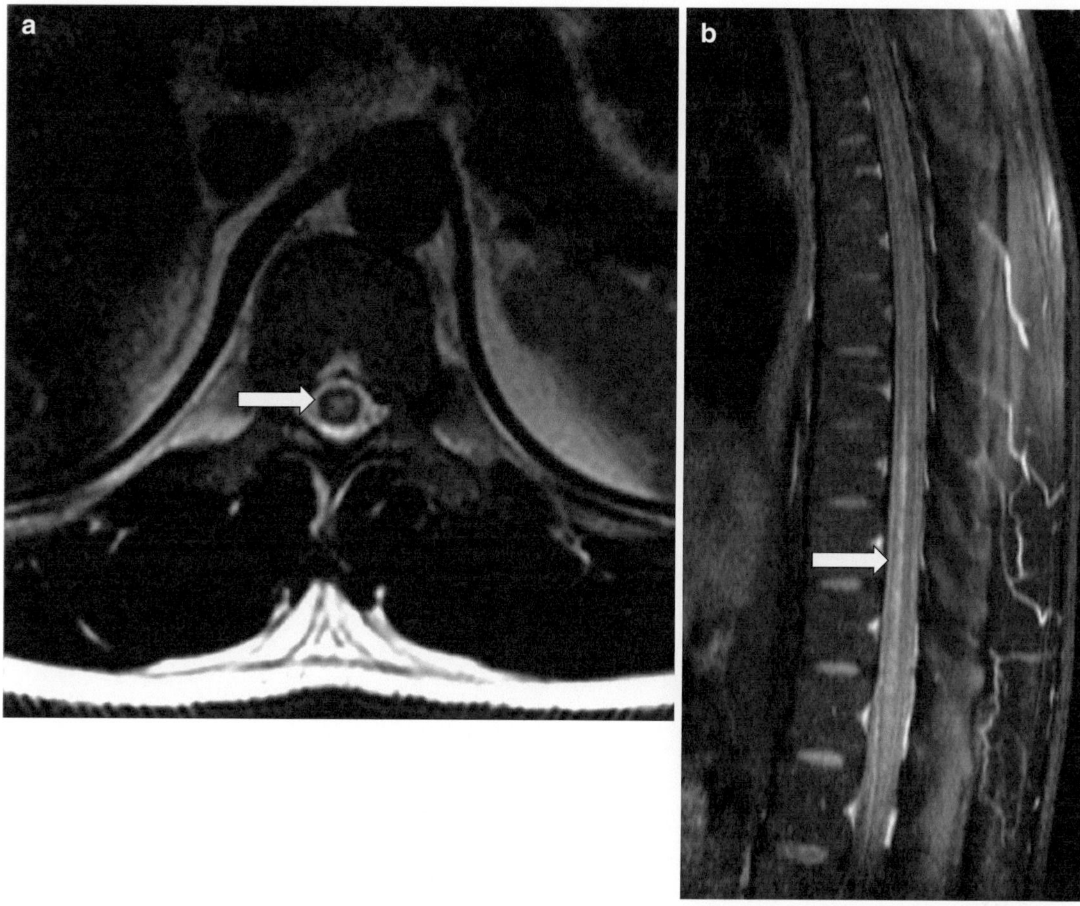

Fig. 48.3 Subacute spinal cord infarction. (**a**) Axial T2WI demonstrates a hyperintense lesion centrally located within the spinal cord at the level of the gray matter. (**b**) Midsagittal postcontrast fat-suppression T1WI shows a pencil-like intramedullary enhancement in the spinal cord. Note that the typical location of the abnormality on the sagittal image is at the junction of the anterior one-third and posterior two-thirds

Myelitis: In the acute phase, inflammatory myelitis is characterized by high signal intensity on T2WI and contrast enhancement on T1WI in about 62–84 % of patients [1, 45] which is not seen in acute stages of SCI. However, in the subacute and chronic stages, the findings are similar for both entities, and the differential diagnosis usually relies on clinical and laboratory basis.

- Viral: Similar imaging findings are described in acute flaccid paralysis related to viral agents that demonstrate tropism to the anterior horns such as enterovirus and poliovirus as well as some flavivirus. In these particular settings, the diagnosis usually relies on clinical, epidemiological, and laboratory results [1, 45].
- Myelitis related to systemic inflammatory diseases such as systemic lupus erythematosus or Sjogren's disease [49].
- Other vascular causes: Even though the clinical presentation is different and usually not abrupt, other vascular diseases such as spinal dural arteriovenous fistula should also be considered [1, 45].

Demyelinating diseases: In this category, neuromyelitis optica and multiple sclerosis should be considered [49]. Different from SCI, MRI shows abnormal signal intensity

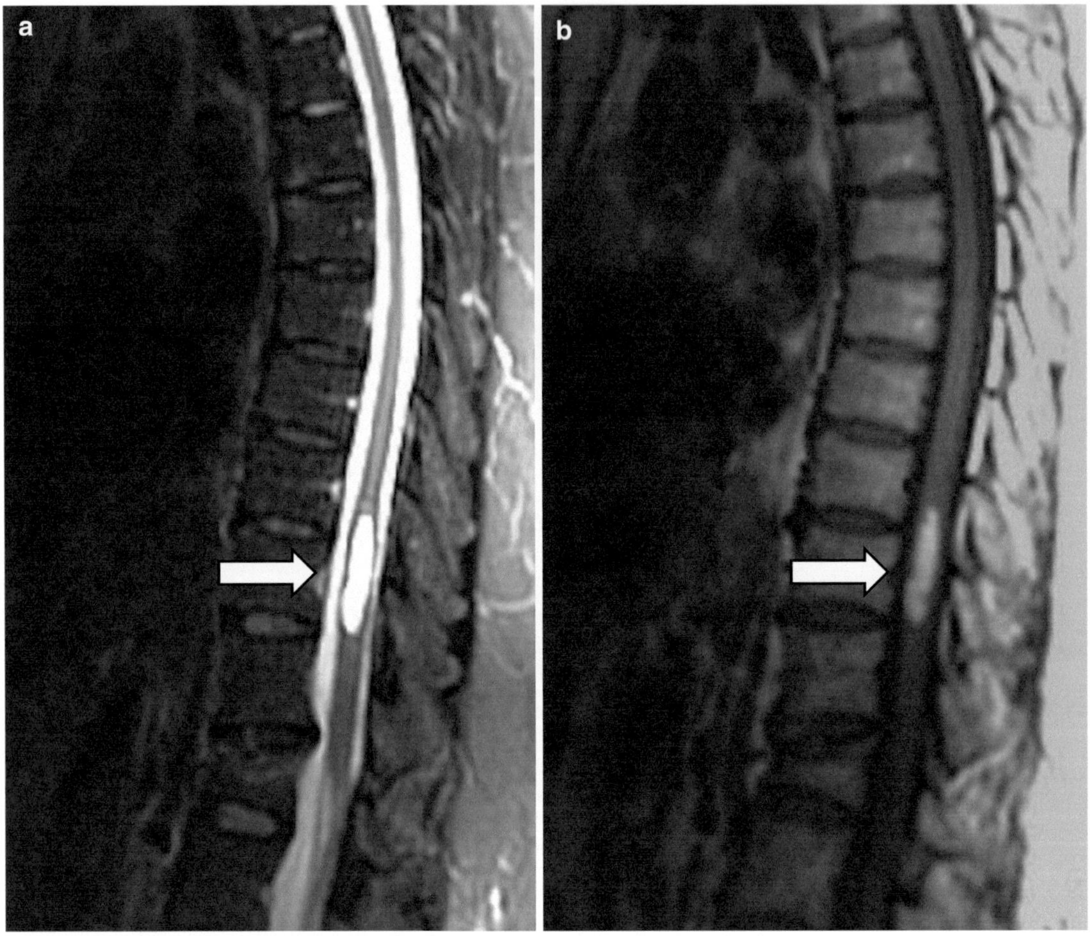

Fig. 48.4 Subacute hemorrhagic necrosis. (**a**) Sagittal fat-suppression T2WI reveals a hyperintense ovoid lesion in the distal spinal cord and conus medullaris (*arrow*). (**b**) Midsagittal T1WI depicts increased signal intensity within the lesion (*arrow*)

on T2WI and variable-associated gadolinium enhancement in the acute stage. Clinical (acute vs. insidious onset) and laboratory findings as well as the distribution of the signal abnormalities in the CNS permit to reach a diagnosis. SC lesions in multiple sclerosis patients are typically peripheral, sharply marginated, well circumscribed, and generally not respecting boundaries between white and gray matter, and the length of cord involvement is typically less than two vertebral bodies (multifocal short and ovoid lesions). On the other hand, neuromyelitis optica usually presents with longitudinal extensive transverse myelitis, hyperintense on T2WI, extending across >3 vertebral segments, usually affecting the spinal central gray matter, and frequently demonstrating higher T2WI hyperintense areas, the so-called bright spotty lesions [8, 37, 50–52].

Lower motor neuron syndromes: Hirayama disease and cervical spondylotic amyotrophy may display variable, unilateral, asymmetric, or bilateral hyperintensities in the anterior horns in axial T2WI similar to the changes seen in SCI. However, in Hirayama disease, imaging studies demonstrate displacement of the posterior cervical dura upon neck flexion with resultant cord

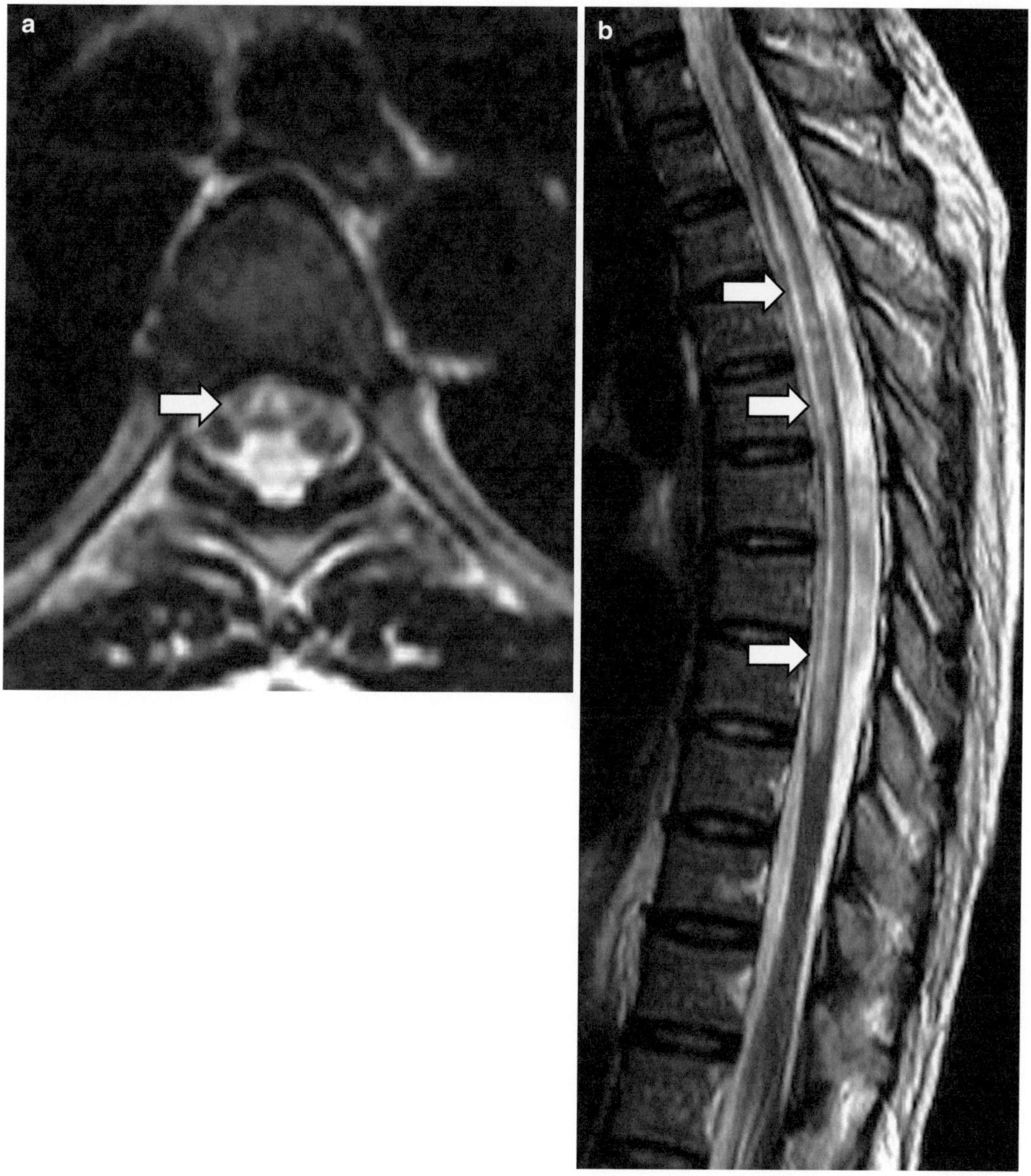

Fig. 48.5 Extensive spinal cord infarction due to hypoperfusion. (**a**) Axial T2WI shows the "owl eye" or "snake eye" sign (*arrow*). (**b**) Sagittal T2WI reveals a longitudinally extensive lesion in the thoracic spinal cord with the typical "pencil-like" appearance (*arrows*)

compression and/or venous congestion. The clinical course of these patients is slow and progressive and characterized by a pure motor focal amyotrophy usually involving the spinal muscles innervated by C7, C8, and T1 [53]. In spondylotic amyotrophy, SC compression is readily demonstrated on imaging, and the clinical presentation is characterized by upper extremity weakness and atrophy, affecting either proximal or distal musculature without sensory impairment or lower extremity dysfunction [54, 55].

Table 48.1 Spinal cord ischemia syndromes

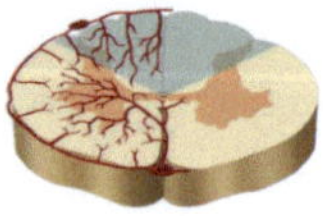	**Syndrome**	**Imaging**	**Clinical presentation**
A. 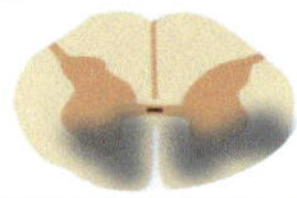	Anterior spinal artery infarct	Limited to the anterior horns and the surrounding white matter	Bilateral motor deficit with spinothalamic sensory deficit (centromedullary infarct syndrome)
B. 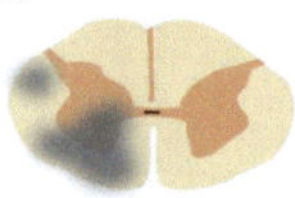	Spinal sulcal artery infarct	Unilateral involvement of one anterior horn	Hemiparesis with contralateral spinothalamic sensory deficit
C. 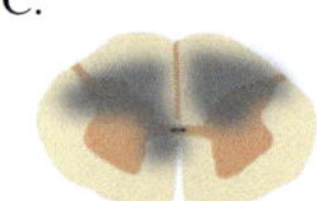	Posterior spinal artery infarct	Bilateral posterolateral involvement	Bilateral motor deficit with lemniscal sensory deficit
D. 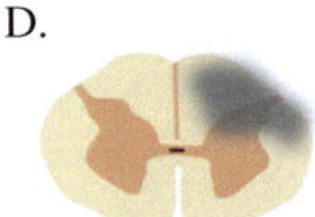	Posterior unilateral infarct	Restricted to one posterior column or extends into the ipsilateral posterolateral region	Hemiparesis with homolateral lemniscal sensory deficit
E. 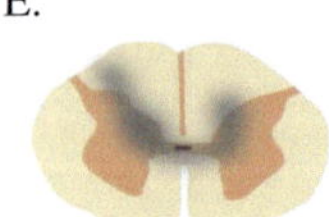	Central infarct	Limited around the anterior sulcus with a crescent shape	Bilateral sensory deficit without motor deficit
F. 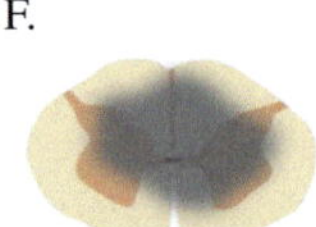	Transverse infarct	Involves the anterior and posterior columns and extends into both anterolateral and posterolateral regions	Complete transverse spinal cord syndrome

Fig. 48.6 "Owl eye" or "snake eye" typical appearance of acute spinal cord infarction. Axial T2WI demonstrates hyperintense lesions affecting exclusively the anterior horns of the spinal cord (Courtesy of Lazaro Amaral, Sao Paulo, Brazil)

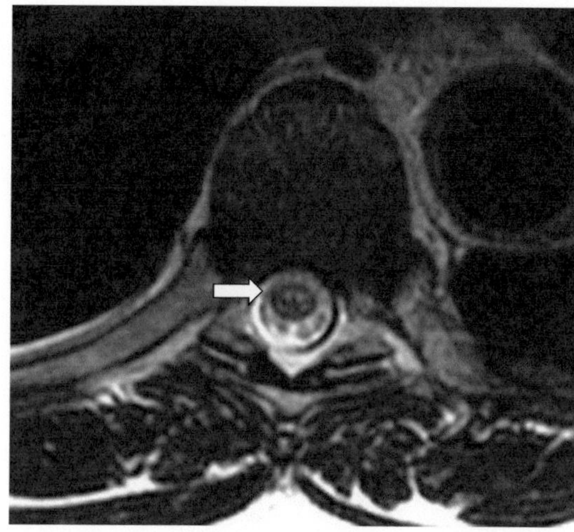

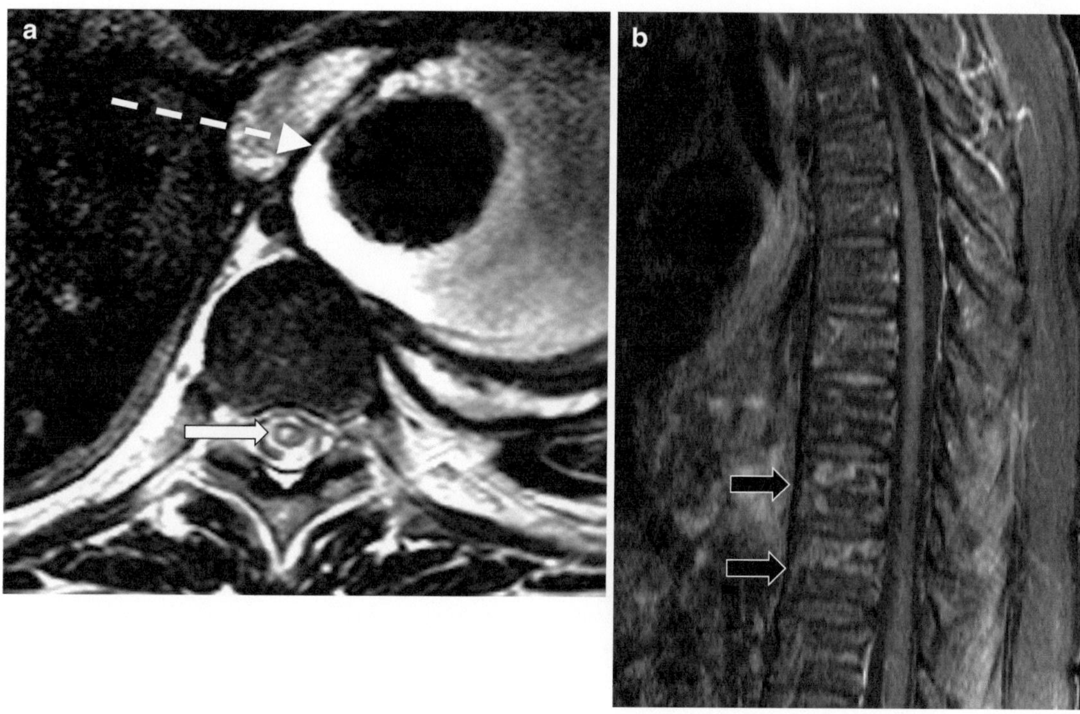

Fig. 48.7 Unilateral spinal cord ischemia associated with vertebral body infarcts. (**a**) Axial T2WI shows hyperintense lesion in the right anterior horn due to unilateral involvement of the spinal cord (*solid arrow*) and a large aortic aneurysm (*dashed arrow*). (**b**) Midsagittal postcontrast fat-suppression T1WI demonstrates abnormal bone marrow enhancement involving multiple vertebrae, especially T11 and T12 levels (*arrows* on **b**), predominantly in areas near the end plates and at the same level as the spinal cord abnormality

Tips

- The key for the diagnosis of SCI is its sudden onset and rapid progression within less than 4 h of the ictus. At times, a stepwise progression may occur.
- Conventional MRI is usually normal in the hyperacute phase, but it is recommended in all cases of acute myelopathy and not only for the diagnosis but also to exclude other treatable causes of cord lesions (e.g., acute compression). Acutely, the diagnosis of SCI may be confirmed using DWI.
- Typical imaging findings of ischemia compromising ASA territories include hyperintense intramedullary lesions confined to the anterior horn area with the classic *owl eye or snake eye* appearance on axial images.
- Remember to look for arterial dissection (aorta and vertebral arteries).
- The common vascularization of the vertebral body, disk, and SC may result in concomitant SC and vertebral body infarcts.

References

1. De Seze J, Stojkovic T, Breteau G, Lucas C, Michon-Pasturel U, Gauvrit JY, et al. Acute myelopathies: clinical, laboratory and outcome profiles in 79 cases. Brain. 2001;124(Pt 8):1509–21. [cited 2015 Mar 24] Available from: http://www.ncbi.nlm.nih.gov/pubmed/11459743.
2. Sandson TA, Friedman JH. Spinal cord infarction. Report of 8 cases and review of the literature. Medicine (Baltimore). 1989;68(5):282–92. [cited 2015 Mar 24]. Available from: http://www.ncbi.nlm.nih.gov/pubmed/2677596.
3. Larsson EM, Desai P, Hardin CW, Story J, Jinkins JR. Venous infarction of the spinal cord resulting from dural arteriovenous fistula: MR imaging findings. Am J Neuroradiol. 1991;12(4):739–43.
4. Weidauer S, Nichtweiß M, Hattingen E, Berkefeld J. Spinal cord ischemia: aetiology, clinical syndromes and imaging features. Neuroradiology. 2014;57(3):241–57. Available from: http://link.springer.com/10.1007/s00234-014-1464-6.
5. Lynch K, Oster J, Apetauerova D, Hreib K. Spinal cord stroke: acute imaging and intervention. Case Rep Neurol Med. 2012;2012:706780. [cited 2015 Mar 30]. Available from: http://www.pubmedcentral.nih.gov/articlerender.fcgi?artid=3420482&tool=pmcentrez&rendertype=abstract.
6. Romanes GJ. The arterial blood supply of the human spinal cord. Paraplegia. 1965;2:199–207. [cited 2015 Mar 31]. Available from: http://www.ncbi.nlm.nih.gov/pubmed/14261502.
7. Lazorthes G, Poulhes J, Bastide G, Roulleau J, Chancholle AR. Arterial vascularization of the spine; anatomic research and applications in pathology of the spinal cord and aorta. Neurochirurgie. 1958;4(1):3–19. [cited 2015 Mar 31]. Available from: http://www.ncbi.nlm.nih.gov/pubmed/13552909.
8. Vargas MI, Gariani J, Sztajzel R, Barnaure-Nachbar I, Delattre BM, Lovblad KO, et al. Spinal cord ischemia: practical imaging tips, pearls, and pitfalls. AJNR Am J Neuroradiol. [Internet]. 2014 Oct 16 [cited 2015 Mar 31]; Available from: http://www.ncbi.nlm.nih.gov/pubmed/25324492.
9. Backes WH, Nijenhuis RJ. Advances in spinal cord MR angiography. Am J Neuroradiol. 2008;29:619–31.
10. Turnbull IM, Brieg A, Hassler O. Blood supply of cervical spinal cord in man. A microangiographic cadaver study. J Neurosurg. 1966;24(6):951–65. [cited 2015 Mar 31]. Available from: http://www.ncbi.nlm.nih.gov/pubmed/5936484.
11. Gailloud P. The artery of von Haller: a constant anterior radiculomedullary artery at the upper thoracic level. Neurosurgery. 2013;73(6):1034–43.
12. Skalski JH, Zembala M. Albert Wojciech Adamkiewicz: the discoverer of the variable vascularity of the spinal cord. Ann Thorac Surg. 2005;80(5):1971–5. [cited 2015 Mar 31]. Available from: http://www.ncbi.nlm.nih.gov/pubmed/16242505.
13. Koshino T, Murakami G, Morishita K, Mawatari T, Abe T. Does the Adamkiewicz artery originate from the larger segmental arteries? J Thorac Cardiovasc Surg. 1999;117(5):898–905. [cited 2015 Mar 31]. Available from: http://www.ncbi.nlm.nih.gov/pubmed/10220681.
14. Kumral E, Polat F, Güllüoglu H, Uzunköprü C, Tuncel R, Alpaydin S. Spinal ischaemic stroke: clinical and radiological findings and short-term outcome. Eur J Neurol. 2011;18(2):232–9. [cited 2015 Mar 4]. Available from: http://www.ncbi.nlm.nih.gov/pubmed/20402756.
15. Novy J, Carruzzo A, Maeder P, Bogousslavsky J. Spinal cord ischemia: clinical and imaging patterns, pathogenesis, and outcomes in 27 patients. Arch Neurol. 2006;63(8):1113–20. [cited 2015 Mar 4] Available from: http://www.ncbi.nlm.nih.gov/pubmed/16908737.
16. Kaneki M, Inoue K, Shimizu T, Mannen T. Infarction of the unilateral posterior horn and lateral column of the spinal cord with sparing of posterior columns: demonstration by MRI. J Neurol Neurosurg Psychiatry. 1994;57(5):629–31. [cited 2015 Mar 30]. Available from: http://www.pubmedcentral.nih.gov/

articlerender.fcgi?artid=1072931&tool=pmcentrez&rendertype=abstract.
17. Pullicino P. Bilateral distal upper limb amyotrophy and watershed infarcts from vertebral dissection. Stroke. 1994;25(9):1870–2. [cited 2015 Apr 2]. Available from: http://www.ncbi.nlm.nih.gov/pubmed/8073471.
18. Gelfan S, Tarlov IM. Differential vulnerability of spinal cord structures to anoxia. J Neurophysiol. 1955;18(2):170–88. [cited 2015 Apr 2]. Available from: http://www.ncbi.nlm.nih.gov/pubmed/14354454.
19. Berg D, Müllges W, Koltzenburg M, Bendszus M, Reiners K. Man-in-the-barrel syndrome caused by cervical spinal cord infarction. Acta Neurol Scand. 1998;97(6):417–9. [cited 2015 Apr 2]. Available from: http://www.ncbi.nlm.nih.gov/pubmed/9669478.
20. Weidauer S, Nichtweiß M, Hattingen E, Berkefeld J. Spinal cord ischemia: aetiology, clinical syndromes and imaging features. Neuroradiology. 2014;57(3):241–57. [cited 2015 Feb 6]. Available from: http://www.ncbi.nlm.nih.gov/pubmed/25398656.
21. Stapf C, Mohr JP, Straschill M, Mast H, Marx P. Acute bilateral arm paresis. Cerebrovasc Dis. 2000;10(3):239–43. [cited 2015 Apr 2]. Available from: http://www.ncbi.nlm.nih.gov/pubmed/10773652.
22. Hsu C-Y, Cheng C-Y, Lee J-D, Lee M, Huang Y-C, Wu C-Y, et al. Clinical features and outcomes of spinal cord infarction following vertebral artery dissection: a systematic review of the literature. Neurol Res. 2013;35(7):676–83. [cited 2015 Mar 31]. Available from: http://www.ncbi.nlm.nih.gov/pubmed/23562138.
23. Ghandehari K, Gerami Sarabi MR, Maarufi P. Clinical evaluation of patients with spinal cord infarction in Mashhad, Iran. Stroke Res Treat. 2010;2010:942417. [cited 2015 Mar 31]. Available from: http://www.pubmedcentral.nih.gov/articlerender.fcgi?artid=2964906&tool=pmcentrez&rendertype=abstract.
24. Oh JY, Kapoor S, Koh RK, Yang EW, Hee H-T. Spinal cord ischemia secondary to hypovolemic shock. Asian Spine J. 2014;8(6):831–4. [cited 2015 Mar 31]. Available from: http://www.pubmedcentral.nih.gov/articlerender.fcgi?artid=4278991&tool=pmcentrez&rendertype=abstract.
25. Mikulis DJ, Ogilvy CS, McKee A, Davis KR, Ojeman RG. Spinal cord infarction and fibrocartilaginous emboli. AJNR Am J Neuroradiol. 1992;13(1):155–60. [cited 2015 Mar 31]. Available from: http://www.ncbi.nlm.nih.gov/pubmed/1595434.
26. Ii Y, Maki T, Furuta T, Kuzuhara S. Cervical spinal cord infarction in a patient with cervical spondylosis triggered by straining during bowel movement. J Clin Neurosci. 2009;16(1):106–7. [cited 2015 Mar 31]. Available from: http://www.ncbi.nlm.nih.gov/pubmed/19013809.
27. Mateen FJ, Monrad PA, Leep Hunderfund AN, Robertson CE, Sorenson EJ. Clinically suspected fibrocartilaginous embolism: clinical characteristics, treatments, and outcomes. Eur J Neurol. 2011;18(2):218–25.
28. Márquez JC, Granados AM, Castillo M. MRI of cervical spinal cord infarction in a patient with sickle cell disease. Clin Imaging. 2012;36(5):595–8. [cited 2015 Mar 31]. Available from: http://www.ncbi.nlm.nih.gov/pubmed/22920369.
29. Lyders EM, Morris PP. A case of spinal cord infarction following lumbar transforaminal epidural steroid injection: MR imaging and angiographic findings. AJNR Am J Neuroradiol. 2009;30(9):1691–3. [cited 2015 Mar 31]. Available from: http://www.ncbi.nlm.nih.gov/pubmed/19369604.
30. Weidauer S, Nichtweiss M, Lanfermann H, Zanella FE. Spinal cord infarction: MR imaging and clinical features in 16 cases. Neuroradiology. 2002;44(10):851–7. [cited 2015 Mar 31]. Available from: http://www.ncbi.nlm.nih.gov/pubmed/12389137.
31. Katramados AM, Rabah R, Adams MD, Huq AHMM, Mitsias PD. Longitudinal myelitis, aseptic meningitis, and conus medullaris infarction as presenting manifestations of pediatric systemic lupus erythematosus. Lupus. 2008;17(4):332–6. [cited 2015 Apr 2]. Available from: http://www.ncbi.nlm.nih.gov/pubmed/18413416.
32. Chang CWJ, Donovan DJ, Liem LK, O'Phelan KH, Green DM, Bassin S, et al. Surfers' myelopathy: a case series of 19 novice surfers with nontraumatic myelopathy. Neurology. 2012;79(22):2171–6.
33. Marcel C, Kremer S, Jeantroux J, Blanc F, Dietemann J-L, De Sèze J. Diffusion-weighted imaging in noncompressive myelopathies: a 33-patient prospective study. J Neurol. 2010;257(9):1438–45. [cited 2015 Mar 31]. Available from: http://www.ncbi.nlm.nih.gov/pubmed/20425119.
34. Sagiuchi T, Iida H, Tachibana S, Kusumi M, Kan S, Fujii K. Case report: diffusion-weighted MRI in anterior spinal artery stroke of the cervical spinal cord. J Comput Assist Tomogr. 2003;27(3):410–4. [cited 2015 Mar 31]. Available from: http://www.ncbi.nlm.nih.gov/pubmed/12794607.
35. Fujikawa A, Tsuchiya K, Takeuchi S, Hachiya J. Diffusion-weighted MR imaging in acute spinal cord ischemia. Eur Radiol. 2004;14(11):2076–8. [cited 2015 Mar 31]. Available from: http://www.ncbi.nlm.nih.gov/pubmed/15022011.
36. Andre JB, Zaharchuk G, Saritas E, Komakula S, Shankaranarayan A, Banerjee S, et al. Clinical evaluation of reduced field-of-view diffusion-weighted imaging of the cervical and thoracic spine and spinal cord. Am J Neuroradiol. 2012;33(10):1860–6.
37. Alblas CL, Bouvy WH, Lycklama À, Nijeholt GJ, Boitena J. Acute spinal-cord ischemia: evolution of MRI findings. J Clin Neurol (Korea). 2012;8:218–23.
38. Hyodoh H, Shirase R, Kawaharada N, Hyodoh K, Sato T, Onodera M, et al. MR angiography for detecting the artery of Adamkiewicz and its branching level from the aorta. Magn Reson Med Sci. 2009;8(4):159–64. [cited 2015 Jun 9]. Available from: http://www.ncbi.nlm.nih.gov/pubmed/20035124.
39. Mordasini P, El-Koussy M, Schmidli J, Bonel HM, Ith M, Gralla J, et al. Preoperative mapping of arterial

spinal supply using 3.0-T MR angiography with an intravasal contrast medium and high-spatial-resolution steady-state. Eur J Radiol. 2012;81(5):979–84. [cited 2015 Jun 9]. Available from: http://www.ncbi.nlm.nih.gov/pubmed/21377307.

40. Yamamoto S, Kanaya H, Kim P. Spinal intraarterial computed tomography angiography as an effective adjunct for spinal angiography. J Neurosurg Spine. 2015;29:1–8. [cited 2015 Jun 10]. Available from: http://www.ncbi.nlm.nih.gov/pubmed/26023900.
41. Nishii T, Kono AK, Negi N, Hashimura H, Uotani K, Okita Y, et al. The feasibility of a 64-slice MDCT for detection of the Adamkiewicz artery: comparison of the detection rate of intravenous injection CT angiography using a 64-slice MDCT versus intra-arterial and intravenous injection CT angiography using a 16-slice MDCT. Int J Cardiovasc Imaging. 2013;29 Suppl 2:127–33. [cited 2015 Jun 9]. Available from: http://www.ncbi.nlm.nih.gov/pubmed/24081485.
42. Yuh WT, Marsh EE, Wang AK, Russell JW, Chiang F, Koci TM, et al. MR imaging of spinal cord and vertebral body infarction. AJNR Am J Neuroradiol. 1992;13(1):145–54.
43. Ghosh PS, Mitra S. Owl's eye in spinal magnetic resonance imaging. Arch Neurol. 2012;69(3):407–8. [cited 2015 Apr 1]. Available from: http://www.ncbi.nlm.nih.gov/pubmed/22410453.
44. Zhang Z, Wang H. Is the "snake-eye" MRI sign correlated to anterior spinal artery occlusion on CT angiography in cervical spondylotic myelopathy and amyotrophy? Eur Spine J. 2014;23(7):1541–7. [cited 2015 Apr 1]. Available from: http://www.ncbi.nlm.nih.gov/pubmed/24823850.
45. Nowak DA, Mutzenbach S, Fuchs HH. Acute myelopathy. Retrospective clinical, laboratory, MRI and outcome analysis of 49 cases. J Clin Neurosci. 2004;11(2):145–52. [cited 2015 Apr 1]. Available from: http://www.ncbi.nlm.nih.gov/pubmed/14732373.
46. Faig J, Busse O, Salbeck R. Vertebral body infarction as a confirmatory sign of spinal cord ischemic stroke: report of three cases and review of the literature. Stroke. 1998;29(1):239–43. [cited 2015 Apr 1]. Available from: http://www.ncbi.nlm.nih.gov/pubmed/9445357.
47. Amoiridis G, Ameridou I, Mavridis M. Intervertebral disk and vertebral body infarction as a confirmatory sign of spinal cord ischemia. Neurology. 2004;63(9):1755. [cited 2015 Apr 1]. Available from: http://www.ncbi.nlm.nih.gov/pubmed/15534280.
48. Duprez TP, Danvoye L, Hernalsteen D, Cosnard G, Sindic CJ, Godfraind C. Fibrocartilaginous embolization to the spinal cord: serial MR imaging monitoring and pathologic study. Am J Neuroradiol. 2005;26(3):496–501.
49. Hess CW. Non-traumatic acute transverse spinal cord syndromes. Praxis (Bern 1994). 2005;94(30–31):1151–9. [cited 2015 Apr 1]. Available from: http://www.ncbi.nlm.nih.gov/pubmed/16117470.
50. Grayev AM, Kissane J, Kanekar S. Imaging approach to the cord T2 hyperintensity (myelopathy). Radiol Clin N Am. 2014;52(2):427–46. [cited 2015 Mar 30]. Available from: http://www.ncbi.nlm.nih.gov/pubmed/24582348.
51. Rathnasabapathi D, Elsone L, Krishnan A, Young C, Larner A, Jacob A. Solitary sclerosis: progressive neurological deficit from a spatially isolated demyelinating lesion: a further report. J Spinal Cord Med [Internet]. 2015 Jan 23 [cited 2015 Apr 1]; Available from: http://www.ncbi.nlm.nih.gov/pubmed/25615515.
52. Yonezu T, Ito S, Mori M, Ogawa Y, Makino T, Uzawa A, et al. "Bright spotty lesions" on spinal magnetic resonance imaging differentiate neuromyelitis optica from multiple sclerosis. Mult Scler. 2014;20(3):331–7. [cited 2015 Apr 1]. Available from: http://www.ncbi.nlm.nih.gov/pubmed/23828869.
53. Foster E, Tsang BK-T, Kam A, Storey E, Day B, Hill A. Hirayama disease. J Clin Neurosci. 2015;22(6):951–4. [cited 2015 May 10]. Available from: http://www.ncbi.nlm.nih.gov/pubmed/25766368.
54. Gebere-Michael SG, Johnston JC, Metaferia GZ, Wuhib MZ, Fernandez HH. Bilaterally symmetric cervical spondylotic amyotrophy: a novel presentation and review of the literature. J Neurol Sci. 2010;290(1–2):142–5. [cited 2015 Jun 10]. Available from: http://www.ncbi.nlm.nih.gov/pubmed/20045121.
55. Kong L-D, Wang L-F, Zhang J-T, Zhang Y-Z, Ding W-Y, Shen Y. Predictive factors relating to prognosis of anterior decompressive surgery for proximal-type cervical spondylotic amyotrophy. J Back Musculoskelet Rehabil. 2015;28(2):261–6. [cited 2015 May 24]. Available from: http://www.ncbi.nlm.nih.gov/pubmed/25096308.

Spinal Cord Masses in Adults

49

Marcio Marques Moreira and
Lázaro Luís Faria do Amaral

Abstract

Intramedullary spinal cord neoplasms are rare central nervous system tumors. Despite their rarity, these lesions are important to the radiologist and imaging is performed to narrow the clinical differential diagnosis and guide surgical resection. Spinal cord ependymomas are the most common type of cord tumors in adults and along with cord astrocytomas constitute up to 70 % of all intramedullary neoplasms. Cord hemangioblastomas are the third most common type of intramedullary spinal tumor. Metastatic disease is characterized by prominent cord edema for the size of the enhancing lesion and is becoming more common as cancer patients survive longer.

Background

Intramedullary spinal cord tumors refer to a subgroup of intradural spinal tumors that arise from cells within the spinal cord. They account for 20 % of all intraspinal tumors in adults [1], with a peak incidence in the fourth to fifth decades of life [2].

The clinical presentation of intramedullary tumors depends on their size and location. Initially, patients often present with mild symptoms, including local or radiating pain. Motor weakness, gait problems, and bowel and bladder dysfunction may present in later stages of the disease. An exception is intramedullary metastases, which are frequently symptomatic [1, 2].

Since most of intramedullary spinal cord tumors are low grade, surgical biopsy and resection are indicated in individuals with progressive neurologic decline. There are no significant benefits with adjuvant radiation and chemotherapy. Generally, such therapies are reserved for malignant gliomas (WHO grades 3–4) [3]. Predictors of a good outcome after surgery for intramedullary

M.M. Moreira, MD
Radiology Department, Medimagem – Hospital Beneficência Portuguesa de São Paulo, Sao Paulo, SP, Brazil
e-mail: moreirammarcio@gmail.com

L.L.F. do Amaral, MD (✉)
Division of Neuroradiology, Medimagem – Hospital Beneficência Portuguesa de São Paulo, Sao Paulo, SP, Brazil

Division of Neuroradiology, Hospital Santa Casa de Misericórdia de São Paulo, Rua Dr. Cesário Motta Junior 112, Vila Buarque, Sao Paulo, SP 01221-020, Brazil
e-mail: lazden@terra.com.br

R. Hoffmann Nunes et al. (eds.), *Critical Findings in Neuroradiology*,
DOI 10.1007/978-3-319-27987-9_49

spinal cord tumors are the complete removal of the lesion and a good neurological status before surgery [4].

Key Points

Etiology

The majority of spinal cord neoplasms encountered in routine practice are glial tumors, making up for about 95 % of all intramedullary tumors with ependymoma being the most frequent (40–60 %) followed by astrocytoma. Hemangioblastoma is the third most frequent intramedullary tumor in adults [2, 5].

Ependymoma: These tumors arise from the ependymal cells that line the spinal central canal. They are centrally located within the spinal cord and are well circumscribed although not encapsulated. Cyst formation and hemorrhage are common especially at the tumor margins. Calcification is uncommon in contrast to intracranial ependymomas which often calcify. Ependymal cells with uniform hyperchromatic nuclei arranged in perivascular pseudorosettes are typical findings on histologic examination. The cellular type is the most common histology and is often located in the cervical spine. Myxopapillary ependymomas occur almost exclusively in the conus medullaris and filum terminale [5]. Tanycytic ependymoma is a rare subtype that is distinct and contains more fibrillar cells; these tumors are usually more eccentrically located [6].

Astrocytoma: Spinal cord astrocytomas are usually eccentrically located, characterized by ill-defined diffuse and fusiform enlargement of the cord. Hypercellularity without a surrounding capsule and an infiltrative pattern suggests this histological type. Almost two-thirds of spinal cord astrocytomas are low grade (pilocytic and fibrillary astrocytomas) [2]. At the time of diagnosis, they usually involve several segments and the thoracic cord as the most common site followed by the cervical cord. Cysts are a common feature, with polar and intratumoral ones, whereas calcifications and hemorrhages are rare [7]. Few spinal cord astrocytomas are anaplastic in nature. Glioblastomas represent about 7.5 % of all intramedullary gliomas and 1–3 % of all spinal cord tumors [8].

Hemangioblastoma: The majority of spinal cord hemangioblastomas are intramedullary, occur in the cervical or thoracic levels, are usually subpial in location, and often have enlarged feeding arteries and draining veins [9, 10]. They occur sporadically or in association with von Hippel–Lindau disease. The presence of a small superficially located tumor with a large syrinx is considered a characteristic imaging pattern. The presence of vascular flow voids are observed in or around medium-sized to larger tumors [10, 11].

Metastases: Intramedullary spinal cord metastases are rare and portray poor prognosis with short median survival (3–4 months) after diagnosis. Lung cancer is the most common primary tumor followed by breast cancer [12, 13].

Others spinal cord tumors: Spinal paragangliomas are neoplasms of neuroendocrine origin, highly vascular lesions, usually found in the conus medullaris, cauda equina, or filum terminale [7]. Intramedullary lymphomas may present as focal or multifocal lesions and with less cord enlargement than seen with other intramedullary tumors [9].

Best Imaging Modality

The imaging modality of choice for the evaluation of spinal cord tumors is Magnetic Resonance Imaging (MRI) which allows determination of location and characteristics of the mass without ionizing radiation [5].

Computed tomography (CT) often fails to reveal the true extent of intramedullary spinal neoplasms until gross expansion of the spinal canal has occurred. Myelography, either with radiography or CT, reveals an intramedullary mass as well as a complete or partial block to the flow of intrathecal contrast material, a nonspecific finding [5].

The administration of intravenous paramagnetic MRI contrast agent allows for the identification of the solid portions of the lesion and associated cysts as well as other features that help narrow the differential diagnosis. Mapping the location of the solid-enhancing portions of a tumor is vital as their extent dictates the need for number of laminectomies employed [5, 14].

Radiography and CT are considered useful to detect skeletal abnormalities such as mild scoliosis, widened interpedicular distance, and scalloping of the dorsal surface of the vertebral bodies. The MRI protocol must include T1-weighted images (T1WI) and T2-weighted images (T2WI) in the sagittal and axial plane, followed by contrast material-enhanced T1WI in at least two planes. Gradient-echo T2* is sensitive in detecting hemorrhage, calcification, and flow voids.

For any spinal cord mass, the visualized lungs should be scrutinized because lung cancer is a common cause for cord metastases [13].

Conventional or MR angiography may be used as supplementary techniques for characterizing vascular flow voids [10].

Diffusion-weighted imaging (DWI) and diffusion-tensor imaging (DTI) have been applied to the spinal cord particularly for presurgical planning. Spinal cord DTI may aid to differentiate astrocytomas from ependymomas, because of the typical infiltrating nature of astrocytomas as compared with ependymomas, which tend to displace rather than disrupt white matter tracts [15].

Major Findings

The essential imaging criterion for an intramedullary neoplasm is cord expansion. Almost all neoplasms, including low-grade forms, enhance after intravenous contrast material [5].

Associated cysts are common findings. Nontumoral cysts, also called polar cysts, do not enhance and probably represent a reactive dilatation of the central canal. Tumoral cysts are contained within the mass itself and frequently show peripheral enhancement [5].

Ependymoma: It is a central located and well-circumscribed mass commonly hyperintense on T2WI. Intramedullary ependymomas are usually hypo- or isointense to spinal cord on T1WI, whereas those of the myxopapillary subtype present with mild high signal on T1WI. All demonstrate intense and variable contrast enhancement. Cystic formation and hemorrhage are common particularly in larger ones. Some ependymomas demonstrate the "cap sign," especially seen on T2WI, with hypointensity rostral and caudal of the tumor representing hemosiderin deposits secondary to hemorrhage (Fig. 49.1) [5, 7, 9].

Astrocytoma: This tumor is seen as an eccentric mass with poorly defined margins, cystic components, and associated edema and syrinx. Typically, the tumor affects fewer than four segments of the spinal cord in length. They are usually iso- to hypointense relative to the spinal cord on T1WI and hyperintense on T2WI, showing enhancement in a patchy, irregular fashion. Nonenhancing intramedullary astrocytomas are uncommon but must be included in the differential diagnosis of a prominent mass with cord expansion [9, 16]. Intramedullary glioblastoma has a predilection to develop in the cervical region in most cases (Fig. 49.2). Some patients develop hydrocephalus which is thought to be due to increased protein concentration in CSF. Seeding by an intracranial glioblastoma of the spine occurs in some patients, but the reverse process is extremely uncommon [8].

Hemangioblastoma: Small hemangioblastomas (<10 mm) are mostly isointense on T1WI and hyperintense on T2WI and show homogeneous enhancement. Larger hemangioblastomas tend to be hypointense or mixed hypo- and isointense on T1WI images and heterogeneous on T2WI images with intermixed flow voids and show heterogeneous contrast enhancement. Extensive spinal cord swelling is also common. The presence of cysts and/or syringohydromyelia is commonly reported (Figs. 49.3 and 49.4) [10].

Metastases: Spinal cord swelling, with extensive spinal cord T2 hyperintensity, often disproportional when compared with the enhancing portion of the lesion is a typical imaging finding (Fig. 49.5). Intratumoral hemorrhage and cystic/necrotic changes are rare in cord metastases [13]. Two enhancement features on MRI have been described as suggestive of spinal cord metastasis compared with primary cord masses including a more intense thin rim of peripheral enhancement around an enhancing lesion (rim sign) and an ill-defined flame-shaped region of enhancement at the superior/inferior margins (flame sign) [17].

Imaging Follow-Up

Recommended follow-up and prognosis is dependent upon histology. Generally 4- to 6-month follow-up MRI is recommended for intramedullary tumors. In a postoperative assessment, a contrast-enhanced MRI is useful for establishing the presence of residual/recurrent tumor [4, 5, 18].

Patients should be followed clinically and by imaging. The vast majority of patients will have some degree of new proprioceptive dysfunction post operatively that may require physical therapy. Immediate postoperative imaging is usually not performed, and most clinicians delay imaging for a period of months after surgery unless acute complications ensue. Routine interval imaging is required for years thereafter even after gross total resection. If neurological function worsens, immediate reimaging is warranted. Residual tumor can undergo repeat resection, radiation therapy, or observation. If tumor recurrence is noted, imaging the entire neuraxis is warranted to rule out distant seeding through CSF [4, 18].

For hemangioblastomas, complete surgical resection of sporadic cases is usually curative. Patients with von Hippel–Lindau are at risk of developing new lesions and must have their entire neuraxis imaged annually [4, 5, 18].

Regarding astrocytoma, the literature is confusing and often contradictory regarding the role of surgery, radiation, and prognosis in general. Undoubtedly, the prognosis for astrocytoma is worse than that of ependymoma because astrocytomas are infiltrative and impossible to resect completely [4, 5, 18].

Surgical series of ependymomas report low recurrence rates. Factors associated with recurrence include initial partial resection and the presence of histological anaplasia. Unlike the findings seen in patients with cord ependymomas, the amount of resected astrocytoma seems not to have an effect on survival. Even in cases of gross total resection, patients with astrocytomas have higher mortality rates than those with ependymomas. This poor prognosis is likely a reflection of the infiltrative nature of astrocytomas and is due to the fact that neoplastic astrocytes extend far beyond the apparent gross tumor margins and provide a source of tumor progression postoperatively. Second, because malignant cells may extend along the network of normal axonal processes, removal of all neoplastic tissues invariably will also necessitate resection of normal functioning cord tissues which increases the likelihood of postoperative neurological deficits [5].

Fig. 49.1 Ependymoma, different histological subtypes. (**a–c**) Cellular ependymoma in a 33-year-old man. Sagittal T1WI and T2WI (**a**, **b**) demonstrate a cervicothoracic cord mass displaying small polar cysts (*arrows*). Sagittal postcontrast fat-suppressed T1WI (**c**) shows an intense and well-defined homogeneously enhancing mass centrally located in the cord. (**d**, **e**) "Cap sign" demonstrated in a 55-year-old man with a cellular ependymoma. Sagittal T1WI and T2WI demonstrate a heterogeneous cervical cord mass with hemosiderin deposits located superiorly and inferiorly (*dashed arrows*) which is a common finding in ependymomas. (**f–h**) Tanycytic ependymoma in a 48-year-old man presenting with a progressive spinal cord syndrome. Sagittal and coronal T2WI (**f**, **g**) reveal an eccentric lesion in upper thoracic spinal cord. Sagittal postcontrast fat-suppressed T1WI (**h**) shows peripheral and heterogeneous contrast enhancement (*arrow*) in the inferior tumor margin. (i–**l**) Myxopapillary ependymoma in a 37-year-old man presenting with low back pain. Sagittal T1WI, T2WI, and postcontrast fat-suppressed T1WI (**i–k**) depict a large heterogeneous-enhancing intradural mass extending from the conus medullaris to the level of S2, expanding the spinal canal, and causing scalloping of the vertebral bodies. In addition, midsagittal postcontrast fat-suppressed T1WI (**l**) demonstrates multiple enhancing nodular lesions in the thoracic level due to CSF dissemination

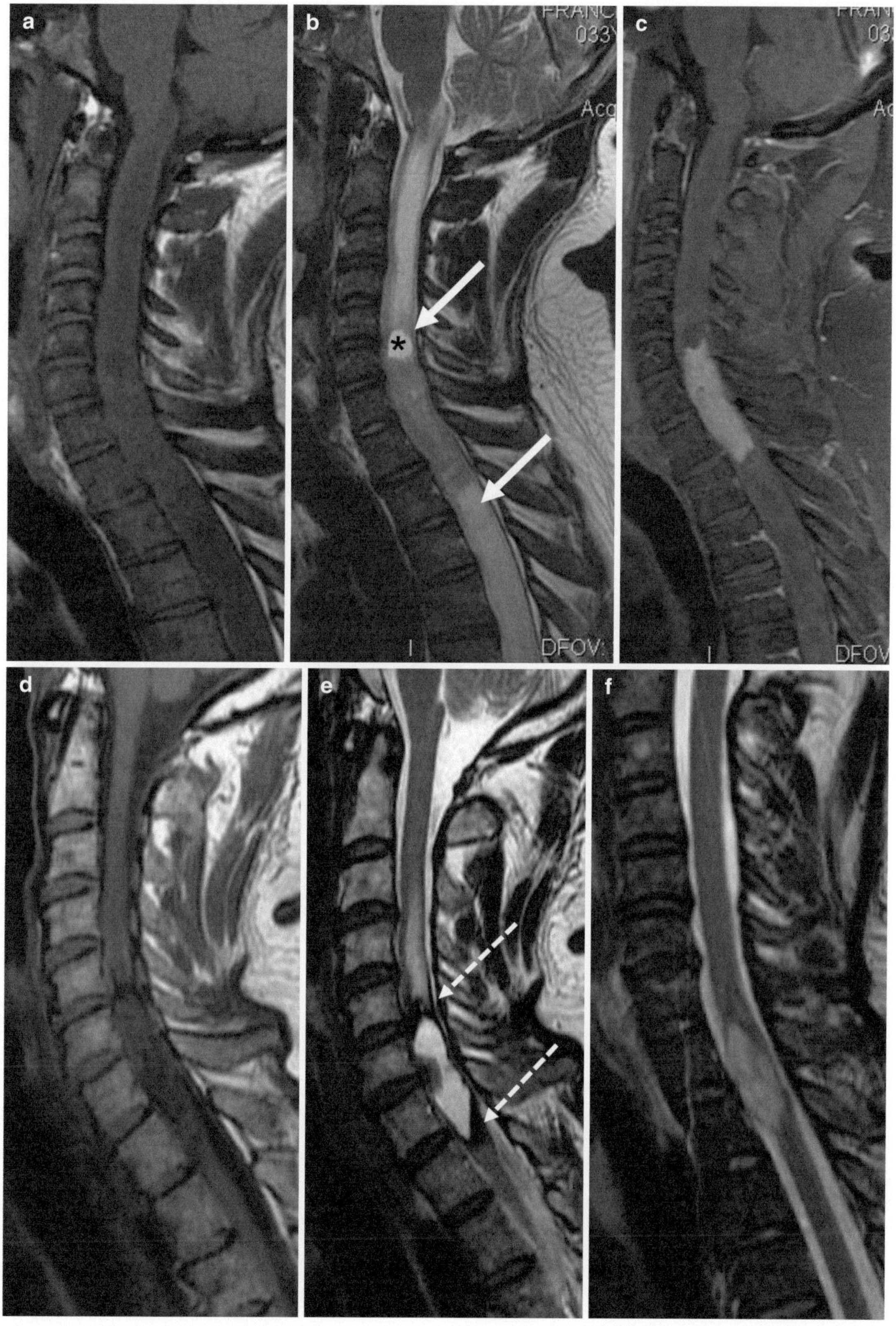
a
b
c
d
e
f
*
DFOV:
Acq

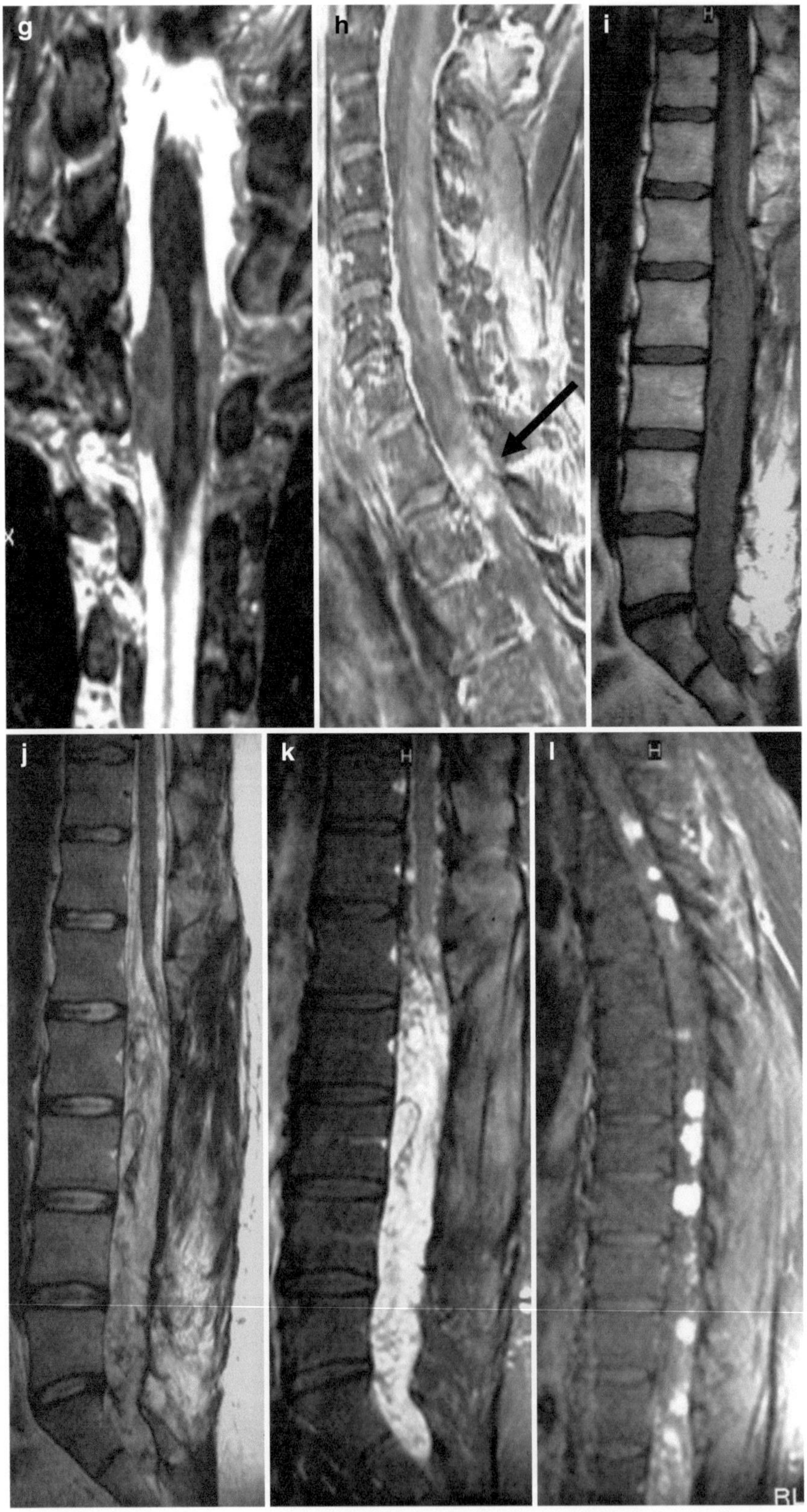

Fig. 49.1 (continued)

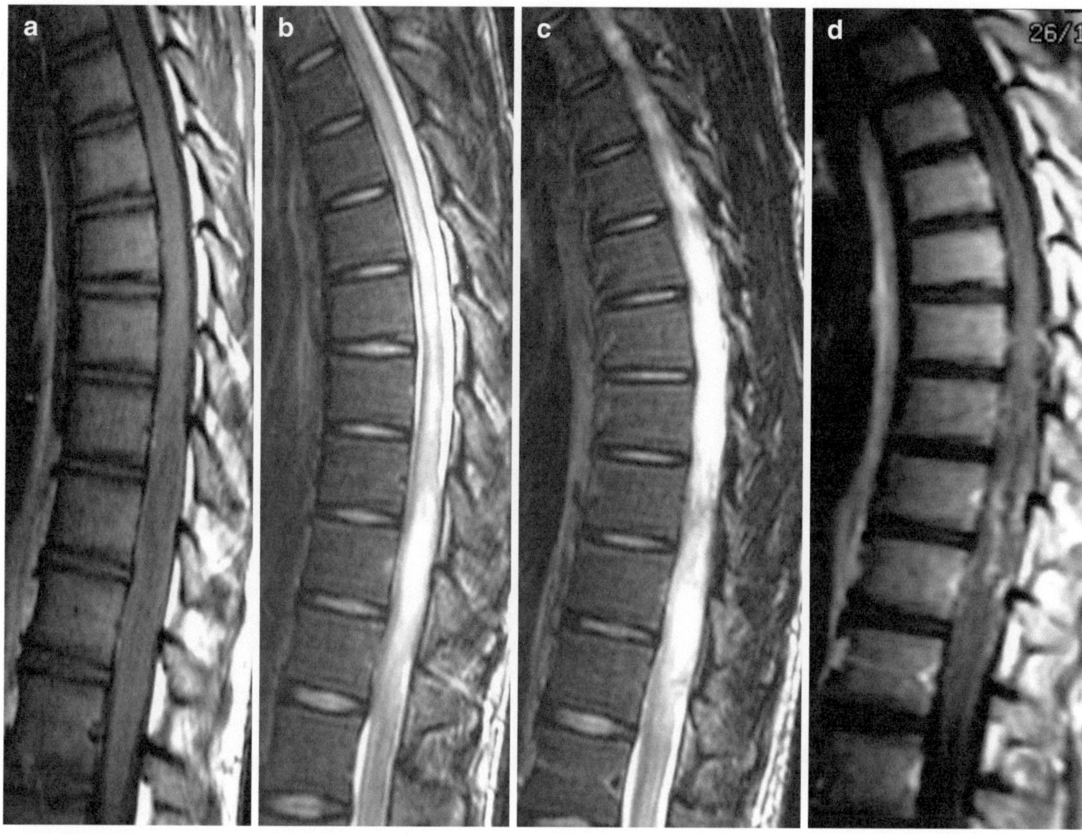

Fig. 49.2 Spinal cord glioblastoma. A 27-year-old woman presenting with fast and progressive paraparesis. (**a–c**) Sagittal T1WI (**a**) and T2WI (**b**, **c**) show spinal cord expansion at the lower thoracic level. (**d**) Sagittal postcontrast fat-suppression T1WI reveals a heterogeneous and patchy enhancing cord lesion associated with extensive edema

Main Differential Diagnosis

Nonneoplastic lesions may present with spinal cord expansion, such as tumefactive demyelinating lesions, NMO, vascular malformations, transverse myelitis, cord contusion, and cord infarction. They differ from most spinal cord tumors in their clinical presentation that is usually more acute and with a more abrupt onset of neurological deficits and symptoms. Congenital and infectious lesions should also be included in the differential diagnosis.

Cavernous malformations: Cavernomas are seen as rounded regions of heterogeneous signal intensity on T1WI and T2WI due to blood products of varying ages ("popcorn appearance") presenting a low-signal intensity rim on T2WI (hemosiderin) and hypointense "blooming" on susceptibility imaging. Minimal cord expansion or edema is seen unless there has been recent hemorrhage in which case, cord expansion is the rule [19].

Dural arteriovenous fistula: In the presence of an AVF, the spinal cord may be normal in size or slightly enlarged. Edema and prominent vessels (flow voids) on the posterior surface of the cord are usually present and are typically located in the dorsal aspect of the lower thoracic cord and conus medullaris. Cord contrast enhancement may occur [20].

Spinal cord infarction: In this condition, the spinal cord is usually enlarged and hyperintense on T2WI, and contrast enhancement may or may not be present. Symptoms onset is usually abrupt. The presence of restricted diffusion and signal abnormality limited to the central gray matter may aid in the imaging differential diagnosis as both findings are typical of infarctions [21].

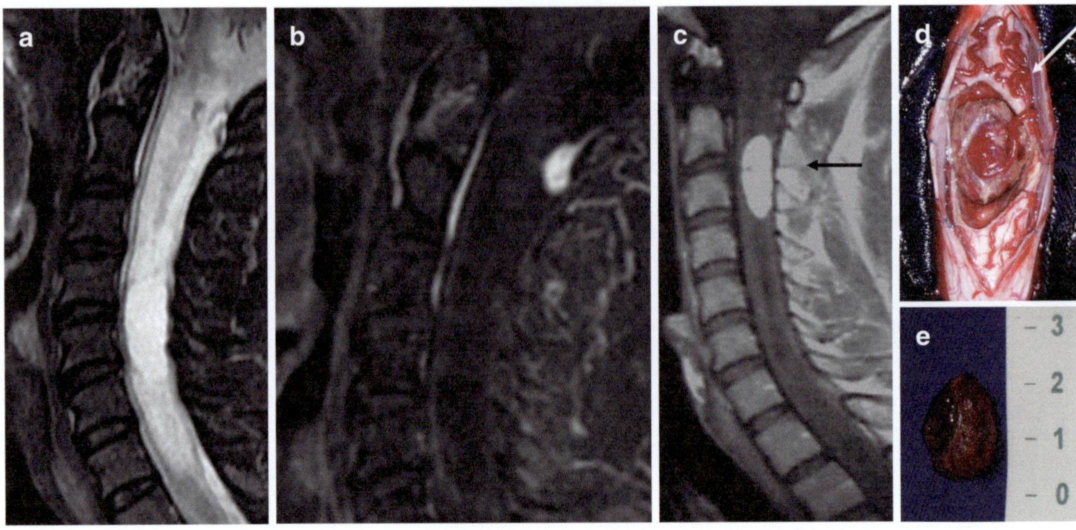

Fig. 49.3 Cervical spinal cord sporadic hemangioblastomas. A 28-year-old man presenting with progressive bilateral pain and numbness in his shoulders. (**a** and **b**) Sagittal T2WI (**b**) shows an enlarged cervicothoracic cord due to extensive edema and sirynx. Sagittal postcontrast fat-suppressed T1WI (**b**) reveals an avid and well-demarcated solid mass in the periphery of the cord at the C2 level. A 39-year-old man presenting with history of slow progressive bilateral numbness in his shoulders and upper back. (**c–e**) Sagittal postcontrast fat-suppressed T1WI (**c**) reveals an avid and well-demarcated solid mass (*arrow*) at the C2 level. Intraoperative photograph (**d**) and macroscopic specimen picture (**e**) demonstrate a reddish lesion associated with prominent surrounding vessels (*arrow*). There were no other systemic findings associated with von Hippel–Lindau disease (Courtesy of Helder Tedeschi, MD)

Demyelination/inflammatory: Neuromyelitis optica usually presents with longitudinal extensive myelitis, hyperintense on T2WI, extending across >3 vertebral segments, usually affecting the spinal central gray matter and frequently demonstrating higher T2WI hyperintense areas, the so-called bright spotty lesions. The enhancement correlates with acute lesion activity, and in most patients, additional brain lesions typically distributed in the periventricular areas and near the optic chiasm and the hypothalamus aid in the differential diagnosis [22].

Transverse myelitis: May present with variable enlargement and contrast enhancement patterns (none, diffuse, patchy, peripheral). Its acute clinical course may help in the differentiation from a neoplastic process [23].

Spinal cord abscess: It is characterized by the presence of a typical rim-enhancing lesion and restricted diffusion centrally [19, 24].

Tips

- One must report the presence of cord expansion as it is considered an essential imaging criterion for the diagnosis of a spinal cord tumor, although some inflammatory lesions also expand the cord.
- Mentioning if the intramedullary neoplasm is solid or associated with neoplastic or nonneoplastic cysts is important as neoplastic cysts are removed surgically. Nonneoplastic cysts may be drained and aspirated but not resected.
- Describe extent of edema and the enhancement pattern of the lesion. Enhanced areas probably represent more cellular portions of the tumors and may be potential sites for biopsy if resection is not feasible.

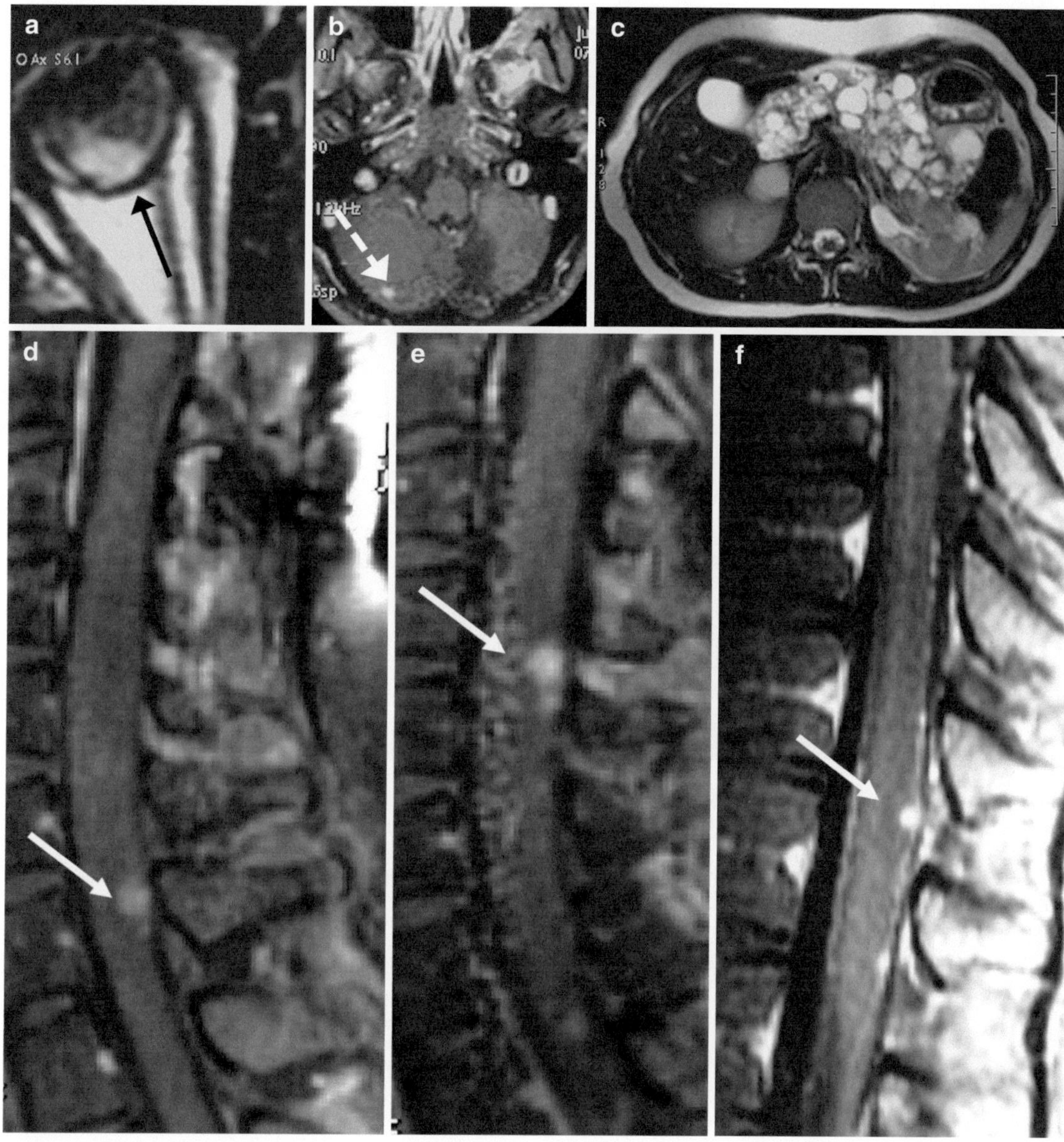

Fig. 49.4 Von Hippel–Lindau disease. A 25-year-old man presenting with painless decrease of vision in the right eye, ataxia, and paresthesia. A left cerebellar hemangioblastoma was surgically removed 5 years ago. (**a**) Axial postcontrast T1WI shows a retinal lesion in the right eye (*arrow*) consistent with hemangioblastoma. (**b**) A small right cerebellar nodular enhancing lesion is depicted on axial postcontrast fat-suppressed T1WI (*dashed arrow*) consistent with residual/recurrent hemangioblastoma. (**c**) Pancreatic cysts were also revealed on axial T2WI. (**d–f**) Sagittal postcontrast fat-suppressed T1WI demonstrate multiple nodular enhancing lesions along the spinal cord (*arrows*), consistent with multiple hemangioblastomas

- A central location within the spinal cord, presence of a cleavage plane, and intense homogeneous enhancement are imaging features that favor an ependymoma.

- Intramedullary astrocytomas are usually eccentrically located within the cord, are ill defined, and have patchy enhancement after gadolinium administration.

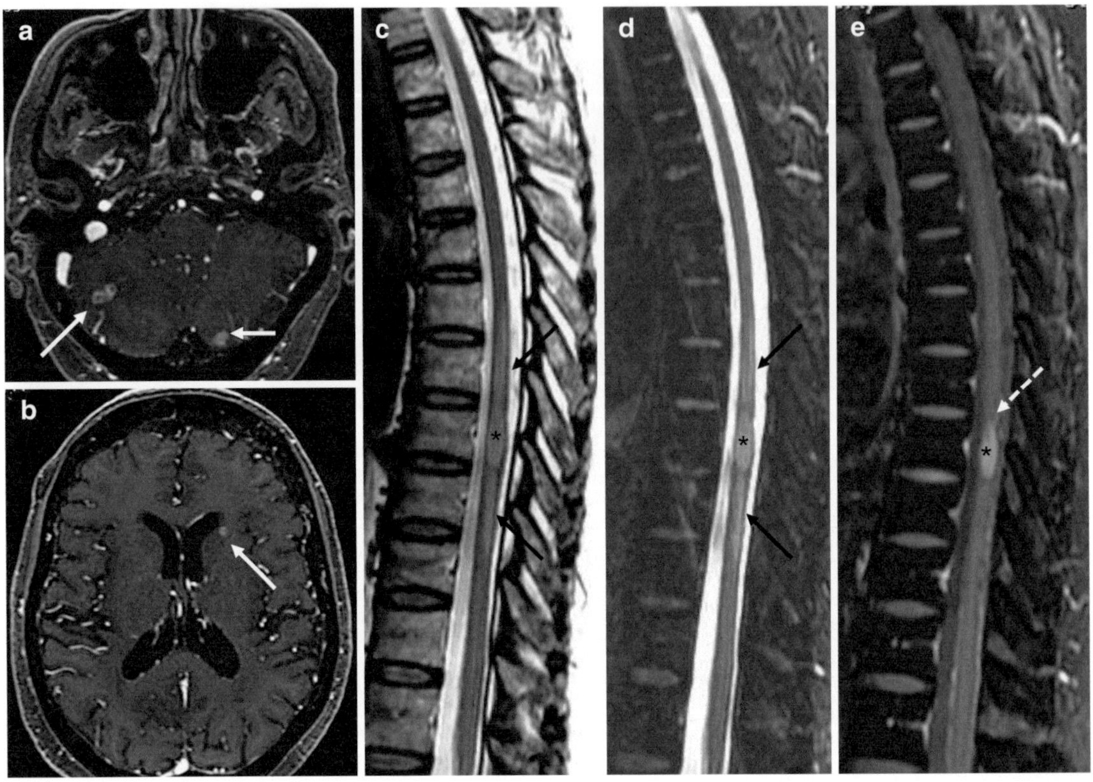

Fig. 49.5 Spinal cord metastases. A 36-year-old woman with breast cancer (lobular invasive) presenting with rapid onset paraparesis and severe mid-back pain. (**a**, **b**) Axial postcontrast fat-suppressed T1WI reveal nodular enhancing brain lesions consistent with metastases (*arrows*). (**c**–**e**) Sagittal T2WI (**c**), short-tau inversion recovery (STIR, **d**) and postcontrast T1 images of the thoracic spine demonstrate intramedullary spinal cord metastasis at T10. The enhancing lesion (*) is associated with edema (*arrows* on **c**, **d**). Note a subtle flame sign (*dashed arrow* on **e**)

References

1. Constantini S, Houten J, Miller DC, Freed D, Ozek MM, Rorke LB, Allen JC, Epstein FJ. Intramedullary spinal cord tumors in children under the age of 3 years. J Neurosurg. 1996;85(6):1036–43. doi:10.3171/jns.1996.85.6.1036.
2. Traul DE, Shaffrey ME, Schiff D. Part I: spinal-cord neoplasms-intradural neoplasms. Lancet Oncol. 2007;8(1):35–45. doi:10.1016/S1470-2045(06)71009-9.
3. Harrop JS, Ganju A, Groff M, Bilsky M. Primary intramedullary tumors of the spinal cord. Spine (Phila Pa 1976). 2009;34(22 Suppl):S69–77. doi:10.1097/BRS.0b013e3181b95c6f.
4. Raco A, Esposito V, Lenzi J, Piccirilli M, Delfini R, Cantore G. Long-term follow-up of intramedullary spinal cord tumors: a series of 202 cases. Neurosurgery. 2005;56(5):972–81; discussion 972–81.
5. Koeller KK, Rosenblum RS, Morrison AL. Neoplasms of the spinal cord and filum terminale: radiologic-pathologic correlation. Radiogr: Rev Publ Radiol Soc N Am Inc. 2000;20(6):1721–49. doi:10.1148/radiographics.20.6.g00nv151721.
6. Krisht KM, Schmidt MH. Tanycytic ependymoma: a challenging histological diagnosis. Case Rep Neurol Med. 2013;2013:170791. doi:10.1155/2013/170791.
7. Van Goethem JW, van den Hauwe L, Ozsarlak O, De Schepper AM, Parizel PM. Spinal tumors. Eur J Radiol. 2004;50(2):159–76. doi:10.1016/j.ejrad.2003.10.021.
8. Morais N, Mascarenhas L, Soares-Fernandes JP, Silva A, Magalhaes Z, Costa JA. Primary spinal glioblastoma: a case report and review of the literature. Oncol Lett. 2013;5(3):992–6. doi:10.3892/ol.2012.1076.
9. Abul-Kasim K, Thurnher MM, McKeever P, Sundgren PC. Intradural spinal tumors: current classification and MRI features. Neuroradiology. 2008;50(4):301–14. doi:10.1007/s00234-007-0345-7.
10. Chu BC, Terae S, Hida K, Furukawa M, Abe S, Miyasaka K. MR findings in spinal hemangioblastoma: correlation with symptoms and with angiographic and surgical findings. AJNR Am J Neuroradiol. 2001;22(1):206–17.

11. Neumann HP, Eggert HR, Weigel K, Friedburg H, Wiestler OD, Schollmeyer P. Hemangioblastomas of the central nervous system. A 10-year study with special reference to von Hippel-Lindau syndrome. J Neurosurg. 1989;70(1):24–30. doi:10.3171/jns.1989.70.1.0024.
12. Lee SS, Kim MK, Sym SJ, Kim SW, Kim WK, Kim SB, Ahn JH. Intramedullary spinal cord metastases: a single-institution experience. J Neurooncol. 2007;84(1):85–9. doi:10.1007/s11060-007-9345-z.
13. Diehn FE, Rykken JB, Wald JT, Wood CP, Eckel LJ, Hunt CH, Schwartz KM, Lingineni RK, Carter RE, Kaufmann TJ. Intramedullary spinal cord metastases: prognostic value of MRI and clinical features from a 13-year institutional case series. AJNR Am J Neuroradiol. 2015;36(3):587–93. doi:10.3174/ajnr.A4160.
14. Lowe GM. Magnetic resonance imaging of intramedullary spinal cord tumors. J Neurooncol. 2000;47(3):195–210.
15. Setzer M, Murtagh RD, Murtagh FR, Eleraky M, Jain S, Marquardt G, Seifert V, Vrionis FD. Diffusion tensor imaging tractography in patients with intramedullary tumors: comparison with intraoperative findings and value for prediction of tumor resectability. J Neurosurg Spine. 2010;13(3):371–80. doi:10.3171/2010.3.SPINE09399.
16. Seo HS, Kim JH, Lee DH, Lee YH, Suh SI, Kim SY, Na DG. Nonenhancing intramedullary astrocytomas and other MR imaging features: a retrospective study and systematic review. AJNR Am J Neuroradiol. 2010;31(3):498–503. doi:10.3174/ajnr.A1864.
17. Rykken JB, Diehn FE, Hunt CH, Eckel LJ, Schwartz KM, Kaufmann TJ, Wald JT, Giannini C, Wood CP. Rim and flame signs: postgadolinium MRI findings specific for non-CNS intramedullary spinal cord metastases. AJNR Am J Neuroradiol. 2013;34(4):908–15. doi:10.3174/ajnr.A3292.
18. Bostrom A, Kanther NC, Grote A, Bostrom J. Management and outcome in adult intramedullary spinal cord tumours: a 20-year single institution experience. BMC Res Notes. 2014;7:908. doi:10.1186/1756-0500-7-908.
19. Kharkar S, Shuck J, Conway J, Rigamonti D. The natural history of conservatively managed symptomatic intramedullary spinal cord cavernomas. Neurosurgery. 2007;60(5):865–72. doi:10.1227/01.NEU.0000255437.36742.15; discussion 865–72.
20. Lee SK, Willinsky RA, Montanera W, terBrugge KG. MR imaging of dural arteriovenous fistulas draining into cerebellar cortical veins. AJNR Am J Neuroradiol. 2003;24(8):1602–6.
21. Masson C, Pruvo JP, Meder JF, Cordonnier C, Touze E, De La Sayette V, Giroud M, Mas JL, Leys D, Study Group on Spinal Cord Infarction of the French Neurovascular S. Spinal cord infarction: clinical and magnetic resonance imaging findings and short term outcome. J Neurol Neurosurg Psychiatry. 2004;75(10):1431–5. doi:10.1136/jnnp.2003.031724.
22. Chang KH, Lyu RK, Chen CM, Wu YR, Chang HS, Huang CC, Kuo HC, Chu CC, Hsu WC, Ro LS. Distinct features between longitudinally extensive transverse myelitis presenting with and without anti-aquaporin 4 antibodies. Mult Scler. 2013;19(3):299–307. doi:10.1177/1352458512451659.
23. DeSanto J, Ross JS. Spine infection/inflammation. Radiol Clin N Am. 2011;49(1):105–27. doi:10.1016/j.rcl.2010.07.018.
24. Murphy KJ, Brunberg JA, Quint DJ, Kazanjian PH. Spinal cord infection: myelitis and abscess formation. AJNR Am J Neuroradiol. 1998;19(2):341–8.

Spinal Cord Masses in Children 50

Marcio Marques Moreira
and Lázaro Luís Faria do Amaral

Abstract

Intramedullary spinal cord tumors refer to a subgroup of intradural spinal tumors that arise from cells within the spinal cord. They account for 35–40 % of all intraspinal tumors in children. Low-grade histology tumors predominate in all age groups, producing a slowly progressive clinical course with pain being the most common and earliest symptom. Astrocytomas predominate in younger children and decrease in frequency in adulthood when ependymomas become the predominant type. The prognosis for pediatric patients is favorable with sustained functional improvement expected in a significant proportion of them on long-term follow-up.

Background

Intramedullary spinal cord tumors refer to a subgroup of intradural spinal tumors that arise from cells within the spinal cord. They account for 35–40 % of all intraspinal tumors in children [1].

Low-grade histology predominates in all age groups [2], producing a slowly progressive clinical course with pain being the most common and earliest symptom.

Astrocytomas predominate in younger children and decrease in frequency in adulthood when ependymomas become the predominant type. No ependymomas were reported in a series of intramedullary spinal cord tumors in patients under 3 years of age [3].

M.M. Moreira, MD
Radiology Department, Medimagem – Hospital Beneficência Portuguesa de São Paulo, Rua Maestro Cardim 476 apt 12, Liberdade, 01323-000 Sao Paulo, SP, Brazil
e-mail: moreirammarcio@gmail.com

L.L.F. do Amaral, MD (✉)
Division of Neuroradiology, Medimagem – Hospital Beneficência Portuguesa de São Paulo, Rua Luiz Gottschal, 151, apt. 111 MS, Vila Mariana, 04008-070 Sao Paulo, SP, Brazil

Division of Neuroradiology, Hospital Santa Casa de Misericórdia de São Paulo, Rua Dr. Cesário Motta Junior 112, Vila Buarque, Sao Paulo, SP 01221-020, Brazil
e-mail: lazden@terra.com.br

R. Hoffmann Nunes et al. (eds.), *Critical Findings in Neuroradiology*,
DOI 10.1007/978-3-319-27987-9_50

There is an association between spinal cord tumor and neurofibromatosis. Astrocytomas occur more often in patients with NF1 and ependymomas occur in those with NF2 [4].

The radical resection of intramedullary spinal cord tumors has become safer and more effective with the advent of microsurgical techniques, imaging, and intraoperative electrophysiology. The functional outcome after surgery is determined by the preoperative status; therefore, surgery should ideally be performed prior to the onset of severe motor deficits. Adjuvant radiation and chemotherapy are reserved for malignant or inoperable intramedullary tumors [1, 5].

The prognosis for pediatric patients is favorable with sustained functional improvement expected in a significant proportion of them on long-term follow-up. Long-term survival at 10 years (75 %) and 20 years (64 %) is related to resection [1, 5].

Key Points

Etiology

Astrocytomas: Astrocytomas are slow-growing tumors that are eccentrically located often with associated polar or intratumoral cysts [7, 8]. Hypercellularity and absence of a surrounding capsule leading to an infiltrative pattern are characteristic [9]. Low grade (pilocytic and fibrillary astrocytomas) represent the majority (90 %) of intramedullary astrocytomas in children [10]. Glioblastoma (WHO grade IV) is uncommon in the spinal cord, accounting for only 0.2–1.5 % of all intramedullary primary tumors [9]. They are predominantly located in the cervicothoracic or thoracic regions and usually extended multiple levels. True holocord involvement, from the cervicomedullary junction to the conus, is rare but may occur, especially with pilocytic astrocytoma and ganglioglioma in children [11].

Ganglioglioma: Gangliogliomas account for up to 15 % of intramedullary tumors in the pediatric age group [7]. They are composed of a mixture of neoplastic neurons (neurons or ganglion cells) and glial cells (primarily neoplastic astrocytes). Cervicothoracic or thoracic levels are the most common sites, and these tumors often span multiple segments. These tumors are commonly eccentric in location and may contain cysts. Calcification is a suggestive feature of gangliogliomas. Contrast enhancement is variable and nonspecific [12].

Ependymoma: Ependymomas arise from the ependymal cells lining the central canal, displacing the fiber tracts rather than interrupting them. They are centrally located within the spinal cord and are well circumscribed often showing a cleavage plane separating them from normal cord. Associated cysts and hemorrhages are common especially at tumor margins. Ependymal cells with uniform hyperchromatic nuclei arranged in perivascular pseudorosettes are typical findings at histologic examination [9].

Other spinal cord tumors: Spinal cord primitive neuroectodermal tumors (PNETs) are rare and aggressive tumors. Most cases involving the spinal axis are secondary to metastatic spread through cerebrospinal fluid (CSF) from a primary intracranial tumor [9]. They can be intramedullary, extramedullary intradural, or extradural in location. Spinal PNETs in children occur at an older age than those that occur intracranially and are most commonly found in young adults. Hemangioblastomas are also intramedullary tumors occurring in the cervical or thoracic levels, usually subpial in location and often have large feeding arteries and draining veins. The tumor nodule abuts the central ependymal or the peripheral pia. When associated with von Hippel-Lindau disease, they can occur in younger patients, even in children, and tend to be solid and multiple. Hemangioblastomas become symptomatic due to cyst growth [13, 14].

Best Imaging Modality

Radiographs are a good initial diagnostic tool for the evaluation of back pain in children but not for adults. Patients with skeletal abnormalities of the spine seen on radiographs and presenting with a spinal cord symptoms should undergo magnetic resonance imaging (MRI) [6], which is the imaging modality of choice for the evaluation of all spinal cord abnormalities [14, 15].

Computed tomography (CT) often fails to reveal intramedullary spinal neoplasms until gross expansion of the spinal canal has occurred. MRI allows for the identification of internal abnormalities of the spinal cord, such as cysts, syringohydromyelia, hemorrhage, and edema, and is routinely used in the setting of suspected intramedullary spinal masses [16].

The administration of intravenous paramagnetic agents allows for the identification of the solid portions of a tumor, to determine presence associated cysts and other features that often narrow the differential diagnosis and determine surgical management. Identification of the location of the solid enhancing portions of a tumor is vital because current neurosurgical techniques allow for laminotomies or laminectomies limited only to the zone where the tumor is located thereby decreasing surgical morbidity [2, 16].

Conventional radiography and CT are considered useful to detect associated skeletal abnormalities, such as mild scoliosis, widened interpedicular distance, and scalloping of posterior margins of the vertebral bodies. MRI protocol must include T1-weighted images (T1WI) and T2-weighted images (T2WI) in the sagittal and axial plane, followed by contrast-enhanced T1WI in at least two planes. Gradient echo (T2*) is sensitive in detecting hemorrhage, calcification, and flow voids [16].

Diffusion tensor imaging (DTI) can be performed in pediatric intramedullary spinal cord neoplasms as an adjunct to conventional structural imaging to help determine the location of tumor margins as well as the presence and degree of deflection and infiltration of the white matter tracts. DTI documents splaying versus disruption of fibers allowing determination of whether it is safe to attempt resection or whether biopsy is more appropriate [15].

Imaging of the entire neuraxis is indicated because CSF dissemination has been reported, especially with the higher-grade astrocytomas [16].

Major Findings

Astrocytoma: These tumors are commonly seen as an ill-defined eccentrically located mass that typically spans fewer than four vertebral levels, characterized by hypo- to isointense on T1WI and hyperintense on T2WI. Cysts are a common feature, with both polar and intratumoral types observed [17]. The majority of spinal astrocytomas enhance with a uniform or heterogeneous enhancement patterns although lack of enhancement has been reported (Fig. 50.1) [18, 19].

Ganglioglioma: These tumors tend to be eccentrically located, extending for multiples segments. Calcification and small cysts are common. Characteristically, the solid portions have mixed iso-hypointensity on T1WI. On T2WI, they present iso-hyperintensity. Contrast enhancement can be focal or patchy, or occasionally absent (Fig. 50.2) [20, 21].

Ependymoma: These tumors are centrally located well-circumscribed lesions with a cleavage planes separating them from the adjacent normal cord. Usually they are iso- or hypointense lesions on T1WI and iso- or hyperintense on T2WI. Some degree of enhancement is typically seen. Cyst formation and hemorrhage are common. A rim of low signal rostral and caudal of the solid neoplasm is referred to as the "cap sign" and seen on T2WI and represents hemosiderin deposition secondary to intratumoral hemorrhages [18]. Holocord ependymomas are extremely rare; most have mixed solid and cystic components (Fig. 50.3) [22].

Hemangioblastoma: Small hemangioblastomas (<10 mm) are mostly isointense on T1WI and hyperintense on T2WI and show homogeneous contrast enhancement. Larger hemangioblastomas tend to be hypointense or mixed hypo- and isointense on T1WI images, heterogeneous on T2WI images with intermixed focal flow voids, presenting heterogeneous enhancement. Extensive spinal cord swelling is also a common imaging feature. The presence of cysts and/or syringohydromyelia is commonly reported (Fig. 50.4). A central or peripheral location of the enhancing tumor nodules is typical [16].

PNET: These are rare and aggressive spinal cord tumors. Most cases involving the spinal cord are secondary to metastatic spreading through CSF from a primary intracranial tumor. They can be intramedullary, extramedullary intradural, or extradural in location. Spinal PNETs in children

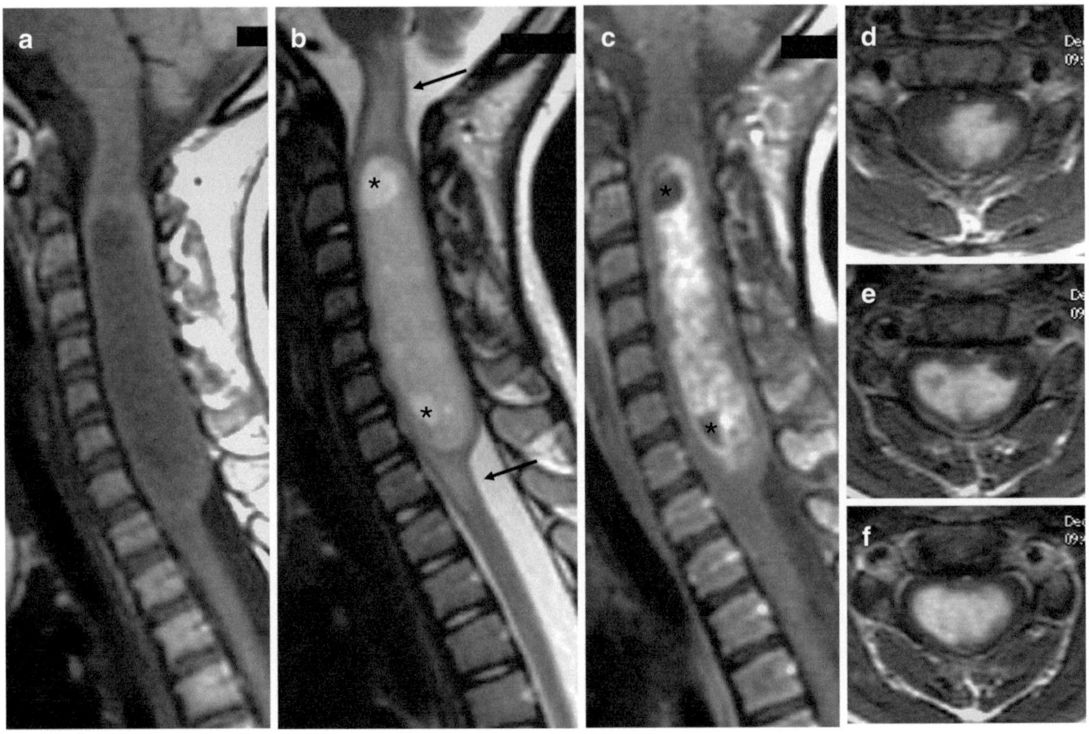

Fig. 50.1 Pilocytic astrocytoma. A 3-year-old boy with motor and sensory deficits and gait disturbances. (**a**, **b**) Sagittal T1WI and T2WI show a hypointense lesion resulting in expansion of the cervical cord and bony spinal canal as well as narrowing the adjacent CSF spaces and associated with rostral and caudal edema (*arrows*). Cystic areas (*) are present inside the tumor. (**c–f**) A heterogeneous enhancement is seen on sagittal and axial postcontrast fat-suppression T1WI

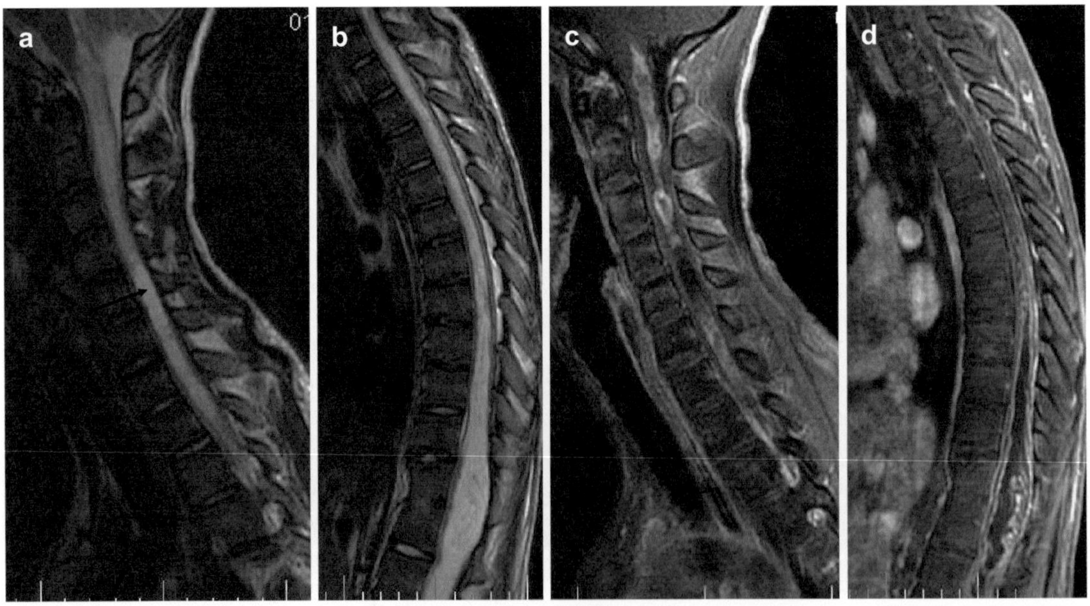

Fig. 50.2 Holocord ependymoma. A 17-year-old boy with scoliosis and flaccid paraplegia. (**a**, **b**). Sagittal T2WI of the cervical and thoracic spine show a diffusely enlarged spinal cord with cystic areas (*arrow*) (**c**, **d**). A diffuse heterogeneous pattern of enhancement characterized by a central thick enhancement following the region of the central canal is demonstrated on sagittal postcontrast fat suppression

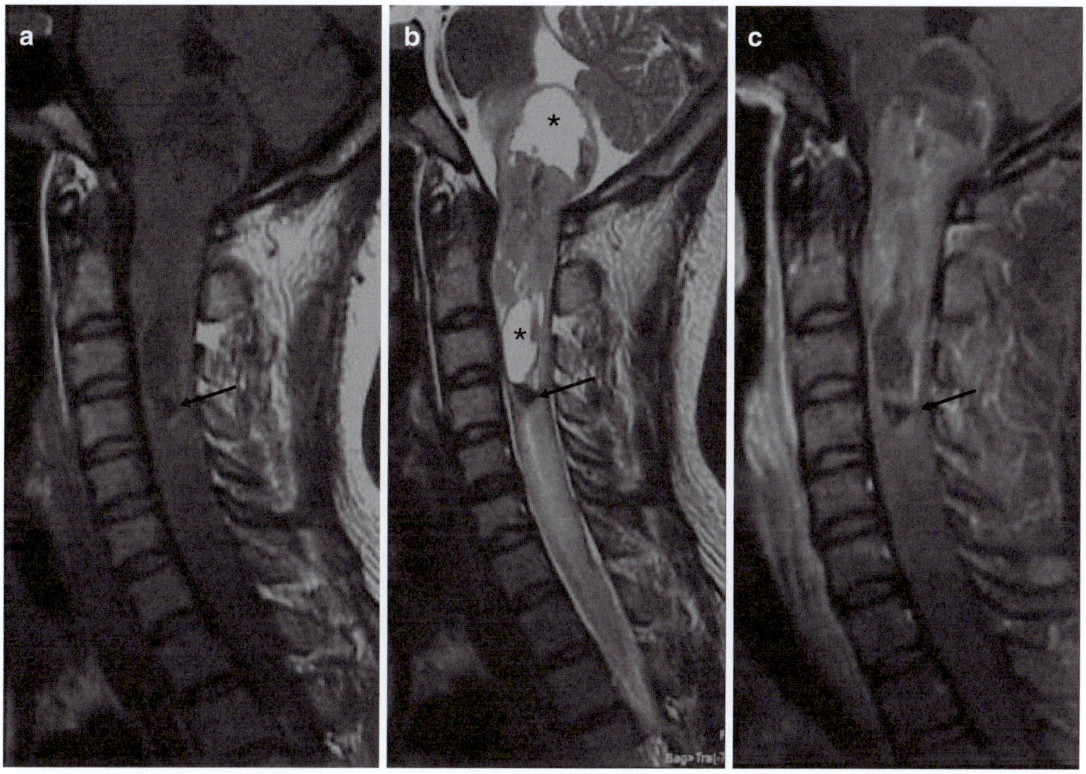

Fig. 50.3 Ganglioglioma. A 19-year-old girl presenting with neck pain, upper limb paresthesia, and mild quadriparesis. (**a**, **b**) Sagittal T1WI and T2WI of the cervical spine show a heterogeneous intramedullary tumor affecting the medulla and the upper cervical spinal cord. Rostral, caudal, and intratumoral cysts are seen on (**b**) (*stars*). (**c**) Sagittal postcontrast fat-suppression T1WI shows irregular enhancement. A low signal foci inside the lesion demonstrated in all sequences (*arrows*) suggests calcifications which are described in gangliogliomas

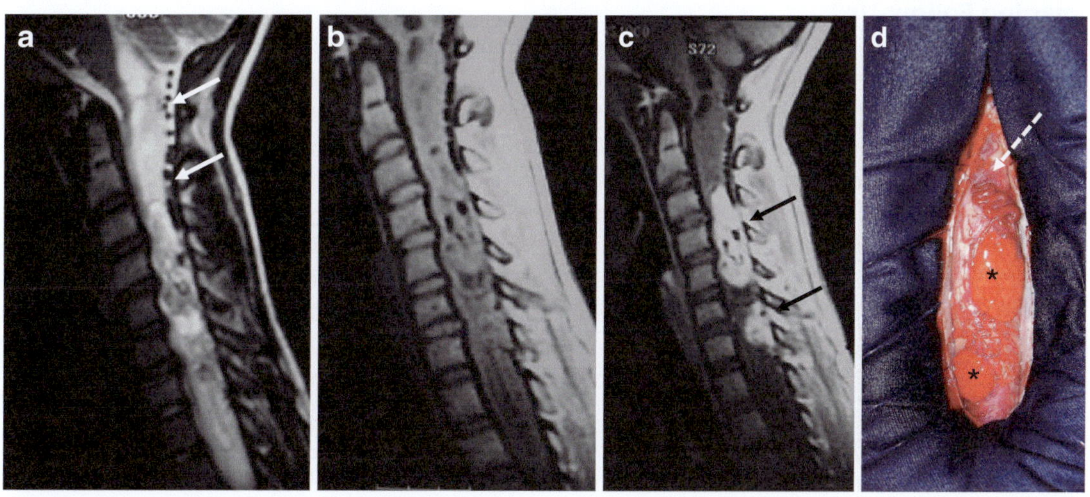

Fig. 50.4 Hemangioblastoma. A 13-year-old girl presenting with progressive cervical pain and incomplete tetraplegia. (**a**, **b**) Sagittal T2WI and T1WI reveal a heterogeneous lesion along the entire cervical spinal cord. Adjacent flow voids are seen on (**a**) (*arrows*). (**c**) Sagittal postcontrast fat suppression shows areas of avid enhancement (*arrows*) corresponding to the solid portions of the tumor. (**d**) Intraoperative photograph displays red lesions (*stars*) with associated prominent surrounding vessels (*dashed arrow*) (Courtesy of Helder Tedeschi, MD)

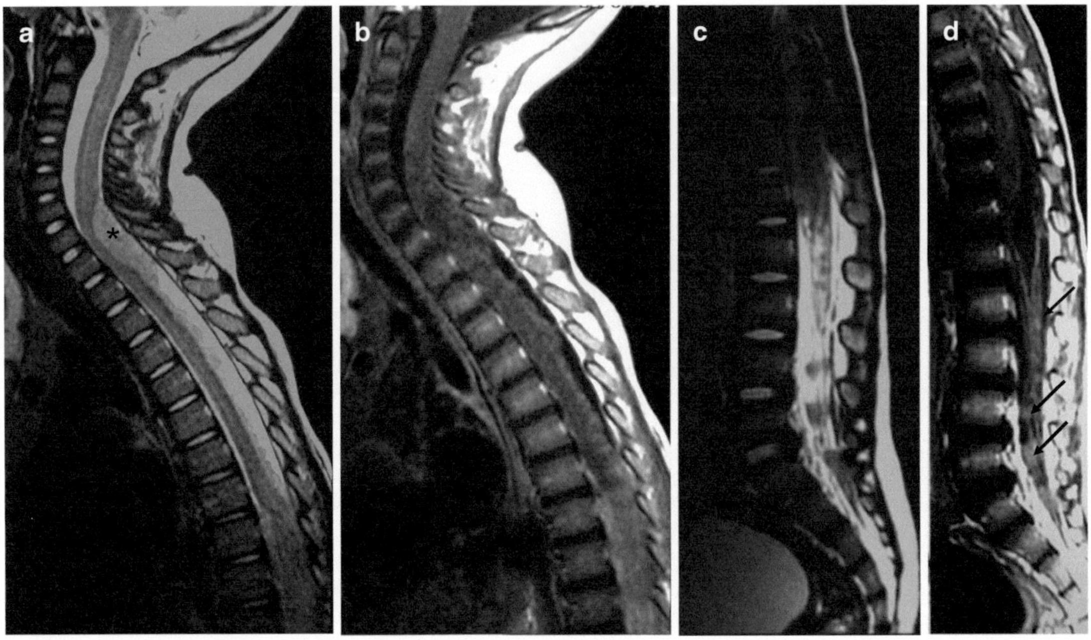

Fig. 50.5 PNET. A 4-year-old girl presenting with thoracic and low back pain, bilateral lower extremity weakness, as well as bowel and bladder involvement. (**a–d**) Sagittal T2WI and postcontrast T1WI demonstrate a primary spinal intramedullary and exophytic PNET (*) involving the cervicothoracic spinal cord and extending inferiorly to the conus medullaris. In addition, there is diffuse intradural enhancement in the distal thecal sac due to CSF spread (*arrows* on **d**)

occur at an older age than those that occur intracranially and are most commonly found in young adults (Fig. 50.5) [9].

Imaging Follow-Up

Recommended follow-up and prognosis is dependent on tumor histology. Generally, biannual follow-up MRI is recommended for intramedullary tumors. In a postoperative assessment, the contrast-enhanced MRI is useful for establishing the presence of recurrent/residual tumor [7, 23, 24].

Children with either low-grade astrocytomas or gangliogliomas treated with radical surgery have a relatively good prognosis [5]. Therefore, patients are usually followed clinically and by MRI for years [5]. Most clinicians delay imaging for a period of months after the initial surgery. If neurological function worsens, immediate re-imaging is warranted. Residual tumor can lead to repeat resection, radiation therapy, or just observation. If tumor recurrence is noted, imaging the entire neuraxis is warranted to rule out distant seeding through CSF [23, 24].

Main Differential Diagnosis

Nonneoplasic spinal cord lesions may present in adults and children and include demyelinating disease, granulomatous disease, vascular malformations, and infection. They differ from most spinal cord tumors by their clinical presentations which are commonly more abrupt [25–29].

Ventriculus terminalis: Ventriculus terminalis is a cavity situated at the level of the conus medullaris surrounded by ependymal tissue. The ventriculus terminalis may be visualized as a cystic lesion in the conus medullary and represents a transient finding in children under 5 years of age. It typically appears on MRI as a small, round cavity with regular borders containing no septations and is filled with fluid of the same intensity of CSF on all sequences and shows no contrast enhancement [30].

Tips

When facing a spinal cord lesion in a child, one should report the presence of cord expansion and mention if the intramedullary neoplasm is solid or associated with neoplastic or nonneoplastic cysts. Neoplastic cysts must be removed surgically. Nonneoplastic cysts can be drained and aspirated but not resected.

It is also important to describe the presence of edema and the enhancement pattern. Enhanced areas probably represent more active portions of the tumors and may indicate potential sites for biopsy if resection is not feasible.

References

1. Jallo GI, Freed D, Epstein F. Intramedullary spinal cord tumors in children. Childs Nerv Syst. 2003;19(9):641–9. doi:10.1007/s00381-003-0820-3.
2. Lowe GM. Magnetic resonance imaging of intramedullary spinal cord tumors. J Neuro Oncol. 2000;47(3): 195–210.
3. Constantini S, Houten J, Miller DC, Freed D, Ozek MM, Rorke LB, Allen JC, Epstein FJ. Intramedullary spinal cord tumors in children under the age of 3 years. J Neurosurg. 1996;85(6):1036–43. doi:10.3171/jns.1996.85.6.1036.
4. Lee M, Rezai AR, Freed D, Epstein FJ. Intramedullary spinal cord tumors in neurofibromatosis. Neurosurgery. 1996;38(1):32–7.
5. Ahmed R, Menezes AH, Awe OO, Torner JC. Long-term disease and neurological outcomes in patients with pediatric intramedullary spinal cord tumors. J Neurosurg Pediatr. 2014;13(6):600–12. doi:10.3171/2014.1.PEDS13316.
6. Rodriguez DP, Poussaint TY. Imaging of back pain in children. AJNR Am J Neuroradiol. 2010;31(5): 787–802. doi:10.3174/ajnr.A1832.
7. Van Goethem JW, van den Hauwe L, Ozsarlak O, De Schepper AM, Parizel PM. Spinal tumors. Eur J Radiol. 2004;50(2):159–76. doi:10.1016/j.ejrad.2003.10.021.
8. Rossi A, Gandolfo C, Morana G, Tortori-Donati P. Tumors of the spine in children. Neuroimaging Clin N Am. 2007;17(1):17–35. doi:10.1016/j.nic.2006.11.004.
9. Koeller KK, Rosenblum RS, Morrison AL. Neoplasms of the spinal cord and filum terminale: radiologic-pathologic correlation. Radiographics: Rev Publ Radiol Soc N Am Inc. 2000;20(6):1721–49. doi:10.1148/radiographics.20.6.g00nv151721.
10. Traul DE, Shaffrey ME, Schiff D. Part I: spinal-cord neoplasms-intradural neoplasms. Lancet Oncol. 2007;8(1):35–45. doi:10.1016/S1470-2045(06)71009-9.
11. Schittenhelm J, Ebner FH, Tatagiba M, Wolff M, Nagele T, Meyermann R, Mittelbronn M. Holocord pilocytic astrocytoma – case report and review of the literature. Clin Neurol Neurosurg. 2009;111(2): 203–7. doi:10.1016/j.clineuro.2008.09.014.
12. Jallo GI, Freed D, Epstein FJ. Spinal cord gangliogliomas: a review of 56 patients. J Neuro Oncol. 2004;68(1):71–7.
13. Abul-Kasim K, Thurnher MM, McKeever P, Sundgren PC. Intradural spinal tumors: current classification and MRI features. Neuroradiology. 2008;50(4): 301–14. doi:10.1007/s00234-007-0345-7.
14. Chu BC, Terae S, Hida K, Furukawa M, Abe S, Miyasaka K. MR findings in spinal hemangioblastoma: correlation with symptoms and with angiographic and surgical findings. AJNR Am J Neuroradiol. 2001;22(1):206–17.
15. Choudhri AF, Whitehead MT, Klimo Jr P, Montgomery BK, Boop FA. Diffusion tensor imaging to guide surgical planning in intramedullary spinal cord tumors in children. Neuroradiology. 2014;56(2):169–74. doi:10.1007/s00234-013-1316-9.
16. Nemoto Y, Inoue Y, Tashiro T, Mochizuki K, Oda J, Kogame S, Katsuyama J, Hakuba A, Onoyama Y. Intramedullary spinal cord tumors: significance of associated hemorrhage at MR imaging. Radiology. 1992;182(3):793–6. doi:10.1148/radiology.182.3.1535896.
17. Smith AB, Soderlund KA, Rushing EJ, Smirniotopolous JG. Radiologic-pathologic correlation of pediatric and adolescent spinal neoplasms: part 1, Intramedullary spinal neoplasms. AJR Am J Roentgenol. 2012;198(1):34–43. doi:10.2214/AJR.10.7311.
18. Seo HS, Kim JH, Lee DH, Lee YH, Suh SI, Kim SY, Na DG. Nonenhancing intramedullary astrocytomas and other MR imaging features: a retrospective study and systematic review. AJNR Am J Neuroradiol. 2010;31(3):498–503. doi:10.3174/ajnr.A1864.
19. Tortori-Donati P, Rossi A, Biancheri R. Tumors of the spine and spinal cord. In: Tortori- Donati P, editor. Pediatric neuroradiology. 2005th ed. Berlin: Springer Verlag; 2005. p. 11609–51.
20. Patel U, Pinto RS, Miller DC, Handler MS, Rorke LB, Epstein FJ, Kricheff II. MR of spinal cord ganglioglioma. AJNR Am J Neuroradiol. 1998;19(5): 879–87.
21. Castillo M. Gangliogliomas: ubiquitous or not? AJNR Am J Neuroradiol. 1998;19(5):807–9.
22. Aryan S, Ghosal N, Aziz ZA, Hegde AS, Dadlani R. Infantile holocord cellular ependymoma with communicating hydrocephalus: unusual presentation of a rare case. Brain Tumor Pathol. 2014;31(1):47–50. doi:10.1007/s10014-013-0145-1.

23. Bostrom A, Kanther NC, Grote A, Bostrom J. Management and outcome in adult intramedullary spinal cord tumours: a 20-year single institution experience. BMC Res Notes. 2014;7:908. doi:10.1186/1756-0500-7-908.
24. Raco A, Esposito V, Lenzi J, Piccirilli M, Delfini R, Cantore G. Long-term follow-up of intramedullary spinal cord tumors: a series of 202 cases. Neurosurgery. 2005;56(5):972–81. discussion 972-981.
25. Kharkar S, Shuck J, Conway J, Rigamonti D. The natural history of conservatively managed symptomatic intramedullary spinal cord cavernomas. Neurosurgery. 2007;60(5):865–72. doi:10.1227/01.NEU.0000255437.36742.15. discussion 865–872.
26. Lee SK, Willinsky RA, Montanera W, terBrugge KG. MR imaging of dural arteriovenous fistulas draining into cerebellar cortical veins. AJNR Am J Neuroradiol. 2003;24(8):1602–6.
27. Masson C, Pruvo JP, Meder JF, Cordonnier C, Touze E, De La Sayette V, Giroud M, Mas JL, Leys D, Study Group on Spinal Cord Infarction of the French Neurovascular S. Spinal cord infarction: clinical and magnetic resonance imaging findings and short term outcome. J Neurol Neurosurg Psychiatry. 2004;75(10):1431–5. doi:10.1136/jnnp.2003.031724.
28. Chang KH, Lyu RK, Chen CM, Wu YR, Chang HS, Huang CC, Kuo HC, Chu CC, Hsu WC, Ro LS. Distinct features between longitudinally extensive transverse myelitis presenting with and without anti-aquaporin 4 antibodies. Mult Scler. 2013;19(3):299–307. doi:10.1177/1352458512451659.
29. DeSanto J, Ross JS. Spine infection/inflammation. Radiol Clin N Am. 2011;49(1):105–27. doi:10.1016/j.rcl.2010.07.018.
30. Celli P, D'Andrea G, Trillo G, Roperto R, Acqui M, Ferrante L. Cyst of the medullary conus: malformative persistence of terminal ventricle or compressive dilatation? Neurosurg Rev. 2002;25(1–2):103–6.

Spondylodiscitis

51

Francisco Jose Medina

Abstract

Spondylodiscitis is a term that includes vertebral osteomyelitis, infection of the intervertebral disk and/or the soft tissues of the extradural spine. The most common route of infection is hematogenous spread from a distant infection focus and is considered primarily a monomicrobial infection, most frequently caused by *Staphylococcus aureus*. Although the diagnostic suspicion is based on clinical, laboratory, and imaging findings, definite diagnosis is achieved by bacteriological examination of the infected tissue.

MRI is the most useful modality for any imaging spine infection, demonstrating bone marrow, endplate, and disk involvement and allowing the direct visualization of the neural structures. Sometimes non-pyogenic spondylitis, degenerative changes, dialysis spondyloarthropathy, and neuropathic spine are difficult to differentiate from pyogenic spondylitis and CT and radionuclide imaging are useful as adjunct techniques.

Background

Spondylodiscitis is a term that includes infection of the bony spinal column (vertebral osteomyelitis), the intervertebral disk (discitis), and/or the ligaments of the extradural spine, which are considered different manifestations of the same pathological process. Although a wide range of organisms have been associated with spondylodiscitis (bacterial, mycobacterial, fungal, and parasitic), it remains primarily a monomicrobial bacterial infection [1, 2]. Between 30 and 80 % of all spinal infections are caused by *Staphylococcus aureus. Mycobacterium tuberculosis* is particularly common in HIV-positive patients [3].

The incidence of spine infections varies between 1:100,000 and 1:250,000 in developed countries, and its estimated mortality rate ranges between 2 and 4 %. Numerous studies refer to a bimodal distribution with a peak below 20 years and another between 50 and 70 years of age. A 2:1–5:1 male to female ratio has been reported.

F.J. Medina, MD
Departamento de Imágenes Diagnosticas Fundación Valle del Lili, Calle 15 # 122-151 Apt 101D, Cali, Colombia
e-mail: fjmedinav@yahoo.es

R. Hoffmann Nunes et al. (eds.), *Critical Findings in Neuroradiology*, DOI 10.1007/978-3-319-27987-9_51

Known predisposing risk factors include previous spine surgery, a distant infection focus, diabetes mellitus, advanced age, immunosuppression, oncologic history, renal failure, rheumatological diseases, and liver cirrhosis [3].

Diagnosis is based on clinical, laboratory, and imaging features. Nonspecific back or neck pain are usually the first clinical symptoms. Fever is less common and occurs in only about half of the patients. Spinal tenderness is the most common sign detected on physical examination, often associated with paravertebral muscle spasm. Neurological deficits are more likely to be associated with epidural abscess, delayed diagnosis, cervical lesions, and tuberculosis infection. Laboratory findings include elevated erythrocyte sedimentation rate, white cell count, and C-protein values. The definitive diagnosis however only can be achieved by microscopic or bacteriological examination of the infected tissues [1, 3].

Treatment includes antibiotic therapy, which preserves or restores spinal stability and decompression of the spinal canal in the presence of neurological deficits or epidural abscess [3].

Key Points

Etiology

Pathogens can infect the spine via three routes: hematogenous, direct external inoculation, and spread from contiguous tissues. Hematogenous spread is the most common source of infection, typically via an arterial route. In children, intraosseous arteries display extensive anastomose, and vascular channels penetrate the disk. Therefore, a septic embolus is unlikely to produce a substantial osseous infarct, and the resulting infection spreads to the disk. By contrast in adults, the disk is avascular, and the intraosseous anastomoses involute, meaning that a septic embolus results in a larger infarct. Extensive infarction leads to wedging, cavitation, and compression fractures. Uncontrolled infection can breach the bone and track into the surrounding soft tissues, causing paravertebral or psoas abscess and spread posteriorly into the spinal canal, forming an epidural abscess with further risk of subdural abscess and meningitis [1].

Best Imaging Modality

Magnetic Resonance Imaging (*MRI*). It is the most useful modality for imaging spine infection, allowing the demonstration of bone marrow and disk involvement in addition to direct visualization of the spinal canal and neural structures. It has a reported sensitivity of 96 %, specificity of 93 %, and accuracy of 94 % for identification of spinal infections [6]. Fat-suppressed T2-weighted images (T2WI) and postgadolinium T1-weighted images (T1WI) sequences increase the conspicuity of the lesions [2].

Computed Tomography (*CT*). It is considered the best modality for evaluation of bony changes, including endplate erosions, destruction of the vertebral bodies, and sequestra formation. Effacement of paravertebral fat and hypodensity of the intervertebral disk may be seen at the beginning of an infection [4].

CT is useful when MRI is contraindicated or not available and routinely used to guide percutaneous biopsy and aspiration/drainage of fluid collections (Fig. 51.1).

Radionuclide Imaging. Conventional radionuclide imaging tests suffer from poor spatial resolution and lack sensitivity, specificity, or both. Among the radionuclide procedures, the combination of ^{67}Ga-SPECT with bone scintigraphy is still considered as the radionuclide gold standard for diagnosing spinal infection. [^{18} F]-FDG PET and PET/CT are emerging adjunct imaging techniques in patients in whom the diagnosis is inconclusive by other means (Fig. 51.2) [5].

Radiography. The earliest radiographic sign of infectious spondylitis are not seen until 2–3 weeks following beginning of the infection. They include subchondral radiolucency, frequently anteriorly, followed by loss of definition of the endplate and low intervertebral disk height. The progression of the infection is characterized

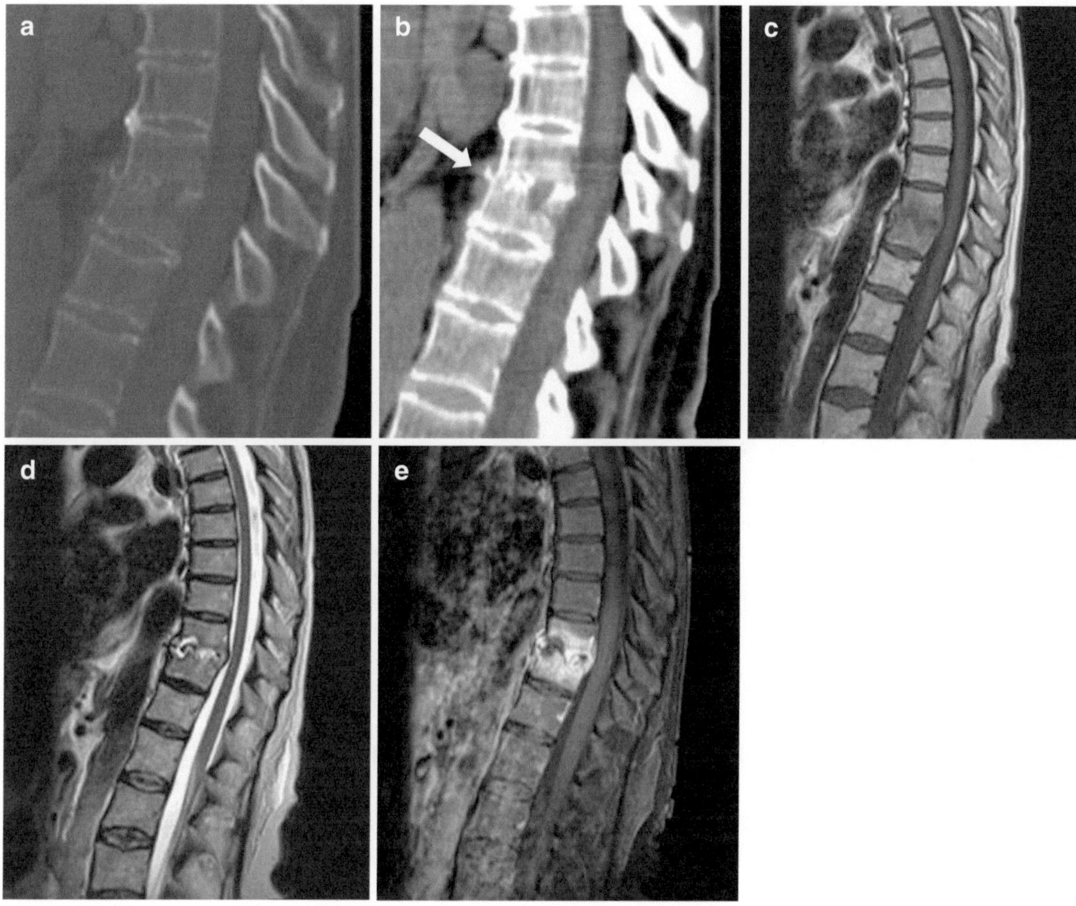

Fig. 51.1 CT and MRI imaging findings in spondylodiscitis. (**a**) CT sagittal reformatted bone window image shows loss of disk space height at level T10–T11 associated to endplate destruction. (**b**) CT sagittal reformatted soft tissue window image demonstrates increased prevertebral soft tissue density (*arrow*). (**c**) Sagittal T1WI shows loss of the normal endplate cortical hypointensity and bone marrow signal hypointensity. (**d**) Sagittal T2WI demonstrates increased signal, similar to fluid signal within the intervertebral disk. (**e**) Sagittal contrast-enhanced fat-saturated T1WI shows bone marrow enhancement and irregular intervertebral disk enhancement with an intradiscal abscess (nonenhancing regions). There is solid enhancement of the prevertebral and epidural inflammatory tissue

by destruction of the vertebral body with involvement of the opposite endplate. Paraspinal bulging and loss of soft tissue planes may be seen, although the soft tissue contrast of conventional radiography is poor (Fig. 51.3) [4, 6].

Major Findings

Vertebral Osteomyelitis. The earliest sign of infection in the vertebral body is bone marrow edema (T1 hypointensity, T2 hyperintensity, and contrast enhancement), typically located in the anterior aspect of the end plate region. Bone marrow edema are frequently seen in the opposite vertebral body endplate [6, 7].

A more specific early finding is erosion or destruction of the endplates with loss of the hypointense line of the endplates on non-enhanced T1WI which presumably represents cortical bone. Progression of the disease is characterized by the appearance of fibrovascular

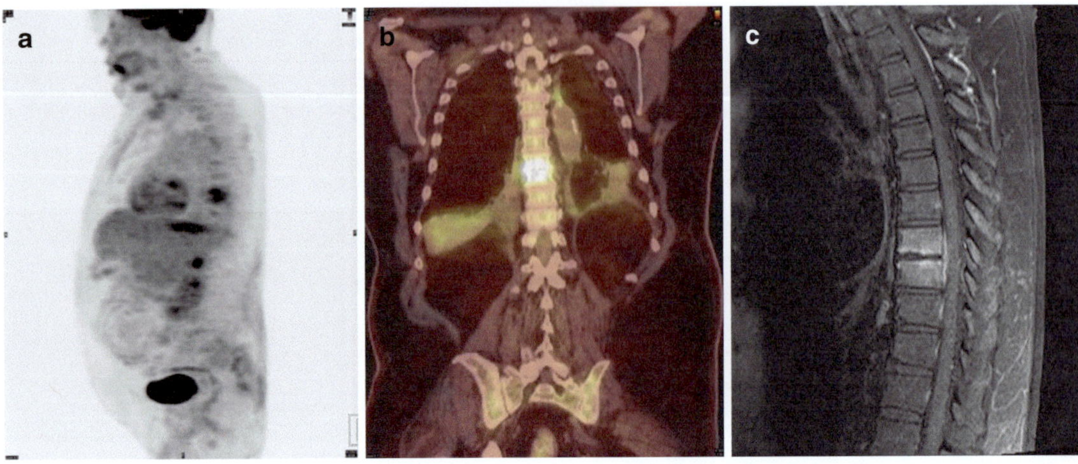

Fig. 51.2 [[18] F]-FDG PET and PET/CT detecting early spinal infection in a patient with a prolonged fever. (**a**) Sagittal view PET imaging shows increased FDG uptake at level T8–T9. (**b**) Coronal PET/CT imaging better demonstrates the anatomic localization of the site of uptake. (**c**) Sagittal contrast-enhanced fat-saturated T1WI shows vertebral bodies and disk enhancement compatible with early spondylodiscitis (Courtesy of Ana Melissa Álvarez MD, Cali – Colombia)

tissue at the periphery of erosions and necrotic areas [4, 7].

Discitis: Typically infected disks show height loss, decreased signal intensity on T1WI, and high signal, almost fluid-signal intensity, on T2WI. Loss of the normal intranuclear cleft has been reported to be indicative of early spinal infection, but it is rarely visible in the cervical and thoracic spine, limiting its clinical use [6–8]. The enhancement pattern of the infected disk can be variable, from thick patchy enhancement, to linear and peripheral enhancement [7, 8].

Paraspinal soft tissue involvement: Extension of the inflammatory process to the paraspinous soft tissues is often seen in spinal infection, helping considerably in establishing the diagnosis. Involved paraspinal soft tissues may show a homogeneous edema-type enhancement (cellulitis/myositis) or ring enhancement indicating true abscesses [7, 8].

Epidural abscess: Early diagnosis and treatment of epidural abscess is of paramount importance because delay on treatment may cause permanent neurological deficits or death. On MRI, epidural abscesses are shown as epidural space masses, hypo- or isointense to the spinal cord on T1WI and hyperintense on T2WI. On postgadolinium T1WI there may be homogeneous or peripheral enhancement reflecting phlegmonosus granulation tissue or necrotic abscess respectively. Demonstration of an abscess cavity may influence clinical and surgical approaches [9, 10]. Other patterns of contrast enhancement related to epidural abscess include linear enhancement along the dura mater and engorgement of the epidural or basivertebral veins [10]. Diffusion-weighted images (DWI) may show high signal intensity in the abscess, with the corresponding low signal intensity on apparent diffusion coefficient maps (ADC map) (Fig. 51.4) [11].

Imaging Follow-Up

MRI is not recommended for short-term routine follow-up to monitor acute response to treatment in patients with spine infections. Although resolution of gadolinium uptake and restoration of bone with increase of T1 bone marrow signal, corresponding with fatty replacement, are more chronic changes compatible with resolution of the infection, their appearance is delayed by several weeks or even months after clinical improvement [12]. In early stages, some patients may show improvement of paraspinal tissue

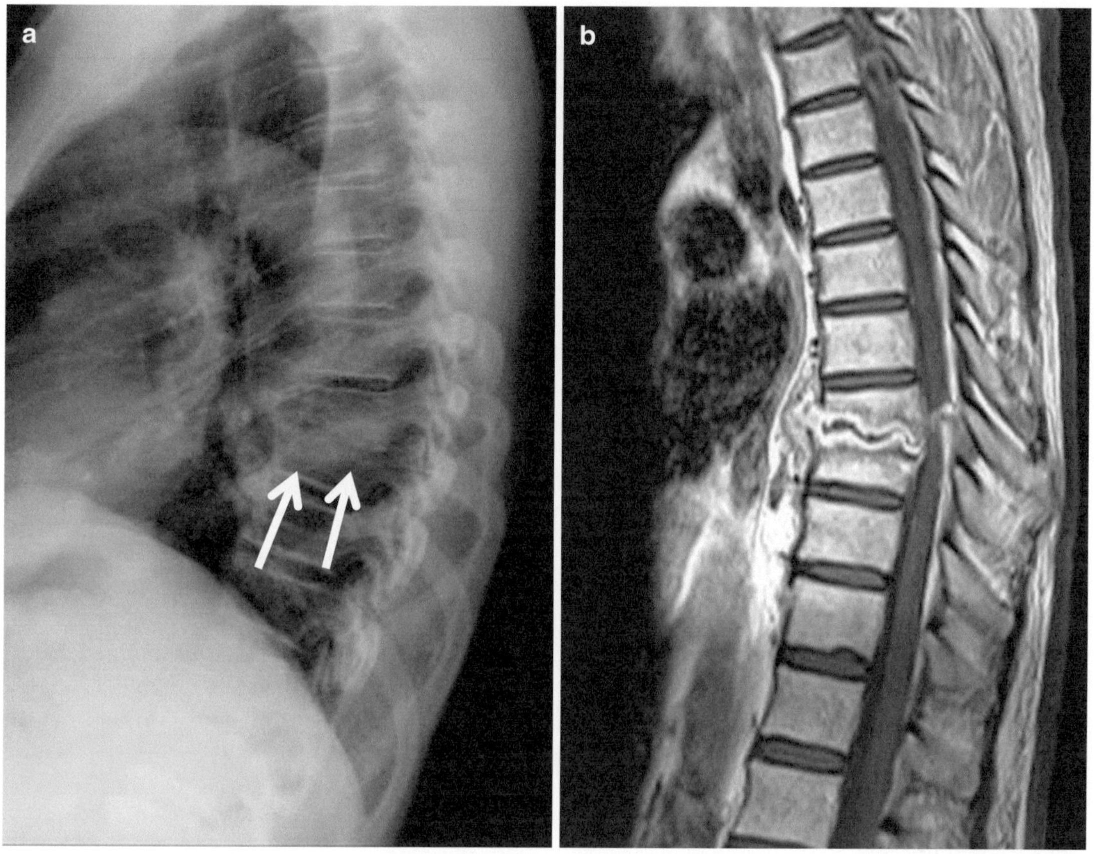

Fig. 51.3 Radiographic findings of spondylodiscitis. (**a**) Lateral thoracic spine radiography shows loss of definition of endplates at T9–T10 with decreased intervertebral disk space height (*arrows*). (**b**) Sagittal contrast-enhanced T1WI demonstrate endplate destruction and irregular peripheral disk enhancement with paraspinal soft tissue involvement. Note compression of the spinal cord

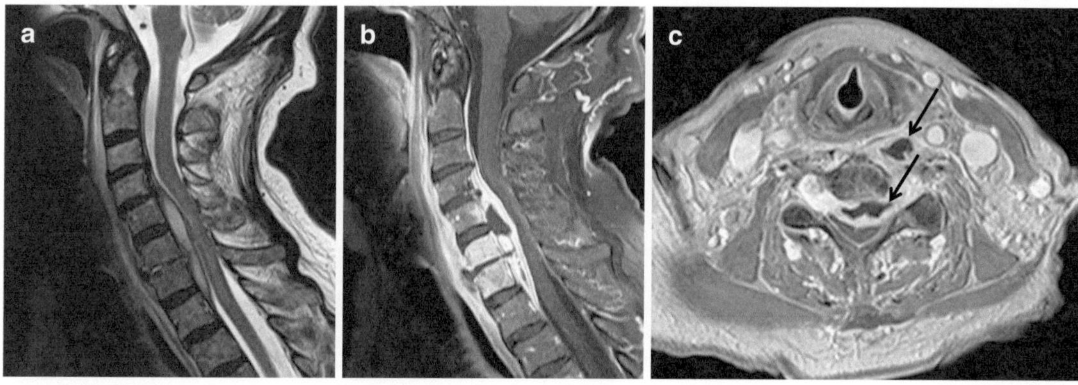

Fig. 51.4 Epidural abscess. (**a**). Sagittal T2WI show high signal intensity and loss of disk space height at C6–C7 with paraspinal and epidural abscesses and mass effect on the spinal cord. (**b**) Sagittal contrast-enhanced fat-saturated T1WI demonstrate homogeneous enhancement of the vertebral bodies and peripheral enhancement of the epidural collection, confirming a necrotic pus-filled abscess. (**c**) Axial contrast-enhanced T1WI show paraspinal and epidural rim enhancing abscesses (*arrows*) with spinal cord compression

inflammation; however, the imaging extension of disk and bone involvement and destruction may progress, including involvement of new levels, not necessarily denoting treatment failure [12, 13].

Epidural abscess follow-up findings correlate better with clinical improvement or deterioration. Response to therapy is manifested by diminished contrast enhancement and better visualization of the subarachnoid space. Persistent contrast enhancement can be observed at the sites of surgical drainage and decompression surgery and may not indicate treatment failure [10].

Main Differential Diagnosis

Tuberculous spondylitis (*TS*). Many times it is difficult to differentiate pyogenic spondylitis and TS clinically and by imaging. The relatively late presentation and chronic course of TS and the lack of proteolytic enzymes in the *Mycobacterium* as compared with pyogenic infection have been proposed as the causes for the different MRI findings between pyogenic and TS [14, 15].

Findings suggestive of TS rather than pyogenic spondylitis are a well-defined paraspinal abnormal signal: a thin and smooth abscess wall, subligamentous spread to three or more vertebral levels, and multiple vertebral or entire vertebral body involvement [14]. TS most commonly involves the thoracic spine and less often the lumbar spine. The presence of skip lesions and relative preservation of the intervertebral disk is also suggestive of TS. MRI is less sensitive than CT for identifying pathological calcifications, which are a distinctive imaging feature of TS (Table 51.1) (Fig. 51.5) [14–16].

Degenerative disk and Modic type 1 changes. Modic type 1 degenerative signal changes, representing vascularized bone marrow and edema, may mimic MRI findings associated with infection. Imaging features that may help distinguishing pyogenic spondylitis from Modic type 1 changes are the presence of endplate destruction, blurred margins of marrow signal alterations on T1WI, and the presence of paraspinal soft tissue abnormalities all of them seen in infections. Useful features that can suggest degenerative changes are stability over time and a disk space vacuum sign [2, 17]. On DWI, a well-marginated, linear region of high signal situated between the interface of normal and abnormal bone marrow is highly suggestive of degeneration (called the "claw" sign) [18].

Hyperintensity of the disks on T2WI and disk enhancement are not specific to infectious spondylitis; however, it is important to note that the areas of enhancement related to disk degeneration correspond with the areas of high T2 signal intensity, representing inflammation and not an abscess (Table 51.2) [17].

Dialysis spondyloarthropathy: Destructive spondyloarthropathy is considered a serious complication of chronic hemodialysis and may closely resemble spondylodiscitis on imaging. It shows a predilection for the lower portion of the cervical spine, although the craniocervical junction, and occasionally the thoracic and lumbar spine, may also be affected. Imaging findings are nonspecific, but decrease signal intensity in the affected vertebral endplates and intervertebral disks on T2WI and the absence of paraspinal masses suggest this rare condition [19]. This disease is a diagnosis of exclusion.

Neuropathic spine: Repeated trauma in the setting of diminished protective sensation leads

Table 51.1 Imaging finding of tuberculous and pyogenic spondylodiscitis

	Pyogenic	Tuberculous
Spine segment	Lumbar	Thoracic/thoracolumbar
Paraspinal/epidural space involvement	Small abscesses with thick and irregular enhancement	Large, well defined, with thin and smooth wall Subligamentous spread
Vertebral body	Endplate destruction, homogeneous enhancement	Intravertebral osseous abscess, heterogeneous enhancement, high bone destruction
Multilevel involvement	$\leq$2 vertebral bodies	Common, skip lesions
Disk space involvement	Intradiscal abscess, collapse, and destruction	Variable, from normal to severe destruction
Posterior elements	Rare	More frequently

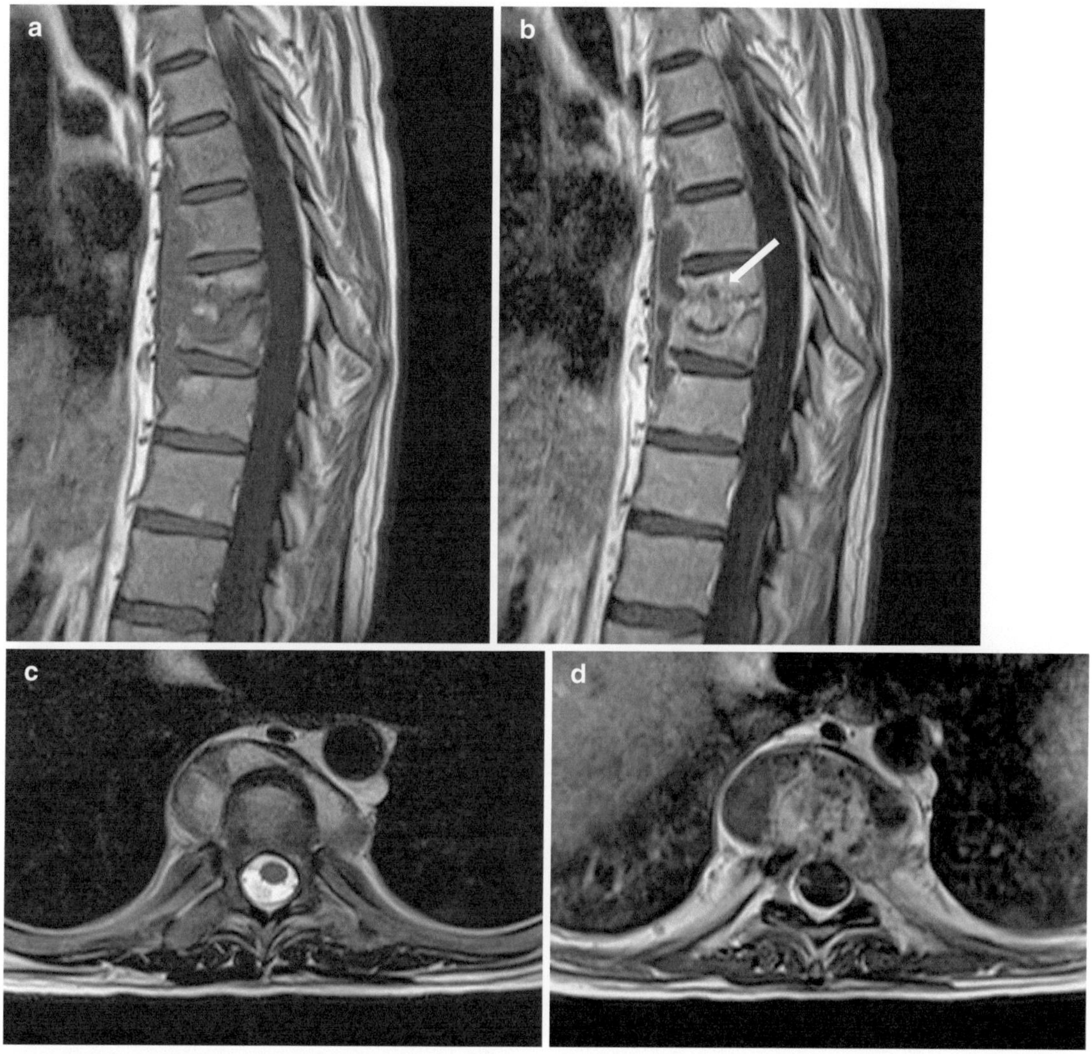

Fig. 51.5 Tuberculous spondylodiscitis. (**a**) Sagittal T1WI show heterogeneous signal in T8–T9 vertebral bodies with paraspinal mass and subligamentous spread from T6 to T10. (**b**) Sagittal contrast-enhanced T1WI demonstrate heterogeneous disk enhancement and intraosseous abscesses (*arrow*). (**c**) Axial T2WI and (**d**) axial contrast-enhanced T1WI show well-defined paraspinal collections with a thin and smooth rim enhancement

Table 51.2 Degenerative changes and pyogenic spondylitis imaging findings

	Degenerative	Spondylodiscitis
Disk space signal	T2 hypointensity	T2 hyperintensity
	Severe degenerated disks can be T2 hyperintense	
Disk enhancement	May be present	Typically present
Vacuum sign	Often present	Absent
Vertebral endplates	Irregularity with preservation of cortical T1 hypointense signal	Destruction with loss of cortical T1 hypointense signal
Bone marrow	Sharp margins of the signal alterations	Blurred definition between normal and abnormal signal
Location	Related to biomechanical stress	Anterior
Paraspinal tissue	Normal	Inflammation/abscess
Temporal evolution	Stability	Rapid progression

to vertebral fractures followed by bone sclerosis, formation of large osteophytes, and loss of the disk space. On T2WI, the disk space and surrounding marrow have lower signal intensity in the neuropathic spine than in spondylodiscitis. Vacuum phenomenon and facet involvement are other common findings suggestive of spinal neuropathic arthropathy [16].

Tips

- Immediately report the presence of epidural abscess to allow for rapid surgical intervention.
- The presence of a necrotic cavity related to an abscess influences the clinical approach and identifies drainable areas.
- Spinal deformity and possible spinal instability should be mentioned, because surgical intervention to stabilize the spine may be indicated.
- CT can be useful confirming degenerative findings suspected on MRI, demonstrating better the vacuum phenomenon and lack of destructive changes. DWI is useful in confirming degenerative findings and confirming the presence of abscess.

References

1. Gouliouris T, Aliyu SH, Brown NM. Spondylodiscitis: update on diagnosis and management. J Antimicrob Chemother. 2010;65 Suppl 3:iii11–24.
2. Diehn FE. Imaging of spine infection. Radiol Clin N Am. 2012;50:777–98.
3. Duarte RM, Vaccaro AR. Spinal infection: state of the art and management algorithm. Eur Spine J. 2013; 22(12):2787–99.
4. Jetvic V. Vertebral infection. Eur Radiol. 2004;14: E43–52.
5. Gemmel F, Rijk PC, Collins JM, et al. Expanding role of ^{18}F-fluoro-D-deoxylgucose PET and PET/CT in spinal infections. Eur Spine. 2010;19:540–51.
6. Modic MT, Feiglin DH, Pirano DW, et al. Vertebral osteomyelitis: assessment using MR. Radiology. 1985;157:157–66.
7. Ledermann HP, Schweitzer ME, Morrison WB, et al. MR imaging findings in spinal infections: rules or myths? Radiology. 2003;228:506–14.
8. Dagirmanjian A, Schils J, McHenry M, et al. MR imaging of vertebral osteomyelitis revisited. AJR Am J Roentgenol. 1996;167:1539–43.
9. Sandhu FS, Dillon WP. Spinal epidural abscess: evaluation with contrast-enhanced MR imaging. AJNR Am J Neuroradiol. 1991;12:1087–93.
10. Numaguchi Y, Rigamonti D, Rothman M, et al. Spinal epidural abscess: evaluation with gadolinium enhanced MR imaging. Radiographics. 1993;13:545–59.
11. Eastwood JD, Vollmer RT, Provenzale JM. Diffusion-weighted imaging in a patient with vertebral and epidural abscesses. AJNR Am J Neuroradiol. 2002;23:496–8.
12. Kowalski TJ, Layton KF, Berbari EF. Follow-up MR imaging in patients with pyogenic spine infections: lack of correlation with clinical features. AJNR Am J Neuroradiol. 2007;28:693–9.
13. Gilliams AR, Chaddha B, Carter AP. MR appearances of the temporal evolution and resolution of infectious spondylitis. AJR Am J Roentgenol. 1996;166:903–7.
14. Jung NY, Jee WH, Ha KY, et al. Discrimination of tuberculous spondylitis from pyogenic spondylitis on MRI. AJR Am J Roentgenol. 2004;182:1405–10.
15. Lee KY. Comparison of pyogenic spondylitis and tuberculous spondylitis. Asian Spine J. 2014;8(2):216–23.
16. Hong SH, Choi JY, Lee JW, et al. MR Imaging assessment of the spine: infection or and imitation? Radiographics. 2009;29:599–612.
17. Kwon JW, Yoon YC, Choi SH, et al. MR imaging for the differentiation of early infectious spondylitis and Modic type I change in the lumbar spine. J Korean Soc Radiol. 2010;62:563–70.
18. Patel KB, Poplawski MM, Pawha PS, et al. Diffusion-weighted MRI "claw sign" improves differentiation of infectious from degenerative Modic type 1 signal changes of the spine. AJNR Am J Neuroradiol. 2014;35(8):1647–52.
19. Theodorou DJ, Theodorou SJ, Resnick D. Imaging in dialysis spondyloarthropathy. Semin Dial. 2002;15(4): 290–6.

Spinal Fractures in Adults

52

Denise Tokeshi Amaral,
Rodrigo Sanford Damasceno,
and Lázaro Luís Faria do Amaral

Abstract

Traumatic spinal fractures typically occur in younger patients generally following a high-energy motor vehicle accidents or falls. In a poly-traumatized patient, the precise mechanism of a complex spinal injury may be difficult to elicit, but recognition of a fracture pattern may lead the radiologist to infer the likelihood of soft tissue and/or neurological injuries and/or instability. The advent of multi-detector CT has allowed a rapid assessment of the spine and to expedite management and reduce patient morbidity.

Background

Trauma to spinal vertebrae may result in isolated spinal column or spinal cord injuries. These lesions often result in profound and long-term disabilities that have a devastating effect from the physical, psychological, and socioeconomic points of view. Traumatic vertebral fractures predominantly affect young men and elderly women. The average age is 32 years old and 55 % of patients are between 16 and 30 years of age. Approximately one half of spinal injuries occur in the cervical spine. Motor vehicle accidents are their main cause (40 %), and other common causes include falls, followed by acts of violence and sporting activities [1, 2].

Clinical manifestations include pain, tenderness, or/and neurological deficits. Since the majority of spine injuries are not a result of direct force impact, external signs of trauma may not be present. Some clinical factors may be con-

D.T. Amaral, MD (✉)
Radiology Department, Hospital Sírio-Libanês,
Rua Luiz Gottschal, 151, apt. 111 MS, Vila Mariana,
04008-070 Sao Paulo, SP, Brazil
e-mail: denitok@gmail.com

R.S. Damasceno, MD
Division of Musculoskeletal Radiology,
Hospital Sírio-Libanês, Rua Antonio Carlos,
196, apt 107A, 001309-010 Sao Paulo, SP, Brazil
e-mail: sanfordrsd@yahoo.com

L.L.F. do Amaral, MD
Division of Neuroradiology at Medimagem,
Hospital Beneficência Portuguesa de São Paulo,
Rua Luiz Gottschal, 151, apt. 111 MS, Vila Mariana,
04008-070 Sao Paulo, SP, Brazil

Division of Neuroradiology,
Hospital Santa Casa de Misericórdia de São Paulo,
Rua Dr. Cesário Motta Junior 112,
Vila Buarque, Sao Paulo,
SP 01221-020, Brazil
e-mail: lazden@terra.com.br

R. Hoffmann Nunes et al. (eds.), *Critical Findings in Neuroradiology*,
DOI 10.1007/978-3-319-27987-9_52

sidered as risks of spinal fracturs, optimizing imaging strategies. The National Emergency X-Radiography Utilization Study (NEXUS) is a decision tool that comprises five criteria of low-risk cervical spine injury [3]:

- No posterior midline cervical tenderness
- No focal neurological deficit
- Patient is alert
- No intoxication
- No painful distracting injuries elsewhere

The Canadian cervical spine rule (CCS) identifies patients at low risk when the subject, age 16–65 years, is able to turn the head 45° in both directions [4]. High-risk patients according to the "Harbourview Criteria" are those involved in high energy trauma (>50 km/h, fall from more than 3 m height, motor vehicle crash with death at scene) or that have high-risk clinical parameters such as significant head injuries, neurological signs referable to the cervical spine, and pelvic or multiple extremity fractures [5]. Treatment can be conservative if stability is preserved and surgery is necessary for unstable injuries or when significant deformities are present [1, 2].

Key Points

Etiology

Axial loading, hyperflexion, hyperextension, distraction, and rotational stress [6] represent the main mechanisms of spinal injuries. The cervical spine is highly susceptible to traumatic injury because it is extremely mobile, has relatively small vertebral bodies, and supports the relatively heavy head. Spinal column injuries have a bimodal age distribution with a first peak in young adults (traumatic fractures) and a second peak in adults older than 65 years of age (osteoporotic fractures) (See Chap. 44) [1, 2].

Best Imaging Modality

Computed tomography (CT) is the modality of choice for acute spinal trauma screening. However, radiographs may be used as the primary choice for assessing cervical spinal trauma in low-risk group patients (see flow chart). If the results are unclear, CT or magnetic resonance imaging (MRI) must be performed. The advantages of radiographs are their low cost, wide availability, and the broad experience available with this method [2]. A radiographic study of the cervical spine should consist of at least three images, a lateral view (from skull base to T1), an open-mouth odontoid, and an anteroposterior view. Dynamic views (flexion and extension) are relatively contraindicated in the acutely traumatized spine and unconscious high-risk patients [7, 8].

High-risk patients must undergo a multidetector CT study (see flow chart) [2]. CT depicts the bony anatomy of the spinal canal, bony fragments within the spinal canal, disk herniations, and epidural hemorrhage. Its limitation is the inability to provide appropriate screening for ligamentous injury and spinal cord lesions [2]. The CT protocol involves scanning the entire cervical spine (above foramen magnum to T2), without contrast, collimation of 0,6 mm and 2 mm axial section thickness with a 1 mm reconstruction interval. Coronal and sagittal reformations are recommended, and contiguous acquisition of images is desirable as disk-space-targeted axial images decrease the detection of fractures [9].

MRI is the preferred technique for the detection of bone contusions, spinal cord lesions, disk herniations, spinal ligamentous injuries, and intramedullary hemorrhage [2]. MRI is indicated regardless of CT findings when there is clinical evidence of progressive neurological deficits, incomplete neurological deficit, and/or severe pain [9]. The typical MRI protocol includes sagittal T1-weighted imaging (T1WI), T2-weighted imaging (T2WI), fluid-sensitive MR images that includes short inversion time inversion recovery (STIR) or fat-saturated T2-weighted sequences as well as at least axial gradient echo images which tend to accentuate the artifacts caused by blood products allowing an easier identification of hematomas. Sagittal fluid-sensitive images are particularly important for the evaluation of the integrity of the posterior ligamentous complex, detection of fluid within the facet capsules, or edema in the interspinous regions. If a pathological fracture is suspected, sagittal and axial fat-suppressed post-contrast T1WI are recommended [2, 9].

CT angiography may be considered when vascular involvement such as arterial dissection/occlusion is suspected, and CT myelography may be used in cases which MRI is not available or contraindicated [2, 9].

Major Findings

The major imaging finding related to a fracture is the presence of a cortical bone discontinuity. In acute fractures, there may be an associated paravertebral soft tissue component seen on CT and MRI, and the affected bone shows increased signal on T2WI and STIR images corresponding to bone and bone marrow edema [2, 9, 10].

Specific Fractures

Burst (Jefferson) fractures: This is an unstable fracture that occurs due to axial compression transmitted through the lateral masses of C1 causing fractures of both its anterior and posterior arches. Lateral displacement of the lateral masses of C1 over the lateral masses of C2 of >7 mm implies instability due to tearing of transverse ligament and atlantoaxial instability (Fig. 52.1) [7].

C1 posterior arch fractures: An extension mechanism can lead to the compression of the posterior arch of C1 only by the occiput and spinous process of C2. It is considered stable since the anterior arch and transverse ligament are intact [10].

C2 pedicle fractures: It is also known as "hangman fracture" and is an unstable traumatic spondylolysis of C2 caused by extreme hyperextension compromising both pedicles of C2 [10]. It is imperative to visualize the entire cervical spine to prevent missing multilevel spine injuries which are overlooked in 23 % of all spine injuries (Fig. 52.2) [11].

Odontoid fractures: These are caused by forceful flexion or extension of the head in the sagittal plane, classified into three types as follows: [12]

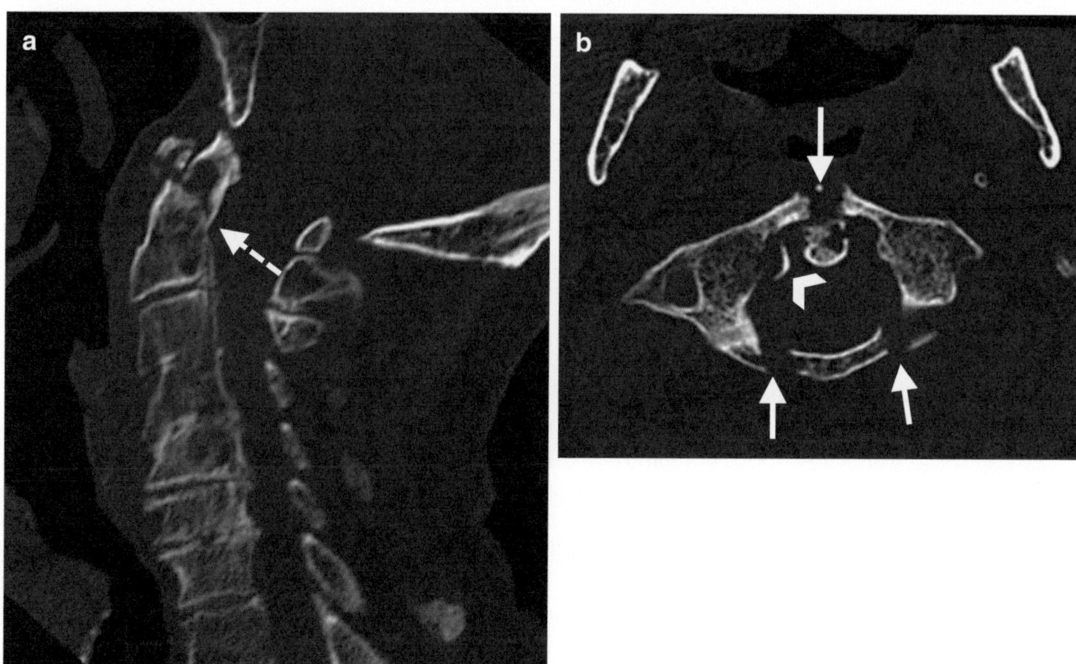

Fig. 52.1 A 76-year-old man with C2 odontoid and Jefferson type fractures. Sagittal (**a**) and axial (**b**) CT images demonstrate a fracture at the base of the odontoid process (type II injury) with posterior distal fragment angulation (*dashed arrow*). Fractures of the anterior and posterior arches of C1 (*arrows*) and rupture of right transverse and alar ligament with osseous avulsion on the right (*arrowhead*) are also seen

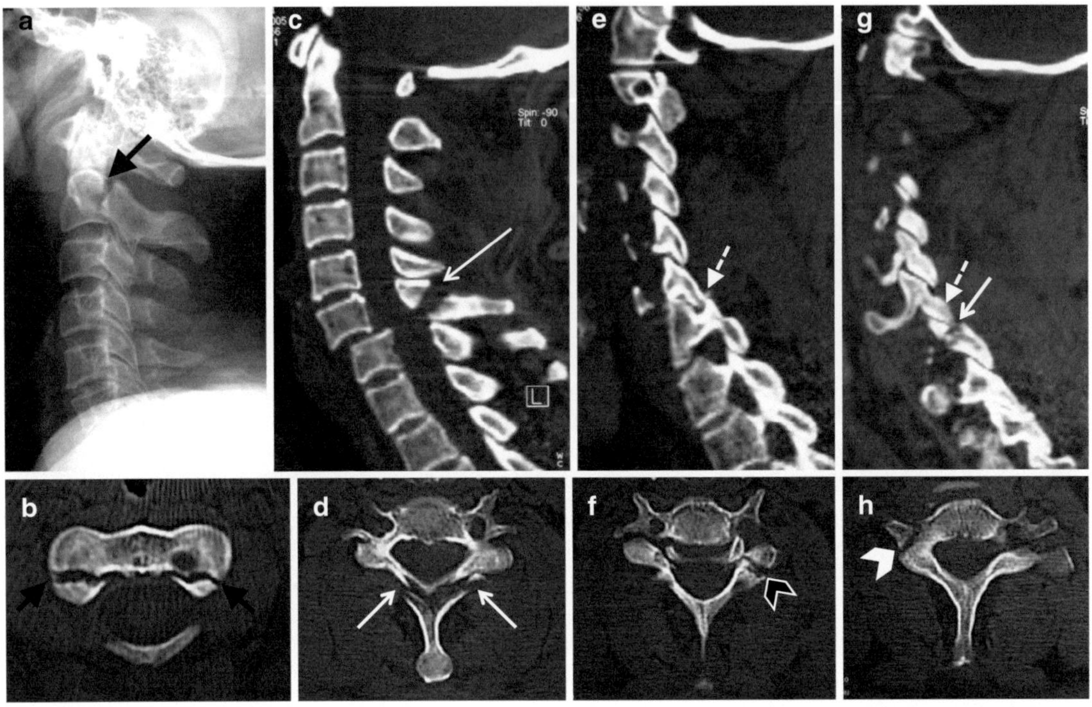

Fig. 52.2 A 52-year-old man after a motor vehicle accident presenting with left upper limb paresis and paresthesia. (**a**) Lateral cervical spine radiograph image demonstrates fractures of the pedicles of C2 (*arrow*). Note that the C6–C7 level is not properly evaluated. (**b**) Axial CT image confirms fractures of both pedicles of C2 (*arrows*). Sagittal (**c**) and axial (**d**) CT images show anterolisthesis of the vertebral body of C6 (*star*) as well as a fracture of the spinous process at the same level (*arrows* on **c** and **d**). (**e–h**) Series of sagittal and axial CT images reveal bilateral facet dislocations with "locked" appearances (*dashed arrows* on **e** and **g**) and fractures of the left superior articular (*arrowhead* on **f**) and right transverse processes of C7 (*white arrowhead* on **h**)

- Type I: It is an avulsion fracture of the tip of the dens which is stable and occurs above the transverse ligament.
- Type II fracture: It is the most common fracture of the dens, is unstable and involves the base of the odontoid process (Fig. 52.1).
- Type III fracture: It occurs when the fracture extends into the upper part of the C2 vertebral body and heals well with external immobilization but can cause spinal canal compromise [13, 14].

Teardrop fracture: This injury is the result of abrupt neck extension which causes the anterior longitudinal ligament to avulse the inferior border of the vertebral body. It results in instability at hyperextension. Flexion teardrop fractures result from a combination of forceful flexion and axial compression. The intervertebral disk, the facet joint capsules, and the posterior ligamentous structures are disruptured, and thus, it is highly unstable (Fig. 52.3) [15].

Facet Dislocations

- Bilateral facet dislocations: These occur due to a combined flexion and anterior dislocation, causing disruption of the annulus fibrosus of the intervertebral disks and of the anterior longitudinal ligament. The inferior articulating facets of the upper vertebra lie superior to the articulating facets of the lower vertebra resulting in anterior displacement of the spine and disruption of the posterior ligament complex. The lesion is extremely unstable and often results in complete spinal cord injury (Fig. 52.2) [16].
- Unilateral facet dislocation: This injury is due to flexion and rotation of one of the facet joints with dislocation occurring in the contralateral joint [16].

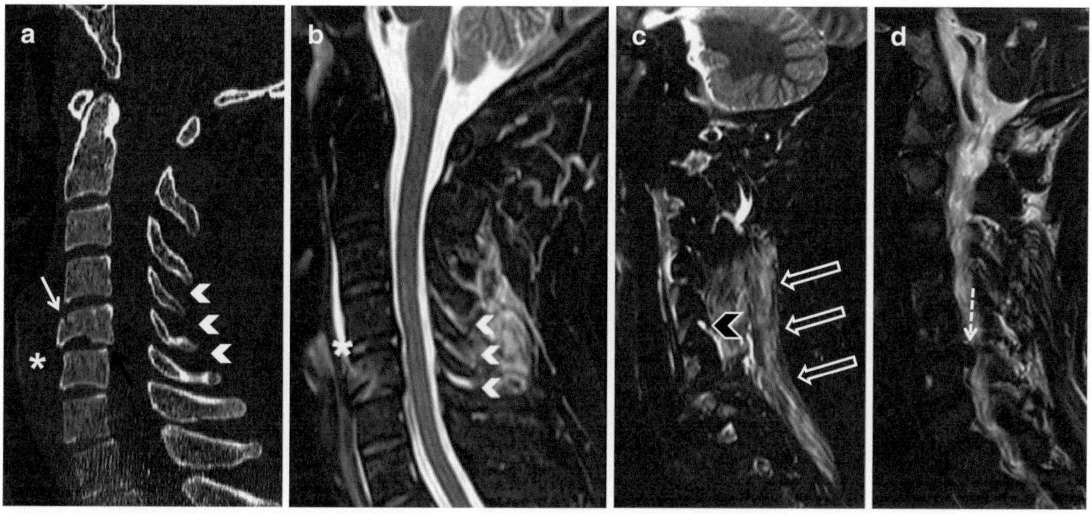

Fig. 52.3 A 33-year-old man who sustained chest injuries and a flexion teardrop fracture after being ejected from a car. (**a**) Sagittal CT image demonstrates a fracture of the anterior C5 vertebral body (*white arrow*) with anterior soft tissue swelling (*star*), subtle retrolisthesis of C5 on C6 (*black arrow*), and no evidence of diastasis of the spinous processes (*arrowheads*), although there is abnormal high signal from the posterior spinal soft tissues. (**b–d**) Series of sagittal STIR images depict a small fluid collection in the anterior paravertebral space (*) and increased signal intensity of the interspinous ligaments from C3 to C6 (*white arrowheads*). There are also signs of a rupture of the facet joint capsule of C5–C6 (*black arrowhead*), marked edema of the posterior paravertebral musculature (*open white arrows*), and a disk extrusion at C5–C6 (*dashed arrow*)

Spinous process fractures: These are isolated fractures of one or more spinous processes of a lower cervical vertebrae and are stable lesions generally caused by motor vehicle accidents involving sudden deceleration and forced neck flexion (Fig. 52.2) [10].

Compression and burst fractures: Compression fractures may be either anterior or lateral and result from failure of the anterior spine column under compression with the middle column acting as a hinge and therefore being spared. Burst fractures also arise from the same mechanism; however, the involvement of the middle column differentiates a burst from a compression fracture (Fig. 52.4). In the latter, there is often bony retropulsion into the spinal canal and the interpedicular distance may be widened on frontal images. With the growing use of MRI in spinal trauma, injury to the posterior ligamentous complex is often seen in cases of burst fractures. Compression and burst fractures are seen in approximately 10 % of patients with calcaneal fractures when axial forces are transmitted through to the spine [10].

Chance fractures: They consist of compression and flexion injuries to the anterior portion of the vertebral body and a transverse fracture through the posterior elements of the vertebra. Most occur in the thoracolumbar junction (T12–L2) and are accompanied by aorta or visceral injuries [10].

Vascular injuries: The incidence of vertebral artery injuries is between 17 % and 46 %, and most are caused by direct trauma from bone fragments or from excessive stretching that accompanies fractures and dislocations [9].

Important radiological signs of *cervical spine trauma on radiographs* related to instability are as follows:[7, 17]

- Widened interspinous space or facet joint of more than 50 %
- Anterior listhesis greater than 3.5 mm
- Narrowed or widened disk spaces
- Focal angulation of more than 11°
- Vertebral compression of more than 50 %
- Widened retropharyngeal space (distance from pharyngeal air column to the anterior aspect of the body of C2 exceeding 7 mm)
- Widened retrotracheal space (distance from the posterior tracheal wall to the body of C6

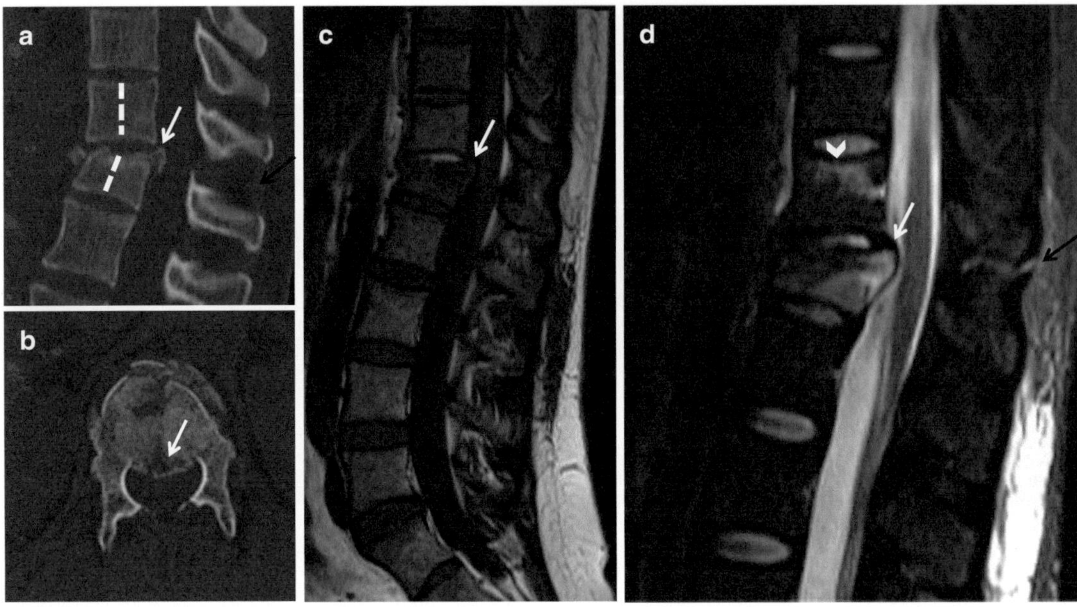

Fig. 52.4 A 32-year-old man presenting with a burst fracture of L1 following a high-speed motor vehicle accident. Sagittal (**a**) and axial (**b**) CT images demonstrate a burst fracture of the L1 vertebral body with a less than 50 % height loss (*white dashed lines* on **a**) and bony fragment retropulsion into the spinal canal (*white arrows* on **a** and **b**). An increased interspinous distance of T12 and L1 (*black arrow* on **a**) is also depicted. Sagittal T1WI (**c**) and STIR (**d**) images confirm the L1 fracture and the fragment retropulsion into the spinal canal (*white arrows*) that impinges on the conus medullaris. A compression fracture of the superior end plate of the vertebral body of T12 (*white arrowhead*) and an increased interspinous distance of T12 and L1 are also seen as well as high signal intensity within the posterior ligamentous complex (*black arrow* on **d**) which is probably due to rupture of the supraspinous and interspinous ligaments making this an unstable fracture

exceeding 14 mm in children and 22 mm in adults)
- Widened middle atlantoaxial joint (more than 3 mm in adults and 5 mm in children)
- Widened apophyseal joints of over 2 mm

Classification of Vertebral Fractures [18, 19]

Historically, the Denis three-column theory [20] classified spinal instability as disruption of two of the three columns [8]. Nowadays, thoracolumbar and cervical spine injuries are preferably classified using the *TLICS* (thoracolumbar injury classification and severity score – Table 52.1) and the *SCSIC* (subaxial cervical spine injury classification system –Table 52.2) schemes which provide a numerical score that can help predict the need for surgical intervention as follows:

The anatomic components of discoligamentous complex comprise the intervertebral disks and the anterior and posterior ligamentous structures. The most reliable signs of posterior ligamentous complex injury are the disruption of the posterior low-signal-intensity black line seen on sagittal T1- or T2-weighted MRI, indicating a supraspinous ligament or ligamentum flavum tear, as well as fluid in the facet capsules or edema in the interspinous region, representing a capsular or interspinous ligament injury, respectively (Fig. 52.4). The neurological status of the patient includes nerve root injury and complete and partial spinal cord injuries.

A thoracolumbar injury with a score higher than 4 requires intervention; meanwhile one with a score less than 4 is treated conservatively. A score of 4 indicates an intermediate zone where surgical or nonsurgical treatment may be equally appropriate. The need for cervical spine surgical intervention is 76 % in patients with a score of 7 [18, 19].

Table 52.1 The thoracolumbar injury classification and severity (TLICS) score

Feature	No. of points
Injury morphology	
Compression (axial, lateral)	1
Burst	2
Translational or rotational (unilateral, bilateral facet dislocation)	3
Distraction (flexion, extension)	4
Posterior ligamentous complex	
Suspected or indeterminate	2
Injured	3
Neurological status	
Nerve roots	2
Complete cord injury	2
Incomplete cord injury	3
Cauda equina	3

Table 52.2 The subaxial (C3–7) cervical injury classification (SLICS) system

Feature	No. of points
Injury morphology	
Compression (axial, lateral)	1
Burst	2
Distraction (perch facet, hyperextension)	3
Rotational or translational (severe flexion or compression injury, facet dislocation, teardrop)	4
Discoligamentous complex	
Indeterminate	1
Disrupted (widening of anterior disk space, perch facet or dislocation, kyphotic deformity)	2
Neurological status	
Root injury	1
Complete cord injury	2
Incomplete cord injury	3

Imaging Follow-Up

Imaging follow-up of vertebral fractures is controversial. Imaging can be obtained to assess healing at 2–3 months when a callus should be visualized on radiographs (earlier on CT). Dynamic evaluation with flexion and extension radiographs for identification of instability is not helpful in the acute stage because of muscle spam, but it has a role in patients with persistent neck pain treated initially with a collar and a normal neurological examination, CT and MRI. These patients should be able to self-achieve flexion and extension during studies to assess stability before discontinuing the use of the collar generally 1–2 weeks after the injury and when muscle spasm has resolved. MRI is sometimes performed within 48 h (Fig. 52.5) to avoid keeping patients in collars for unnecessarily long periods which may lead to complications and because by this time many patients have recovered to the point that a reliable neurological examination may be performed [21].

Main Differential Diagnosis

Benign Versus Malignant Fracture

Signs of a benign fracture on MRI:

- Low-signal-intensity band within a vertebral body on T1WI and T2WI representing the fracture line
- Sparing of the bone marrow signal intensity in the fractured vertebra
- Retropulsion of a posterior bone fragment and multiple compression fractures at other levels [22]

Signs of malignant compression fractures:

- A convex posterior border of the fractured vertebral body (due to expansion of the vertebral body secondary to underlying tumor)
- A compression fracture involving the inferior end plate with normal superior end plate should raise suspicion for a pathologic fracture
- Abnormal bone marrow signal intensity extending to the pedicles and posterior elements
- Presence of epidural, encasing epidural. and/or paraspinal soft tissue mass [22]

Congenital anomalies:

- Congenital alterations such as *os odontoideum*, occult *spina bifida*, and lack of segmentation are usually seen in children but may also be identified in adult patients and must not be interpreted as pathological [7, 9, 13].

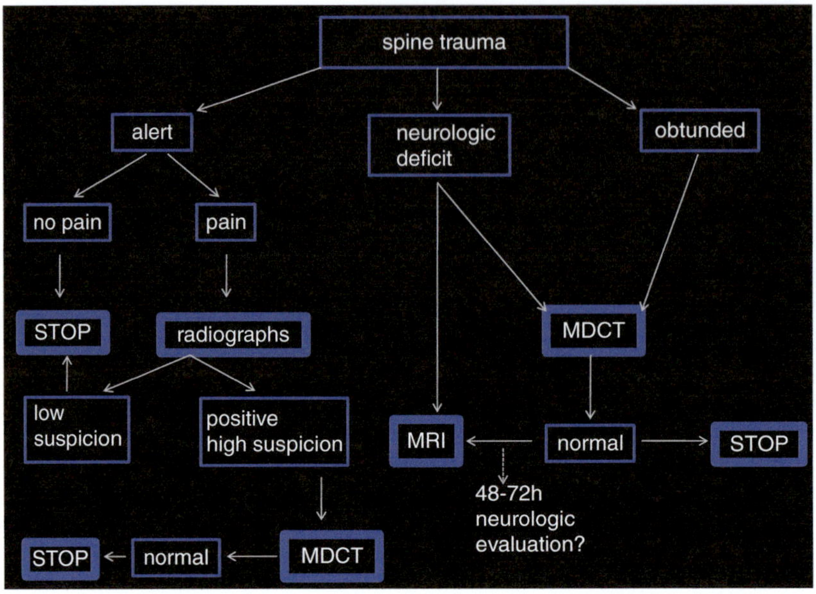

Fig. 52.5 Spine trauma imaging approach

Tips

- Application of the clinical prediction rules as NEXUS and CCS dramatically decreases the rate of unnecessary cervical spine imaging.
- Look for bone fragments in the spinal canal, vertebral dislocations, or other signs of potential cord compression and report them immediately.
- Multiple vertebral fractures of vertebrae are common. Examine each one of them for evidence of subtle fractures, particularly in the facets, transverse, and spinous processes which are frequently missed.
- Recent fractures tend to be associated with impaction of bone trabeculae (seen on radiographs), bone marrow edema (seen only on MRI), pre- and paravertebral hemorrhage (seen on MRI and CT), epidural hemorrhage (better seen on MRI but also detectable by CT), and spinal cord edema (seen only on MRI).
- Search for signs of pathologic fractures, such as replacement of the normal fatty (bright T1) bone marrow signal intensity and paraspinal/epidural soft tissue mass.
- Report involvement of the transverse foramina that may be associated with vertebral artery dissection in the cervical spine.

References

1. Hu R, Mustard CA, Burns C. Epidemiology of incident spinal fracture in a complete population. Spine (Phila Pa 1976). 1996;21(4):492–9.
2. Parizel PM, van der Zijden T, Gaudino S, Spaepen M, Voormolen MH, Venstermans C, et al. Trauma of the spine and spinal cord: imaging strategies. Eur Spine J. 2010;19 Suppl 1:S8–17.
3. Hoffman JR, Mower WR, Wolfson AB, Todd KH, Zucker MI. Validity of a set of clinical criteria to rule out injury to the cervical spine in patients with blunt trauma. National Emergency X-Radiography Utilization Study Group. N Engl J Med. 2000;343(2):94–9.
4. Stiell IG, Wells GA, Vandemheen KL, Clement CM, Lesiuk H, De Maio VJ, et al. The Canadian C-spine rule for radiography in alert and stable trauma patients. JAMA. 2001;286(15):1841–8.

5. Hanson JA, Blackmore CC, Mann FA, Wilson AJ. Cervical spine injury: a clinical decision rule to identify high-risk patients for helical CT screening. AJR Am J Roentgenol. 2000;174(3):713–7.
6. Vollmer DG, Gegg C. Classification and acute management of thoracolumbar fractures. Neurosurg Clin N Am. 1997;8(4):499–507.
7. Ehara S, el-Khoury GY, Clark CR. Radiologic evaluation of dens fracture. Role of plain radiography and tomography. Spine (Phila Pa 1976). 1992;17(5): 475–9.
8. Freemyer B, Knopp R, Piche J, Wales L, Williams J. Comparison of five-view and three-view cervical spine series in the evaluation of patients with cervical trauma. Ann Emerg Med. 1989;18(8):818–21.
9. Munera F, Rivas LA, Nunez Jr DB, Quencer RM. Imaging evaluation of adult spinal injuries: emphasis on multidetector CT in cervical spine trauma. Radiology. 2012;263(3):645–60.
10. Hockerberg RS, Kaji AH. Spinal column injuries. In: Marx J, Hockberger R, Walls R, editors. Rosen's emergency medicine: concepts and clinical practice, vol. 6. Philadelphia: Mosby; 2006.
11. Wittenberg RH, Hargus S, Steffen R, Muhr G, Botel U. Noncontiguous unstable spine fractures. Spine (Phila Pa 1976). 2002;27(3):254–7.
12. Anderson LD, D'Alonzo RT. Fractures of the odontoid process of the axis. J Bone Joint Surg Am. 1974;56(8):1663–74.
13. Dreizin D, Letzing M, Sliker CW, Chokshi FH, Bodanapally U, Mirvis SE, et al. Multidetector CT of blunt cervical spine trauma in adults. Radiographics: Rev Publ Radiol Soc N Am Inc. 2014;34(7):1842–65.
14. Koivikko MP, Kiuru MJ, Koskinen SK, Myllynen P, Santavirta S, Kivisaari L. Factors associated with nonunion in conservatively-treated type-II fractures of the odontoid process. J Bone Joint Surg (Br). 2004;86(8): 1146–51.
15. Kim KS, Chen HH, Russell EJ, Rogers LF. Flexion teardrop fracture of the cervical spine: radiographic characteristics. AJR Am J Roentgenol. 1989;152(2): 319–26.
16. Woodring JH, Goldstein SJ. Fractures of the articular processes of the cervical spine. AJR Am J Roentgenol. 1982;139(2):341–4.
17. Clark W, Gehweiler Jr J, Laib R. Twelve significant signs of cervical spine trauma. Skelet Radiol. 1979;3(4):201–5.
18. Khurana B, Sheehan SE, Sodickson A, Bono CM, Harris MB. Traumatic thoracolumbar spine injuries: what the spine surgeon wants to know. Radiographics: Rev Publ Radiol Soc N Am Inc. 2013;33(7): 2031–46.
19. Vaccaro AR, Lehman Jr RA, Hurlbert RJ, Anderson PA, Harris M, Hedlund R, et al. A new classification of thoracolumbar injuries: the importance of injury morphology, the integrity of the posterior ligamentous complex, and neurologic status. Spine (Phila Pa 1976). 2005;30(20):2325–33.
20. Denis F. The three column spine and its significance in the classification of acute thoracolumbar spinal injuries. Spine (Phila Pa 1976). 1983;8(8): 817–31.
21. Daffner RH, Weissman BN, Wippold II FJ, Angtuaco EJ, Appel M, Berger KL, et al. Expert panels on musculoskeletal and neurological imaging. ACR appropriateness criteria® suspected spine trauma. Reston: American College of Radiology (ACR); 2012. [online publication]. 2012 [updated 2012; cited 2015]. Available from: http://www.acr.org/~/media/f579c123f999479c88390a3df976be77.pdf.
22. Jung HS, Jee WH, McCauley TR, Ha KY, Choi KH. Discrimination of metastatic from acute osteoporotic compression spinal fractures with MR imaging. Radiographics: Rev Publ Radiol Soc N Am Inc. 2003;23(1):179–87.

53 Adult Spinal Ligamentous Injuries

Joana Ramalho and Mauricio Castillo

Abstract

Ligamentous injuries may lead to clinical instability of the spine which occurs when the spinal ligaments and bones lose their ability to maintain the normal alignment between vertebral segments under a physiologic load. Instability poses risks to the spinal cord and nerve roots and is a critical factor in treatment planning. Ligaments can only be directly visualized on MRI, although CT and radiographs may show indirect signs of ligamentous injury especially when flexion and extension views are used.

Background

Spine ligaments are strong fibrous bands that connect the vertebrae together, providing support, flexibility, and stability to the spine. Ligaments prevent excessive movement such as hyperflexion or hyperextension during physiologic or traumatic motion helping to protect the spine and its contents.

Spine stability is defined as the ability to prevent the development of neurologic injury and progressive deformity in response to physiologic loading within a normal range of movement. Spine stability relies on the integrity of both bone and ligamentous components and injuries to either or both can result in instability. Instability can lead to further injury, pain, or deformity and may require surgical stabilization.

Ligamentous injuries are invariably associated with trauma. Motor vehicle-related accidents are the leading cause of spinal injuries, and speeding, alcohol intoxication, texting, and failure to use seat belts are the major compounding risk factors. Other common causes include falls, followed by acts of violence and sport activities.

Spinal column injuries are more common in males and have a bimodal age distribution with a first peak in young adults between 15 and 29 years of age and a second peak in adults older than 65 years of age [1]. The prevalence of unstable

J. Ramalho, MD (✉)
Radiology Department, University of North Carolina at Chapel Hill, Chapel Hill, NC, USA

Neuroradiology Department, Centro Hospitalar de Lisboa Central, Lisbon, Portugal
e-mail: Joana-ramalho@netcabo.pt

M. Castillo, MD, FACR
Division of Neuroradiology, University of North Carolina, Chapel Hill, NC, USA
e-mail: mauricio_castillo@med.unc.edu

R. Hoffmann Nunes et al. (eds.), *Critical Findings in Neuroradiology*,
DOI 10.1007/978-3-319-27987-9_53

ligamentous injuries in survivors of trauma has been estimated at 0.9 % by flexion–extension radiographs [2] and at 23 % by MRI studies. However, MRI does not directly assess stability, but rather ligamentous structural integrity, and the clinical implication of such findings remains uncertain [3].

Clinical manifestations include pain, tenderness, or/and neurological deficits. Since the majority of spine injuries are not a result of a direct force impact, external signs of trauma such as abrasions or contusions are relatively infrequent [4]. Unreliable patients with altered level of consciousness represent a particular diagnostic challenge, since only approximately one-half of patients with ligamentous injury present with neurological deficits [4]. Treatment and prognosis depend on the severity and stability of the lesion. Unstable lesions usually require surgical fixation.

The main ligaments of the spine are the anterior longitudinal ligament (ALL), posterior longitudinal ligament (PLL), and posterior ligamentous complex (PLC) that include the supraspinous and interspinous ligaments, articular facet capsules, and ligamentum flavum. The PLC serves as the posterior "tension band" of the spinal column and protects it from excessive flexion, rotation, translation, and distraction (Table 53.1).

Table 53.1 Ligaments of the spine

The *ALL* runs vertically along the anterior aspect of the vertebral body, firmly attached to the periosteum and disks (anterior annulus), extending from the anterior tubercle of the atlas to the anterior aspect of the upper sacrum. It limits extension of the spine and reinforces anteriorly the annulus fibrosus
The *PLL* runs vertically along the posterior aspect of the vertebral body, loosely attached to the vertebral body and firmly attached to the disks (posterior annulus), extending from the posterior aspect of the axis (C2) body to the posterior aspect of the sacrum. It limits flexion, reinforces posteriorly the annulus fibrosus, and is thick in its central portion, which helps to prevent disk herniation
The *interspinous ligament* is a relatively weak fibrous tissue ligament that runs from the lower edge of one spinous process to the upper edge of the next one. It fuses with supraspinous ligament
The *supraspinous ligament* merges with the interspinous ligaments, running the whole length of the vertebral column connecting the tips of the spinous processes
Articular facet capsule is a connective tissue that surrounds the sinovial facet joints
The *ligamentum flavum* lies on the front of the laminae extending from one lamina to the next, all the way down the spine. It is made of yellowish fibroelastic tissue, thus named yellow ligament

The anatomic and biomechanical properties of the craniocervical junction (CCJ) are unique and distinct from those of the subaxial (C2) spine. The CCJ is composed of two joints (the atlantooccipital and atlantoaxial joints) and a complex network of ligaments that allow significant mobility while simultaneously maintain the stability that is essential to protect its contents [5]. From this network, three CCJ ligaments are considered the major stabilizers: transverse ligament, alar ligaments, and tectorial membrane (Table 53.2) [6].

Key Points

Etiology

Axial loading, hyperflexion, hyperextension, distraction, and rotational stress [7] represent the main mechanisms of spinal injuries. The cervical spine is highly susceptible to traumatic injury because it is extremely mobile with relatively small vertebral bodies and supports the relatively heavy head. Within the cervical spine, the most commonly injured vertebrae are the axis (C2) and the regions of C5, C6, and C7. Typically, ligamentous injuries are associated with vertebral fractures, but pure ligamentous injuries may occur and are commonly associated with abnormal anatomic alignment (dislocation, subluxation, or listhesis).

A hyperflexion mechanism leads to disruption of the PLC that progress from posterior to anterior, beginning with disruption of the supraspinous ligament, interspinous ligaments, capsular ligaments, and ligamentum flavum. Alone, PCL injury is insufficient to generate spinal instability [8]. Anterior subluxation reflects further hyperflexion with disruption of the posterior longitudinal ligament and posterior disk annulus (middle of column of Denis), which leads to instability [8]. Hyperextension spine injuries result predominantly in ligamentous disruptions that progress

Table 53.2 Ligaments of the craniocervical junction

The *transverse ligament of the atlas* (C1) is the horizontal component of the *cruciform ligament*. It is the largest, strongest, and thickest craniocervical ligament (mean height/thickness 6–7 mm). It runs posterior to the odontoid process of C2 and attaches to the lateral tubercles of C1, bilaterally locking the odontoid process anteriorly against the posterior aspect of the anterior arch of C1. The superior and inferior limbs of the cruciform ligament, which attaches to the clivus and to the C2 body, respectively, are extremely thin and offer no known craniocervical stability [5]
The *alar ligaments* connect the lateral aspect of the odontoid process to the foramen magnum or occipital condyles, attaching the axis to the base of the skull [5]. They limit axial rotation at the occipito-atlantoaxial complex [6]
The *tectorial membrane* is composed of 2–3 distinct layers that run posterior to the cruciform ligament extending from the body of the axis (where it fuses with the PLL) to the posterior surface of the clivus (where it blends with the cranial dura mater)
The *apical ligament*, also known as the middle odontoid ligament or suspensory ligament, attaches the tip of the odontoid process to the basion [5]
The *transverse occipital ligament* attaches to the inner aspect of the occipital condyles and extends horizontally across the foramen magnum [5]
The *accessory atlantoaxial ligament* inserts medially onto the dorsal surface of the axis and courses laterally and superiorly to insert on the lateral mass of the atlas [5]
The *anterior atlantooccipital membrane* is a thin structure that attaches the anterior aspect of the atlas to the anterior rim of the foramen magnum [5]
The *posterior atlantooccipital membrane* is a broad, thin ligament that attaches the posterior arch of the atlas inferiorly to the posterior rim of the foramen magnum superiorly. It is continuous inferiorly with the ligamentum flavum [5]
The *nuchal ligament* is the cephalic extension of the supraspinous ligament extending from the C7 spinous process to the union of the occipital bone [5]
The *Barkow ligament* is a horizontal band attaching onto the anteromedial aspect of the occipital condyles anterior to the attachment of the alar ligaments, running anterior to the superior aspect of the odontoid process

from anterior to posterior, beginning with the anterior longitudinal ligament and anterior annulus fibrosus extending through the posterior annulus, posterior longitudinal ligament, and ligamentum flavum [8].

Best Imaging Modality

Computed tomography (CT): It is the modality of choice for acute spinal trauma screening [7]. In the setting of acute spinal trauma, axial data acquisition followed by sagittal multiplanar reformations (generally sagittal and coronal) is the mainstay of initial evaluation. Coronal reformations are also useful for visualization of the craniocervical junction as well as for the remainder of the spinal axis if scoliosis is present. If cervical fractures are detected, most patients will proceed to CT angiography to exclude vascular (especially vertebral artery) injuries [9, 10].

Magnetic resonance imaging (MRI): Although ligamentous injuries may be inferred from CT by using measurements, disruption of the ligaments can only be directly visualized on MRI. This capability suggests that MRI could be the preferred diagnostic study for ligamentous injury. However, several disadvantages of MRI prevent its widespread adoption of this purpose. Unlike radiographs and CT, MRI may be difficult to perform in the acute setting. Its long acquisition time makes unstable patients inappropriate candidates for MRI. Patients that require ventilator support and head trauma patients with intracranial pressure monitoring devices may not be appropriate candidates especially when imaged at 3.0 Tesla [4]. Furthermore, despite the high sensitivity of MRI for detecting ligamentous injuries, a recent study [11] raised concerns regarding the relative lack of agreement between specific MRI-detected abnormalities and corresponding intraoperative findings, suggesting that it may falsely overestimate the degree and extent of disruptive injuries [11].

Despite the lack of well-established criteria for MRI and its difficulty in distinguishing significant from inconsequential abnormalities, this technique has become part of the standard imaging protocol for patients with acute cervical spine injury in three main clinical scenarios: (1) patients with negative radiographs and negative CT who have neurologic symptoms or persistent neck pain [11], (2) patients with a high-energy mechanism of injury and an unreliable neurological examination with or without evidence CT abnormalities [5], and (3) patients with fractures or unstable injuries noted on radiographs and/or CT workup in whom MRI is needed for preoperative planning [11]. MRI allows direct evaluation of spinal cord, nerve roots, and ligamentous and soft tissue injuries.

The standard spine MRI protocol comprises sagittal and axial T1-weighted images (T1WI), T2-weighted images (T2WI), and fluid-sensitive MR images (which includes short inversion time inversion recovery (STIR) or fat-saturated T2-weighted sequences) as well as at least axial gradient-echo images (which tend to accentuate the artifacts caused by blood products and make identification of hematomas easier).

Radiographs: Active flexion and extension radiographs of the cervical spine have been used for identification of ligamentous injuries and instability. In unreliable patients, physicians may impart maximum flexion and extension to the patient's neck without concurrent knowledge of its consequences [4]. In this setting, some authors prefer to use MRI rather than dynamic radiographs [12–15]. Flexion and extension radiographs may be useful in evaluating potential ligamentous injury in patients who have equivocal MRI examinations such as when MRI demonstrates abnormal signal in spinal ligaments without definite disruptions. However, muscle spasm following an acute injury frequently results in poor degrees of flexion or extension limiting the use of MRI and radiographs in the acute setting.

Major Findings

As stated before, ligamentous injuries can be indirectly diagnosed or suspected based on CT or radiographic findings or directly assessed on MRI. Ligaments are visualized on MRI as continuous bands of hypointense T1 and T2 signal intensities. Therefore, ligament tears are visible as anatomical disruptions of these stripes with high signal intensity on T2WI. Partial tears are seen as focus of ill-defined soft tissue hyperintensity on T2WI or STIR images [7].

Subaxial hyperflexion injuries comprise different levels of severity of PLC disruption. Disruption of the PLC may be inferred on radiographs, CT, or MRI by the splaying of the spinous processes (widening of the interspinous space with resulting high T2 signal), avulsion fractures of the superior or inferior aspects of contiguous spinous processes, widening of the facet joints, empty ("naked") facet joints, perched or dislocated facet joints, or vertebral body translations or rotations. In this setting the PLC must be directly assessed using MRI regardless of the severity of vertebral body injury seen at CT. Fluid in the facet joint capsules or edema in the interspinous regions on fluid-sensitive MR images (STIR or fat-saturated T2-weighted sequences) reflects a capsular or interspinous ligament injuries.

Hyperextension injuries range from stable hyperextension sprains to the highly unstable hyperextension–dislocations. Hyperextension–dislocation injuries may be seen on lateral radiographs and sagittal CT reformations as mild anterior intervertebral disk space widening, anterior vertebral body avulsion fragments, and facet malalignment (V-shaped facet joints that are wide anteriorly and tapered posteriorly). MRI directly demonstrates ligamentous disruptions, soft tissue edema, disk protrusions, and associated spinal cord injuries [8] (Figs. 53.1, 53.2, 53.3, 53.4, 53.5, and 53.6).

The CCJ is susceptible to a wide range of fractures, dislocations, and ligamentous injuries. Jefferson fractures are mechanically and neurologically stable if the transverse ligament is intact. Transverse separation of fracture fragments by 7 mm or more indicates transverse ligament injury and instability. This measurement, known as the rule of Spence, is obtained axial CT images but is applicable only in the presence of a fracture. Other signs of instability include avulsion of the C1 tubercle (transverse ligament insertion), two anterior C1 ring fractures, and an atlantodental interval greater than

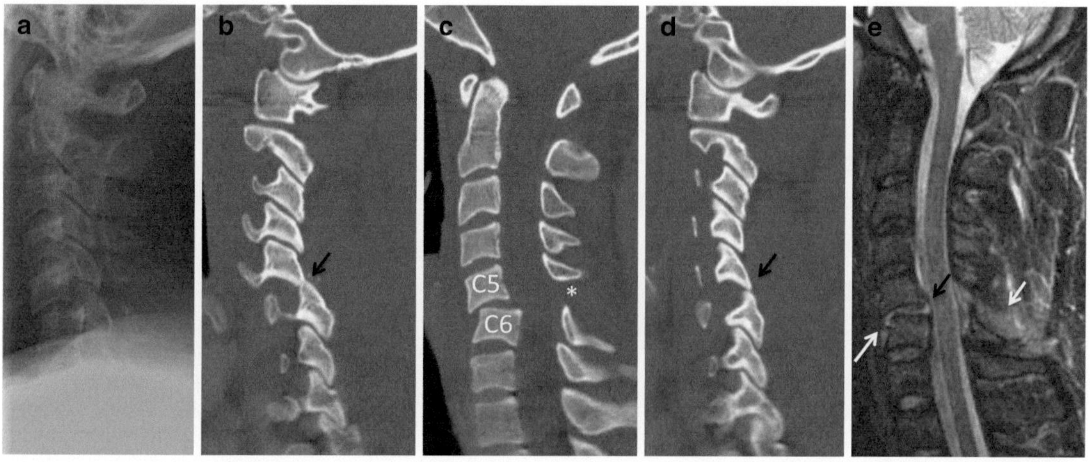

Fig. 53.1 Multiple ligament injury with bilateral facet joint dislocation. Lateral plain film (**a**), sagittal CT at the level of the right facets (**b**), at midline (**c**), and at the level of the left facets (**d**) show traumatic anterolisthesis of C5 on C6, widening of the interspinous space (*) and bilateral perched facets (*arrows*), indirect signs of ligamentous injury. The midline sagittal STIR (**e**) MRI shows the posterior ligamentous complex and anterior and posterior longitudinal ligament injury (*arrows*) at the level of C5–C6

3 mm in adults or 5 mm in children. MRI is highly sensitive for the diagnosis of transverse ligament rupture by directly visualizing this ligament [8].

The normal tectorial membrane and transverse ligament are routinely seen on MRI, whereas the normal alar ligaments are difficult to visualize because of lack of contrast from adjacent tissues and their small size [6]. However, blood or edema adjacent to an acute alar ligament tear improves the visualization of these ligaments. Secondary evidence of ligamentous injury to one of the alar ligaments is displacement of the dens to the contralateral side [6] (Figs. 53.7, 53.8, and 53.9).

Imaging Follow-Up

Dynamic evaluation with flexion and extension radiographs for identification of ligamentous injury and instability may not be helpful in the acute stage because of muscle spam, but it has a role in patients with persistent neck treated initially with collar and normal neurologic examination and normal CT and MRI [8]. These patients should be able to perform flexion and extension studies to assess stability before discontinuing the collar generally 1–2 weeks after injury and when muscle spasm has resolved [3, 8].

MRI is sometimes performed within 48 h to avoid keeping patients in collars for unnecessarily long periods of time to avoid complications of the collar and because many patients recover to the point that a reliable neurologic examination may be then performed [3].

Imaging is part of the routine follow-up of all patients after spinal surgery and instrumentation [16]. Radiography with anteroposterior, lateral, oblique, and flexion–extension views is the primary imaging modality for postoperative evaluation [16]. CT is the best to optimize postoperative assessment of implants. It can also be used to evaluate spinal alignment and integrity, exact position of implants, and progress of bone fusion and bone graft incorporation. MRI plays a major role in diagnosing complications such as infection. MRI may be limited by metal artifacts which can be reduced by positioning the hardware as closely as possible to parallel to the direction of the main magnetic field and by using fast spin-echo sequences rather than gradient-echo sequences [17].

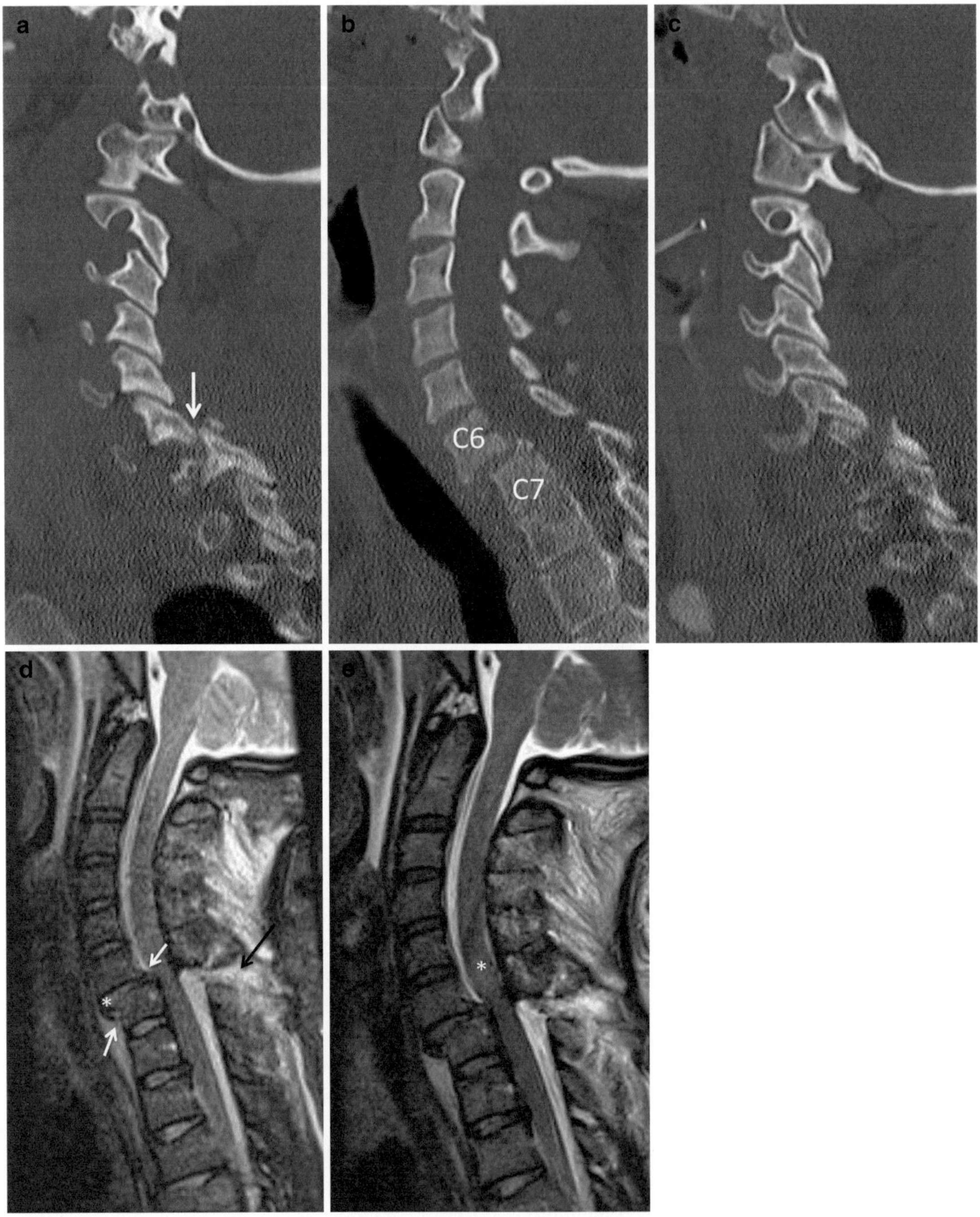

Fig. 53.2 Cervical fracture with severe ligament injury and spinal cord compression. Sagittal CT at the level of the right facets (**a**), at midline (**b**), and at the level of the left facets (**c**) show comminuted fracture of the C7 vertebral body with grade 2 anterolisthesis of C6 on C7 (**b**) that extends to the posterior arch involving the articular facets and C6–C7-locked facet joins on the right (*arrow* on **a**). Midline sagittal T2WI (**d**) and STIR (**e**) MRI show complete disruption of the posterior ligamentous complex (*arrows* in **d**), anterior and posterior longitudinal ligaments at the level of C6–C7 (*arrows*) resulting in traumatic anterolisthesis of C6 on C7. Note the disk space narrowing at C6–C7 with anterior displacement and slight inferior migration of the intervertebral disk (* on **d**). There is severe spinal canal stenosis and abnormal spinal cord signal at this level (* on **e**)

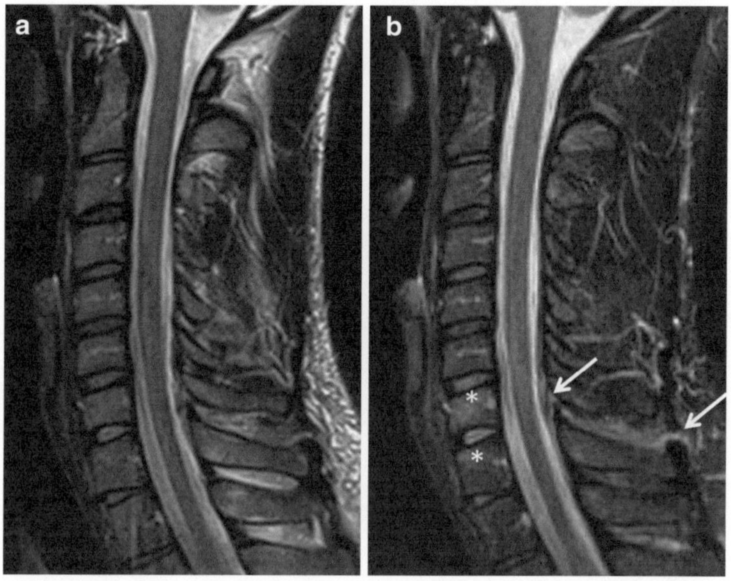

Fig. 53.3 Posterior ligament complex injury. Midline sagittal T2WI (**a**) and STIR (**b**) MR images show an increased STIR signal in the superior end plates of C7 and T1 vertebral bodies compatible with microtrabecular fracture (*), difficult to depict on T2WI. Note also the focal disruption of the interspinous ligament at the C7–T1 level and ligamentum flavum (*arrows*). The anterior and posterior ligaments are intact

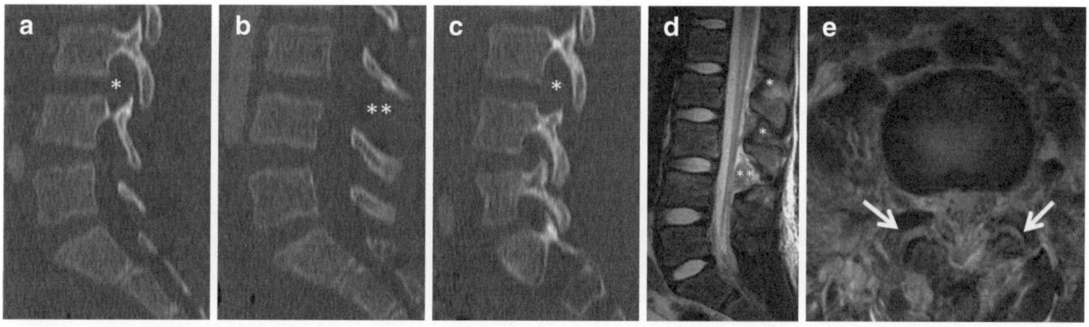

Fig. 53.4 Interspinous ligament disruption secondary to distraction injury in the lumbar spine. Sagittal CT at the level of the right facets (**a**), at midline (**b**), and at the level of the left facets (**c**) show superior distraction of the L3 vertebral body relative to L4 vertebral body with marked widening of the interspinous space (**) and neural foramina (*) on both sides suggesting underlying ligamentous injury. Midsagittal STIR (**d**) MRI shows abnormal high signal involving the L3 vertebral body and superior end plate of L4 consistent with microtrabecular fractures and edema. There is abnormal increased STIR signal involving the interspinous ligament L1–L2 and L2–L3 and L3–L4 (* on **d**) and a hematoma in the anterior interspinous L3–L4 space (**). (**e**) Axial T2WI at L3–L4 space shows widening of the bilateral facets consistent with underlying ligamentous injury (*arrows*)

Main Differential Diagnosis

Degenerative changes may be confused with traumatic subluxations. In contrast to traumatic anterior subluxation, retrolisthesis is the usual consequence of spondylosis. An accurate clinical history that specifies injury mechanism and location of pain is essential for accurately interpreting subtle findings in the presence of degenerative disk disease [8].

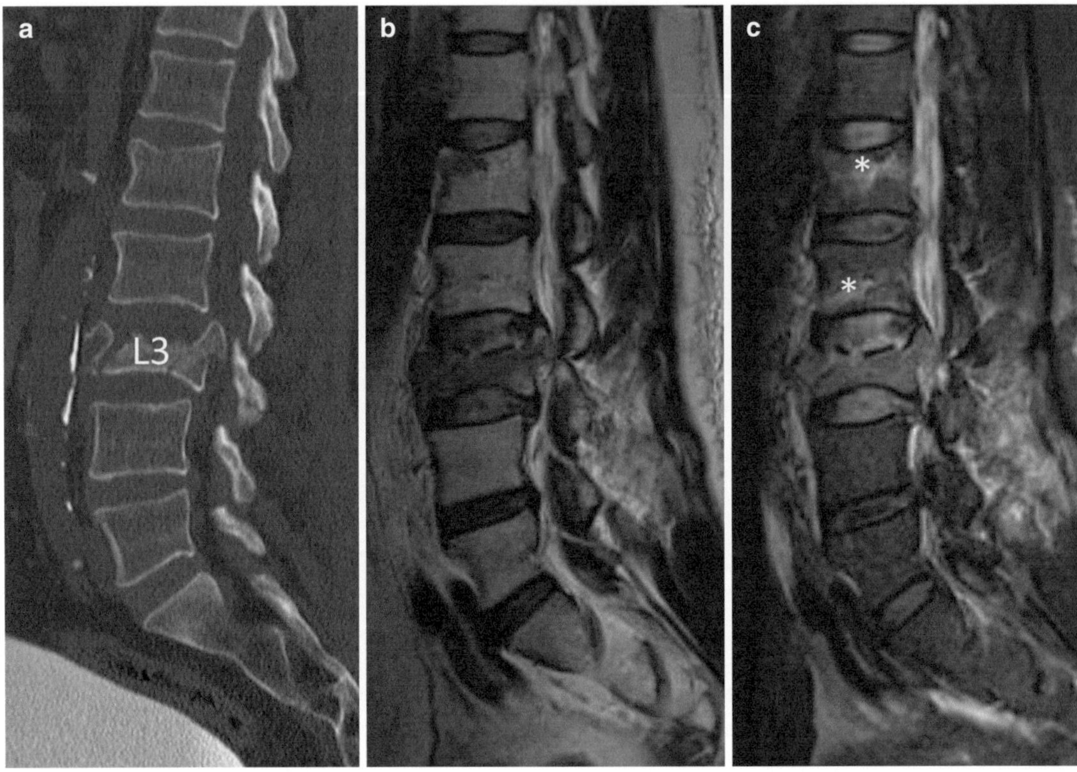

Fig. 53.5 Extensive ligamentous damage – burst fracture related. Midline sagittal CT (**a**), midline sagittal T2WI (**b**), and STIR (**c**) MRI show burst fracture of L3 with retropulsion resulting in severe canal stenosis and likely cauda equina compression. There is disruption of the posterior longitudinal ligament and ligamentum flavum at L3–L4 level and microtrabecular fractures involving L1 and L2 seen as areas of high STIR signal without height loss (*)

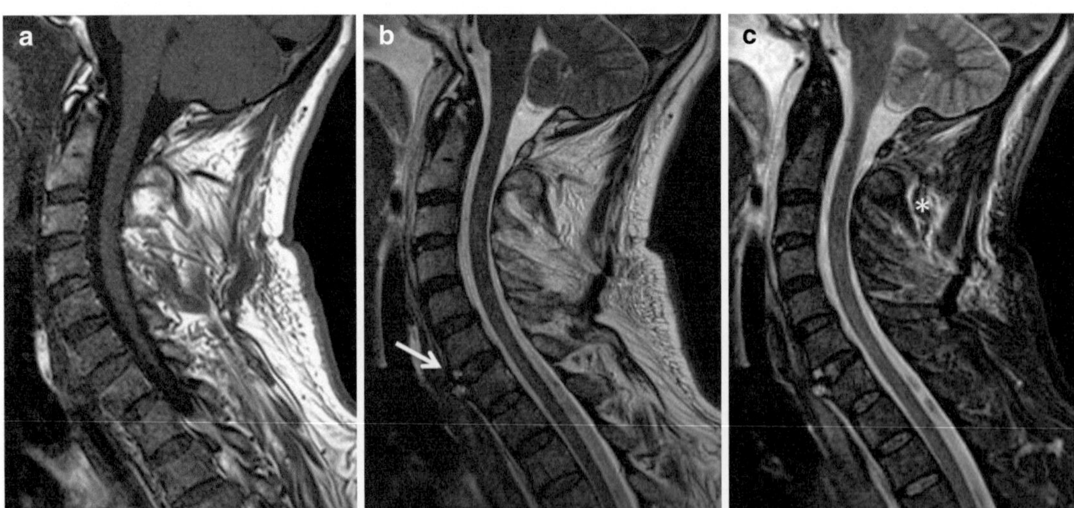

Fig. 53.6 ALL and PLC injuries in the cervical spine. Sagittal T1WI (**a**), T2WI (**b**), and STIR (**c**) MRI show abnormal widening of the anterior C6–C7 intervertebral disk space with apparent discontinuity of the anterior longitudinal ligament at this level (*arrow*). The posterior longitudinal ligament appears to be intact. There is abnormal T2 signal within the posterior soft tissues in the region of the ligamentum nuchae and interspinous ligament extending from C1 to C6 suggesting ligamentous injury (*)

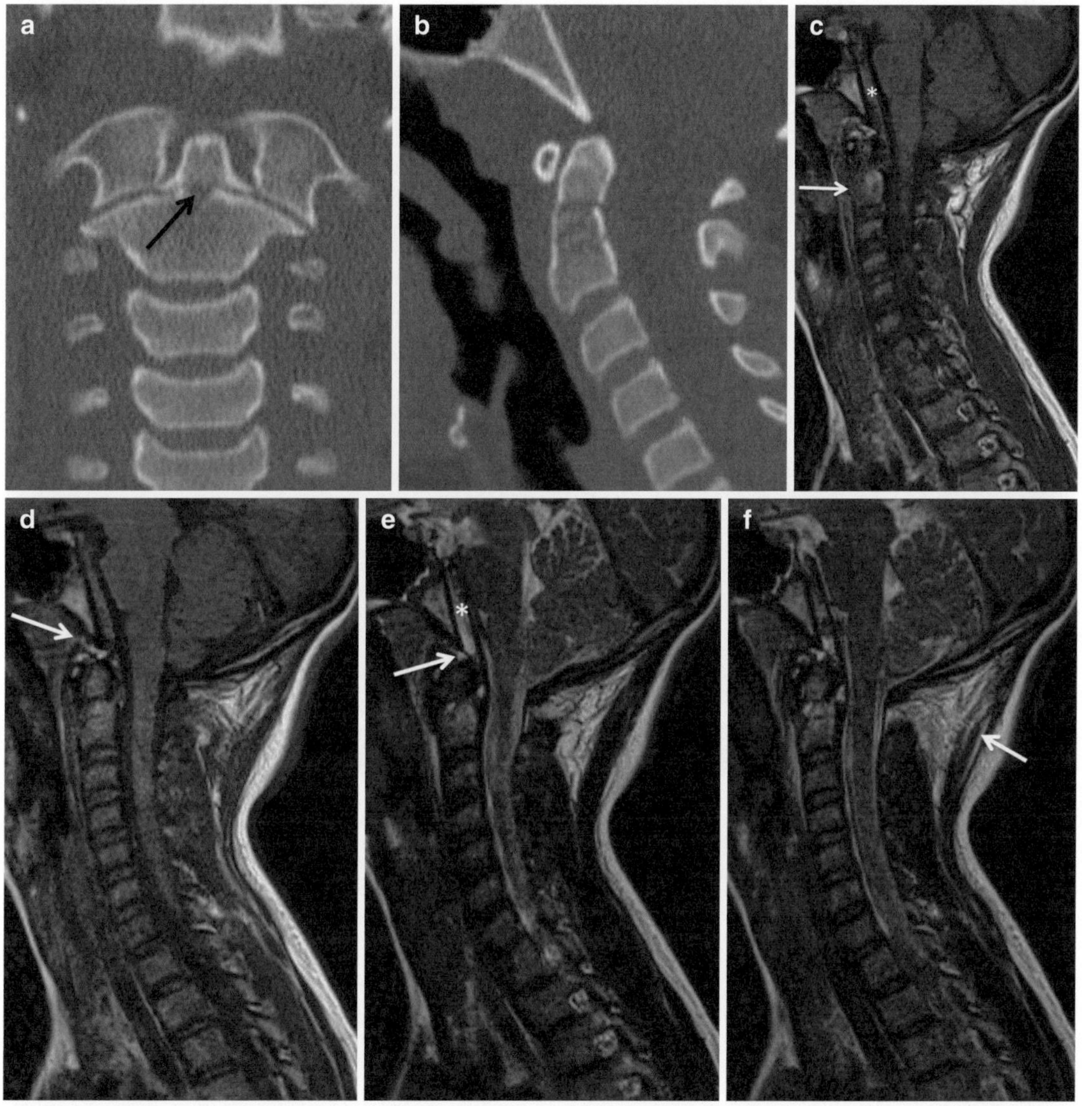

Fig. 53.7 Dens fracture and ligament injury. Coronal (**a**) and midline sagittal CT (**b**) show type II odontoid fracture (*arrow*), with mild anterior subluxation of the superior portion of the dens. Sagittal T1WI (**c**, **d**) and T2WI (**e**, **f**) MRI show disruption of the anterior longitudinal ligament between C1 and C2 (*arrow* on **c**) as well as at the C1–clivus junction (*arrow* on **d**). The tectorial membrane is stripped off of the clivus by an epidural hematoma (*). The apical dental ligament appears intact (*arrow* on **e**). Sagittal T2WI shows abnormal increased T2 signal within the nuchal ligament extending from the occiput to approximately C4 (*arrow* on **f**)

Extensive soft tissue injury and osseous displacement occur at the moment of impact but may be reduced by muscle spasm and immobilization with placement of a hard collar which may mask instability by maintaining vertebral alignment resulting in an apparently normal spine examination [8]. These patients usually have pain and/or neurologic findings despite good alignment.

Soft tissue injuries and ligamentous edema are common after significant trauma, and many of these lesions do not lead to mechanical instability [3].

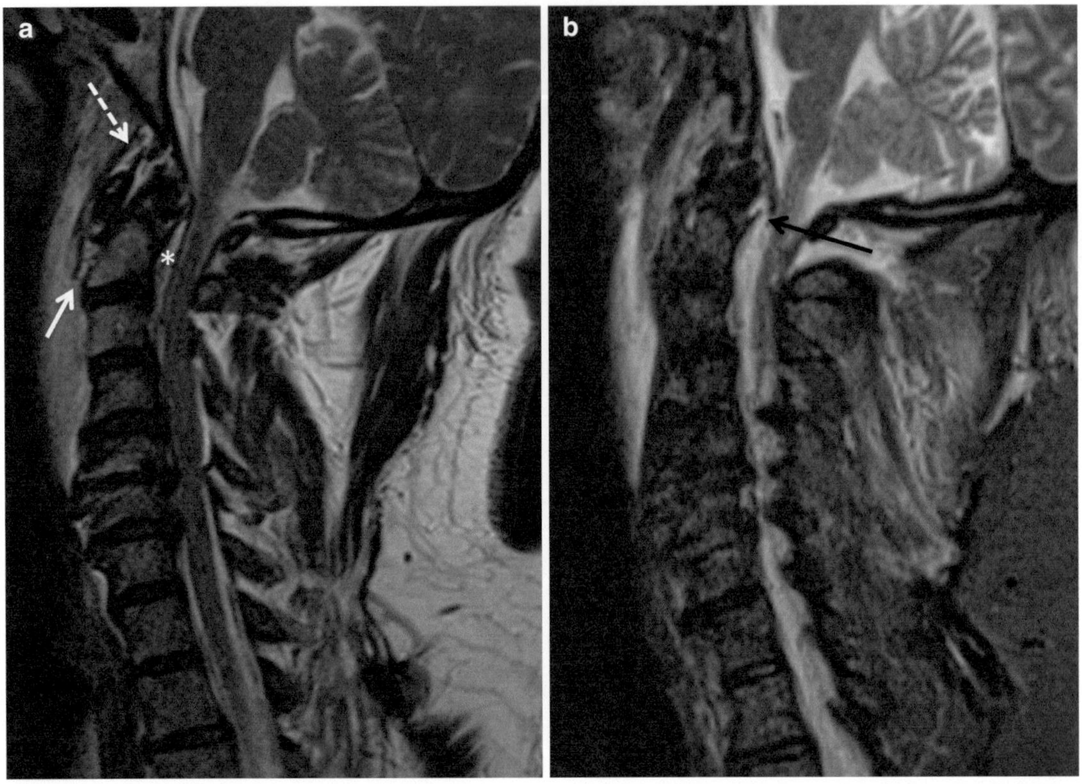

Fig. 53.8 ALL and craniocervical ligament injury. Midline sagittal T2WI (**a**) and off-midline STIR (**b**) MRI show disruption of the anterior longitudinal ligament (*arrow* in **a**), the anterior atlantooccipital membrane (*dashed arrow* on **a**), tectorial membrane (*arrow* in **b**), and an epidural hematoma (*) without compression of the spinal cord

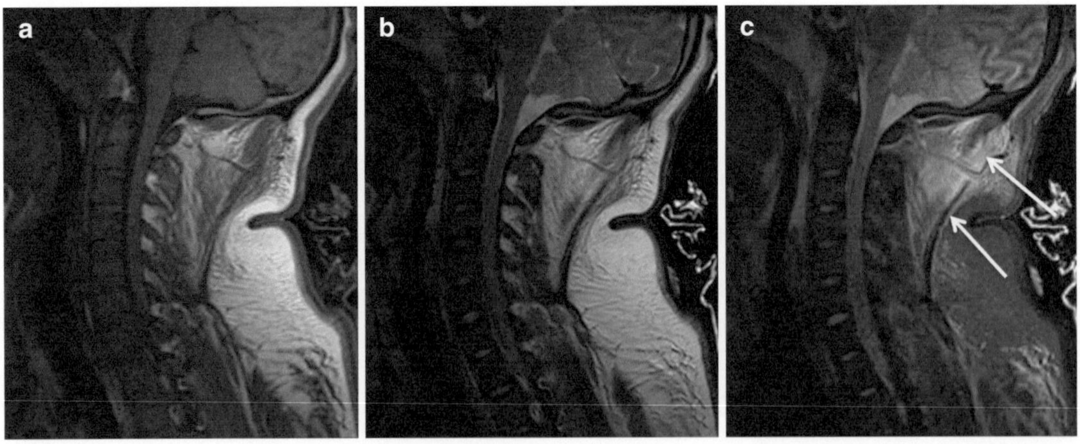

Fig. 53.9 Nuchal ligament injury. Sagittal T1WI (**a**), T2WI (**b**), and STIR (**c**) show edema within the suboccipital soft tissues with disruption of the nuchal ligament (*arrows*)

Tips

- Measurements are not able to accurately rule out ligamentous instability, and thus a normal CT does not exclude significant and unstable ligamentous injury; however, it is unlikely to have a major ligament injury in face of completely normal CT.
- CT abnormalities associated with ligamentous injuries may be subtle but should not be missed. They should be carefully described in the report since ligamentous injury is often an indication for surgical stabilization.
- Close attention should be given to facet alignment, interspinous space, anterior and posterior disk spacing, and other indirect signs of ligamentous disruptions.
- Disks and anterior ligamentous structures should always be assessed before surgery for posterior fusion because these patients are at risk for progressive cord compression [18, 19].
- The transverse ligament must be carefully assessed, since its integrity is the key for atlantoaxial stability.
- Isolated posttraumatic alar ligament tears should be reported because they are clinically significant and because hypermobility at the atlantoaxial joint can reduce blood flow in the contralateral vertebral artery potentially leading to brain ischemia [6].

References

1. Kaji A, Hockberger RS. Spinal column injuries in adults: definitions, mechanisms, and radiographs. http://www.uptodate.com/contents/spinal-column-injuries-in-adults-definitions-mechanisms-and-radiographs.
2. Sliker CW, Mirvis SE, Shanmuganathan K. Assessing cervical spine stability in obtunded blunt trauma patients: review of medical literature. Radiology. 2005;234(3):733–9.
3. Daffner RH, Hackney DB. ACR Appropriateness Criteria on suspected spine trauma. J Am Coll Radiol. 2007;4(11):762–75.
4. Chiu WC, Haan JM, Cushing BM, et al. J Trauma. 2001;50:457–64.
5. Roy AK, Miller BA, Holland CM, et al. Magnetic resonance imaging of traumatic injury to the craniovertebral junction: a case-based review. Neurosurg Focus. 2015;38(4):E3.
6. Benedetti PF, Fahr LM, Kuhns LR, Hayman LA. MR imaging findings in spinal ligamentous injury. AJR Am J Roentgenol. 2000;175:661–5.
7. Goldberg AL, Kershah SM. Advances in imaging of vertebral and spinal cord injury. J Spinal Cord Med. 2010;33(2):105–16.
8. Bernstein MP, Baxter AB. Cervical spine trauma: pearls and pitfalls. ARRS Categorical Course syllabus. (ed Anderson, S) 2010. p. 21–5.
9. Sliker CW. Blunt cerebrovascular injuries: imaging with multidetector CT angiography. Radiographics. 2008;28(6):1689–708; discussion 1709–10.
10. Eastman AL, Chason DP, Perez CL, McAnulty AL, Minei JP. Computed tomographic angiography for the diagnosis of blunt cervical vascular injury: is it ready for primetime? J Trauma. 2006;60(5):925–9.
11. Goradia D, Linnau KF, Cohen WA, et al. Correlation of MR imaging findings with intraoperative findings after cervical spine trauma. AJNR Am J Neuroradiol. 2007;28:209–15.
12. Ryken TC, Aarabi B, Dhall SS, et al. Management of isolated fractures of the atlas in adults. Neurosurgery. 2013;72 Suppl 2:127–31.
13. Ryken TC, Hadley MN, Aarabi B, et al. Management of acute combination fractures of the atlas and axis in adults. Neurosurgery. 2013;72 Suppl 2:151–8.
14. Ryken TC, Hadley MN, Aarabi B, et al. Management of isolated fractures of the axis in adults. Neurosurgery. 2013;72 Suppl 2:132–50.
15. Ryken TC, Hadley MN, Walters BC, et al. Radiographic assessment. Neurosurgery. 2013;72 Suppl 2:54–72.
16. Hayashi D, Roemer FW, Mian A, et al. Imaging features of postoperative complications after spinal surgery and instrumentation. AJR Am J Roentgenol. 2012;199:W123–9.
17. LeBlang SD, Nunez Jr DB. Helical CT of cervical spine and soft tissue injuries of the neck. Radiol Clin North Am. 1999;37(3):515–32, v–vi.
18. Robertson PA, Ryan MD. Neurological deterioration after reduction of cervical subluxation. Mechanical compression by disc tissue. J Bone Joint Surg Br. 1992;74:224–7.
19. Mahale YJ, Silver JR, Henderson NJ. Neurological complications of the reduction of cervical spine dislocations. J Bone Joint Surg Br. 1993;75:403–9.

Pediatric Vertebral Fractures

54

Mariana Cardoso Diogo
and Carla Ribeiro Conceição

Abstract

Vertebral fractures are relatively rare in children, and their clinical and imaging features are determined by the degree of skeletal maturity. Trauma is the main cause of vertebral fractures across all age groups, but other etiologies such as infections and neoplasms have to be included in the differential diagnosis when they occur in children. There are specific patterns of injuries that change with spinal maturity. Fractures of ossified structures are rare below 8 years of age, and as the spine matures, the types of fractures become similar to those seen in adults. Special attention must be paid not to mistake normal synchondroses and other vertebral development variants as fractures. Epiphyseal involvement may later impair growth and cause spine deformities. Radiographs, CT, and MRI play a role in the evaluation of pediatric vertebral fractures.

Background

Vertebral fractures are relatively rare in children representing 1–3 % of all pediatric fractures [1]. They may involve the body of the vertebra, the neural arch, or both. Trauma is the main culprit across all age groups, with motor vehicle accidents playing a major role. Nontraumatic vertebral collapse in children and adolescents can be secondary to infectious, neoplastic, metabolic disorders or osseous dysplasias [2]. A specific pattern of injury, normally seen in adolescent athletes is isthmic spondylolysis resulting from chronic microtrauma to the pars interarticularis. Over two-thirds of spinal injuries in children under 8 years of age occur in the cervical spine. The incidence of thoracolumbar spine fractures increases with age [1].

Lesions affecting the epiphyses or the disks may later impair vertebral growth and cause focal kyphosis or scoliosis.

M.C. Diogo, MD
Departamento de Neurorradiologia, Hospital de São José, Centro Hospitalar de Lisboa Central,
Rua José António Serrano, 1150 Lisboa, Portugal
e-mail: Mariana_cdiogo@hotmail.com

C.R. Conceição, MD (✉)
Departamento de Neurorradiologia, Hospital Dona Estefânia, Centro Hospitalar de Lisboa Central,
Rua Jacinta Marto, 1169-045 Lisboa, Portugal
e-mail: cribeiroconceicao@gmail.com

R. Hoffmann Nunes et al. (eds.), *Critical Findings in Neuroradiology*,
DOI 10.1007/978-3-319-27987-9_54

Treatment can be conservative if stability is preserved, and surgical for unstable injuries or when significant deformities are present.

Key Points

Etiology

Fractures of ossified vertebral structures are rare below age 8 years with their incidence progressively increasing and approaching an adult distribution in adolescents [3]. Across all age groups, the most common cause of vertebral fractures is traffic-related incidents followed by falls in young children and sports-related injuries in adolescents [4, 5]. Birth trauma is a rare but well-recognized cause of cervical spine and cervicothoracic transition vertebral injuries with up to 75 % occurring after complicated breech deliveries [6].

Cervical Spine

Fractures of the cervical vertebrae have two distinct patterns of distribution depending on age: they commonly involve the C1–C3 levels in children under 8 years old and the C5–C6 levels in older children [4]. The high prevalence of upper cervical spine injuries in young children is related to the developmental anatomy of this region, a proportionately larger head, and increased laxity of their ligaments. The high mobility and flexibility of the cervical spine protects against fractures, and until the synchondroses close, fractures through the cartilaginous end plates are the most common type found. On the other hand, in the younger age groups, the presence of a fracture implies a higher-energy mechanism of injury predisposing to other coexisting traumatic lesions [1].

Congenital fusions of the spine, such as Klippel–Feil anomalies, predispose a child to vertebral fractures by reducing spinal flexibility and concentrating stresses at the residual mobile segments.

Because of developmental and structural differences, injuries of the cervical spine are divided into those occurring in craniovertebral junction (CVJ) and those of the subaxial regions as follows [7].

CVJ fractures are unusual in preadolescent children and tend to be stable. Dens fractures through the subdental synchondroses (type 3 dens fracture) which fuse at 5–7 years of age are the most common type of dens fracture in children (Fig. 54.1) [8]. Twenty-five to fifty percent of young children with this type of fracture have concurrent head injuries [2].

Subaxial injuries are typical of adolescents. Common mechanisms of injury include whiplash (flexion/distraction) associated with motor vehicle accidents and hyperextension and/or hyperflexion associated with head-first falls and dives (Fig. 54.2).

Thoracic and Lumbar Spine

Traumatic fractures: Injuries at these levels are more common in the pediatric age group than previously thought. The most frequently injured levels are T4–T12 followed by T12–L2 [9]. Seatbelt-related injuries, combining distraction and flexion, are common and followed in incidence by compression fractures (typically caused by falls) (Fig. 54.3). Lumbar apophyseal ring avulsions are characteristic of adolescents, typically affecting the L4 and L5. In them, there is detachment of the ring apophyses with intervertebral disk herniations.

Spondylolysis: Injuries of the pars interarticularis are a common cause of back pain in adolescents, especially in young athletes [10]. The L5 vertebra is the most affected and lesions are often bilateral. The etiology of spondylolysis is multifactorial, but repetitive microtrauma is probably the most important underlying factor. MRI grading in 5 grades (0–4) has been developed by Hollenberg and colleagues [11] and should be used whenever possible to convey the severity of the disease (Table 54.1) (Fig. 54.4).

Pathological fractures: Disease processes weakening the vertebrae are a rare cause of spinal fractures in children unlike adults in whom they are relatively common. Pathological fractures may be associated with infection, benign lesions (such as aneurysmal bone cysts), malignancies, and metabolic disorders, congenital or acquired,

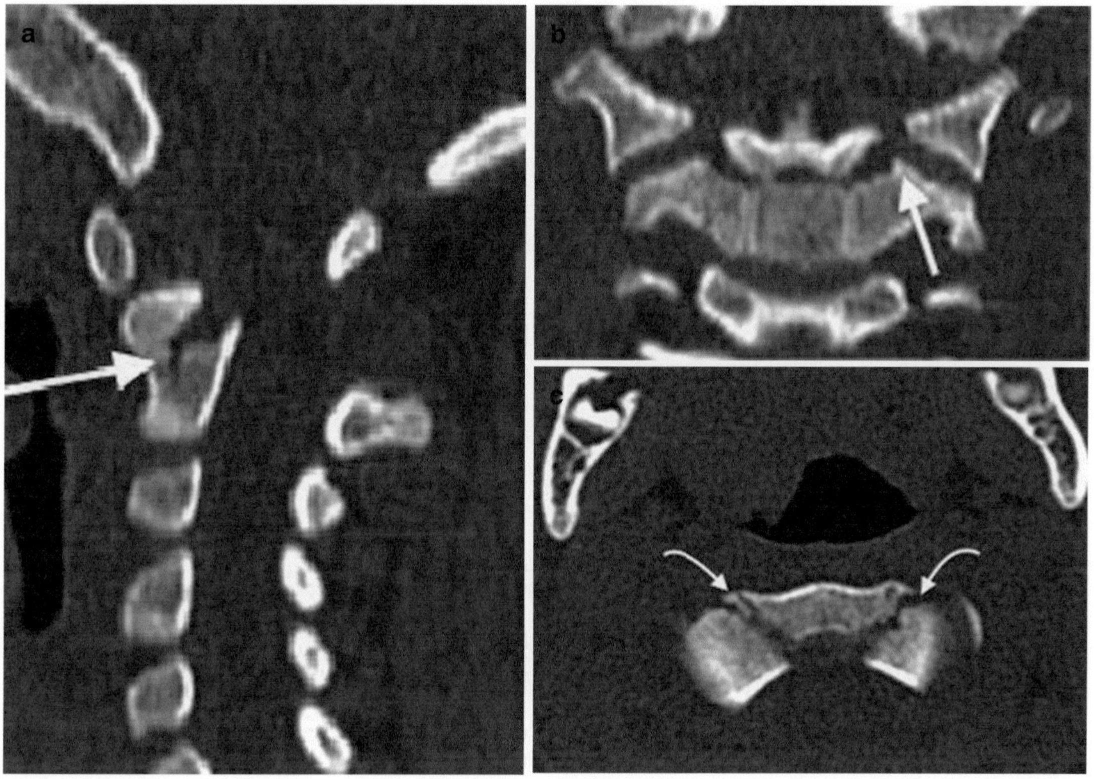

Fig. 54.1 Dens fracture. C2 fracture in a 4-year-old boy, involving the subdental synchondroses and C2 vertebral body. CT acquisition with reformations in the sagittal (**a**), coronal (**b**), and axial (**c**) shows diastasis of the synchondroses more prominent in the left side (*arrows*). In the sagittal view, (**a**) the *arrow* points the anteriorly displaced dens

such as in chronic intake of corticosteroids [12]. Malignant tumors infiltrating vertebral bodies vary with age, lymphoma being a main culprit across all age groups (Fig. 54.5).

Best Imaging Modality

Radiographs: Are the preferred initial evaluation of a child under age 14 years for two main reasons: the relatively low incidence of fractures in this age group and the need to limit radiation exposure dose which can be relatively high with CT. Radiographs should include a minimum of two views: anteroposterior (AP) and lateral. In the cervical spine, AP open-mouth views may be added but may be difficult to obtain in children [13, 14].

Computed tomography (*CT*): This is the modality of choice for patients over age 14 years and those with moderate to severe injuries. Multiple injuries are frequent [6, 13, 14]. Volumetric CT acquisition with multiplanar reformations using bone and soft tissue algorithm is recommended. Coronal reformations are advised to visualize the dens. Contiguous acquisition of images is desirable as disk space-targeted axial images decrease the detection of fractures [4]. Dose-limiting techniques should always be employed.

Magnetic resonance imaging (*MRI*): It is indicated in patients with neurological deficits and is useful in distinguishing anatomic variants (such as anterior vertebral body wedging) from acute fractures or when pathological fractures are suspected. Sagittal T1-weighted image (T1WI) and

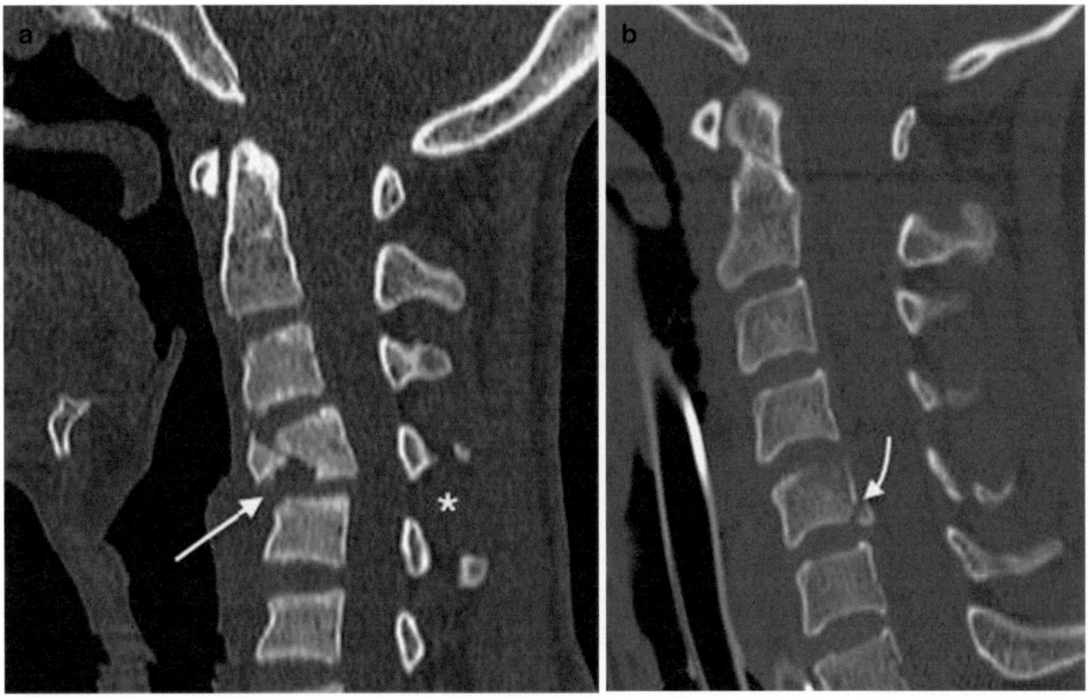

Fig. 54.2 Subaxial cervical fractures in two different adolescents. Sagittal CT images. In (**a**) there is a compression/hyperflexion fracture of C4 with inversion of the cervical curvature (*arrow*), retrolisthesis of C4, and widening of the interspinous C4–C5 space (*), indicating posterior ligamentous injury. In (**b**) there is a C5 vertebral body fracture with a bone fragment detached from posterior aspect of the body, slightly displaced into the cervical canal (*arrow*)

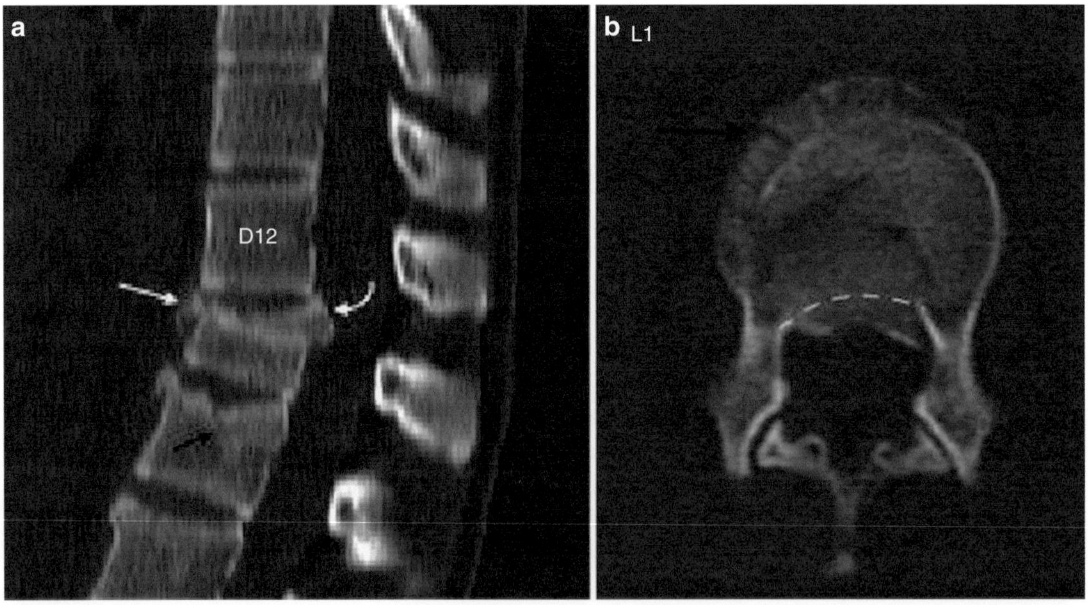

Fig. 54.3 Lumbar compression fractures in a 13-year-old girl. CT with sagittal (**a**) and axial (**b**) reconstructions in bone windows. There is loss of vertebral height of L1 and L2 more prominent in the anterior aspects of the vertebral bodies. L1 shows a bursting aspect of the vertebral body (*arrow*) and retropulsion of the posterior aspect (*dashed line* shows expected course of normal posterior cortex), thus a "burst fracture." L2 shows a simple compression fracture (*black arrow*)

T2-weighted image (T2WI) fat suppressed or short tau inversion recovery (STIR) and axial T2*WI should be obtained. If malignancy is suspected, sagittal and axial T1WI fat suppressed after gadolinium are recommended.

CT angiography should be considered when vascular involvement such as arterial dissection is suspected.

Major Findings

The major imaging finding is the presence of a discontinuity in the vertebral cortical bone. In acute fractures, there may be a paravertebral soft tissue component seen on CT and MRI. The affected vertebra shows hyperintensity on T2WI and STIR images corresponding to bone and marrow edema.

Table 54.1 MRI classification of lumbar pars interarticularis abnormalities [11]

Grade	MRI abnormalities
0	Normal
1	T2 signal abnormalities of the pars interarticularis with or without signal changes in the adjacent pedicle or articular process
2	T2 signal abnormalities and thinning, fragmentation, or irregularity of the pars interarticularis visible on T1- and/or T2WI
3	Visible complete unilateral or bilateral spondylolysis with associated abnormal T2 signal
4	Complete spondylolysis without abnormal T2 signal

A *hangman's fracture* involves a bilateral lamina and pedicle fractures at C2, usually associated with anterolisthesis of C2.

In a simple *wedged compression vertebral fracture*, there is a reduction of height of the anterior body which is generally an isolated failure of the anterior column (Fig. 54.2a). For a compression fracture to be classified as a *burst fracture*, there needs to be retropulsion of bone fragments into the spinal canal associated with a "bursting" aspect of the vertebral body on axial CT (Fig. 54.3). These injuries may be stable or unstable (when there is associated disruption of the posterior column) as disruption of the middle column is always present in these patients. Differentiating a simple compression from a burst fracture is important as the latter has a higher frequency of neurological deficits, is unstable, and requires surgical management. A *Jefferson fracture* is a burst fracture of C1, involving the anterior and posterior arches, and a distance between the C1 lateral mass and the odontoid process ≥6 mm is suggestive of transverse ligament disruption and instability [5].

Chance fractures consist of a compression injury to the anterior portion of the vertebral body and a transverse fracture through the posterior elements of the vertebra. Most occur in the thoracolumbar junction (T12–L2).

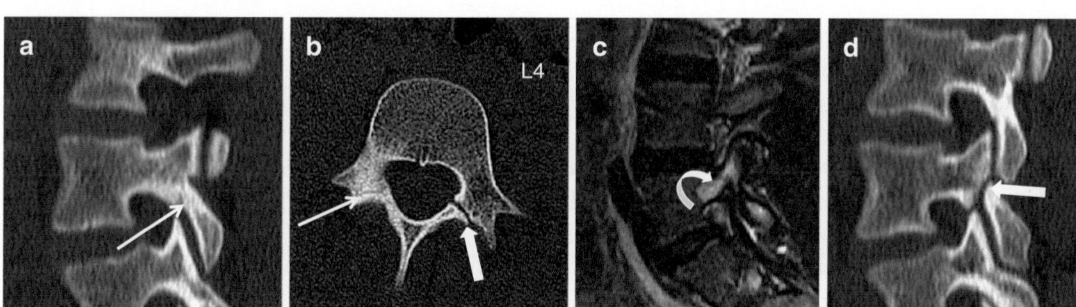

Fig. 54.4 Bilateral L4 spondylolysis in a 14-year-old soccer player. Sagittal (**a**) and axial CT (**b**) show sclerosis without thinning or fragmentation of the right pars interarticularis of L4 (*thin arrows*). However, a clear cleft is seen in the opposite pars (*thick arrow*). Sagittal STIR (**c**) depicts bone edema without cortical defect (*arrow*) compatible with spondylolysis grade 1 in the right side. (**d**) Sagittal CT on the left side. There is a cleft compatible with spondylolysis grade 4 (*arrow*)

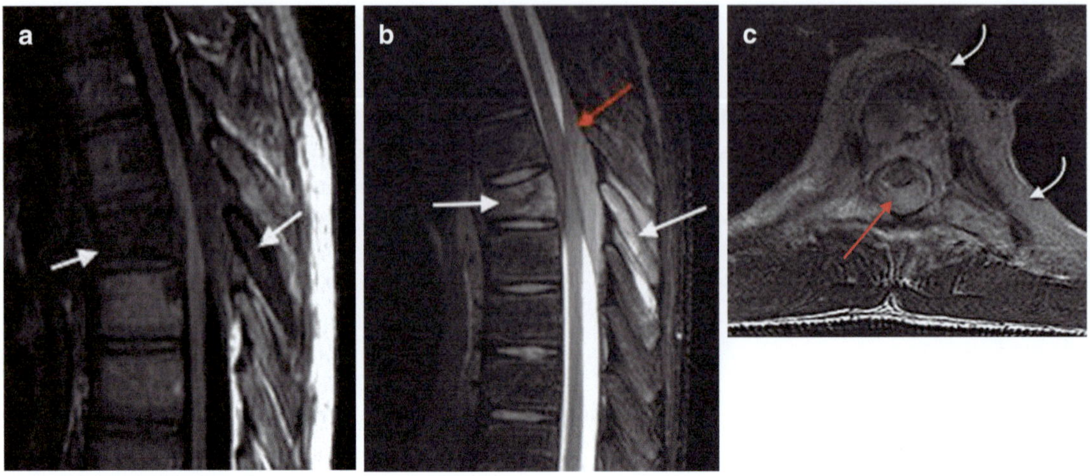

Fig. 54.5 Pathological fracture of T8 in a 16-year-old boy with lymphoblastic B-cell lymphoma. (**a**) Sagittal T1WI, (**b**) sagittal T2WI, and (**c**) axial T2WI. There is anterior wedging of the vertebral body and abnormal diffuse hypointense and hyperintense signal in the vertebra on T1 and T2WI respectively (*white arrows* in **a** and **b**) with associated soft tissue paravertebral and epidural mass (*red* and *white curved arrows* in **b** and **c**). The axial T2WI better depicts paravertebral component. Cord compression and edema is present

Imaging Follow-Up

Imaging follow-up of vertebral fractures is controversial. Imaging can be obtained to assess healing at 2–3 months when a callus should be visualized on radiographs or earlier on CT. In fractures treated acutely by immobilization such as cervical collars, dynamic studies should be obtained at the time of device removal to rule out instability.

Main Differential Diagnosis

Anatomic variants: Several common pediatric variants can be confused with pathologic conditions and these include:

Subdental synchondrosis may be mistaken for a dens fracture before its fusion by age 7. Conversely, fractures through synchondroses may be misinterpreted as normal variants.

Anterior wedging of vertebral bodies is normal during the first decade of life, and it may be misinterpreted as a compression/hyperflexion fracture.

Pseudosubluxation of cervical spine is frequent until 8 years of age, mainly at C2–C3.

Secondary ossification centers must not be confused with avulsion fractures. *Ring apophysis* usually appears between 10 and 12 years of age and should not be mistaken for fractures [6].

Congenital anomalies: Congenital alterations such as os odontoideum, occult spina bifida, and lack of segmentation should not be interpreted as pathological.

Tips

- Check alignment on midsagittal bone window CT slice by using the anterior/posterior spinal lines and the spinolaminar line. Same measurements can be used in radiographs.
- Look for bone fragments in the spinal canal, vertebral dislocations, or other signs of potential cord compression.
- Look for subtle fractures in the facets, transverse, and spinous processes.
- Multiple fractures of vertebrae are common. Examine each adjacent vertebra for evidence of subtle fractures [13].

MRI may be needed for this purpose because all fractures are accompanied by edema.

- Always look for anomalies suggestive of underlying disease (pathological fractures).
- Report involvement of the transverse foramina which may be associated with vertebral artery injuries in the cervical spine.
- Dens fractures can be classified according to the schema proposed by Anderson in three types.
- Always look for cord compression and report it immediately.
- Always report signs of disruption of the posterior ligament complex as these injuries are highly unstable.

References

1. Leonard M, Sproule J, McCormack D. Paediatric spinal trauma and associated injuries. Injury Int J Care Injured. 2007;38:188–93.
2. Lustrin ES, Karakas SP, Ortiz AO, et al. Pediatric cervical spine: normal anatomy, variants, and trauma. Radiographics. 2003;23:539–60.
3. Easter JS, Barkin R, Rosen CL, Ban K. Cervical spine injuries in children, part I: mechanism of injury, clinical presentation and imaging. J Emerg Med. 2011;41:142–50.
4. Bilston LE, Brown J. Pediatric spinal injury type and severity are age and mechanism dependent. Spine. 2007;32:2339–47.
5. Polk-Williams A, Carr BG, Blinman TA, et al. Cervical spine injury in young children: a National Trauma Data Bank review. J Pediatr Surg. 2008;43: 1718–21.
6. Antevil JL, Sise MJ, Sack DI, et al. Spiral computed tomography for the initial evaluation of spine trauma: a new standard of care? J Trauma. 2006;61:382–7.
7. Leonard JA. Cervical spine injury. Pediatr Clin N Am. 2013;60:1123–37.
8. Gore PA, Chang S, Theodore N. Cervical spine injuries in children: attention to radiographic differences and stability compared to those in the adult patient. Semin Pediatr Neurol. 2009;16:42–58.
9. Lubicky JP, Gussous YM. Thoracolumbar spine injuries in children and adolescents. Semin Spine Surg. 2010;22:44–9.
10. DeLuigi AJ. Low back pain in the adolescent athlete. Phys Med Rehabil Clin N Am. 2014;25:763–88.
11. Hollenberg GM, Beattie PF, Meyers SP, et al. Stress reactions of the lumbar pars interarticularis: the development of a new MRI classification system. Spine. 2002;27:181–6.
12. Codd PJ, Riesenburger RI, Klimo P, Slotkin JR, Smith ER. Vertebra plana due to an aneurysmal bone cyst of the lumbar spine. Case report and review of the literature. J Neurosurg. 2006;105:490–5.
13. Daffner RH, Weissman BN, Wippold II FJ, Angtuaco EJ, et al. ACR appropriateness criteria: suspected spine trauma. Reston: American College of Radiology (ACR); 2012.
14. Rogers LF, West OC. Imaging skeletal trauma, 4th ed. Philadelphia: Saunders, an imprint of Elsevier Inc; 2015.

Pediatric Spinal Ligamentous Injuries

55

Mariana Cardoso Diogo
and Carla Ribeiro Conceição

Abstract

Spinal ligamentous injuries can affect children of any age and are almost invariably secondary to trauma. These injuries differ from those of adults due to the particular anatomic and biomechanical features of the developing/maturing spine. Correct diagnosis of spinal ligamentous injury is essential as spinal stability may be compromised and further injury to the spinal cord may ensue. Indirect signs of spinal instability must be recognized on computed tomography or radiographs and distinguished from normal anatomical variants in children. Magnetic resonance imaging is the only imaging modality that can directly visualize spinal ligamentous and cord injuries, making it the gold standard if such lesions are suspected.

Background

Spinal ligamentous injury (SLI) refers to lesions affecting the connective tissue bands that interconnect the vertebrae and is almost invariably secondary to trauma. Spinal ligaments provide stability, preventing excessive joint movement. Damage to these structures must be reported to avoid further injury to the spine and/or spinal cord. SLI can affect children of any age with patterns varying as the spine matures [1].

The most common presenting symptom is pain, sometimes associated with functional limitations. Treatment and prognosis are determined by the severity of the injury, and minor and stable lesions need no treatment and have excellent outcomes, while more significant unstable lesions

M.C. Diogo, MD
Departamento de Neurorradiologia,
Hospital de São José,
Centro Hospitalar de Lisboa Central,
Rua José António Serrano, 1150 Lisboa, Portugal
e-mail: Mariana_cdiogo@hotmail.com

C.R. Conceição, MD (✉)
Departamento de Neurorradiologia,
Hospital Dona Estefânia,
Centro Hospitalar de Lisboa Central,
Rua Jacinta Marto, 1169-045 Lisboa, Portugal
e-mail: cribeiroconceicao@gmail.com

R. Hoffmann Nunes et al. (eds.), *Critical Findings in Neuroradiology*,
DOI 10.1007/978-3-319-27987-9_55

may need immobilization or surgical fixation. If the spinal cord is affected, severe neurological deficits (depending on the affected level) and even death may occur [2].

Key Points

Etiology

Spinal injuries in children differ from those in adult due to increased ligamentous laxity, a relatively large head mass, shallow angulations of facet joints, developing ossification of vertebrae with partial cartilaginous composition, and immature musculature. These features seen particularly in younger children bestow increased musculoskeletal elasticity which dissipates the kinetic energy during trauma predisposing to a higher incidence of SLI as opposed to vertebral fractures [3]. This increased flexibility is not shared by the spinal cord, and this fact may lead to spinal cord injury without radiological abnormality (SCIWORA).

Spinal ligaments, unlike ossified structures, are present from birth and can be divided into two major areas which are anatomically and functionally distinct as follows: the craniovertebral junction (CVJ) and the subaxial spine (below C2).

Craniovertebral Junction Injuries

Spinal injury in children less than 8 years old occurs mainly in the CVJ/cervical spine (C1–C2 level) and is associated with a high risk of neurological damage [4].

Atlantoaxial subluxation: Results from traumatic rupture of the transverse ligament and is rare in children as the more vulnerable odontoid usually fails before the ligament does. The atlas moves forward on C2, increasing the distance between the anterior arch and the odontoid (>5 mm) and reducing spinal canal amplitude.

Atlantoaxial rotatory fixation: This is a fundamentally pediatric disorder presenting with painful torticollis. There is an alteration of the normal rotational relationship between C1 and C2 and clinically the condition ranges from significant limitation of motion to complete fixation.

Table 55.1 Classification of atlantoaxial rotatory fixation [5]

Type	Findings
1	Rotatory fixation without anterior displacement of the atlas (displacement of 3 mm or less) and the odontoid acting as the pivot
2	Rotatory fixation with anterior displacement of the atlas of 3–5 mm and one lateral articular process acting as the pivot
3	Rotatory fixation with anterior displacement of more than 5 mm
4	Rotatory fixation with posterior displacement

Trauma, upper respiratory infections, and head and neck surgery are the main causes of this condition. It was classified in 4 types by Fielding and Hawkins (Table 55.1) [5]. Types II, III, and IV are easily defined on computed tomography (CT) and magnetic resonance imaging (MRI) and usually require surgical stabilization of the atlantoaxial complex [6].

Subaxial Ligamentous Injuries

Subaxial spine injuries represent a broad set of injury patterns and degrees of instability.

The main ligaments of the spine are the anterior longitudinal ligament (ALL), posterior longitudinal ligament (PLL), and posterior ligamentous complex that include the supraspinous and interspinous ligaments, articular facet capsules, and ligamentum flavum.

- *The anterior longitudinal ligament (ALL)* extends from the skull base to the sacrum. It is seen as a dark band adjacent to bright retropharyngeal fat [7] and may be indistinguishable from bone cortex and annuli.
- *Posterior longitudinal ligament (PLL)* is variable in width, being widest at the intervertebral disk level, thinner behind the vertebral bodies, and sometimes appearing discontinuous on sagittal MRI. It extends through the spinal length.
- *Ligamentum flavum* and *interspinous ligaments* form strips of fibroelastic tissues that bridge adjacent laminae and spinous processes, respectively. They are the principal ligaments of the posterior column, acting as check ligaments to

oppose hyperflexion and distraction of the posterior elements and today are thought to play a major role in spine stability [8].

Injuries to the subaxial cervical spine are rare in children aged <8 years. As the pediatric spine matures toward adult-like biomechanics, subaxial injuries become more common with an increasing proportion of bony rather than ligamentous injuries.

Hyperextension typically results in injury to ligaments of the anterior column or to both the anterior and middle columns [9]. Hyperflexion may result in injury to ligaments of the middle and posterior columns. Injury to any two adjacent columns results in instability.

The severity of subaxial soft tissue and ligamentous injuries varies, and minor forms may present without any abnormality on computed tomography (CT) or dynamic radiographs. Severe interspinous ligament injury may be associated with widening of facet joints or interspinous spaces, widening or collapse of the disk spaces, and ultimately dislocations/dissociations (Figs. 55.1 and 55.2).

Best Imaging Modality

Magnetic resonance imaging (MRI): MRI is the only modality that can directly visualize SLI, making this condition an underdiagnosed entity as imaging methods used in acute trauma setting are usually limited to radiographs and/or computed tomography [8]. MRI is the imaging choice when SLI is suspected [1, 2, 8]. The optimal time for MRI is controversial, but it should probably be performed within 72 h of injury as beyond this

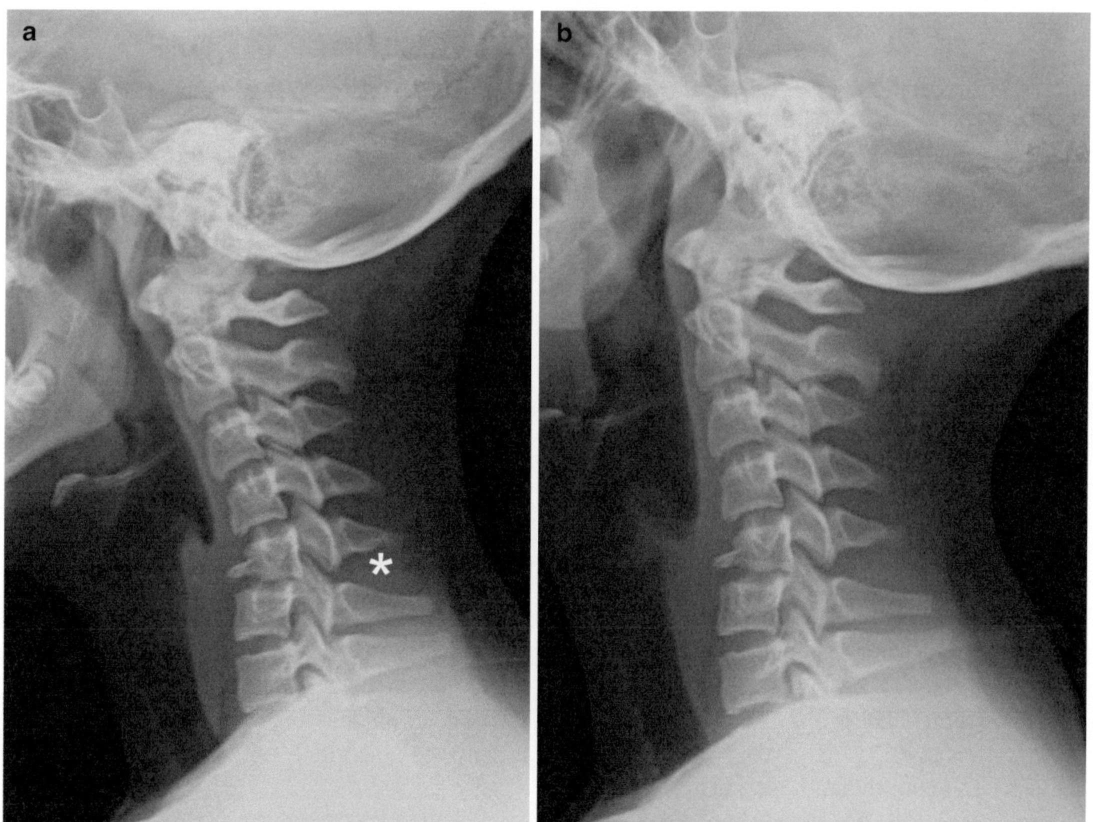

Fig. 55.1 Radiographs of a 14-year-old boy following a car accident. In the neutral position lateral view, (**a**) there is inversion of the cervical curvature, maintained in the hyperextension lateral film (**b**), as well as loss of posterior vertebral alignment of C5. A compression fracture of the body of C5 is seen as well as a widening of the C5–C6 facets and interspinous space (*). These findings suggest anterior and posterior ligamentous injuries

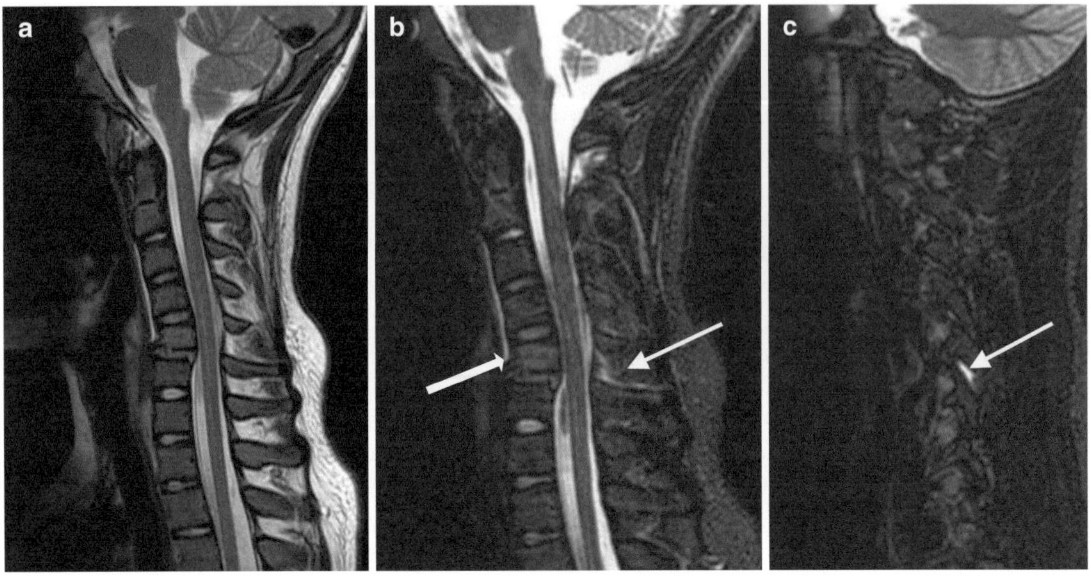

Fig. 55.2 MRI of the same patient seen in Fig. 55.1. Sagittal T2WI (**a**) and STIR images (**b**, **c**) show inversion of the cervical curvature and grade 1 retrolisthesis of C5. STIR images better depict the vertebral body edema of C5 (*thick arrow*), ligament edema, and intra-articular effusion (*thin arrows*)

time edema and/or hemorrhage reduces sensitivity of MRI to detect these injuries [9]. T2-weighted image (T2WI) MRI fat saturation and suppression – short tau inversion recovery (STIR) or fat-saturated (FS) images – are the best sequences to evaluate ligamentous injury. Both sagittal (for ALL, PLL, and ligamentum flavum) and axial (ligamentum flavum and interspinous ligament) images should be obtained [2, 9]. Gradient-echo images (GRE) should also be acquired (usually in the axial plane) for detection of blood products.

Computed tomography (CT): As MRI is not always available and may be impracticable or impossible in the acute trauma setting, CT may be performed and indirect signs of SLI should be recognized (Fig. 55.3). A normal CT virtually excludes the presence of significant ligament injuries calling to question the use of MRI in such instances.

Radiographs: These are of limited benefit in the assessment of SLI. If they are the only available imaging method, lateral films in flexion and extension should be obtained with the patient carefully monitored for symptoms of cord compression during the examination.

Major Findings

Ligaments are composed of fibroelastic tissues with little water content and therefore appear as continuous thin lines that are relatively hypointense to other structures on all MRI pulse sequences. The following should be remembered when evaluating the ligaments:

- When injury is present, there is a discontinuity of the affected ligaments and increased signal intensity on T2WI, indicative of edema, hemorrhage, and/or inflammation (Fig. 55.2) [2].
- There may be edema of the surrounding tissues or associated fractures or dislocations. Fractures may be missed acutely on MRI; look for indirect signs of bone or soft tissue edema on T2WI or STIR (Figs. 55.2 and 55.4).
- All ligaments are better depicted on sagittal images; ligamentum flavum focal discontinuity may be identified on parasagittal images (Fig. 55.5).
- Widening of the interspinous space between C1 and C2 of more than 10 mm may also suggest ligamentous instability.

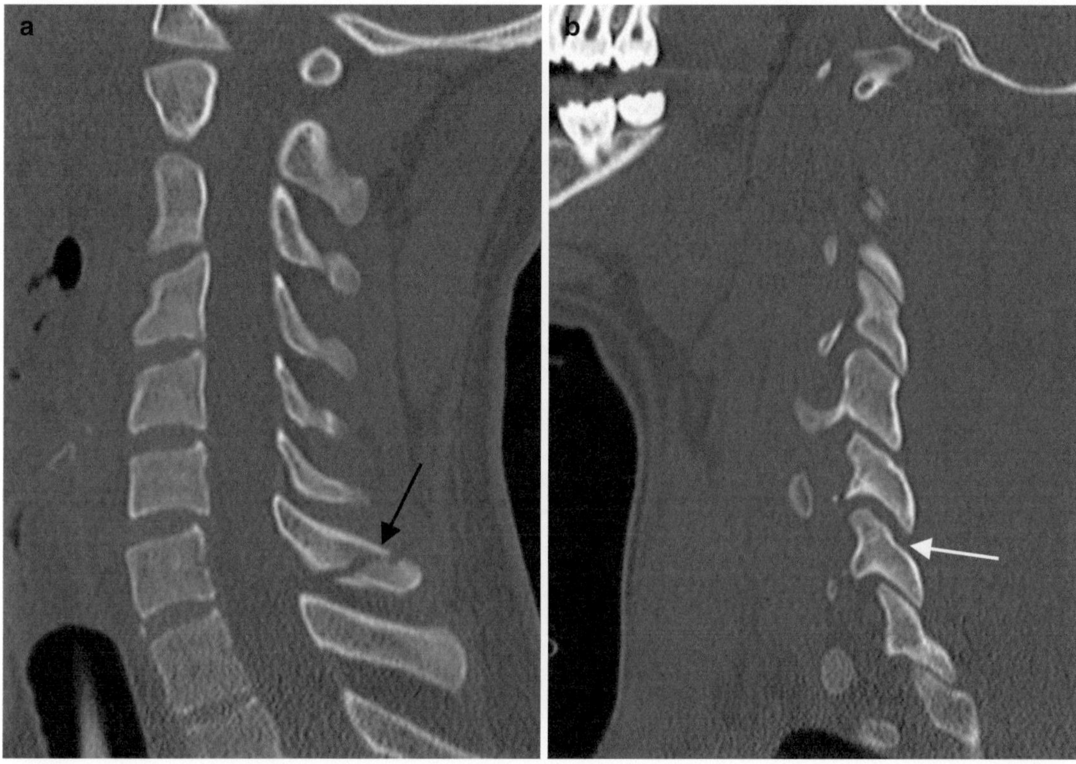

Fig. 55.3 Sagittal CT images show C7 spinous process fracture (*arrow* in **a**) and grade 1 retrolisthesis of C6 on C7. A more lateral view (**b**) shows widening of the right C6–C7 facet joint (*arrow*). In the setting of loss of vertebral body alignment (*middle column*) and facet joint anomalies (posterior column), ligamentous injury with instability should be suspected. A small bony fragment is seen anterior to the C6–C7 disk space, suggesting ALL injury

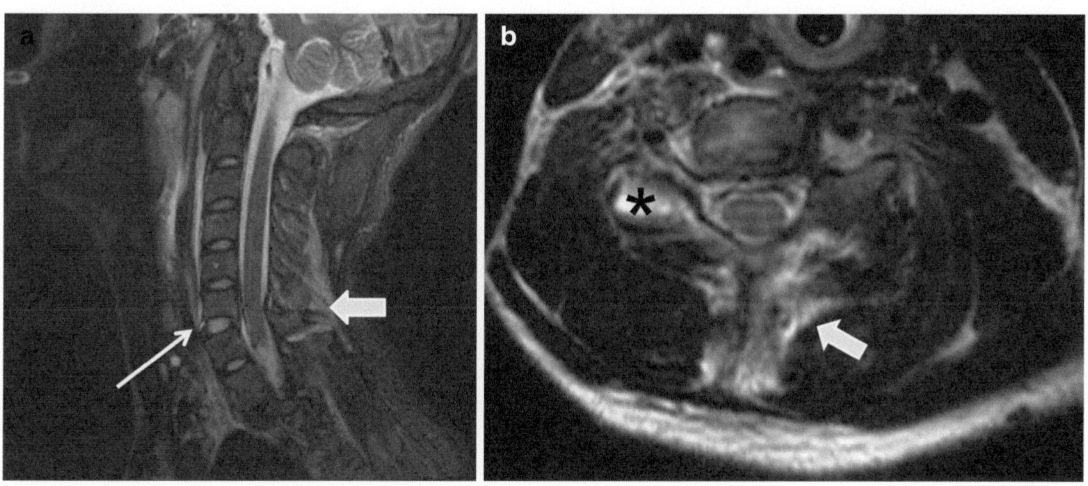

Fig. 55.4 MRI of the same patient seen in Fig. 55.3. Sagittal STIR (**a**) and axial T2WI (**b**). There is a torn ALL and avulsion of the anterior disk from the C6 inferior end plate (*thin white arrow* in **a**), as well as edematous changes in the interspinous ligament and posterior muscle/adipose planes (*thick white arrows* in **a** and **b**) in the C6–C7 level. There is an articular effusion in the C6–C7 right facet joint (*asterisk* in **b**)

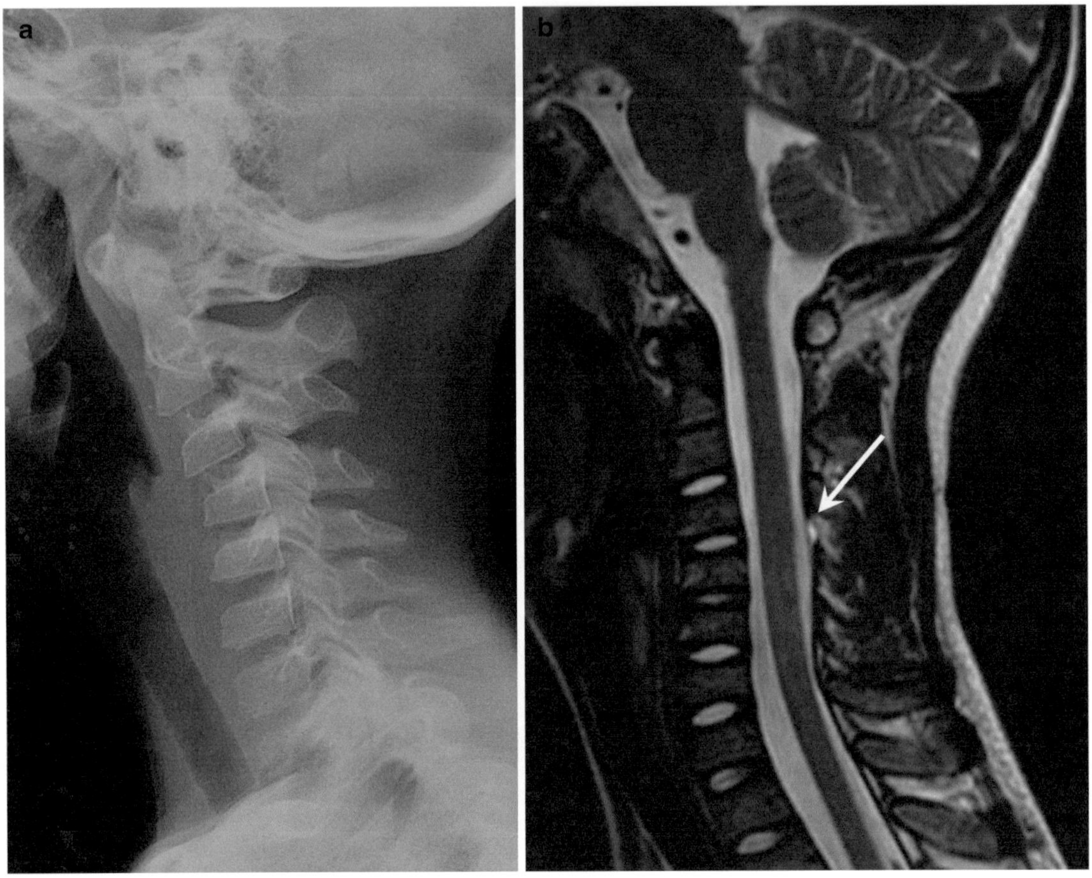

Fig. 55.5 Images of a 12-year-old boy with neck pain following a fall while playing rugby 1 week earlier. Lateral radiograph in neutral position (**a**) shows inversion of the cervical curvature centered at the C3–C4 level, loss of vertebral body and spinolaminar line alignment. MRI performed the same day (**b**, T2WI) shows a small lesion of the ligamentum flavum at level C3–C4 (*arrow*) and slight edema of the C3, C4, and C5 vertebral bodies which appear minimally compressed. The ALL and PLL appear intact. Symptoms resolved with conservative treatment

Imaging Follow-Up

Follow-up is generally clinical and imaging is not needed. If surgical fixation is performed, imaging (radiographs and/or CT) is done intraoperatively and after the first few days after intervention to assess position of fixation material and related complications.

Main Differential Diagnosis

Pseudosubluxation of C2: It is present in up to 24 % of normal pediatric static cervical spine radiographs [2, 7]. Fourteen percent of normal children also have a pseudosubluxation of C3. Complete reduction on extension studies suggests a pseudosubluxation rather than true instability. On MRI, both ALL and PLL should be intact in a pseudosubluxation.

Loss of cervical lordosis, which can indicate injury in adults, is normal and seen in up to 14 % of children.

Apparent superior subluxation of the C1 anterior arch is caused by incomplete ossification of odontoid tip. Absence of ossification of the anterior arch of C1 in first year of life may also suggest ligamentous instability but constitutes a normal variant. Atlanto-dens interval up to 4.5 mm in child <8 years old is a normal finding.

Tips

- Always report any signs of instability to avoid (further) neurological deficits.
- Look for signs of SLI on radiographs and/or CT such as widened interspinous and interarticular distances, widening of the intervertebral disk spaces, and non-parallel end plates.
- Cord compression is a surgical emergency and must be always sought out and reported. If there are signs of cord contusion/hemorrhage, prognosis is not favorable.
- Ligamentum flavum lesions are often associated with fractures of the posterior elements.

References

1. Hohl JB, Devin CJ, Fedorka CJ, Lee JY. Cervical, thoracic, and lumbar spinal trauma of the immature spine. In: Herkowitz HN, Garfin SR, Eismont FJ, Bell GR, Balderston RA, editors. Rothman-Simeone the spine. 6th ed. Philadelphia: Saunders; 2011. p. 486–504.
2. Easter JS, Barkin R, Rosen CL, Ban K. Cervical spine injuries in children, part I: mechanism of injury, clinical presentation, and imaging. J Emerg Med. 2011;41:142–50.
3. Leonard M, Sproule J, McCormack D. Paediatric spinal trauma and associated injuries. Injury Int J Care Injured. 2007;38:188–93.
4. Roche C, Carty H. Spinal trauma in children. Pediatr Radiol. 2001;31:677–700.
5. Fielding WJ, Hawkins RJ. Atlanto-axial rotatory fixation (Fixed rotatory subluxation of the atlanto-axial joint). J Bone Joint Surg. 1977;59-A:37–44.
6. Gore PA, Chang S, Theodore N. Cervical spine injuries in children: attention to radiographic differences and stability compared to those in the adult patient. Semin Pediatr Neurol. 2009;16:42–58.
7. Keiper MD, Zimmerman RA, Bilaniuk LT. MRI in the assessment of the supportive soft tissues of the cervical spine in acute trauma in children. Neuroradiology. 1998;40:359–63.
8. Flanders AE, Schwartz ED. Spinal trauma. In: Atlas SW, editor. Magnetic resonance imaging of the brain and spine. 4th ed. Philadelphia: Lippincott Williams & Wilkins; 2009. p. 1564–623.
9. Benedetti PF, Fahr LM, Kuhns LR, Hayman LA. MR imaging findings in spinal ligamentous injury. AJR Am J Roentgenol. 2000;175:661–5.

Traumatic Spinal Cord Injuries

56

Ana Lorena Abello

Abstract

Spinal cord injury results from direct trauma to the cord itself or by indirect damage to the bones and soft tissues surrounding it. Motor vehicle accidents account for the greatest number of spinal cord injuries. Acute spinal cord injury is a two-step process involving primary and secondary mechanisms (combination of the initial impact and subsequent persisting compression as well as hypoperfusion leading to spinal shock). Spinal MRI is the modality of choice to image and classify the injury and allows to predict prognosis for functional recovery.

Background

The annual incidence of spinal cord injury (SCI) in developed countries varies from 11.5 to 53.4 per million. Typically, young male patients comprise the majority of victims, injuries peaking in the third and fourth decades of life in most countries. In about 55 % of cases, the cervical spine is the most affected region [1].

Injuries are classified in terms of being neurologically "complete" or "incomplete" based upon the sacral sparing definition. "Sacral sparing" refers to the presence of sensory or motor function in the most caudal sacral segments as determined by clinical examination. A complete injury is defined as the absence of sacral sparing, whereas an incomplete injury is defined as the presence of sacral sparing. The American Spinal Injury Association (ASIA) Impairment Scale designation is used in grading the degree of impairment [2]. Other incomplete syndromes not included in the ASIA scale have been described such as the central cord syndrome, Brown–Sequard syndrome, anterior cord syndrome, cauda equina syndrome, and conus medullaris syndrome [2].

Forty years ago, approximately two-thirds of SCIs were complete, whereas today approximately 45 % are complete. The reasons are multiple and include improved initial care, greater awareness of the importance of immobilization after injury, use of restraints and air bags in motor vehicles, and hospital maneuvers that limit secondary injuries [1].

A.L. Abello, MD
Department of Radiology,
University of North Carolina, Chapel Hill, NC, USA
e-mail: anaabellop@hotmail.com

R. Hoffmann Nunes et al. (eds.), *Critical Findings in Neuroradiology*,
DOI 10.1007/978-3-319-27987-9_56

Treatment consists of medical support in the intense care unit and early surgical stabilization. The use of steroids acutely is controversial [3].

Key Points

Etiology

Spinal cord contusion is a damage to the spinal cord that results from direct trauma to the cord itself or by indirect damage to the bones and soft tissues surrounding it. Most of injuries occur by hyperflexion mechanisms [4].

Traffic accidents account for the greatest number of SCIs, typically 50 % of all such injuries. Violence-related injuries show alarming increases mostly in developing nations where violence is common. Many of these injuries are penetrating in nature [1, 5].

Pathophysiology

It is now generally accepted that acute SCI is a two-step process involving primary and secondary mechanisms.

Primary mechanism: It is most commonly a combination of the initial impact as well as subsequent persisting compression. This will typically occur with fracture dislocations, burst fractures, missile injuries, and acutely ruptured disks. Clinical scenarios where impact alone occurs without ongoing compression may include severe ligamentous injuries in which the spinal column dislocates and then spontaneously reduces [1].

Secondary mechanism: After the injury, hypoperfusion develops in gray matter and extends to the surrounding white matter slowing or completely blocking propagation of action potentials along axons, leading to spinal shock. Although this term has been used for over 150 years, the pathophysiology of spinal shock remains poorly understood. Several new important concepts of secondary injury have recently emerged. Damaged cells, axons, and blood vessels release toxic chemicals that affect intact neighboring cells. One chemical, glutamate, plays a key role in a highly disruptive process known as excitotoxicity [5].

Subacute progressive ascending myelopathy following spinal cord injury (SPAM): Described several years ago, this rare, but well-recognized, entity represents a neurological complication of SCI. After an insult to any part of the spinal cord, patients present with an ascending neurological deficit within 3 weeks of the initial SCI. Clinically, the neurological deterioration may extend at least two segments above the level established at the initial insult. Most patients make a good recovery, but there is a reported mortality of up to 10 %, particularly, if the injury ascends to the level of the brainstem. The cause for this neurological deterioration is not understood. Hypotheses include vascular injury, further mechanical insult, infection, and immune-mediated injury, including apoptosis [6].

Best Imaging Modality

Magnetic resonance imaging (MRI): In the setting of traumatic SCI, MRI provides invaluable and rapid assessment of spinal cord pathology, improves clinical examination (particularly in patients who cannot be fully examined clinically), and helps predict prognosis for functional recovery [4, 5, 7]. The internal architecture of the spinal cord as well as other soft tissue injuries are best visualized with MRI. T2-weighted image (T2WI) appears to be the best sequence to discriminate medullary hemorrhage from edema or the combination of both [8, 9]. Susceptibility weighted-imaging (SWI) is an emerging technique in the spinal cord, and it has been considered more sensitive than other sequences in the detection of blood products in acute injuries [10].

Major Findings

Several MRI signal patterns have been described in the setting of acute phase SCI and correlated with the neurological status at the time of admission and with outcome. Initially three MRI patterns were described: hemorrhage, edema, and contusion (small central hemorrhage surrounded

Table 56.1 SCI patterns, appearance on MRI, and prognosis

SCI pattern	T1	T2	Neurological compromise	Prognosis
Medullary hemorrhage	Usually normal	Central hypointensity with hyperintense halo	Complete	Poor
Medullary edema	Normal or cord enlargement	Hyperintensity	Incomplete syndrome	Favorable prognosis
Contusion	Normal or cord enlargement	Small area of hypointensity with a large hyperintense halo. Usually the hypointense area disappears in few days	Incomplete syndrome	Favorable prognosis
Medullary compression	Anatomy distortion	Anatomy distortion and/or hyperintensity	Complete	Poor
Medullary transection	Gap between spinal cord segments or loss of signal	Gap between spinal cord segments or loss of signal	Complete	Poor
SPAM	Normal or cord enlargement of at least four vertebral segments above the site of the original injury	Hyperintensity at least four vertebral segments above the site of the original injury	Incomplete	Favorable prognosis

by edema). These were better characterized in T2WI than in T1-weighted image (T1WI) in which most of the time the spinal cord was inhomogeneous or normal or sometimes only demonstrated focal cord enlargement [8, 9]. Lately other MRI findings have been described (Table 56.1).

Medullary hemorrhage: It is characterized by an area of mild hypointensity on T2WI in the first 72 h followed by hyperintensity in the peripheral portion of the lesion, while the central portion continues demonstrating hypointensity lasting up to 3–7 days (Fig. 56.1). This pattern is irreversible and represents a severe form of SCI with poor prognosis [8, 9, 11–13].

Medullary edema: This pattern shows hyperintensity in T2WI in the acute phase. Spinal cord edema reflects accumulation of intracellular and interstitial fluid and may be associated with swelling [4, 8, 9]. The edema initially appears patchy, but gradually becomes more extensive and confluent as the secondary injury cascade continues [7]. Follow-up imaging in a few weeks usually demonstrates resolution of the hyperintensity (Fig. 56.2) [4, 8, 9].

Medullary contusion: It is a mixed pattern of signal intensities compared with the first two patterns. In the acute phase, T2WI demonstrates a central area of hypointensity surrounded by a hyperintense area. MRI performed 7–10 days after injury shows the lesion decreasing in size and filling in of the central area by hyperintense signal.

Patients with medullary edema and medullary contusion usually are neurologically normal or have incomplete spinal cord damage and may have significant improvement in neurologic function [8, 9].

Medullary compression: It is a severe obliteration of the spinal canal with spinal cord compression and significant alteration of its morphology. The decrease diameter and encroachment of spinal canal hinder the visualization of the spinal cord internal architecture as well as hemorrhage foci which may explain why it is associated with complete SCI and poor prognosis (Fig. 56.3) [11, 12].

Medullary transection: It is inferred by the presence of a gap between spinal cord segments and a complete loss of spinal cord signal at the site of injury. This is associated with complete SCI and a poor outcome without changes in the

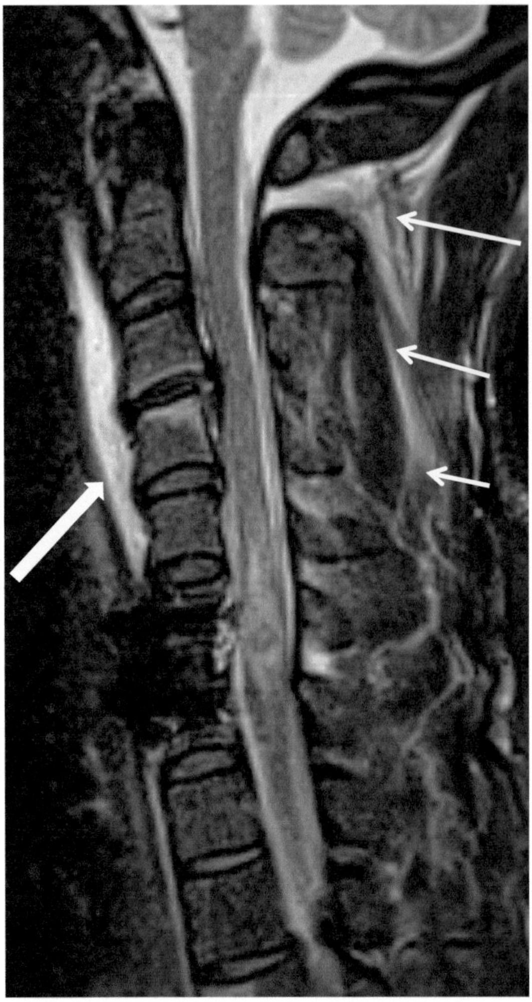

Fig. 56.1 Spinal cord hemorrhage – patient with cervical trauma related to hyperflexion mechanism. Sagittal STIR MRI obtained 3 days after injury shows an intramedullary injury with a hemorrhagic pattern, characterized by central hypointensity and peripheral hyperintensity at the C6 level. Prevertebral edema/hematoma (*thick arrow*) and soft tissue edema in the posterior ligaments (*thin arrows*) are also seen

evaluation in further clinical assessments (Fig. 56.4) [11, 14].

Soft tissues damage: A ligamentum flavum injury has a significant association with the spinal cord lesion length. It is believed that the ligamentum flavum is more elastic and that more pressure is needed to tear it. The force required for this kind of injury is responsible for SCI (Fig. 56.5) [15].

Posttraumatic disk herniation: Acute disk herniation in cervical spine injury is one of the major causes for central cord syndrome, squeezing or pinching of the spinal cord. MRI shows tissue with signal characteristics similar to those of the disk extending beyond the posterior cortical margin of a vertebral body even into the anterior epidural space (Fig. 56.6) [16].

Subacute progressive ascending myelopathy following spinal cord injury (SPAM): Patients demonstrate abnormal signal in T2WI within the cord extending at least four vertebral segments above the site of the original injury. The maximum ascent that has been reported is 11 vertebral segments. The cord changes consist in high signal on T2WI and minimal change on T1WI. Mild cord expansion may be present. Images in the surviving patients following recovery from SPAM demonstrate resolution of the previously described changes and near normalization of the cord cephalic to the primary spinal injury site. This recovery takes between 3 and 14 months; however, complete recover usually does not occur [6].

Imaging Follow-Up

In the setting of trauma, MRI should be considered in every patient with neurological deficits and potential unstable vertebral lesion. In the postoperative of spinal surgery, MRI is useful to rule out neurological complications. Imaging has a major role identifying and confirming the diagnosis of SPAM and others complications in patients with history of SCI and worsen of the symptoms.

Main Differential Diagnosis

Myelopathy secondary to degenerative spinal disease: You should suspect that signal alterations in the cord may be due to degenerative spinal disease instead of posttraumatic injury in a patient with canal stenosis accompanied by cerebrospinal fluid obliteration around the spinal cord and spinal cord deformity. Intense and well-defined T2 hyperintensity more likely represents fixed gliosis

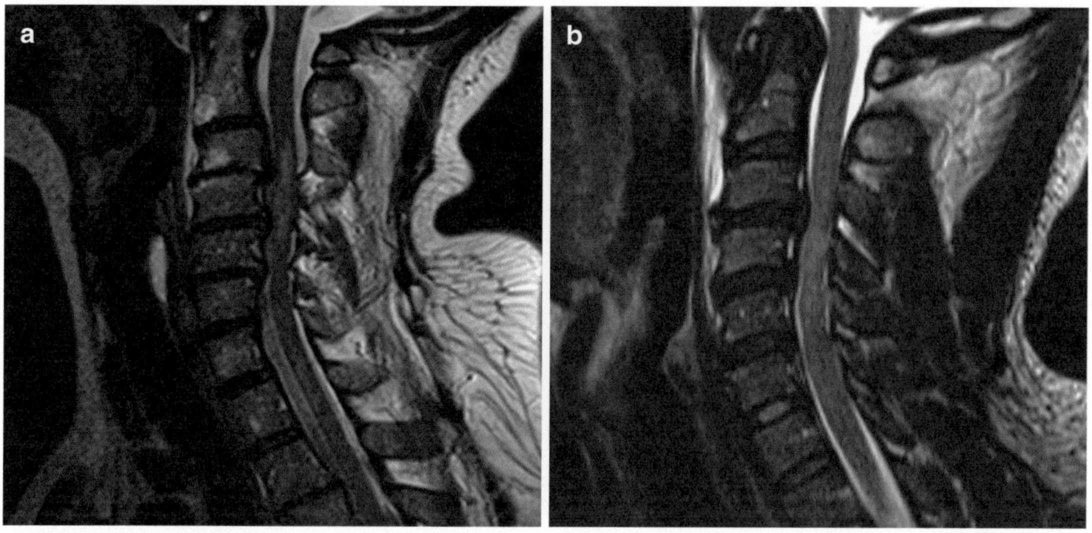

Fig. 56.2 (**a**, **b**) Spinal cord edema – two different patients with acute spinal cord injury and spinal cord edema. Sagittal cervical spine T2WI MRI show high signal in both and swelling of the spinal cord in (**b**). There is spinal canal narrow due to degenerative spinal disease that produces compression and increases the edema in both patients

or cystic necrotic changes due to degenerative disease. In opposite to traumatic SCI in which abnormalities on T1WI are absent, in degenerative spinal disease T1WI may demonstrate hypointensities that represent irreversible necrosis and myelomalacia. Faint and indistinct T2 hyperintensity in the spinal cord is more likely to reflect reversible edema in degenerative disease, and it is inseparable from the edema related to traumatic SCI. However, the two conditions are related, since patients with degenerative changes have a higher risk of SCI due to the decreased volume of their spinal canal (Fig. 56.2) [4, 17].

Truncation artifact is the most important artifact in MRI spine that can mimic SCI. It is manifested as parallel bright or dark lines seen adjacent to borders of abrupt intensity changes, for example, at the interface between bright CSF and the low-signal spinal cord on T2WI. On sagittal T2WI, a central, fine linear signal within the spinal cord due to truncation artifact should be not confused with medullary edema pattern by SCI [4].

Tips

- Make a clear description of the lesion that rules out the presence of hemorrhage taking into account that it implies a poor prognosis.
- Report signs related to spinal instability in order to convey the need for early surgical management.
- Evaluate compression of the spinal canal and spinal cord compression.
- Look for ligament injuries especially of the ligamentum flavum which is commonly associated with SCI.
- Neurological deterioration several days after the traumatic event should raise suspicion for SPAM, and MRI findings may corroborate this diagnosis.
- Always rule out artifacts when accessing SCI. In order to avoid mistakes, review sagittal and axial images to confirm the finding.

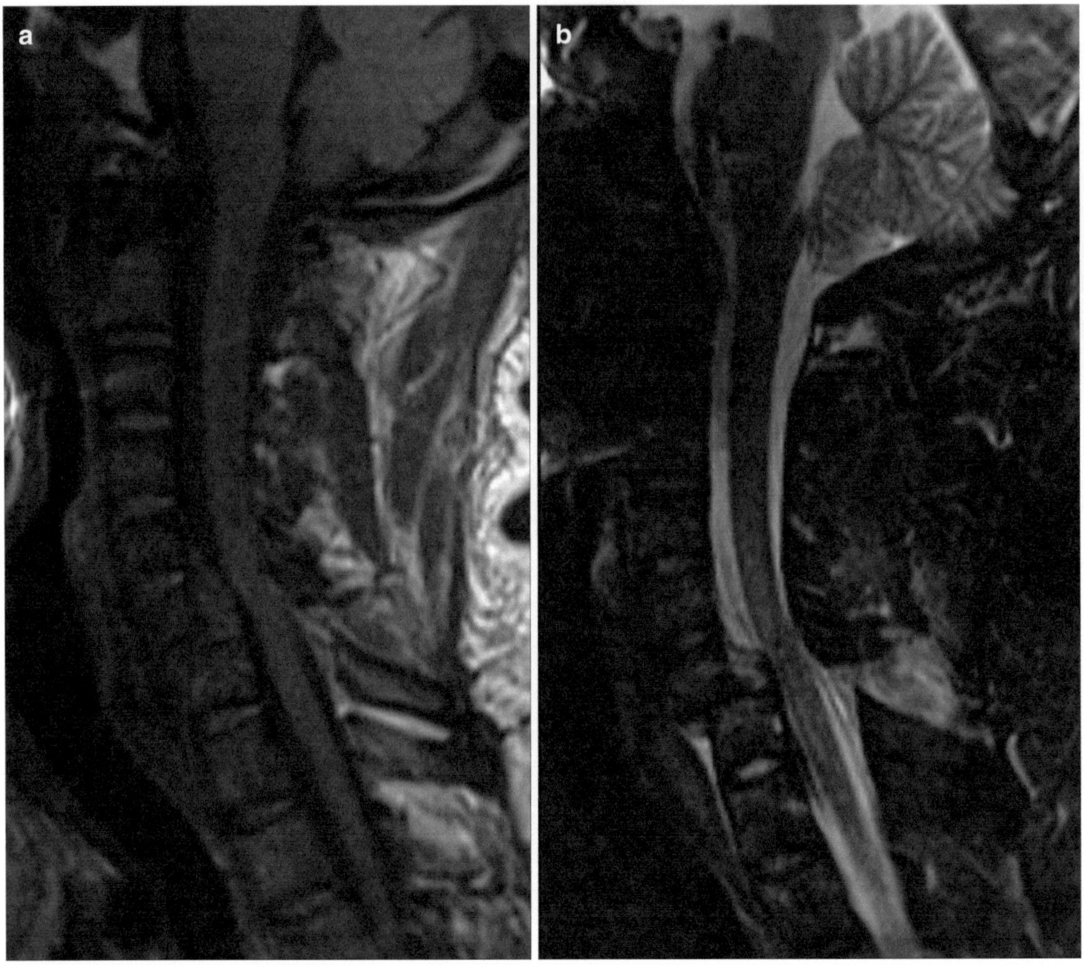

Fig. 56.3 Medullary compression – male patient involved in a motor vehicle accident resulting in a complete SCI secondary to a severe C6–C7 fracture dislocation. Sagittal T1W1 (**a**) and T2WI MRI (**b**) demonstrate a retropulsed posterior wall of the C7 vertebral body. This encroachment of medullary canal produces severe spinal cord compression, spinal cord edema, increasing the difficulty in ruling out hemorrhagic foci

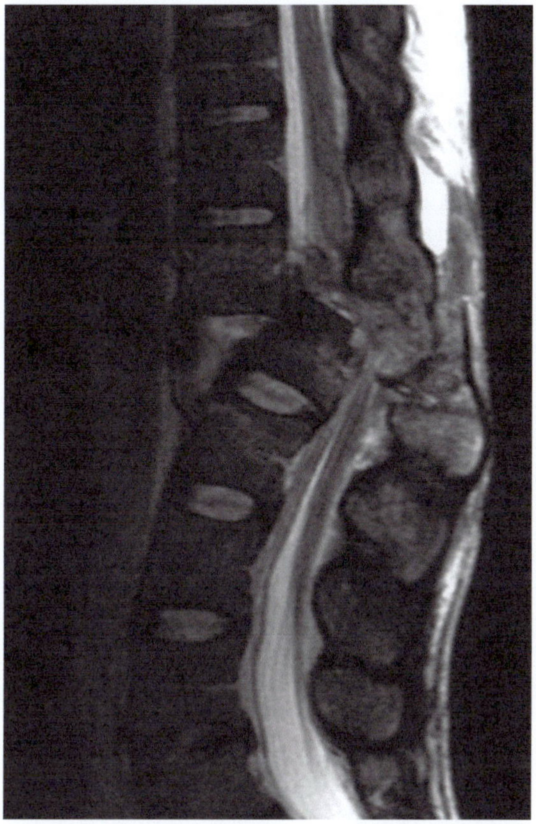

Fig. 56.4 Medullary transection – severe spinal trauma with complete dislocation of T12–L1 and dislocated L1 vertebral body extending into the medullary canal producing transection of the conus medullaris

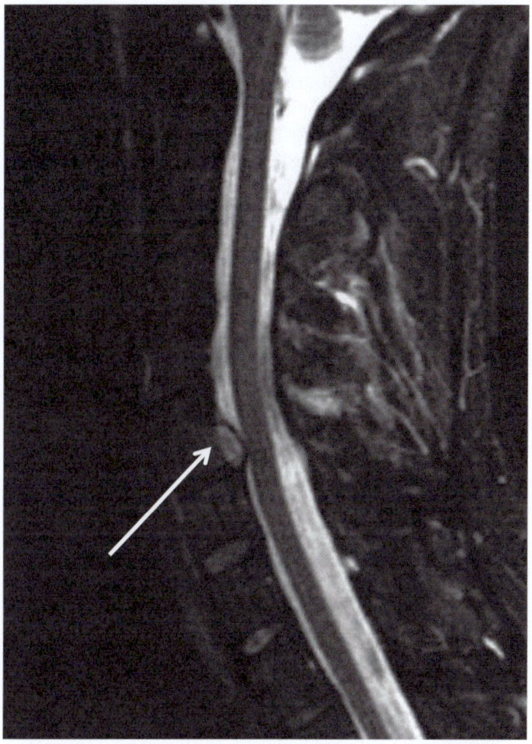

Fig. 56.6 Soft tissue injury – sagittal STIR MRI in a patient with hyperflexion trauma. An acute disk herniation (*arrow*) is shown in C5–C6 level with slight cord compression without detectable edema or hemorrhage. Hyperintensity due to edema and ligament damage in the posterior soft tissues is also seen

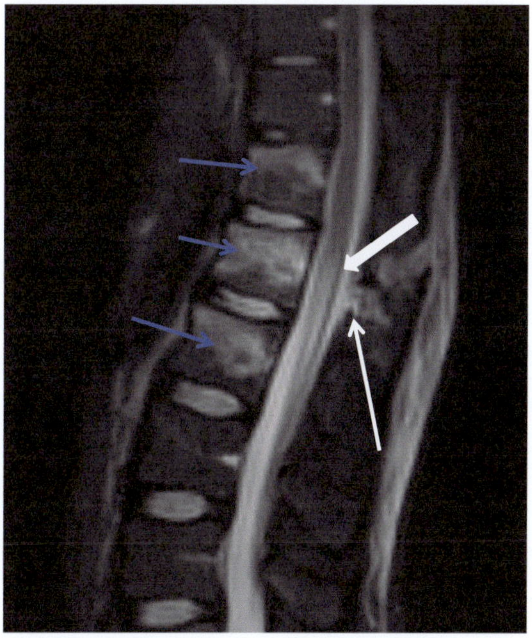

Fig. 56.5 Ligament injury – patient with spinal injury and cauda equina syndrome. Sagittal T2WI MRI shows ligamentum flavum tear (*thin white arrow*), contusion of several vertebral bodies (*blue arrows*), and probable edema of the tip of the conus medullaris (*thick white arrow*)

References

1. Sekhon LH, Fehlings MG. Epidemiology, demographics, and pathophysiology of acute spinal cord injury. Spine. 2001;26(24 Suppl):S2–12.
2. Kirshblum SC, Burns SP, Biering-Sorensen F, Donovan W, Graves DE, Jha A, et al. International standards for neurological classification of spinal cord injury (revised 2011). J Spinal Cord Med. 2011;34(6):535–46.
3. Stahel PF, VanderHeiden T, Finn MA. Management strategies for acute spinal cord injury: current options and future perspectives. Curr Opin Crit Care. 2012;18(6):651–60.
4. Kang HS, Lee JW, Kwon JW, SpringerLink (Online service). Radiology illustrated: spine. Berlin/ Heidelberg: Springer Berlin Heidelberg: Imprint: Springer; 2014. Available from: http://VB3LK7EB4T.search.serialssolutions.com/?V=1.0&L=VB3LK7EB4T&S=JCs&C=TC0001187485&T=marc.
5. McDonald JW, Sadowsky C. Spinal-cord injury. Lancet. 2002;359(9304):417–25.
6. Planner AC, Pretorius PM, Graham A, Meagher TM. Subacute progressive ascending myelopathy following spinal cord injury: MRI appearances and clinical presentation. Spinal Cord. 2008;46(2): 140–4.
7. Leypold BG, Flanders AE, Burns AS. The early evolution of spinal cord lesions on MR imaging following traumatic spinal cord injury. AJNR Am J Neuroradiol. 2008;29(5):1012–6.
8. Bondurant FJ, Cotler HB, Kulkarni MV, McArdle CB, Harris Jr JH. Acute spinal cord injury. A study using physical examination and magnetic resonance imaging. Spine. 1990;15(3):161–8.
9. Kulkarni MV, McArdle CB, Kopanicky D, Miner M, Cotler HB, Lee KF, et al. Acute spinal cord injury: MR imaging at 1.5 T. Radiology. 1987;164(3):837–43.
10. Wang M, Dai Y, Han Y, Haacke EM, Dai J, Shi D. Susceptibility weighted imaging in detecting hemorrhage in acute cervical spinal cord injury. Magn Reson Imaging. 2011;29(3):365–73.
11. Ramon S, Dominguez R, Ramirez L, Paraira M, Olona M, Castello T, et al. Clinical and magnetic resonance imaging correlation in acute spinal cord injury. Spinal Cord. 1997;35(10):664–73.
12. Miyanji F, Furlan JC, Aarabi B, Arnold PM, Fehlings MG. Acute cervical traumatic spinal cord injury: MR imaging findings correlated with neurologic outcome – prospective study with 100 consecutive patients. Radiology. 2007;243(3):820–7.
13. Flanders AE, Spettell CM, Tartaglino LM, Friedman DP, Herbison GJ. Forecasting motor recovery after cervical spinal cord injury: value of MR imaging. Radiology. 1996;201(3):649–55.
14. Kalfas I, Wilberger J, Goldberg A, Prostko ER. Magnetic resonance imaging in acute spinal cord trauma. Neurosurgery. 1988;23(3):295–9.
15. Martinez-Perez R, Paredes I, Cepeda S, Ramos A, Castano-Leon AM, Garcia-Fuentes C, et al. Spinal cord injury after blunt cervical spine trauma: correlation of soft-tissue damage and extension of lesion. AJNR Am J Neuroradiol. 2014;35(5):1029–34.
16. Dai L, Jia L. Central cord injury complicating acute cervical disc herniation in trauma. Spine. 2000;25(3):331–5. discussion 6.
17. Fernandez de Rota JJ, Meschian S, Fernandez de Rota A, Urbano V, Baron M. Cervical spondylotic myelopathy due to chronic compression: the role of signal intensity changes in magnetic resonance images. J Neurosurg Spine. 2007;6(1):17–22.

SCIWORA

57

Jaime Isern Kebschull

Abstract

Spinal cord injury without radiographic abnormality (SCIWORA) is a concept introduced to define "clinical symptoms of traumatic myelopathy with no radiographic or computed tomographic features of spinal fracture or instability." Specific biomechanics of the vertebral column in children allow the musculoskeletal system to move beyond the normal physiological range of motion without the risk of fracture, a feature not shared by the spinal cord. Early diagnosis of spinal cord injury is important to optimize clinical outcome. MRI is the best modality for direct evaluation of the spinal cord, and the main findings of an acute spinal cord injury include edema, hemorrhage, and transection. Spinal cord injury patterns revealed by MRI are important prognostic factors in patients with SCIWORA.

Background

Spinal cord injury without radiographic abnormality (SCIWORA) is a concept first introduced by Pang and Wilberger in 1982 who used the acronym to define "clinical symptoms of traumatic myelopathy with no radiographic or computed tomographic features of spinal fracture or instability" [1]. This clinical–radiological condition does not include spinal cord injury from obstetric complications, congenital spinal anomalies, electric currents, or penetrating injuries to the spinal canal [2]. Even though SCIWORA in adults is an uncommon phenomenon, it has been described in victims of all ages after blunt trauma. Inherent elasticity of the vertebral column due to ligamentous laxity, combined with the large head size, predisposes the pediatric cervical spine to deforming forces [3]. Based on reports from different authors, SCIWORA is responsible for 6–19 % and 9–14 % of spinal injuries in children and adults, respectively [4–6]. Though the most common site of involvement is the cervical spine, the thoracic spinal cord may also be involved [7]. SCIWORA should be suspected in patients subjected to blunt trauma, who report early (nearly immediate) or transient symptoms of neurological deficits or have findings upon initial assess-

J. Isern Kebschull, MD
Department of Radiology,
Radiologist Hospital Universitari Sagrat Cor,
Barcelona, Spain
e-mail: jaimeisernk@gmail.com

R. Hoffmann Nunes et al. (eds.), *Critical Findings in Neuroradiology*,
DOI 10.1007/978-3-319-27987-9_57

ment. Early diagnosis of spinal cord injury is important to optimize outcome. Treatment and prognosis are based upon neurologic presentation and MRI findings [8, 9]. Specific assessments to determine spine injury should include clinical exploration with a special focus on neurological examination. SCIWORA has a wide spectrum of neurological dysfunctions [7, 10]. Neurological deficits, which are usually more severe in the upper extremities, are the most typical clinical presentation in patients with SCIWORA [11]. A delay in the onset of neurological deficits or a delayed neurological deterioration have been reported and can range from hours to 4 days after injury [3, 12, 13]. Since physical examination is limited, clinicians mainly rely on diagnostic imaging when planning treatment for these patients [14].

Key Points

Etiology

Physiopathology: Specific biomechanics of the vertebral column in children allow the musculoskeletal system to move beyond the normal physiological range of motion without the risk of fracture. The injury to the spinal cord is caused by a contusion and/or ischemia due to temporary occlusion of vertebral and/or spinal arteries followed by a spontaneous return of vertebrae to their original position [9]. Pang et al. described four mechanisms of SCIWORA: flexion, hyperextension, longitudinal distraction, and ischemia [1].

The pathophysiology of adult SCIWORA is different from that of the pediatric population. Underlying degenerative changes like spondylosis, ossification of the posterior longitudinal ligament, and spinal canal stenosis correspond with the levels of spinal cord injury, suggesting that degenerative spine conditions predispose to SCIWORA [7]. Bone spur growth at the posterior margins of vertebral bodies, bulging of the ligamentum flavum into the spinal canal, and venous congestion may cause spinal cord compression and impingement. Hyperextension injury can result in a central cord syndrome [10].

Best Imaging Modality

All patients with suspected spine or spinal cord injury generally undergo radiographs of the cervical spine (at least a lateral view) followed by computed tomography (CT) of the cervical spine and/or other region based on physical examination and radiograph abnormalities [7, 12, 15]. When neurological deficits are diagnosed clinically but neither radiographs nor CT show abnormalities, magnetic resonance imaging (MRI) is the method of choice to demonstrate neural and extraneural injuries (Graphic 57.1) [7, 15].

Magnetic resonance imaging: It is the best modality for direct evaluation of the spinal cord. T1-weighted images (T1WI), T2-weighted images (T2WI), and short-time inversion recovery (STIR) sequences are preferred in patients with spinal injuries. Due to the longitudinal anatomy of the spinal cord, its integrity and possible location of injuries can be easily determined in the sagittal plane [15].

Major Findings

MRI findings can be classified according to the affected anatomic levels of the spinal column and according to neural, extraneural, or both types of injuries [15, 17].

Neural Lesions

The main findings of an acute spinal cord injury (SCI) include edema, hemorrhage, and transection [16].

- *Spinal cord edema* is hyperintense on T2WI and is best seen on STIR images (Figs. 57.1, 57.2, and 57.3).
- *Intramedullary hemorrhage* is best identified on T2WI and gradient recall-echo (GRE) sequences. An increase in the concentration of deoxyhemoglobin in fresh hematoma causes a decrease in signal intensity on these sequences. One week or more later, with the organization of the hematoma, resulting from the conversion of deoxyhemoglobin into methemoglobin, such lesions are seen as hyperintense on T1WI

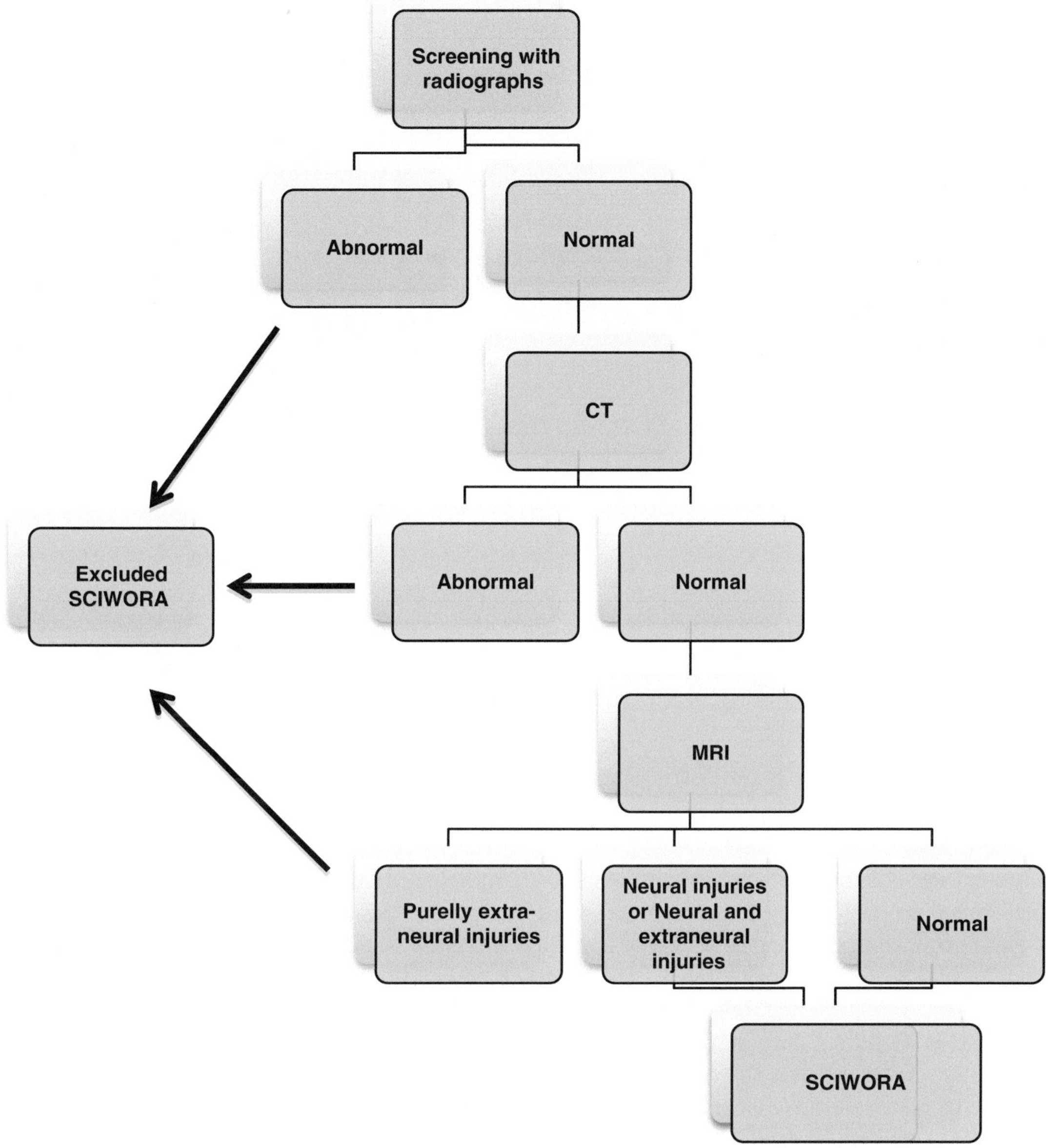

Graphic 57.1 Algorithm for diagnosis of SCIWORA

and eventually bright on T2WI too. Hemorrhages appear hypointense on T2WI due to the presence of hemosiderin in the chronic phase [15, 16].

- *Anatomic transection of spinal cord* is seen as a focal loss of continuity or a cavity filled with cerebrospinal fluid confirmed on both T1WI and T2WI [16].
- *Cord concussion* is characterized by biochemical changes within the spinal cord and is associated with normal MRI. It probably represents SCIWORA in the strictest sense. These cases should be classified as spinal cord injury without neuroimaging abnormality (*SCIWNA*) [17]. Nevertheless, Shen et al. demonstrated the clinical utility of diffusion-weighted imaging (DWI) in evaluation of patients with SCIWNA. Patients with normal MRI findings in conventional sequences had hyperintense lesions on DWI [18].

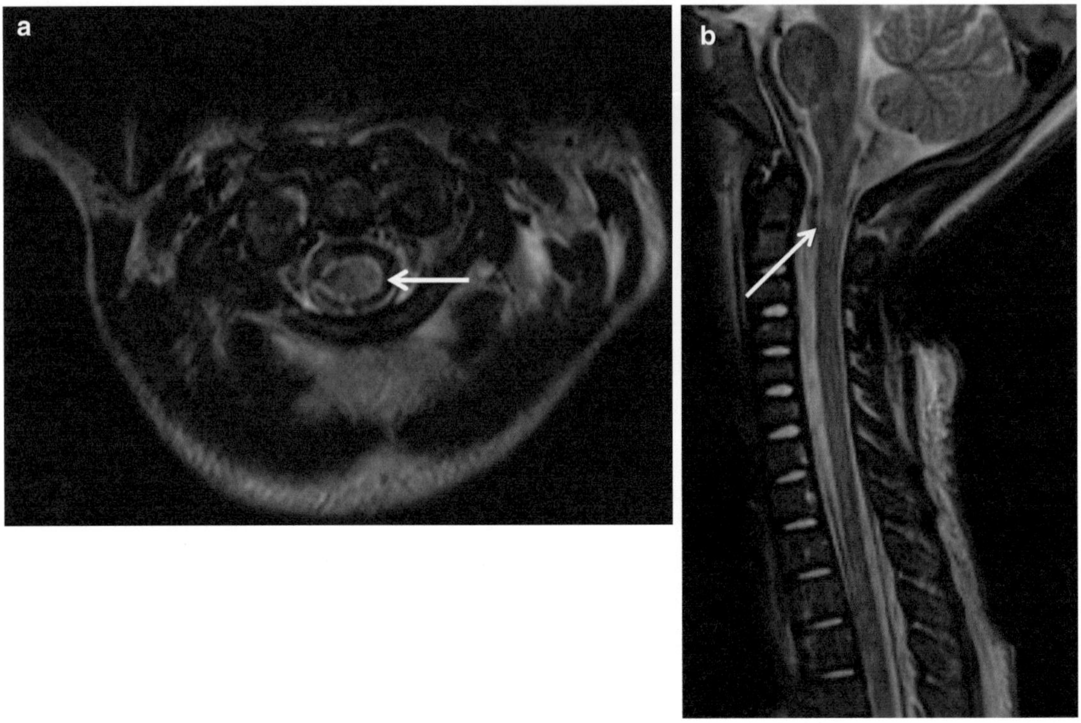

Fig. 57.1 Spinal cord edema. A 6-year-old boy presented hyperflexion injury, manifesting as central cord syndrome. (**a**) Axial and (**b**) sagittal T2WI show a high signal intensity lesion at the level of C2, corresponding with edema (*arrows*). Note the absence of ligament or bone injuries

Extraneural Lesions

Included in SCIWORA are spinal cord pathologies including contusion, edema, transection, as well as extraneural pathologies such as traumatic disk herniation, epidural hematoma, rupture of ligaments, capsules, and muscles (Fig. 57.3) [16, 18]. MRI is useful not only for investigating soft tissue abnormalities, but it also allows for identification of bone marrow edema in injured vertebrae that cannot be seen on CT. STIR, which is used to suppress the signal from fat, is the most valuable MRI sequence in these cases [19]. Imaging features of posttraumatic disk herniations are similar to those of nontraumatic ones. Therefore, it is often impossible to differentiate between these two forms of disk herniations, but the presence of other posttraumatic lesions at the same level(s) may suggest an acute nature [17].

Diffusion tensor imaging (DTI) may also become an important diagnostic tool in patients with SCIWORA due to its ability to assess white matter tract integrity [15].

Imaging Prognostic Factors

Spinal cord injury patterns revealed by MRI are important prognostic factors in patients with SCIWORA. Several authors have correlated the patterns of spinal cord injury with prognosis as follows: (1) worse if there is intramedullary hematoma occupying more than 50 % of the cross-sectional area of the spinal cord, (2) intermediate if the hematoma is minor and associated with edema, (3) better in patients where there is only cord edema, and (4) the best when there are no changes in the spinal cord [20].

Imaging Follow-Up

To assess injuries and their evolution, some clinicians recommend routinely obtaining initial and follow-up MRI scans in all patients with suspected SCIWORA [21].

Follow-up MRI has become important because SCIWORA can recur [7, 21]. Resolution of the

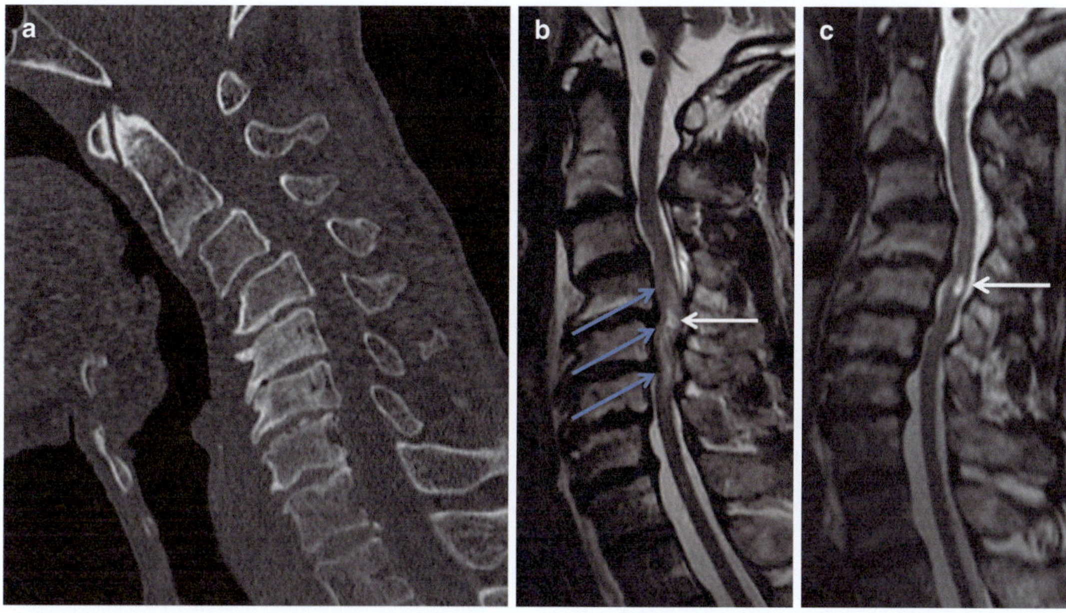

Fig. 57.2 Patient with central cord syndrome after trauma. (**a**) Sagittal CT shows degenerative disease in the cervical spine and narrowing of the spinal canal especially at C4–5. No fractures are seen. (**b**) Sagittal T2WI depicts signal hyperintensity and swelling in spinal cord compatible con edema–trauma related (*blue arrows*). A central round lesion more bright C5 level probably corresponds a prior myelomalacia area due to degenerative disease (*white arrow*). (**c**) Sagittal T2WI 3 months later shows resolution of the edema and the myelomalacia lesion is now better demonstrated (*white arrow*)

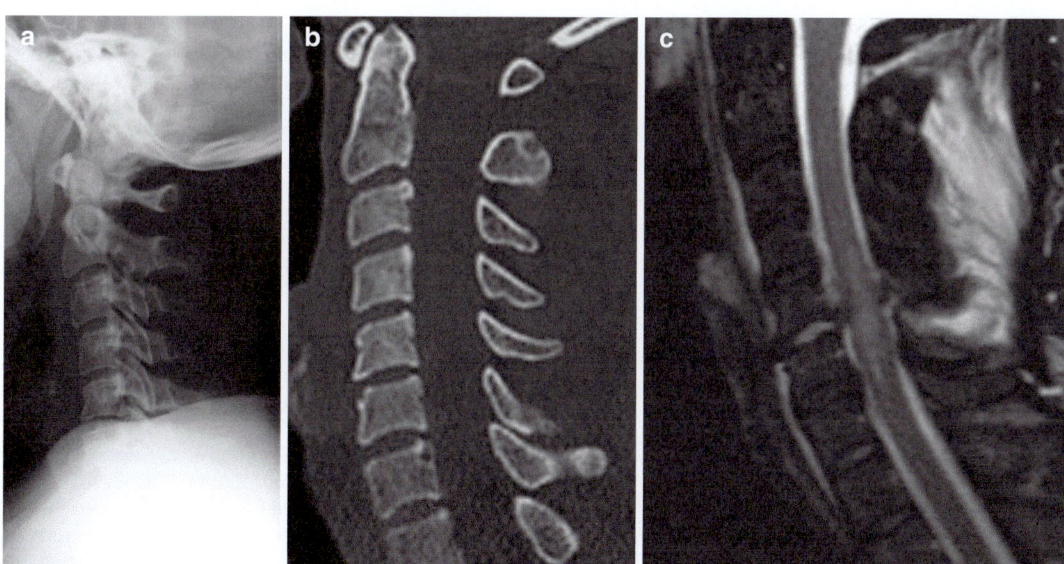

Fig. 57.3 A 45-year-old man with tetraparesia after a motor vehicle accident. (**a**) Sagittal radiograph and (**b**) sagittal CT show no evidence of fractures or lesions. (**c**) Sagittal T2WI shows spinal cord edema centered at C5–6 and ligament injuries at these levels

changes seen on MRI scans predicts almost always a return to normal neurologic function, whereas persistence of spinal cord injury lesions decreases the chances of a good outcome. Recurrent SCIWORA is secondary to early spine mobilization from absent or inadequate treatment and often results in more severe deficits than the initial syndrome [7].

Main Differential Diagnosis

Differential diagnosis should include *infarct* due to the vertebral artery occlusion. *Acute or chronic myelitis* and *myelomalacia* due to degenerative disease (Fig. 57.2) should also be excluded [15].

Tips

- When neurological deficits are diagnosed clinically but neither radiographs nor CT show any abnormality, MRI is the only way to show neural injuries.
- A detailed MRI description of the appearance of the lesion and its measurement can help to determine prognosis. Special attention should be paid to the presence of intramedullary hematoma.
- Soft tissue injuries may affect treatment and help to determine the level of the spine injury as well as possible instability which may have to be managed surgically.
- In the setting of neurology deterioration several days after the traumatic event, suspect delay or recurrent SCIWORA.

References

1. Pang D, Wilberger Jr JE. Spinal cord injury without radiographic abnormalities in children. J Neurosurg. 1982;57(1):114–29.
2. Bruce DA. Efficacy of barbiturates in the treatment of resistant intracranial hypertension in severely head-injured children. Pediatr Neurosci. 1989;15(4):216.
3. Pang D. Spinal cord injury without radiographic abnormality in children, 2 decades later. Neurosurgery. 2004;55(6):1325–42.
4. Eleraky MA, Theodore N, Adams M, et al. Pediatric cervical spine injuries: report of 102 cases and review of the literature. J Neurosurg. 2000;92 Suppl 1:12–7.
5. Kothari P, Freeman B, Grevitt M, Kerslake R. Injury to the spinal cord without radiological abnormality (SCIWORA) in adults. J Bone Joint Surg Br. 2000;82(7):1034–7.
6. Parent S, Mac-Thiong JM, Roy-Beaudry M, et al. Spinal cord injury in the pediatric population: a systematic review of the literature. J Neurotrauma. 2011;28(8):1515–24.
7. Launay F, Leet AI, Sponseller PD. Pediatric spinal cord injury without radiographic abnormality: a meta-analysis. Clin Orthop Relat Res. 2005;433:166–70.
8. Alison Chantal Caviness, MD, MPH, PhD. Spinal cord injury without radiographic abnormality (SCIWORA) in children. http://www.uptodate.com/contents/spinal-cord-injury-without-radiographic--abnormality-sciwora-in-children.
9. Ahmann PA, Smith SA, Schwartz JF, et al. Spinal cord infarction due to minor trauma in children. Neurology. 1975;25:301–7.
10. Kasimatis GB, Panagiotopoulos E, Megas P, Matzaro-Glou C, Gliatis J, Tyllianakis M, Lambiris E. The adult spinal cord injury without radiographic abnormalities syndrome: magnetic resonance imaging and clinical findings in adults with spinal cord injuries having normal radiographs and computed tomography studies. J Trauma. 2008;65(1):86–93.
11. El Masri WS, Kumar N. Traumatic spinal cord injuries. Lancet. 2011;377:972–4.
12. Dickman CA, Zabramski JM, Hadley MN, Rekate HL, Sonntag VKH. Pediatric spinal cord injury without radiographic abnormalities: report of 26 cases and review of literature. J Spinal Disord. 1991;4:296–305.
13. Tiwari MK, Gifti DS, Singh P, Khosla VK, Mathuriya SN, Gupta SK, et al. Diagnosis and prognostication of adult spinal cord injury without radiographic abnormality using magnetic resonance imaging analysis of 40 patients. Surg Neurol. 2005;63:204–9.
14. Bosch A, Stauffer ES, Nickel VL. Incomplete traumatic quadriplegia. A ten-year review. JAMA. 1971;216(3):473–8.
15. Szwedowski D, Walecki J. Spinal cord injury without radiographic abnormality (SCIWORA) – clinical and radiological aspects. Pol J Radiol. 2014;79:461–4.
16. Liao CC, Lui TN, Chen LR, Chuang CC, Huang YC. Spinal cord injury without radiological abnormality in preschool-aged children: correlation of magnetic resonance imaging findings with neurological outcomes. J Neurosurg. 2005;103(1 Suppl):17–23.
17. Yucesoy K, Yuksel KZ. SCIWORA in MRI era. Clin Neurol Neurosurg. 2008;110:429–33.

18. Shen H, Tang Y, Huang L, et al. Applications of diffusion-weighted MRI in thoracic spinal cord injury without radiographic abnormality. Int Orthop. 2007;31(3):375–83.
19. Parizel PM, van der Zijden T, Gaudino S, et al. Trauma of the spine and spinal cord: imaging strategies. Eur Spine J. 2010;19 Suppl 1:S8–17.
20. Tewari MK, Gifti DS, Singh P, et al. Diagnosis and prognostication of adult spinal cord injury without radiographic abnormality using magnetic resonance imaging: analysis of 40 patients. Surg Neurol. 2005;63(3):204–9.
21. Sharma S, Singh M, Wani IH, et al. Adult spinal cord injury without radiographic abnormalities (SCIWORA): clinical and radiological correlations. J Clin Med Res. 2009;1(3):165–72.

Spinal Dural Arteriovenous Fistulas 58

Daniel Varón and Florencia Álamos

Abstract

Spinal dural arteriovenous fistulas are the most commonly encountered vascular malformation of the spinal cord. They are presumably acquired lesions; however, their exact etiology is not known. Most fistulas are located in the thoracolumbar region. The increase in spinal venous pressure leads to decreased drainage of normal spinal veins, venous congestion, and clinical findings of progressive myelopathy. Because presenting clinical symptoms are usually non-specific, the radiologist is often the first to raise the possibility of this diagnosis. On MRI, the combination of cord edema, perimedullary dilated vessels, and cord enhancement is characteristic. There are two treatment options in this patient population: endovascular and surgical occlusion of the shunt.

Background

Spinal dural arteriovenous fistula (SDAVF) is one of the most common of spinal vascular diseases and accounts for about 70 % of all spinal arteriovenous malformations [1, 5].

SDAVF occur at a rate of five to ten cases/year per million population. However, the disease seems to be under diagnosed [4]. Usually, SDAVFs are found in men, and the mean age at diagnosis is 55–60 years [2]. Most fistulas are found in the thoracolumbar region. The AV shunt is located inside the dura mater close to a spinal nerve root where the arterial blood from a radiculomeningeal artery enters a radicular vein at the level where the latter passes through the dura at the dorsal surface of the dural root sleeve in the intervertebral foramen [7]. The increase pressure within the valveless perimedullary venous plexus causes congestion of the radial veins draining the spinal cord, leading to a disturbance of medullary circulation as a result of a decreased arteriovenous pressure gradient [10].

Clinical presentation of SDAVF is usually characterized by a gradual onset of symptoms

D. Varón, MD (✉)
Department of Radiology,
Hospital Universitario del Valle,
Calle 5 No. 36 – 08, Cali, Colombia
e-mail: danielmvaron@hotmail.com

F. Álamos, MD, PhD
Department of Neuroscience School of Medicine,
Universidad Católica de Chile,
Luz Larrain, 3946 Lo Barnechea, Santiago, Chile
e-mail: flopi1987@yahoo.com

R. Hoffmann Nunes et al. (eds.), *Critical Findings in Neuroradiology*,
DOI 10.1007/978-3-319-27987-9_58

that result from venous hypertension and is known as the Foix–Alajouanine syndrome. This insidious onset often leads to delays in diagnosis [7]. The most common initial symptom is gait disturbance, followed by numbness and paresthesias. By the time patients present, most exhibit signs of bladder dysfunction and leg weakness [3]. The slow-flow nature of these lesions makes hemorrhage rare, although this has been reported in the thoracolumbar region [8].

Failure to recognize and treat SDAVF in a timely fashion can result in irreversible neurologic disability, including myelopathy, lower extremity weakness, and bowel, bladder, and sexual dysfunction [6]. Myelopathy that progresses cephalad to involve the medulla may kill the patient.

As this condition can result in permanent spinal cord injury, all patients require treatment. There are two options in the treatment of SDAVFs: surgical occlusion of the intradural vein that receives the blood from the shunt zone and endovascular therapy using liquid embolic agents after selective catheterization of the radiculomeningeal artery supplying the fistula [6].

After complete occlusion of the fistula, the progression of the disease is stopped; however, only two-thirds of patients have a complete regression of their motor symptoms, and only one-third show an improvement in their sensory disturbances [12].

Key Points

Etiology

The etiology of SDAVFs is unknown, but there is evidence suggesting that they are an acquired multifactorial disease. Mechanisms such as infection, syringomyelia, trauma, and surgery are observed in the development of this condition and constitute possible triggers. Unlike cranial dural arteriovenous fistulas where venous sinus thrombosis has been implicated in the pathogenesis and an association with a prothrombotic condition has been demonstrated, thrombophilia has not been established as a factor associated with the development of SDAVF [10].

Best Imaging Modality

Magnetic resonance imaging (*MRI*): The diagnosis of SDAVF rests on MRI. Usually, T2-weighted image (T2WI) sequences are the most helpful, and the combination of cord edema and perimedullary dilated vessels is the characteristic finding that suggests the correct diagnosis [14]. Postcontrast sequences should be obtained as gadolinium increases the conspicuity of the enlarged perimedullary venous plexus and serpiginous longitudinal veins [15, 16]. The coiled or serpentine vascular structures may be better appreciated on myelographic T2WI (such as constructive interference in steady-state [CISS], fast-imaging employing steady-state acquisition [FIESTA], or T2 SPACE) compared with T2WI TSE sequences [7, 18].

Magnetic resonance angiography (*MRA*): MRI allows to suspect or to diagnose an SDAVF; however, routine sequences cannot predict the level of the fistula. SDAVFs may occur anywhere from the level of the foramen magnum to the sacrum; therefore, the noninvasive evaluation of the shunt location is important to guide catheter angiography [20]. Spinal contrast-enhanced MRA (3D or 4D) helps to localize these lesions and helps to avoid unnecessary superselective injections of all possible arterial feeders.

Fast contrast-enhanced MRA (3D fast-spoiled gradient-echo pulse sequence) using a gadolinium bolus technique and a large craniocaudal field of view usually demonstrates the level of the shunt [22–24].

Computed tomography angiography (*CTA*): Spinal CTA can also demonstrate the level of the fistula and may be an alternative to MRI; however, given the large field of view needed, the high dose of ionizing radiation is a possible limitation. Moreover, this study is less reliable than MRA for demonstrating the fistula [18].

Spinal digital subtraction angiography (*spinal DSA*): Spinal catheter angiography is necessary to confirm the diagnosis, to verify the exact level of the fistula, and to identify the feeding artery and possible collateral feeders [6]. Identification of the artery of Adamkiewicz is critical as SDAVFs arising from the same radicular artery pose a treatment challenge and potential complications.

Major Findings

Cord edema: The increase in spinal venous pressure diminishes the AV pressure gradient and leads to decreased venous drainage, venous congestion, and intramedullary edema [25]. MRI findings include enlargement of the cord, primarily in the lower thoracic region and conus, with associated central T2 hyperintensity involving the gray and white matter throughout multiple segments (Fig. 58.1). The periphery of the cord may be of normal signal or reduced T2 signal intensity. Regardless of the location of the fistula, the T2 hyperintensity involves the conus medullary in up to 90 % of cases [13]. The cord may demonstrate contrast enhancement which as a sign of chronic venous congestion [16].

With progression of the disease, there is usually cephalad extension of the cord T2 abnormality. When it reaches the cervicomedullary level, respiratory problems may ensue, and they may be irreversible.

Dilated perimedullary vessels: Venous congestion is demonstrated as prominent and coiled perimedullary vessels along the dorsal aspect of the cord and can be observed on T2 as flow voids. However, if the shunt volume is small, these vessels may only be seen after contrast administration (Fig. 58.2). Heavily weighted T2 sequences may aid in visualizing the flow voids along the dorsal aspect of the cord that may be obscured by pulsation artifact or mass effect in other sequences [18].

Early venous filling can be demonstrated in the first-pass gadolinium-enhanced MRA, thereby confirming the shunt and its location. On spinal DSA, early venous filling and retrograde contrast filling of the radiculomedullary veins are typical [6]. Delayed appearance of the veins is also seen.

Cord atrophy: In the latter course of the disease, the cord becomes atrophic.

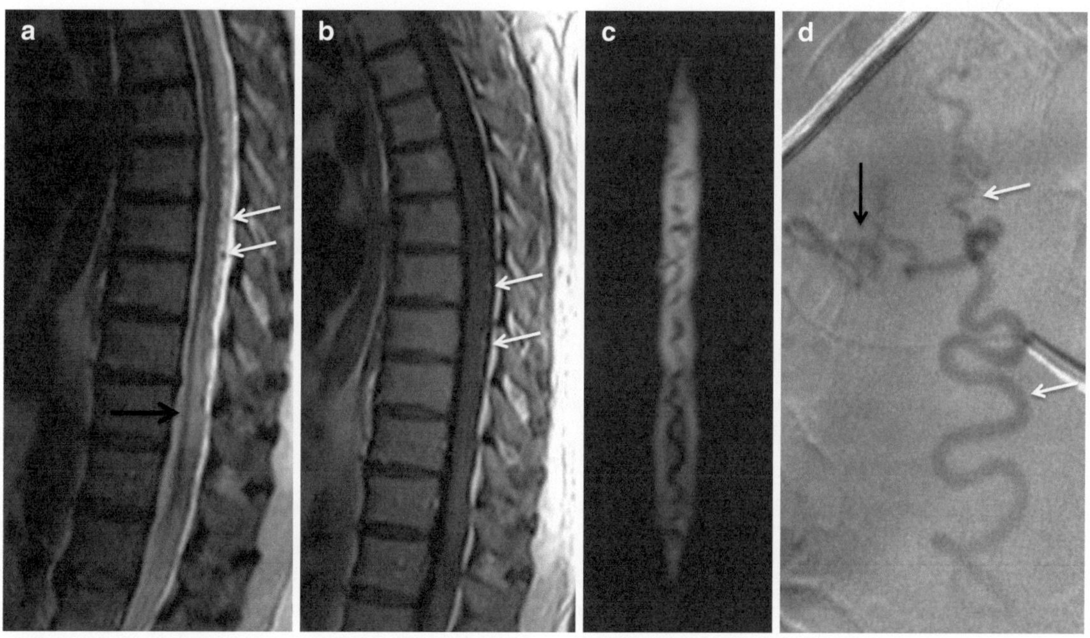

Fig. 58.1 A 63-year-old man with progressive weakness. (**a**) Sagittal T2WI shows perimedullary flow voids along the dorsal aspect of the cord (*white arrows*) with intramedullary T2 hyperintensity (*black arrow*). (**b**) Postcontrast T1WI shows the dilated-enhancing perimedullary veins (*arrows*). (**c**) Coronal reformations from CISS clearly show the flow voids along the dorsal aspect of the cord. (**d**) Spinal DSA of the T8 intercostal artery shows the SDAVF (*black arrow*) and the arterialized dilated perimedullary draining veins (*white arrows*)

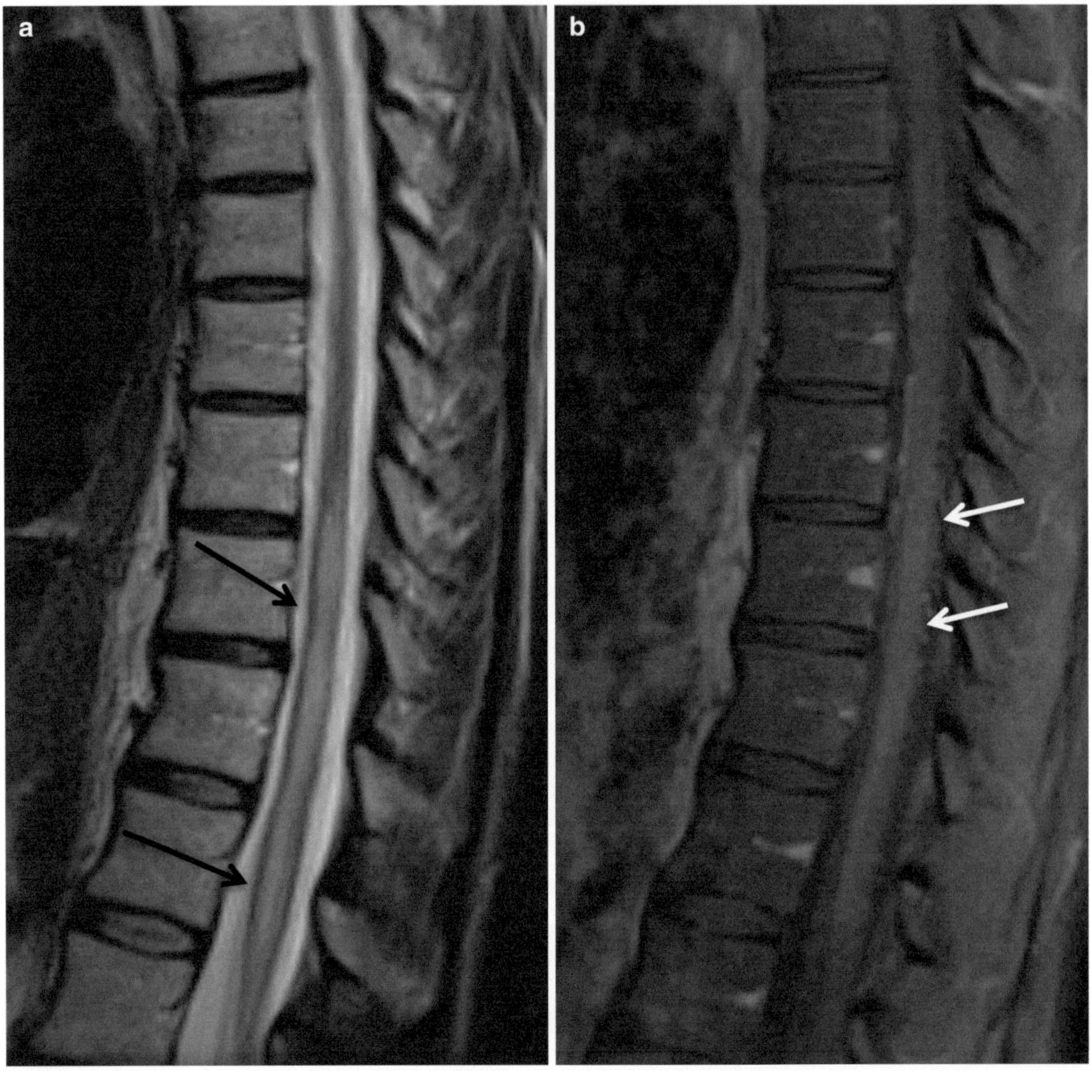

Fig. 58.2 A 67-year-old man with gait disturbance and paresthesias. (**a**) Sagittal T2WI shows intramedullary hyperintensity from T9 to the tip of conus medullary (*arrows*), but the dilated perimedullary veins are not seen. Note that high signal is central in the cord and spares its periphery. (**b**) Postcontrast sagittal T1WI clearly shows the dilated perimedullary blood vessels (*arrows*) with slightly and diffuse enhancement of the spinal cord

Imaging Follow-Up

In patients with improvement or stabilization of symptoms after treatment, the first follow-up can be performed approximately at 2–3 months using MRI with and without gadolinium. In patients with a successfully occluded fistula, the expected postoperative MRI appearance includes diminished cord enlargement and high T2 signal, contrast enhancement, and size and extent of perimedullary serpiginous flow voids [19, 21]. Nevertheless, persistent intramedullary T2 hyperintensity and enhancement can been seen up to 1 year posttreatment even in patients who have undergone successful fistula occlusion, and these findings are not an indication for additional imaging (DSA) and treatment unless there is clinical deterioration [18].

If persistent perimedullary vessels are seen on follow-up studies, recanalization of the fistula should be suspected and additional imaging such as MRA and heavily T2WI myelographic sequences may be obtained. If the MRI findings are inconclusive, or worsening of motor symptoms is present, spinal DSA needs to be performed.

Main Differential Diagnosis

Cerebrospinal fluid flow artifact: This artifact is typically seen on T2WI as signal loss in dorsal thoracic subarachnoid space resulting from turbulent CSF flow. Its margins are ill-defined and there is no cord edema.

Spinal cord infarct: It is usually seen as a long-segment T2 hyperintensity, in the majority of patients involving the central portion (gray matter) of the cord. An abrupt onset and rapid progression of symptoms should make one suspect the correct diagnosis. DWI is confirmatory and shows high signal with restricted diffusion.

Neuromyelitis optica: The clinical course of acute myelitis typically evolves over hours or days and the T2 hyperintensity in the cord may be extensive as that seen in an SDAVF. However, enlarged perimedullary vessels are not seen in myelitis. Contrast enhancement occurs in both entities. Recurrent bouts of myelitis and involvement of the optic nerves should prompt the clinician to ask for the laboratory examinations (aquaporin antibodies) needed to confirm the diagnosis of neuromyelitis optica.

Other vascular lesions: In presence of cord edema together with perimedullary dilated vessels, the only viable imaging differential diagnosis is another type of spinal vascular malformation (radicular AV malformations, epidural AV shunts, or perimedullary AV fistulas) [7]. DSA may be needed for the correct diagnosis.

Tips

- Most common presentation of an SDAVF is progressive lower extremity weakness and sensory changes (Foix–Alajouanine syndrome).
- Classic imaging findings of SDAVF include an enlarged spinal cord with T2 hyperintensity associated and prominent flow voids along the dorsal aspect of the cord. Enlarged vessels may be seen anteriorly and in the nerve roots.
- T2 signal abnormality involving the conus is almost invariably present.
- The sensory level correlates poorly with the level of the fistula; therefore, the entire spine should be examined with MRI when an SDAVF is suspected.
- MRA or CTA should be obtained before catheter angiography to help localize the exact level of the fistula.
- Catheter angiography is the gold standard in the diagnosis of SDAVF.

References

1. Gilbertson JR, Miller GM, Goldman MS, et al. Spinal dural arteriovenous fistulas: MR and myelographic findings. AJNR Am J Neuroradiol. 1995;16(10):2049–57.
2. Jellema K, Tijssen CC, van Gijn J. Spinal dural arteriovenous fistulas: a congestive myelopathy that initially mimics a peripheral nerve disorder. Brain. 2006;129:3150–64.
3. Jellema K, Canta LR, Tijssen CC, et al. Spinal dural arteriovenous fistulas: clinical features in 80 patients. J Neurol Neurosurg Psychiatry. 2003;74(10):1438–40.
4. Grandin C, Duprez T, Stroobandt G, et al. Spinal dural arterio-venous fistula: an underdiagnosed disease? Acta Neurol Belg. 1997;97(1):17–21.
5. Jellema K, Tijssen CC, Sluzewski M, et al. Spinal dural arteriovenous fistulas an underdiagnosed disease. A review of patients admitted to the spinal unit of a rehabilitation center. J Neurol. 2006;253(2):159–62.
6. Krings T, Geibprasert S. Spinal dural arteriovenous fistulas. AJNR Am J Neuroradiol. 2009;30(4):639–48.
7. Fugate JE, Lanzino G, Rabinstein AA. Clinical presentation and prognostic factors of spinal dural arte-

riovenous fistulas: an overview. Neurosurg Focus. 2012;32(5):E17.
8. Koch C, Gottschalk S, Giese A. Dural arteriovenous fistula of the lumbar spine presenting with subarachnoid hemorrhage. Case report and review of the literature. J Neurosurg. 2004;100:385–91.
9. Marcus J, Schwarz J, Singh IP, et al. Spinal dural arteriovenous fistulas: a review. Curr Atheroscler Rep. 2013;15:335.
10. Koch C. Spinal dural arteriovenous fistula. Curr Opin Neurol. 2006;19:69–75.
11. Krings T, Mull M, Gilsbach JM, et al. Spinal vascular malformations. Eur Radiol. 2005;15:267–78.
12. Van Dijk JM, TerBrugge KG, Willinsky RA, et al. Multidisciplinary management of spinal dural arteriovenous fistulas: clinical presentation and long-term follow-up in 49 patients. Stroke. 2002;33:1578–83.
13. Muralidharan R, Saladino A, Lanzino G, et al. The clinical and radiological presentation of spinal dural arteriovenous fistula. Spine. 2011;36(25):1641–7.
14. Koenig E, Thron A, Schrader V, et al. Spinal arteriovenous malformations and fistulae: clinical, neuroradiological and neurophysiological findings. J Neurol. 1989;236:260–6.
15. Minami S, Sagoh T, Nishimura K, et al. Spinal arteriovenous malformation: MR imaging. Radiology. 1988;169(1):109–15.
16. Terwey B, Becker H, Thron AK, et al. Gadolinium-DTPA enhanced MR imaging of spinal dural arteriovenous fistulas. J Comput Assist Tomogr. 1989;13(1): 30–7.
17. Krings T, Lasjaunias PL, Hans FJ, et al. Imaging in spinal vascular disease. Neuroimaging Clin N Am. 2007;17:57–72.
18. Morris JM. Image of dural arterio-venous fistula. Radiol Clin N Am. 2012;50:823–39.
19. Willinsky RA, ter Brugge K, Montanera W, et al. Posttreatment MR findings in spinal dural arteriovenous malformations. AJNR Am J Neuroradiol. 1995;16(10):2063–71.
20. Bowen BC, Fraser K, Kochan JP, et al. Spinal dural arteriovenous fistulas: evaluation with MR angiography. AJNR Am J Neuroradiol. 1995;16:2029–43.
21. Mascalchi M, Ferrito G, Quilici N, et al. Spinal vascular malformations: MR angiography after treatment. Radiology. 2001;219(2):346–53.
22. Farb RI, Kim JK, Willinsky RA, et al. Spinal dural arteriovenous fistula localization with a technique of first-pass gadolinium-enhanced MRangiography: initial experience. Radiology. 2002;222:843–50.
23. Mull M, Nijenhuis RJ, Backes WH, et al. Value and limitations of contrast enhanced MR angiography in spinal arteriovenous malformations and dural arteriovenous fistulas. AJNR Am J Neuroradiol. 2007;28: 1249.
24. Bowen BC, Pattany PM. Contrast-enhanced MRangiography of spinal vessels. Magn Reson Imaging Clin N Am. 2000;8:597–614.
25. Hurst RW, Kenyon LC, Lavi E, et al. Spinal dural arteriovenous fistula: the pathology of venous hypertensive myelopathy. Neurology. 1995;45:1309–13.

Misplaced Spinal Hardware

59

Denise Tokeshi Amaral, Eduardo Luis Bizetto, and Lázaro Luís Faria do Amaral

Abstract

Spinal surgical fusions are performed for a wide spectrum of indications including restoration of anatomic alignment and functional biomechanics. Imaging plays a crucial role in the assessment of the postoperative spine, and adequate evaluation of spinal hardware necessitates a detailed understanding of the initial spinal pathologic condition, the surgical procedure performed, the clinical presentation of the patient, and the time interval from the surgery to the imaging study. Imaging is essential in identifying the location and integrity of surgical implants, in evaluating the success of decompression procedures, in delineating fusion status, and in identifying postoperative complications.

Background

Spinal fusion surgeries are performed for a wide spectrum of indications (i.e., deformities, trauma, infections, and tumors) to restore anatomic alignment and functional biomechanics [1]. In spinal fusion surgeries, surgical implants are used to stabilize the spine, replace resected components, and maintain anatomic alignment during the period osseous fusion occurs [2, 3]. Metallic hardware always serves a temporary purpose, allowing bone fusion to occur.

The surgical approach to spinal fusion can be anterior, posterior, or lateral [3]. The anterior approach is preferred in the cervical spine because of the risk of cord injury. A posterior approach is often preferred in the lumbar spine because the pedicle screws and rods or plates can be placed before dural retraction and dissection of the intervertebral disk, restoring normal disk height and decompressing the neural foramina. The disk space is usually filled with allograft bone blocks or fusion cages [1].

D.T. Amaral, MD (✉) • E.L. Bizetto, MD
Division of Musculoskeletal Radiology,
Hospital Sírio Libanês,
Sao Paulo, SP, Brazil
e-mail: denitok@gmail.com; e.bizetto@gmail.com

L.L.F. do Amaral, MD
Division of Neuroradiology,
Hospital Santa Casa de Misericórdia de
São Paulo, Rua Dr. Cesário Motta
Junior 112, Vila Buarque,
Sao Paulo, SP 01221-020, Brazil
e-mail: lazden@terra.com.br

R. Hoffmann Nunes et al. (eds.), *Critical Findings in Neuroradiology*,
DOI 10.1007/978-3-319-27987-9_59

Commonly used devices are the following:

1. *Rods, plates, and transpedicular screws*: Pedicle screws and rods are most often used to stabilize several vertebral levels, anywhere from the thoracic spine to the sacrum. Rods and transpedicular screws are usually attached to the vertebral bodies in the thoracic and lumbar spine. Lateral mass screws and other screws tend to be used in the cervical spine [2, 4].
2. *Translaminar or facet screws*: These devices can be used when posterior elements are intact to attach the laminae of two adjacent vertebrae [2].
3. *Interbody spacers*: After the removal of a disk, spacers are inserted into the intervertebral spaces with or without additional screws and plates/rods. Cages are usually made of titanium, carbon fiber, polyetheretherketone (PEEK), or cortical or corticocancellous bone grafts. Interbody cages are filled with bone chips/powder and inserted then into the intervertebral space. Most radiolucent cages contain two or more radiopaque markers to identify their position on radiographs [2].
4. *Dynamic stabilization devices*: designed to limit abnormal segmental motion. By altering load-bearing, they help to limit the stress placed on the adjacent segment of level fusion, thus preventing its progressive degeneration [5].
5. *Vertebral body replacement* (*corpectomy*): a vertebral body may require replacement after excision due to tumor, trauma, or infection. The vertebral body replacement hardware often takes the form of an expandable cage filled with bone graft or cement [4].

Key Points

Etiology

Surgical procedures in the spine are typically performed with the following goals [2]:

- Decompression of neural elements via removal of herniated disk material and/or decompression of a stenotic spinal canal or neural foramen (laminotomy, laminectomy, and laminectomy with facetectomy and laminoplasty)
- Stabilization and fusion of movable segments for instability or deformity (such as spondylolisthesis, scoliosis, or posttraumatic injury) or after iatrogenic instability (such as facetectomy or multilevel laminectomies)
- Tumor excision or debridement of infection

Best Imaging Modality

Radiographs allow determination of device position and migration, hardware-related complications, progression of fusion, fracture, and adjacent segment degeneration [6].

Flexion and extension radiographs can be used to evaluate evidence of fusion and signs of motion at the fusion level consistent with incomplete fusion or fusion failure and pseudarthrosis [3].

Computed tomography (CT) is useful for evaluation osteolysis related to polyethylene wear and foreign body soft tissue reactions, fluid collections, and subtle fractures. Three-dimensional reconstructions also help to assess the position of interspinous distraction devices.

Magnetic resonance imaging (MRI) assists in the characterization of fluid collections (Fig. 59.3b), extent of infection, identification of possible epidural communication, and integration of disk replacement [6]. MRI can also be used acutely to exclude intraspinal hematomas. The protocol usually includes axial and/or sagittal T1- and T2-weighted imaging spin-echo sequences as well as axial gradient-echo T2* [1, 6, 7]. Generally, gadolinium administration is recommended when collections, infection, and/or epidural fibrosis is suspected [1, 6, 7]. In the presence of metallic hardware, it is necessary to increase bandwidth and use turbo spin-echo sequences, reducing TE to increase the signal-to-noise ratio, small voxel sizes, and minimize magnetic susceptibility artifacts [6]. A metal artifact reduction sequence is another means of optimizing images. In it, section–selection gradient and bandwidth are increased with a narrow slice thickness and increased read gradient and the view angle tilting is used [7]. In clinically uncomplicated cases, acute MRI is not to be used as the findings can be confusing and appear worse than the preoperative study. Acute MRI should be done only in patients whose clinical status has deteriorated after surgery.

CT myelography is useful to assess the nerve roots and spinal canal in patients with suspicion of hardware impingement, postoperative fibrosis, or CSF leak with contraindications to MRI [6].

Ultrasound can be used for the evaluation of superficial soft tissue collections. However, extension of the process to the spinal canal may be difficult to visualize and generally necessitates MRI [6].

Nuclear medicine is used less often in the evaluation of the postoperative spine. It primarily serves as a complementary modality in the diagnosis of postoperative spine infection [6].

Major Findings

Screws: Optimal screw placement is typically centered in the pedicle and aligned parallel to the superior end plate (neutral position). In general, the tip of the pedicle screw should approach but not breach the anterior cortex of the vertebral body or have contact with blood vessels [1, 3]. The posterior pedicle screws should not extend beyond the anterior margin of the vertebral body or lateral/medial to the pedicle (Fig. 59.1) [8].

Loosening may be seen as a lucency rim around the screw threads (>2 mm) (Fig. 59.2) [9].

Hardware fracture or dislodgment is often associated with regional motion and spinal instability which may be the result of or the cause of pseudarthrosis. In certain cases, fractured hardware may not be displaced, making detection of such complication difficult (Figs. 59.2, 59.3, and 59.4) [4]. The most common clinical manifestations are related to nerve root irritation (secondary to excessive medial angulation of the screw) and violation of the medial bony cortex. Lateral position or migration should be evaluated in the cervical spine where a screw can breach the foramen transversarium and potentially damage the vertebral artery [2, 4].

Interbody spacers: The spacer location can be assessed by the radiopaque markers that should be more than 2 mm from the posterior vertebral body margin to prevent protrusion into the spinal canal (Fig. 59.5) [1, 5].

Cervical cages have potential of nonunion and subsidence (axial migration >3 mm) into vertebral body end plates that may result in narrowing of the neural foramina, nerve root compression, pseudarthrosis, cervical instability, and adjacent segment degeneration (Fig. 59.4) [1, 5].

The lost mobility of the fused segment leads to additional stress on adjacent levels of the vertebral column. There is an increase risk of degenerative changes, ligamentous instability, and even fracture at adjacent levels (Fig. 59.6) [1, 10].

Interspinous spacers are inserted between the spinous process through a small incision along the interspinous ligament in order to reduce foraminal and spinal stenosis. Complications include posterior migration or extrusion of the

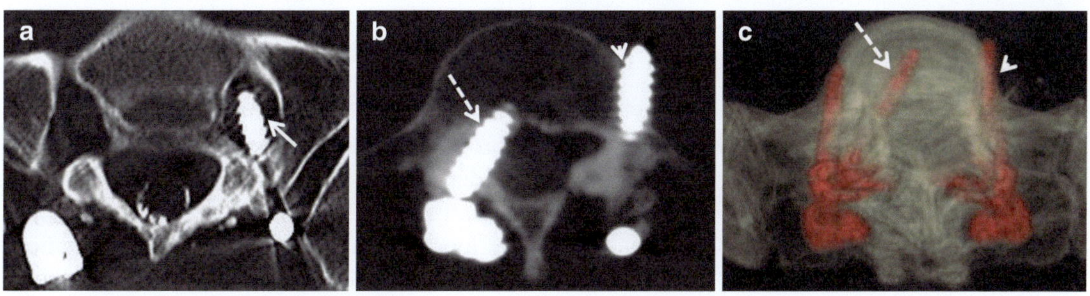

Fig. 59.1 Misplaced pedicle screws. (**a**) Axial CT image of the lumbosacral spine shows a transpedicular screw traversing the left S1 intervertebral foramen (*arrow*). Axial CT (**b**) and 3D (**c**) reformatted images of a different patient demonstrate that the right transpedicular screw violates the pedicle medial margin and is within lateral recess (*dashed arrows*). The left screw violates the anterior margin of the vertebral body (*arrowheads*)

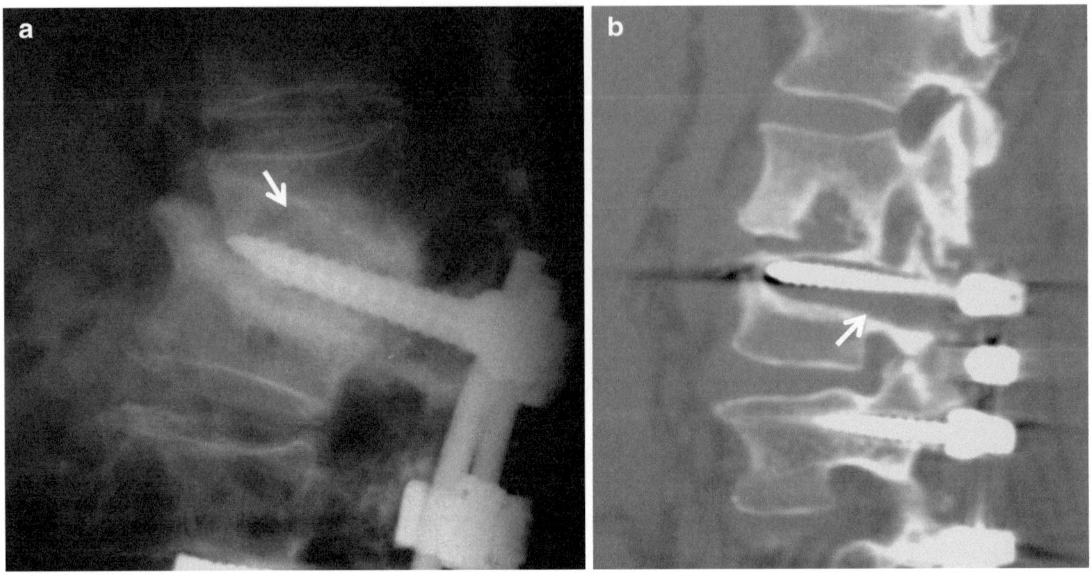

Fig. 59.2 Inadequate fixation with hardware loosening. Lateral lumbar spine radiograph (**a**) and parasagittal CT reformatted image (**b**) reveal transpedicular screw loosening characterized by a rim of lucency >2 mm (*arrows*) associated with erosion of the L1 and L2 end plates

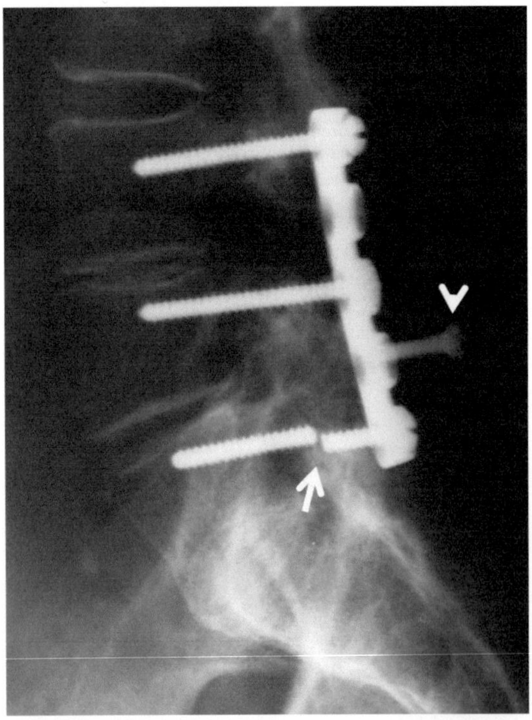

Fig. 59.3 Transpedicular screw fracture. L5 transpedicular screw fracture (*arrow*) is seen on a lateral lumbar spine radiograph, and there is also extrusion of a contralateral screw (*arrowhead*)

device, erosion into the adjacent spinous process, or spinous process fracture [9].

Fusion assessment: Fusion occurs in a series of stages which can be readily identified on thin-section CT scans. Lucency or cystic changes adjacent to hardware should be normally absent, and when present they may be due to persistent motion at the bone–hardware interface, reaction to bone morphogenic protein (BMP), or infection. Trabecular bridging often first occurs outside of the interbody implant. Centrally interrupted bony trabeculation within the interbody space or misalignment of these trabeculations suggests motion, delayed union, and possible early pseudarthrosis formation. A lack of mature trabeculations crossing the disk space at 24 months represents failed fusion and pseudarthrosis formation (Figs. 59.5 and 59.6) [3, 9]. Pseudarthrosis is seen as a linear lucency across the graft material, and it may be a source of pain and loosening or fracture of instrumentation. Early-stage pseudarthrosis may have increased radiotracer uptake on bone scanning or focal high signal intensity on T2-weighted imaging (T2WI) on MRI. Thin-section CT with multiplanar recon-

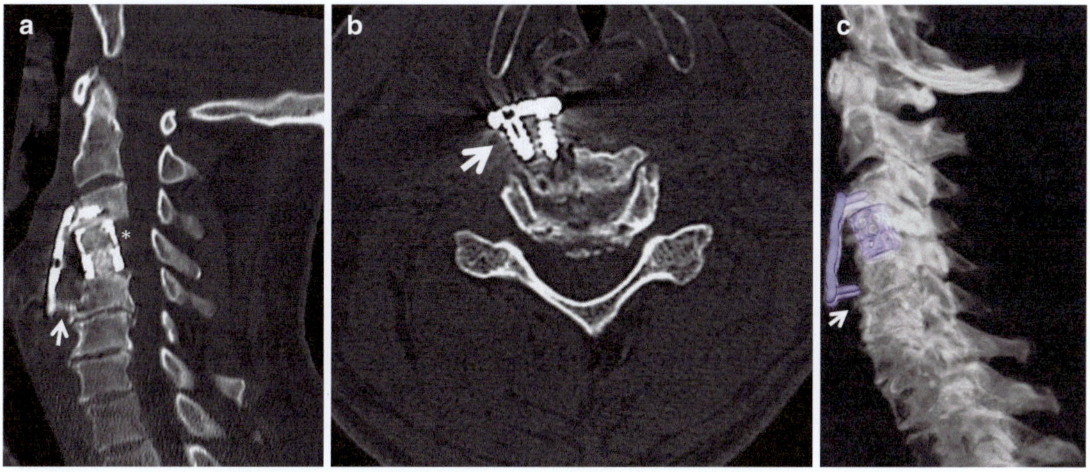

Fig. 59.4 Interbody pseudarthrosis. Sagittal CT reformatted image (**a**) and axial CT image (**b**) demonstrate a C3 corpectomy with cage interposition. Notice that there is no adjacent bone formation what may be related to pseudarthrosis (*). The plate and distal screws are anteriorly and laterally extruded (*arrows*). (**c**) CT 3D reconstruction also depicts the hardware displacement

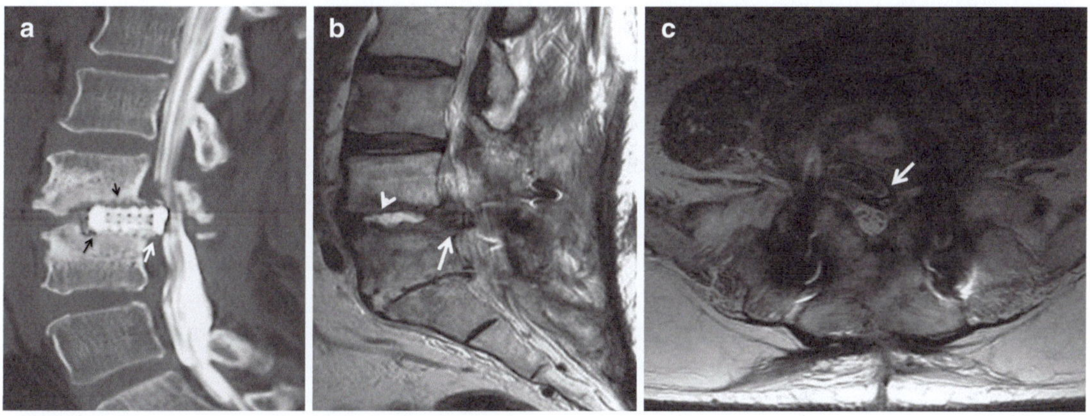

Fig. 59.5 Interbody spacer migration. (**a**) Sagittal CT myelography reformatted image (**a**) displays migration of the L3–L4 cage posteriorly compressing the dural sac (*white arrows*) associated with adjacent vertebral plate lucencies (*black arrows*). Sagittal (**b**) and axial T2WI (**c**) in a different patient show posterior cage migration at the level of L4–L5 compressing the dural sac (*white arrows*). A fluid collection is also depicted in the corresponding intervertebral space (*arrowhead*)

struction is a sensitive and specific imaging modality to detect pseudarthrosis [1].

Various types of bone-graft material (autografts and allografts) and stimulating factors such as BMP may be used to stimulate osseous growth between the vertebral bodies [3]. They produce an initial inflammatory response, followed by a resorptive phase, a bone formation phase, consolidation phase, and, finally, a remodeling phase by osteoclast and osteoblast activity. The intense early inflammatory phase may result in edema, swelling, and abnormal contrast enhancement. In the cervical spine, it may cause dysphagia and even respiratory distress. On MRI, it manifests as an extensive bone signal abnormality with paravertebral soft tissue swelling and signal abnormality in the disk space that may be similar to those seen in discitis/osteomyelitis. Differentiation based exclusively on imaging findings is extremely difficult. On CT, it

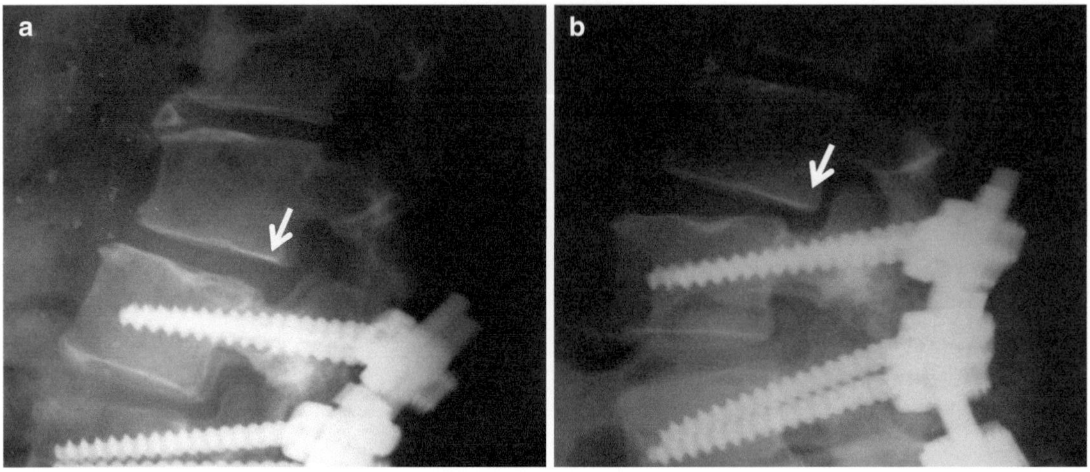

Fig. 59.6 Incomplete fusion. (**a**, **b**) Lateral lumbar spine radiographs in neutral position (**a**) and extension (**b**) show L3 to S1 posterior arthrodesis. There are signs of retrolisthesis of L2 that worsens in extension vertebral end-plate angle deviation >10° (*arrows*)

manifests as cortical irregularity, abnormal bone resorption, and signs of osteolysis [11].

For assessing fusion on radiographs, the following criteria are proposed [12]:

- No motion or less than 3 mm or <10° of intersegmental position change on lateral flexion and extension views
- No lucent area around the implant
- Minimal loss of disk height
- No fracture of the device, graft, or vertebra
- No sclerotic changes in the graft or adjacent vertebra
- Visible bone formation in or about the graft material
- No changes in screw orientation

The temporal changes are as follows:

- At 3 months: increased density around and within the intervertebral implant
- At 6 months: uninterrupted trabecular bony bridging from end plate to end plate
- >12 months: solid cortical bone bridging. No motion or less than 3 mm or 10° of motion angle between the vertebral bodies on lateral flexion and extension views

Imaging Follow-Up

There is no consensus for imaging follow-up schedule in patients with spinal devices. Follow-up depends on the reason for the original surgical procedure. Oncologic patients, for example, need a closer surveillance [1, 6].

Following the immediate postoperative imaging, additional imaging is generally unnecessary as the findings related to healing can be misleading. Expected postoperative findings, such as small epidural fluid collections, granulation tissue, and osteoclastic bone resorption, may be misinterpreted as abnormal [1, 6, 7].

For long-term surveillance following a clinically successful spinal fusion, advanced diagnostic imaging is generally not indicated. In this situation, radiographs are the modality of choice to ascertain hardware position and progression of osseous fusion. However, radiographs do not allow appropriated visualization of the spinal canal and nerve roots or of paravertebral soft tissue fluid collections; therefore, cross-sectional imaging (MRI or CT) is recommended for investigation of unexpected symptoms in all postoperative phases [7].

Main Differential Diagnosis

Discitis/osteomyelitis: The following are signs of infection on radiographs and CT: disk space height loss, end-plate erosion, and vertebral destruction, and paraspinal/epidural phlegmon or abscess are signs of infection. The initial inflammatory response due to bone-graft material and stimulating factors, such as BMP, can have a very similar appearance to discitis/osteomyelitis. Most immediate postoperative fluid collections are seromas and hematomas which may have a complex appearance similar to infection. Clinical and laboratory findings may aid in their differentiation.

Spinal hematoma: Acute onset of neurologic symptoms in the immediate postoperative setting should arouse clinical suspicion for a spinal hematoma which can be characterized using MRI and frequently requires urgent surgical decompression [1].

Tips

- Awareness of the preoperative imaging, the surgical technique and clinical history, clinical problems, and imaging findings that occur at specific time intervals greatly improves the accuracy and value of imaging in patients with spinal fusion.
- In early postoperative studies, besides checking the integrity of the neural foramina, thecal sac, spinal cord, and foramen transversarium, it is important to look for lesions in the major abdominal vessels, psoas musculature, posterior mediastinum, and prevertebral soft tissues.
- Generally, pedicle screws should be centered in the pedicle without cortical breaches or vascular contact and aligned with the superior end plate of the vertebral body.
- An interbody implant spacer location should be no less than 2 mm from the posterior vertebral body margin to prevent protrusion into the spinal canal.
- Any signs of screw malfunction, such as changes in orientation, fractures, pseudarthrosis, subsidence, and surrounding osseous lucencies, must be reported.

References

1. Young PM, Berquist TH, Bancroft LW, Peterson JJ. Complications of spinal instrumentation. Radiographics: Rev Publ Radiol Soc N Am Inc. 2007;27(3):775–89.
2. Thakkar RS, Malloy JP, Thakkar SC, Carrino JA, Khanna AJ. Imaging the postoperative spine. Radiol Clin North Am. 2012;50(4):731–47.
3. Zampolin R, Erdfarb A, Miller T. Imaging of lumbar spine fusion. Neuroimaging Clin N Am. 2014;24(2):269–86.
4. Bittane RM, de Moura AB, Lien RJ. The postoperative spine: what the spine surgeon needs to know. Neuroimaging Clin N Am. 2014;24(2):295–303.
5. Rutherford EE, Tarplett LJ, Davies EM, Harley JM, King LJ. Lumbar spine fusion and stabilization: hardware, techniques, and imaging appearances. Radiographics: Rev Publ Radiol Soc N Am Inc. 2007;27(6):1737–49.
6. Ha AS, Petscavage-Thomas JM. Imaging of current spinal hardware: lumbar spine. AJR Am J Roentgenol. 2014;203(3):573–81.
7. Willson MC, Ross JS. Postoperative spine complications. Neuroimaging Clin N Am. 2014;24(2):305–26.
8. Park JB, Cho YS, Riew KD. Development of adjacent-level ossification in patients with an anterior cervical plate. J Bone Joint Surg Am. 2005;87(3):558–63.
9. Murtagh RD, Quencer RM, Castellvi AE, Yue JJ. New techniques in lumbar spinal instrumentation: what the radiologist needs to know. Radiology. 2011;260(2):317–30.
10. Ray CD. Threaded fusion cages for lumbar interbody fusions. An economic comparison with 360 degrees fusions. Spine. 1997;22(6):681–5.
11. Petscavage-Thomas JM, Ha AS. Imaging current spine hardware: part 1, cervical spine and fracture fixation. AJR Am J Roentgenol. 2014;203(2):394–405.
12. Olsen RV, Munk PL, Lee MJ, Janzen DL, MacKay AL, Xiang QS, et al. Metal artifact reduction sequence: early clinical applications. Radiographics: Rev Publ Radiol Soc N Am Inc. 2000;20(3):699–712.

Index

R. Hoffmann Nunes et al. (eds.), *Critical Findings in Neuroradiology*,
DOI 10.1007/978-3-319-27987-9

R

S

T

MIX
Papier aus verantwortungsvollen Quellen
Paper from responsible sources
FSC® C105338

If you have any concerns about our products,
you can contact us on
ProductSafety@springernature.com

In case Publisher is established outside the EU,
the EU authorized representative is:
Springer Nature Customer Service Center GmbH
Europaplatz 3, 69115 Heidelberg, Germany

Printed by Libri Plureos GmbH
in Hamburg, Germany